The Essential
Herb–Drug–Vitamin
Interaction Guide

ALSO BY BARRY FOX, PH.D.

WITH FREDERIC VAGNINI, M.D.

The Side Effects Bible

WITH JASON THEODOSAKIS AND BRENDA ADDERLY

The Arthritis Cure

The Essential Herb–Drug–Vitamin Interaction Guide

THE SAFE WAY TO USE MEDICATIONS AND SUPPLEMENTS TOGETHER

George T. Grossberg, M.D.,
and Barry Fox, Ph.D.

Broadway Books
New York

PUBLISHED BY BROADWAY BOOKS

Copyright © 2007 by Barry Fox, Ph.D.

Published in the United States by Broadway Books, an imprint of The Doubleday Broadway Publishing Group, a division of Random House, Inc., New York.
www.broadwaybooks.com

BROADWAY BOOKS and its logo, a letter B bisected on the diagonal, are trademarks of Random House, Inc.

This book is not intended to take the place of medical advice from a trained medical professional. Readers are advised to consult a physician or other qualified health professional regarding treatment of their medical problems. Neither the publishers nor the author takes any responsibility for any possible consequences from any treatment, action, or application of medicine, herb, vitamins, or preparation to any person reading the following information in this book.

Book design by Chris Welch

Library of Congress Cataloging-in-Publication Data
Grossberg, George T.
The Essential herb-drug-vitamin interaction guide : the safe way to use medications and supplements together / by George T. Grossberg, and Barry Fox.—1st ed.
p.   cm.
1. Drug interactions. 2. Drug-herb interactions. 3. Drug-nutrient interactions. I. Fox, Barry. II. Title.

RM302.G76   2007
615'.7045—dc22   2006034850

ISBN: 978-0-7679-2277-7

PRINTED IN THE UNITED STATES OF AMERICA

1   3   5   7   9   10   8   6   4   2

First Edition

Dedicated in memory of my father, Henry Grossberg, may he rest in peace, who was always my #1 p.r. person and who never met a vitamin, herb, or prescription medicine he did not like.

Contents

Acknowledgments

I would like to acknowledge Barry Fox, my coauthor, who has the unique ability to make complex things clear to intelligent laypeople, and my wife, Darla, for being such a great mother and wife and enabling me to work on book projects such as this.

How to Use This Book

This is not an "anti-herb" or "anti-medicine" book.

Herbs can be useful as health aids, and medicines can be lifesavers. We're both "pro-herb" and "pro-medicine," and eager to see both types of remedies used properly, safely, and efficaciously, whether taken alone or together. That's why we're offering you the information in this book—not to say you should or should not take a certain medicine or herb, but to help you take both more safely and effectively.

In this book, you'll learn about many of the ways herbs can interact with drugs, vitamins, lab tests, diseases, foods, and other supplements. If you're going to combine an herb with any of these, look up the herb in this book and see if there are any interactions. Then discuss them with your physician.

Simply look up the herb you're taking—they're listed alphabetically in Chapter 2. In the listing for each herb, you'll find a brief introduction to the herb, information about side effects and other matters, then listings of potential interactions: with drugs, laboratory tests, diseases, foods, and other supplements. The drugs are listed alphabetically by generic name, with one or two of the brand names used in the United States or other countries immediately following in parentheses.

As you read through the book you'll see references to Germany's Commission E, the Food and Nutrition Board, RDAs, Adequate Intake, and Tolerable Upper Intake Level. Here's some information on each:

- Germany's Commission E is an official government body charged with investigating and publishing information on the safety and effectiveness of numerous herbs. Some people liken this commission to the U.S. Food and Drug Administration, calling it "an FDA for herbs."
- The Food and Nutrition Board, which is part of the U.S. government's Institute of Medicine, develops and publishes nutritional recommendations, such as the RDAs.
- "RDA" stands for "Recommended Dietary Allowance." The RDA is the amount of a nutrient—such as vitamin C or the mineral selenium—that most healthy people need to consume every day.
- The Adequate Intake (AI) is a recommendation for how much of a nutrient healthy people need to consume every day. It's used in place of an RDA and is like an RDA, but it's an approximation based on less scientific evidence—because the evidence needed to establish an RDA isn't available.
- The Tolerable Upper Intake Level (UL) is the largest amount of a nutrient that can safely be consumed every day by almost everyone in a healthy population.

You'll also come across some words and abbreviations used in the discussions of herbs and nutrients. Here are some quick definitions:

- *Aerial parts* are the parts of the herb that grow above ground.
- The *concentration* is a ratio describing the amount of herb compared to the amount of solvent used to make an herbal preparation. For example, in a tincture with a 1:8 concentration, there's 1 part of the herb (measured in grams) for every 8 parts of the solvent (measured in milliliters).
- *Crude herb* is the raw, unprocessed plant from which a processed herb is produced.
- *Essential oils* are volatile aromatic oils extracted from an herb.
- An *extract* is a concentrated form of the herb, made by mixing the crude herb with water or another solvent, then distilling or evaporating.
- *Gm* stands for gram, a unit of measurement for dry weight.
- An *infusion* is made by steeping the leaves, flowers, or other parts of a plant in water that is just below the boiling point. Tea is an infusion.
- *IU* stands for International Unit, a unit of measurement used for some nutrients such as vitamin E.

- *Mcg* stands for microgram, a unit of measurement for dry weight.
- *Mg* stands for milligram, a unit of measurement for dry weight.
- *Ml* stands for milliliter, a unit of measurement for liquid volume.
- A *poultice* is made by wrapping moistened crushed leaves or other plant parts in a cloth and applying it to the body.
- A *rhizome* is a plant stem that grows in a horizontal pattern underground and produces buds.
- A *tincture* is a liquid herbal extract made by soaking the herb in water, alcohol, or another fluid, then straining the liquid and discarding the plant material.

This book is extensive but by no means complete. It cannot be, for researchers are constantly learning more about herbs, and our knowledge of the ways they interact—for better or worse—with medicines, lab tests, diseases, foods, and other supplements is growing all the time. Given space limitations, we had to confine ourselves to only three hundred herbs and supplements. This book is a good starting point as a basis for discussion with your physician. If you're taking any herbs, ask your physician whether there are any interactions you should know about to ensure that the herbs you take are used properly, safely, and most effectively.

A FINAL NOTE: Sometimes you'll see that an herb increases a medicine's effect, or vice versa. In some cases, that might be beneficial—indeed, some people may take certain herbs as adjuncts to specific medicines. However, we do not indicate which cases may be helpful or not because that depends on many factors—and there's always the possibility that increasing a drug's action may make it too powerful and raise the risk of side effects. That's why we simply indicate which interactions may occur and leave it up to you and your physician to determine if that is helpful, neutral, or harmful.

Chapter One

The Warning You Haven't Heard

Herbs have been used since ancient times to relieve numerous ailments. In the past, people didn't understand how herbs worked; they only knew that they did. Today we know a lot more about herbs, their contents and chemistry, their mechanisms and uses. We know that when used properly, numerous herbs can be useful health aids. We also know that they cannot be indiscriminately mixed with medications, for herbs and drugs do interact, and the interactions can be harmful.

For example, let's say that, like many other people, you take St. John's wort to relieve depression. Then you go to your doctor, who prescribes a medication to deal with a different health issue. No problem, right?

- Not if a birth control pill has been prescribed. Taking birth control pills when you're already taking St. John's wort can cause breakthrough bleeding and unplanned pregnancy.
- Not if an antidepressant, such as Zoloft, has been prescribed. St. John's wort plus Zoloft can trigger serotonin syndrome, which can cause confusion, fever, hallucinations, nausea, shaking, sweating, vomiting—possibly even coma.
- Not if Lanoxin, a medication used to treat heart failure, has been prescribed. St. John's wort can weaken the drug's effectiveness and allow your heart to "fade away."

Suppose you're one of the many people who take echinacea on a regular basis to prevent colds and other upper respiratory tract infections. It's a safe and natural way to ward off a stuffy nose, scratchy throat, and endless bouts of coughing, right?

- Not if you're taking Tylenol for pain, or statin drugs, such as Zocor and Lipitor, for elevated cholesterol. Combining any of these medicines with echinacea can severely damage your liver.
- Not if you ever want to use aspirin, ibuprofen, Celebrex, or other widely used painkillers. Mixing echinacea with these popular pills can increase the likelihood of dangerous uncontrolled bleeding.
- Not if your doctor prescribes Lodine for your arthritis. Lodine plus echinacea can lead to severe gastrointestinal problems, including nausea, vomiting, and gastritis.

Eager to keep your mind sharp and ward off Alzheimer's disease, you diligently take ginkgo biloba every day. A wise precaution, right?

- Not if you ever need to use Glucotrol, DiaBeta, or certain other drugs to treat diabetes. Ginkgo biloba can interfere with the action of these medicines and send your blood sugar out of control.
- Not if you ever need to take antidepressants like Elavil or Norpramin, or antibiotics such as Cipro. Mixing any of these drugs with ginkgo biloba makes you more likely to have a seizure.

Herbs can be wonderful health aids. But dire results may ensue when certain herbs and standard medications are mixed. Odds are you're not aware of the thousands of herb–drug combinations that can be harmful. And, unfortunately, your doctor may not be aware of the risks either.

It's Not a Trivial Problem

It's estimated that 60 million Americans are taking herbs for their headaches, back pain, arthritis, menstrual difficulties, insomnia, depression, anxiety, menopausal symptoms, sexual difficulties, and numerous other problems. Millions of these people are also taking medications with their herbs.

The frightening truth is that an estimated 15 million Americans are at risk of dangerous herb–drug interactions. But who's informing them of the potential dangers? Typically, no one. An article appearing in the *Journal of the American College of Cardiology* in 2002 noted that one-third of patients use herbs, "yet most practicing physicians have little knowledge of herbal remedies or their effects."

The Vital Information Few Health Professionals Know

An alarm has been quietly ringing for years. Articles warning of potentially dangerous interactions between common herbs and standard drugs—both prescription and over-the-counter—periodically appear in cardiology journals, cancer journals, family practice journals, anesthesia journals, nursing journals, emergency medicine journals, pharmacology journals, even dental journals. Over and over again, the authors of these articles emphasize the problems that can arise when drugs are prescribed for people who take herbs, then lament the fact that most doctors know so little about herbs and what happens when they are mixed with medicines. But few seem to be listening.

What exactly can go wrong? Herbs can "harm" drugs by interfering with their absorption, reducing their effectiveness inside the body, increasing their effectiveness (which is like taking a drug overdose), and/or boosting their harmful side effects. They can also:

- combine with drugs (or other herbs) to create new side effects
- alter the results of many laboratory tests
- worsen existing diseases
- trigger potentially dangerous interactions with foods and other supplements

Yet most people are completely unaware of this.

If You're Taking an Herb, Beware the Medicine

If you're taking chaparral, comfrey, echinacea, kava kava, or scullcap, an alarm bell should ring if your doctor prescribes a statin drug for your elevated cholesterol. Mixing Lipitor with any of these herbs can trigger potentially fatal liver damage.

If you're taking chamomile, feverfew, garlic, ginger, or passion flower, beware of using NSAIDs for your arthritis pain. Combining NSAIDs with any of these herbs can cause intestinal bleeding.

If you're taking borage seed oil, fennel oil, ginkgo biloba, St. John's wort, or wormwood, think twice before taking antidepressants. When antidepressants are mixed with any of these herbs, your risk of seizures can increase markedly.

If you're taking aloe, buckthorn, cascara, Chinese rhubarb, licorice, or senna, beware if your doctor prescribes Vascor for your angina. Adding Vascor to any of these herbs can trigger an irregular heartbeat, which is a potentially fatal condition.

And There's More You Need to Know

Herb–drug interactions are only the beginning of what you need to know to use herbs safely. Many herbs can also alter the outcome of lab tests and interact in harmful ways with existing diseases, foods, and other supplements.

Herbs and Lab Tests

Taking certain herbs can cause various lab values to rise or fall—and even if it's only a minor, temporary change, it can distort a doctor's diagnosis or treatment plan. Here are just a few of the herbs that can alter the results of lab tests.

- Black psyllium, used for constipation, can lower the results of tests of blood sugar levels.
- Bladderwrack, used for arthritis and thyroid disorders, can increase the results of tests of thyroid-stimulating hormone levels.
- Cascara, used as a laxative, can discolor urine, interfering with tests dependent on the color of urine when it's exposed to various substances.
- Green tea, used for stomach upset, diarrhea, and headaches, can increase bleeding time and prompt false-positive results on tests for serum urate and certain cancers.
- Juniper, used for stomach upset, heartburn, and urinary tract infections, can interfere with urine tests by discoloring the urine.
- Lavender, used for insomnia and loss of appetite, can depress the results of cholesterol tests.
- Maté, used for depression, ulcers, and inflammation, causes false readings in laboratory tests of uric acid and creatinine in the blood, and tests for the tumors known as neuroblastoma and pheochromocytoma.
- Motherwort, used for heart problems, can lower the results of thyroid tests.

Herbs and Diseases

And what if you're already sick? Did you know that taking herbs might make your condition worse? For example:

- Capsicum (cayenne), which is often used to improve digestion, can irritate the gastrointestinal tract. This makes the herb potentially dangerous for those with infectious or inflammatory gastrointestinal problems, such as irritable bowel syndrome.

- Echinacea, used for colds, viruses, and other problems, can pump up the autoimmune process. This makes the herb potentially harmful for those suffering from multiple sclerosis and other diseases involving immune system reactions and inflammation. Echinacea can also be detrimental to those with diabetes, HIV infections, or allergies.
- Guarana, used for weight loss and fatigue, may aggravate gastric and duodenal ulcers.
- Licorice root, used for ulcers, bronchitis, colic, and numerous other ailments, can make it harder for diabetics to keep their blood sugar under control, rob potassium stores, and worsen both hypertension and erectile dysfunction.
- Panax ginseng, used for anxiety, nerve pain, and insomnia, can lower blood sugar, which may be dangerous for diabetics. The herb can also interfere with blood coagulation, which can be detrimental to those with bleeding conditions, such as hemophilia. Siberian ginseng can increase blood pressure, which is harmful to those who already have hypertension, and it can increase the severity of both mania and schizophrenia.

Herbs and Foods

Then there are herb–food interactions that can harm you in subtle ways. For example:

- Blond psyllium, used for constipation, can decrease the absorption of nutrients from the foods you eat by speeding food through the digestive tract and cutting back on the time available for nutrient absorption.
- Guar gum, used as a laxative and a cholesterol-reducing agent, can also interfere with the absorption of nutrients.
- Kava kava, used to relieve anxiety and insomnia, can become toxic when mixed with alcohol. Symptoms of kava kava toxicity include headache, dizziness, and stomach upset.

Herbs and Other Supplements

Finally, there are potential problems when herbs are mixed with other supplements. For example:

- Angelica root, used as a diuretic, can cause increased bleeding when taken with bogbean, capsicum, chamomile, clove, feverfew, garlic, ginger, ginkgo, licorice, passion flower, or red clover.
- Butternut, used for hemorrhoids and gallbladder diseases, can deplete potassium stores when taken with black root, cascara, jalap root, senna leaves, or wild cucumber.
- Mixing catnip, which is used for migraines, insomnia, colds, and flu, with capsicum, sassafras, Siberian ginseng, St. John's wort, stinging nettle, or valerian can increase the odds of suffering from the typical side effects seen with any of these herbs.
- Eucalyptus oil, used for cough and inflammation of the respiratory tract, can increase the toxicity of borage, coltsfoot, comfrey, and hound's tooth.

It's a rare physician who truly understands the dangers that can arise when herbs are combined with medicines, diseases, foods, and other supplements. Most likely, you're on your own.

Which Herbs, Which Medicines?

Hundreds of herbs interact with hundreds of medicines. And even popular and seemingly safe herbs such as St. John's wort, kava kava, valerian, ginkgo biloba, echinacea, ginseng, garlic, aloe, and green tea can become dangerous when combined with certain common drugs.

A host of lesser-known but widely used herbs can also cause dangerous herb–drug interactions, including apple cider vinegar, basil, black cohosh, borage seed oil, cayenne, chamomile, clove, dandelion, feverfew, gotu kola, hawthorn, kombucha tea, lavender, lemon balm, licorice, mistletoe, onion, oregano, passion flower, red clover, red yeast rice, rose hip, saw palmetto, and wheatgrass.

Which drugs do they interact with? So far, studies have shown that over three hundred prescription and nonprescription medicines may interact with herbs, including:

- Advil, Motrin, and aspirin, taken for pain, inflammation, and fever
- Aleve, taken for arthritis and menstrual difficulties
- Allegra, taken for allergies
- Ambien, Halcion, and Restoril, taken for insomnia

- Benadryl, Sominex, and Sudafed, taken for allergies and to promote sleep
- Celebrex, taken for arthritis
- Celexa, taken for depression
- Cipro, taken for anthrax and various infections
- Claritin, taken for seasonal allergies
- Colchicine, taken for gout
- Concerta and Ritalin, taken for attention deficit hyperactivity disorder
- Coumadin, taken to prevent blood clots
- Demerol, taken for pain
- Dilantin and Thorazine, taken for schizophrenia and seizures
- Estrogen, used in birth control pills
- Flagyl, used for protozoal and bacterial infections
- Lescol, used to lower cholesterol
- Lithium, taken for bipolar disorder
- Orudis, used for painful menstruation and arthritis
- Pepcid and Mylanta, taken for stomach upset and ulcers
- Pepto-Bismol, taken for nausea and diarrhea
- Plavix, taken as a blood thinner/to prevent blood clots
- Prevacid, taken for stomach acid
- Prilosec, taken for gastroesophageal reflux disease
- Propecia, taken for male pattern baldness
- Proscar, taken for prostate enlargement
- Prozac, taken for depression and bulimia nervosa
- Rheumatrex, taken for arthritis, psoriasis, and cancer
- Tegretol, taken for seizures
- Valium, taken for anxiety
- Xanax, taken for anxiety and panic disorder
- Zocor, taken for elevated cholesterol
- Zoloft, taken for depression

And many, many more.

Close-up on St. John's Wort

We know more about the way medicines interact with St. John's wort than with any other herb. St. John's wort is one of the best-selling herbs in the United States, used to treat depression, anxiety, fatigue, insomnia, mood disturbances linked to menopause, migraines, and numerous other ailments. It's apparently safe when used properly and by itself, but adding medicines to the mix can create potentially serious problems.

St. John's Wort in the Medical Literature

Here's a sample of the warnings that have appeared in medical journals.

Data from human studies and case reports indicate that St. John's wort decreased blood concentrations of amitriptyline, cyclosporine, digoxin, fexofenadine, indinavir, methadone, midazolam, nevirapine, phenprocoumon, simvastatin, tacrolimus, theophylline and warfarin . . . St. John's wort caused breakthrough bleeding and unplanned pregnancies when used concomitantly with oral contraceptives. It also caused serotonin syndrome when co-administered with selective serotonin-reuptake inhibitors (e.g., sertraline and paroxetine)—*Journal of Psychopharmacology*, 2004

St. John's wort significantly induced apparent clearance of both S-warfarin and R-warfarin, which in turn resulted in a significant reduction in pharmacological effect of rac-warfarin.—*British Journal of Pharmacology*, 2004

When combined with serotonin reuptake inhibitor antidepressants (e.g., sertraline, paroxetine, nefazodone) or buspirone, St. John's wort can cause serotonergic syndrome.—*International Journal of Clinical Pharmacological Therapy*, 2004

St. John's wort can participate in potential pharmacokinetic interactions with anticancer drugs.—*Journal of Clinical Oncology*, 2004

St. John's wort can also reduce the blood concentrations (and thus, potentially, the effectiveness) of numerous medicines, including:

- Allegra (for allergies)
- Coumadin (to thin the blood)
- Crixivan (for HIV)
- Elavil (for depression)
- Lanoxin (to prevent heart failure)
- Methadone (for pain and detoxification)
- Neoral (to prevent organ rejection)
- Pamelor (for depression)
- Prograf (to prevent organ rejection)

- Theo-lair (for asthma, bronchitis, and emphysema)
- Versed (for sedation)
- Viramune (for HIV)
- Zocor (for elevated cholesterol)

If the standard amount of one of these medicines doesn't seem to be effective, your doctor may increase the dosage. Then not only will your risk of side effects increase, but if you stop taking your St. John's wort (or even cut back on it), the blood levels of this medicine will shoot up. Suddenly you can be at risk of a drug overdose!

A second problem with mixing medicines and St. John's wort is serotonin syndrome. This is a potentially serious problem characterized by confusion, agitation, mania, anxiety, muscle rigidity, tremor, restlessness, shivering, changes in blood pressure, seizures, and even coma. These drugs can trigger serotonin syndrome in people taking St. John's wort:

- Amerge (for migraines)
- Celexa (for depression)
- Cymbalta (for depression and diabetic neuropathy pain)
- Effexor (for depression and anxiety)
- Frova (for migraines)
- Imitrex (for cluster headaches and migraines)
- Lexapro (for depression)
- Maxalt (for migraines)
- Paxil (for depression and obsessive-compulsive disorder)
- Prozac (for depression)
- Remeron (for depression)
- Zoloft (for depression, post-traumatic stress disorder, and panic disorder)
- Zomig (for migraines)

Another problem seen in those taking St. John's wort along with certain medications is photosensitivity—a condition in which exposure to sunlight causes allergic and toxic skin reactions. The medications that can cause photosensitivity when combined with St. John's wort include:

- Amaryl (for diabetes)
- Avelox (for pneumonia, bronchitis, and skin infections)
- Bactrim (for infections)

- Cinobac (for urinary tract infections)
- Cipro (for anthrax and other infections)
- DiaBeta (for diabetes)
- Diabinese (for diabetes)
- Dymelor (for diabetes)
- Elavil (for depression)
- Gantrisin (for infections)
- Glucotrol (for diabetes)
- Levaquin (for pneumonia and skin and urinary tract infections)
- Maxaquin (for various infections)
- NegGram (for urinary tract infections)
- Noroxin (for sexually transmitted diseases and urinary tract infections)
- Ocuflox (for eye and other infections)
- Orinase (for diabetes)
- Septra (for infections)
- Sulfadiazine (for infections)
- Tequin (for bronchitis, pneumonia, and other ailments)
- Tetracycline (for acne and various infections)
- Tolinase (for diabetes)
- Trovan (for gynecologic infections)
- Zagam (for pneumonia)

And altered levels of medicine in the blood, serotonin syndrome, and photosensitivity are just a few of the problems that can strike you if you combine St. John's wort with certain medicines.

Millions of people take St. John's wort. And when used properly, it can be very helpful. But who is warning them that the combination of St. John's wort and numerous medicines can be harmful?

A Big Problem That Receives Little Notice

Aloe, apple cider vinegar, basil, black cohosh, borage seed oil, capsicum, chamomile, clove, dandelion, echinacea, feverfew, garlic, ginkgo biloba, ginseng, green tea, kava kava, lavender, licorice, mistletoe, onion, oregano, passion flower, red clover, rose hip, saw palmetto, St. John's wort, valerian, and wheatgrass—these are just some of the herbs that can make medicines dangerous.

Advil, Motrin, aspirin, Aleve, Allegra, Ambien, Halcion, Restoril, Celebrex, Celexa, Cipro, Claritin, Colchicine, Coumadin, Demerol, estrogen, Flagyl, Lescol, lithium, Orudis, Pepcid, Mylanta, Pepto-Bismol, Plavix, Ritalin, Prevacid, Prilosec, Propecia, Proscar, Prozac, Rheumatrex, Ritalin, Concerta, Sudafed, Benadryl, Seminex, Tegretol, Thorazine, Dilantin, Valium, Xanax, Zocor, and Zoloft: this is just a small part of the long list of common medicines that can interact with herbs in dangerous ways.

For your own safety, you must learn about the dangers of herb–drug interactions.

Herbs That May Interact with Common Medicines

Here are more than three hundred herbs, vitamins, and minerals that can interfere with the actions of medicines, interact with supplements or foods, and/or alter or complicate laboratory tests or diseases.

Herb	Drugs	THIS HERB INTERACTS WITH Other Supplements	Foods	Lab Tests	Diseases
Acerola	✔	✔	✔	✔	✔
Adonis	✔	✔			✔
Agrimony	✔				
Ajava seeds	✔	✔		✔	✔
Aletris	✔				✔
Alfalfa	✔	✔		✔	✔
Allspice	✔	✔			
Aloe	✔	✔		✔	✔
Andrographis	✔	✔			✔
Angel's trumpet	✔				✔
Angelica	✔	✔		✔	
Anise	✔			✔	✔
Apple cider vinegar	✔	✔		✔	✔

Herb	Drugs	Other Supplements	Foods	Lab Tests	Diseases
Areca nut	✔			✔	✔
Arnica	✔	✔		✔	✔
Artichoke	✔				✔
Asafoetida	✔				✔
Ashwagandha	✔	✔		✔	✔
Astragalus	✔			✔	✔
Avaram	✔				
Balsam of Peru	✔				
Banaba	✔	✔			✔
Barley	✔	✔		✔	✔
Basil	✔				
Belladonna	✔				✔
Beta-carotene	✔		✔		
Bilberry	✔	✔		✔	
Biotin	✔				
Birch	✔		✔		✔
Birthwort	✔			✔	✔
Bishop's weed	✔	✔		✔	✔
Bitter almond	✔				
Bitter melon	✔	✔		✔	✔
Bitter orange	✔	✔	✔		✔
Black cohosh	✔	✔			✔
Black hellebore	✔	✔			✔
Black mustard	✔				✔
Black pepper	✔	✔		✔	
Black root	✔	✔			✔
Black tea	✔	✔	✔	✔	✔

Herb	Drugs	Other Supplements	Foods	Lab Tests	Diseases
Black walnut	✔	✔			
Bladderwrack	✔				✔
Blessed thistle	✔	✔			✔
Blue cohosh	✔				✔
Blue flag	✔				✔
Bog bean	✔	✔			✔
Boldo	✔				✔
Boneset	✔				
Borage	✔	✔			✔
Borage seed oil	✔	✔		✔	✔
Brewer's yeast	✔			✔	✔
Bromelain	✔	✔	✔		✔
Buchu	✔				✔
Buckthorn	✔	✔	✔	✔	✔
Bugleweed	✔	✔		✔	✔
Burdock	✔				✔
Butcher's broom	✔	✔			
Butterbur	✔	✔		✔	
Butternut	✔	✔			
Cabbage	✔			✔	✔
Caffeine	✔	✔		✔	✔
Calabar bean	✔				✔
Calamus	✔	✔			
Calcium	✔	✔	✔	✔	✔
California poppy	✔	✔	✔		
Calotropis	✔	✔			
Carrageen	✔				

Herb	Drugs	Other Supplements	Foods	Lab Tests	Diseases
Cascara sagrada	✔	✔	✔	✔	✔
Castor oil plant	✔	✔	✔		✔
Cat's claw	✔				✔
Catechu	✔				
Catnip	✔	✔			✔
Cayenne	✔				✔
Cedar leaf	✔	✔			✔
Cedarwood oil	✔	✔			
Celery	✔			✔	✔
Cereus	✔				✔
Chanca piedra	✔				
Chaparral	✔	✔		✔	✔
Chaste tree berry	✔			✔	✔
Cherokee rosehip	✔	✔	✔	✔	✔
Chicory	✔				
Chinese club moss	✔				✔
Chinese cucumber root	✔	✔		✔	✔
Chinese rhubarb	✔	✔	✔	✔	✔
Chlorella	✔				✔
Cinnamon	✔	✔	✔	✔	
Clove	✔	✔		✔	✔
Cocoa	✔	✔	✔	✔	✔
Coffee	✔	✔	✔	✔	✔
Cola nut	✔	✔	✔	✔	✔
Colchicum	✔				✔
Colocynth	✔	✔		✔	✔

Herb	Drugs	Other Supplements	Foods	Lab Tests	Diseases
Colombo	✔				
Colt's foot	✔	✔			✔
Comfrey	✔	✔		✔	✔
Cordyceps	✔			✔	
Coriander	✔				
Corkwood	✔				
Corn silk	✔				✔
Country mallow	✔	✔	✔	✔	✔
Cowhage	✔	✔		✔	✔
Cowslip	✔				
Cubeb	✔				✔
Cucumber	✔				
Cumin	✔				✔
Damiana	✔				✔
Dandelion	✔	✔			✔
Danshen	✔	✔		✔	✔
Deer's tongue	✔	✔			
Devil's claw	✔				✔
Digitalis	✔	✔		✔	✔
Dong quai	✔	✔		✔	✔
Echinacea	✔			✔	✔
Elecampane	✔	✔			✔
English hawthorn	✔	✔			
English lavender	✔			✔	
English plantain	✔				
Ergot	✔	✔			✔
Ethanol	✔	✔	✔	✔	✔

Herb	Drugs	Other Supplements	Foods	Lab Tests	Diseases
Eucalyptus	✔	✔			✔
European elder	✔				
European mistletoe	✔	✔		✔	✔
Evening primrose oil	✔	✔		✔	
Eyebright	✔				
Fennel	✔				✔
Fenugreek	✔	✔	✔	✔	✔
Fever bark	✔			✔	
Feverfew	✔	✔		✔	
Flax	✔			✔	✔
Folic acid	✔		✔	✔	✔
Fo-ti	✔				
Frangula	✔	✔		✔	✔
Fumitory	✔				
Gamboge	✔	✔			✔
Garlic	✔	✔		✔	✔
German chamomile	✔	✔			✔
Ginger	✔	✔		✔	✔
Ginkgo biloba	✔	✔		✔	✔
Ginseng, American	✔	✔	✔	✔	✔
Ginseng, Panax	✔	✔	✔	✔	✔
Ginseng, Siberian	✔	✔		✔	✔
Glucomannan	✔	✔		✔	
Goat's rue	✔	✔		✔	✔
Goldenseal	✔	✔		✔	✔
Gossypol	✔	✔	✔		✔
Gotu kola	✔	✔			✔

Herb	Drugs	Other Supplements	Foods	Lab Tests	Diseases
Grapefruit	✔	✔	✔	✔	
Grape seed	✔				
Green tea	✔	✔	✔	✔	✔
Guarana	✔	✔	✔	✔	✔
Guar gum	✔	✔	✔	✔	✔
Guggul	✔	✔		✔	
Gymnema	✔			✔	✔
Hawaiian baby woodrose	✔	✔			
Heartsease	✔				
Hedge mustard	✔	✔			
Henbane	✔	✔			✔
Hops	✔	✔	✔		✔
Horehound	✔				
Horse chestnut	✔	✔			✔
Horseradish	✔	✔			✔
Horsetail	✔	✔	✔		✔
Hyssop	✔				✔
Iboga	✔				
Indian hemp	✔	✔			
Indian long pepper	✔	✔		✔	
Indian squill	✔	✔			✔
Iron	✔	✔	✔	✔	✔
Jalap	✔	✔			✔
Jimson weed	✔				✔
Juniper	✔			✔	✔
Kava kava	✔	✔	✔	✔	✔

Herb	Drugs	Other Supplements	Foods	Lab Tests	Diseases
Kelp	✔	✔		✔	✔
Khat	✔				
Kudzu	✔	✔		✔	✔
Larch	✔				✔
Laurel	✔				
Lemon balm	✔	✔			
Lesser galangal	✔				
Licorice	✔	✔	✔	✔	✔
Lily-of-the-valley	✔	✔			
Linden	✔				
Lovage	✔				
Lungwort	✔				
Madagascar periwinkle	✔			✔	✔
Magnesium	✔	✔		✔	✔
Ma-huang	✔	✔	✔	✔	✔
Maitake mushroom	✔	✔		✔	✔
Mandrake	✔	✔			✔
Manna	✔	✔			✔
Marijuana	✔	✔	✔	✔	✔
Marshmallow	✔	✔		✔	
Maté	✔	✔	✔	✔	✔
Mayapple	✔	✔	✔	✔	✔
Meadowsweet	✔				
Milk thistle	✔				✔
Motherwort	✔	✔		✔	✔
Myrrh	✔			✔	✔

Herb	Drugs	Other Supplements	Foods	Lab Tests	Diseases
Nerve root	✔				
Niacin	✔	✔	✔	✔	✔
Noni	✔			✔	✔
Northern prickly ash	✔	✔			✔
Nutmeg	✔	✔			
Oak	✔	✔			
Oats	✔			✔	
Oleander	✔	✔			
Olive	✔	✔		✔	✔
Onion	✔	✔		✔	
Oregano	✔				✔
Papaya	✔	✔	✔	✔	✔
Parsley	✔				✔
Passion flower	✔	✔			
Pau d'arco	✔	✔		✔	✔
Pectin	✔	✔	✔	✔	
Perilla	✔				
Pill-bearing spurge	✔				✔
Pineapple	✔				
Pleurisy root	✔	✔			✔
Poke	✔				
Pomegranate	✔	✔			
Poplar	✔				
Poppy	✔			✔	
Potassium	✔			✔	✔
Prickly pear cactus	✔			✔	✔

Herb	Drugs	Other Supplements	Foods	Lab Tests	Diseases
Psyllium	✔	✔		✔	✔
Quassia	✔	✔			✔
Quillaja	✔	✔	✔		✔
Quinine	✔	✔			✔
Raspberry	✔	✔			✔
Rauwolfia	✔	✔		✔	✔
Red clover	✔	✔			✔
Red yeast rice	✔	✔	✔	✔	✔
Reishi mushroom	✔	✔		✔	✔
Riboflavin	✔	✔	✔	✔	✔
Rose hips	✔	✔	✔	✔	✔
Rosemary	✔				✔
Rue	✔				✔
Safflower	✔	✔			✔
Sage	✔	✔		✔	✔
Sarsaparilla	✔	✔			
Sassafras	✔	✔		✔	✔
Saw palmetto	✔			✔	
Schisandra	✔			✔	✔
Scopolia	✔	✔			✔
Scotch broom	✔				✔
Scullcap	✔	✔		✔	✔
Sea buckthorn	✔	✔			
Senega	✔				✔
Senna	✔	✔		✔	✔
Shepherd's purse	✔				✔
Slippery elm	✔				

Herb	Drugs	Other Supplements	Foods	Lab Tests	Diseases
Solomon's seal	✔	✔			
Sorrel	✔	✔	✔		✔
Soybean	✔		✔	✔	✔
Spinach	✔	✔	✔	✔	✔
Squill	✔	✔		✔	✔
Stevia	✔	✔		✔	✔
Stinging nettle	✔	✔			
St. John's wort	✔	✔	✔	✔	✔
Stone root	✔	✔			
Strophanthus	✔	✔			✔
Swamp milkweed	✔	✔			✔
Sweet clover	✔	✔		✔	
Sweet orange	✔				
Sweet vernal grass	✔	✔			
Tamarind	✔				
Thiamin	✔	✔	✔		
Thunder god vine	✔				
Tonka bean	✔				✔
Turmeric	✔	✔			✔
Uva ursi	✔			✔	✔
Uzara	✔	✔			
Valerian	✔	✔	✔	✔	
Vitamin A	✔		✔	✔	✔
Vitamin B_6	✔			✔	
Vitamin B_{12}	✔	✔	✔	✔	✔
Vitamin C	✔	✔		✔	✔
Vitamin D	✔		✔		✔

Herb	Drugs	Other Supplements	Foods	Lab Tests	Diseases
Vitamin E	✔	✔	✔	✔	✔
Vitamin K	✔	✔		✔	
Wahoo	✔	✔			✔
Wallflower	✔	✔			✔
Watercress	✔			✔	
White willow	✔	✔			✔
Wild carrot	✔	✔			✔
Wild cherry	✔				
Wild lettuce	✔	✔			✔
Wild yam	✔				✔
Wintergreen	✔				✔
Witch hazel	✔				✔
Wood betony	✔				
Wormseed	✔				
Wormwood	✔	✔			✔
Yarrow	✔	✔			
Yellow dock	✔	✔	✔	✔	✔
Yellow gentian	✔				
Yew	✔				
Yohimbe	✔	✔	✔		✔
Zinc	✔	✔	✔	✔	

Chapter Two

Herb Effects

AN A-TO-Z LISTING OF HERBS, AND MEDICINES THEY INTERACT WITH

ACEROLA

Acerola is a large, bushy shrub or small tree originating in Central America and currently grown in tropical areas worldwide. Its small, bright red fruits are very high in vitamin C, providing around 1,500 mg of C per 100 gm of fruit, although the green fruits may have twice that amount. A potent antioxidant, acerola can help ward off atherosclerosis by preventing the conversion of LDL "bad" cholesterol to its more dangerous form.

Scientific Name
Malpighia glabra

Acerola Is Also Commonly Known As
Barbados cherry, Puerto Rican cherry, West Indian cherry

Medicinal Parts
Fruit

Acerola's Uses
To treat colds, tooth decay, scurvy, and heart disease; to increase physical performance; to prevent blood clots and collagen disorders.

Typical Dose
There is no typical dose of acerola.

Possible Side Effects
Acerola's side effects include nausea, abdominal cramps, insomnia, sleepiness, and fatigue.

Drugs That May Interact with Acerola
Taking acerola with these drugs may increase drug absorption and effects:

- cyproterone and ethinyl estradiol (Diane-35)
- estradiol (Climara, Estrace)
- estradiol and norethindrone (Activella, CombiPatch)
- estradiol and testosterone (Climacteron)
- estrogens (conjugated A/synthetic) (Cenestin)
- estrogens (conjugated/equine) (Congest, Premarin)

- estrogens (conjugated/equine) and medroxy-progesterone (Premphase, Prempro)
- estrogens (esterified) (Estratab, Menest)
- estrogens (esterified) and methyltestosterone (Estratest, Estratest H.S.)
- estropipate (Ogen, Ortho-Est)
- ethinyl estradiol (Estinyl)
- ethinyl estradiol and desogestrel (Cyclessa, Ortho-Cept)
- ethinyl estradiol and ethynodiol diacetate (Demulen, Zovia)
- ethinyl estradiol and etonogestrel (NuvaRing)
- ethinyl estradiol and levonorgestrel (Alesse, Triphasil)
- ethinyl estradiol and norelgestromin (Evra, Ortho Evra)
- ethinyl estradiol and norethindrone (Brevicon, Ortho-Novum)
- ethinyl estradiol and norgestimate (Cyclen, Ortho Tri-Cyclen)
- ethinyl estradiol and norgestrel (Cryselle, Ovral)
- mestranol and norethindrone (Necon 1/50, Ortho-Novum 1/50)
- polyestradiol

Taking acerola with these drugs may be harmful:
- fluphenazine (Modecate, Prolixin)—decreases levels of drug in blood
- warfarin (Coumadin, Jantoven)—reduces anticoagulant activity of drug

Lab Tests That May Be Altered by Acerola

- May cause false negative results in stool occult blood tests if acerola is ingested 48 to 72 hours before test.
- May cause false decrease in glucose oxidase test (for example, Clinistix) after ingesting more than 500 mg of vitamin C.
- False increases in cupric sulfate test (for example, Clinitest) due to vitamin C in acerola.

Diseases That May Be Worsened or Triggered by Acerola

Acerola contains vitamin C, which may trigger a rise in uric acid levels and possibly increase the risk of gout.

Foods That May Interact with Acerola

Increased gastrointestinal absorption of iron from foods (ferric) but not from supplements (ferrous), due to vitamin C content of acerola.

Supplements That May Interact with Acerola

Increased risk of adverse effects associated with vitamin C when taken with acerola, because acerola contains vitamin C.

ADONIS

> Named for the Greek god Adonis, from whose blood this plant is said to have sprung, adonis is used as a cardiac stimulant that may be effective even when digitalis fails, especially in cases of kidney disease. Because of its sedative action, adonis may also be used to treat irregular or rapid heartbeat.

Scientific Name

Adonis vernalis

Adonis Is Also Commonly Known As

False hellebore, oxeye, pheasant's eye, rose-a-rubie

Medicinal Parts
Leaf, stem, flower

Adonis's Uses
To treat menstrual problems, dehydration, fever, and a weak heart. Germany's Commission E has approved the use of adonis to treat nervous heart complaints and irregular heartbeat.

Typical Dose
A typical daily dose of adonis is approximately 0.6 gm of powder.

Possible Side Effects
❶ Adonis's side effects include nausea and irregular heartbeat. Adonis contains cardiac glycosides, which can help control irregular heartbeat, reduce the backup of blood and fluid in the body, and increase blood flow through the kidneys, helping to excrete sodium and relieve swelling in body tissues. However, a buildup of cardiac glycosides can occur, especially when the herb is combined with certain medications or other herbs that contain cardiac glycosides, causing arrhythmias, abnormally slow heartbeat, heart failure, and even death.

Drugs That May Interact with Adonis
Taking adonis with these drugs may enhance the therapeutic and adverse effects of the drug:
- beclomethasone (Beconase, Vanceril)
- betamethasone (Betatrex, Maxivate)
- budesonide (Entocort, Rhinocort)
- budesonide and Formoterol (Symbicort)
- calcium acetate (PhosLo)
- calcium carbonate (Rolaids Extra Strength, Tums)
- calcium chloride
- calcium citrate (Osteocit)
- calcium glubionate
- calcium gluceptate
- calcium gluconate
- cascara (*Cascara sagrada*)
- cortisone (Cortone)
- deflazacort (Calcort, Dezacor)
- dexamethasone (Decadron, Dexasone)
- digitalis (Digitek, Lanoxin)
- docusate (Colace, Ex-Lax Stool Softener)
- docusate and senna (Peri-Colace, Senokot-S)
- flunisolide (AeroBid, Nasarel)
- fluorometholone (Eflone, Flarex)
- fluticasone (Cutivate, Flonase)
- hydrocortisone (Cetacort, Locoid)
- lactulose (Constulose, Enulose)
- loteprednol (Alrex, Lotemax)
- magnesium citrate (Citro-Mag)
- magnesium hydroxide (Dulcolax Milk of Magnesia, Phillips' Milk of Magnesia)
- magnesium hydroxide and mineral oil (Phillips' M-O)
- magnesium oxide (Mag-Ox 400, Uro-Mag)
- magnesium sulfate (Epsom salts)
- medrysone (HMS Liquifilm)
- methylprednisolone (Depo-Medrol, Medrol)
- polyethylene glycol–electrolyte solution (Colyte, MiraLax)
- prednisolone (Inflamase Forte, Pred Forte)
- prednisone (Apo-Prednisone, Deltasone)
- psyllium (Metamucil, Reguloid)
- quinidine (Novo-Quinidin, Quinaglute Dura-Tabs)
- rimexolone (Vexol)
- sorbitol (Sorbilax)
- triamcinolone (Aristocort, Trinasal)

Taking adonis with this drug may be harmful:

- quinidine (Novo-Quinidin, Quinaglute Dura-Tabs)—may cause electrolyte abnormalities, plus changes in cardiac rhythm and vital signs.

Lab Tests That May Be Altered by Adonis
None known

Diseases That May Be Worsened or Triggered by Adonis
May worsen conditions related to low levels of calcium or potassium.

Foods That May Interact with Adonis
None known

Supplements That May Interact with Adonis
- Increased risk of cardiac glycoside toxicity when used with other herbs that contain cardiac glycosides, such as black hellebore, calotropis, motherwort, and others. (For a list of cardiac glycoside–containing herbs and supplements, see Appendix B.)
- Increased risk of cardiotoxicity due to potassium depletion when taken with cardioactive herbs, such as digitalis, lily-of-the-valley, and squill. (For a list of cardioactive herbs and supplements, see Appendix B.)
- Increased risk of potassium depletion when used in conjunction with licorice or horsetail plant.
- Increased risk of potassium depletion when used with stimulant laxative herbs, such as black root, cascara sagrada, castor oil, and senna. (For a list of stimulant laxative herbs and supplements, see Appendix B.)
- May increase risk of cardiac toxicity when taken with calcium supplements.

AGRIMONY

Agrimony gets its name from the Greek word *argemone*, which means "plants healing to eyes." Indeed, it was used by the ancient Greeks to soothe eye problems, although the Anglo-Saxons found it useful as a treatment for wounds. Today it is used for its anti-inflammatory and astringent properties and also its prowess as a diuretic and a tonic to invigorate and strengthen the body.

Scientific Name
Agrimonia eupatoria

Agrimony Is Also Commonly Known As
Cocklebur, church steeples, common agrimony, liverwort, philanthropos, sticklewort, stickwort

Medicinal Parts
Leaf, flower, stem

Agrimony's Uses
To treat diarrhea, diabetes, kidney and bladder inflammation, poorly healing wounds, psoriasis, and seborrhoeic eczema. Germany's Commission E has approved the use of agrimony to treat diarrhea and inflammation of the mouth, throat, and skin.

Typical Dose
Taken internally, a typical daily dose may range from 3 to 6 gm of the herb. Agrimony can also be applied topically as a poultice.

Possible Side Effects
Agrimony's side effects include constipation and digestive complaints.

Drugs That May Interact with Agrimony

Taking agrimony with these drugs may increase the risk of hypoglycemia (low blood sugar):

- acarbose (Prandase, Precose)
- acetohexamide
- chlorpropamide (Diabinese, Novo-Propamide)
- gliclazide (Diamicron, Novo-Gliclazide)
- glimepiride (Amaryl)
- glipizide (Glucotrol)
- glipizide and metformin (Metaglip)
- gliquidone (Beglynor, Glurenorm)
- glyburide (DiaBeta, Micronase)
- glyburide and metformin (Glucovance)
- insulin (Humulin, Novolin R)
- metformin (Glucophage, Riomet)
- miglitol (Glyset)
- nateglinide (Starlix)
- pioglitazone (Actos)
- repaglinide (GlucoNorm, Prandin)
- rosiglitazone (Avandia)
- rosiglitazone and metformin (Avandamet)
- tolazamide (Tolinase)
- tolbutamide (Apo-Tolbutamide, Tol-Tab)

Taking agrimony with these drugs may increase skin sensitivity to sunlight:
- bumetanide (Bumex, Burinex)
- ciprofloxacin (Ciloxan, Cipro)
- doxycycline (Apo-Doxy, Vibramycin)
- enalapril (Vasotec)
- etodolac (Lodine, Utradol)
- fluphenazine (Modecate, Prolixin)
- fosinopril (Monopril)
- furosemide (Apo-Furosemide, Lasix)

- gatifloxacin (Tequin, Zymar)
- hydrochlorothiazide (Apo-Hydro, Microzide)
- ibuprofen (Advil, Motrin)
- indomethacin (Indocin, Novo-Methacin)
- ketoprofen (Orudis, Rhodis)
- ketorolac (Acular, Toradol)
- lansoprazole (Prevacid)
- levofloxacin (Levaquin, Quixin)
- lisinopril (Prinivil, Zestril)
- loratadine (Alavert, Claritin)
- methotrexate (Rheumatrex, Trexall)
- naproxen (Aleve, Naprosyn)
- nortriptyline (Aventyl HCl, Pamelor)
- ofloxacin (Floxin, Ocuflox)
- omeprazole (Prilosec, Losec)
- phenytoin (Dilantin, Phenytek)
- piroxicam (Feldene, Nu-Pirox)
- prochlorperazine (Compazine, Compro)
- quinapril (Accupril)
- risperidone (Risperdal)
- rofecoxib (Vioxx)
- tetracycline (Novo-Tetra, Sumycin)

Lab Tests That May Be Altered by Agrimony
None known

Diseases That May Be Worsened or Triggered by Agrimony
None known

Foods That May Interact with Agrimony
None known

Supplements That May Interact with Agrimony
None known

AJAVA SEEDS

Used by ancient Egyptians to treat vitiligo, the loss of pigment in the skin, ajava seeds contain 8-methoxypsoralen, which has been shown to stimulate the production of pigment in skin exposed to ultraviolet light. A liquid preparation made by boiling ground-up ajava seeds in water, taken after intercourse, is thought to prevent implantation of a fertilized egg in the uterus.

Scientific Name
Ammi majus

Ajava Seeds Are Also Commonly Known As
Ajowan caraway, ajowan seeds, bishop's weed, bishop's flower, bullwort, flowering ammi, yavani

Medicinal Parts
Seed

Ajava Seed's Uses
To treat asthma, kidney stones, and psoriasis

Typical Dose
A typical dose of ajava seeds has not been established.

Possible Side Effects
Ajava seed's side effects include nausea and headache.

Drugs That May Interact with Ajava Seeds
Taking ajava seeds with these drugs may increase the risk of bleeding or bruising:
- abciximab (ReoPro)
- antithrombin III (Thrombate III)
- argatroban
- aspirin (Bufferin, Ecotrin)
- aspirin and dipyridamole (Aggrenox)
- bivalirudin (Angiomax)
- clopidogrel (Plavix)
- dalteparin (Fragmin)
- danaparoid (Orgaran)
- dipyridamole (Novo-Dipiradol, Persantine)
- enoxaparin (Lovenox)
- eptifibatide (Integrillin)
- fondaparinux (Arixtra)
- heparin (Hepalean, Hep-Lock)
- indobufen (Ibustrin)
- lepirudin (Refludan)
- ticlopidine (Alti-Ticlopidine, Ticlid)
- tinzaparin (Innohep)
- tirofiban (Aggrastat)
- warfarin (Coumadin, Jantoven)

Lab Tests That May Be Altered by Ajava Seeds
- May increase HDL levels.
- May increase liver function tests.

Diseases That May Be Worsened or Triggered by Ajava Seeds
May worsen liver function in people with liver disease.

Foods That May Interact with Ajava Seeds
None known

Supplements That May Interact with Ajava Seeds
- May increase the risk of liver damage when combined with herbs and supplements that can cause hepatotoxicity (destructive effects on the liver), such as bishop's weed, borage, chaparral, uva ursi, and others. (For a list of herbs and supplements that can cause hepatotoxicity, see Appendix B.)
- Increased risk of bleeding when used with herbs

and supplements that might affect platelet aggregation, such as angelica, danshen, garlic, ginger, ginkgo biloba, red clover, turmeric, white willow, and others. (For a list of herbs and supplements with anticoagulant/antiplatelet potential, see Appendix B.)

- May have additive effects when used with herbs and supplements that increase photosensitivity, such as St. John's wort. (For a list of herbs and supplements that increase photosensitivity, see Appendix B.)

ALETRIS

Many Native American tribes considered aletris to be a sacred female herb. The root was used to stimulate menstruation, strengthen the womb, and as an infusion for "female troubles." Today it's known that aletris contains diosgenin, a plant steroid with anti-inflammatory and estrogenic properties that is the basis of many pharmaceutical hormonal preparations.

Scientific Name
Aletris farinosa

Aletris Is Also Commonly Known As
Ague-root, aloe-root, blazing star, colic-root, star-wort, true unicorn star-grass

Medicinal Parts
Rhizome, root

Aletris's Uses
To treat rheumatism, relieve menstrual complaints, and treat infertility

Typical Dose
A typical dose of aletris may range from 0.3 to 0.6 gm of powdered root taken three times daily.

Possible Side Effects
Aletris's side effects include colic and vertigo.

Drugs That May Interact with Aletris
Taking aletris with these drugs may interfere with the action of the drug:

- aluminum hydroxide (AlternaGel, Alu-Cap)
- aluminum hydroxide and magnesium carbonate (Gaviscon Extra Strength, Gaviscon Liquid)
- aluminum hydroxide and magnesium hydroxide (Maalox, Rulox)
- aluminum hydroxide, magnesium hydroxide, and simethicone (Maalox, Mylanta Liquid)
- aluminum hydroxide and magnesium trisilicate (Gaviscon Tablet)
- calcium carbonate (Rolaids Extra Strength, Tums)
- calcium carbonate and magnesium hydroxide (Mylanta Gelcaps, Rolaids Extra Strength)
- cimetidine (Nu-Cimet, Tagamet)
- esomeprazole (Nexium)
- famotidine (Apo-Famotidine, Pepcid)
- famotidine, calcium carbonate, and magnesium hydroxide (Pepcid Complete)
- lansoprazole (Prevacid)
- magaldrate and simethicone (Riopan Plus, Riopan Plus Double Strength)
- magnesium hydroxide (Dulcolax Milk of Magnesia, Phillips' Milk of Magnesia)
- magnesium oxide (Mag-Ox 400, Uro-Mag)
- magnesium sulfate (Epsom salts)

- nizatidine (Axid, PMS-Nizatidine)
- omeprazole (Losec, Prilosec)
- pantoprazole (Pantoloc, Protonix)
- rabeprazole (Aciphex, Pariet)
- ranitidine (Alti-Ranitidine, Zantac)
- sodium bicarbonate (Brioschi, Neut)
- sucralfate (Carafate, Sulcrate)

Lab Tests That May Be Altered by Aletris
None known

Diseases That May Be Worsened or Triggered by Aletris
- May worsen inflammatory or infectious gastrointestinal ailments by irritating the gastrointestinal tract.
- This herb may have estrogen-like effects and should not be used by women with estrogen-sensitive breast cancer or other hormone-sensitive conditions.

Foods That May Interact with Aletris
None known

Supplements That May Interact with Aletris
None known

ALFALFA

Used since the sixth century by the Chinese as a treatment for kidney stones and edema, alfalfa, called the "father of all foods" by the Arabs, is a source of several important nutrients, including beta-carotene, calcium, chlorophyll, magnesium, and potassium. In folk medicine, alfalfa was often used to treat arthritis, asthma, diabetes, and hay fever and to improve the appetite and overall well-being.

Scientific Name
Medicago sativa

Alfalfa Is Also Commonly Known As
Buffalo herb, purple medic, lucerne

Medicinal Parts
Whole herb, flower, leaf, seed

Alfalfa's Uses
To treat malfunctioning thyroid gland, diabetes, and elevated cholesterol levels

Typical Dose
A typical dose of alfalfa is approximately 15mL–20mL liquid extract per day.

Possible Side Effects
Alfalfa's side effects include photosensitivity and lowered levels of potassium in the blood. The seeds of the alfalfa plant contain a toxic amino acid and should not be eaten.

Drugs That May Interact with Alfalfa
Taking alfalfa with these drugs may either reduce or enhance their anticoagulant effects:
- antithrombin III (Thrombate III)
- argatroban
- bivalirudin (Angiomax)
- dalteparin (Fragmin)
- danaparoid (Orgaran)
- enoxaparin (Lovenox)

- fondaparinux (Arixtra)
- heparin (Hepalean, Hep-Lock)
- lepirudin (Refludan)
- tinzaparin (Innohep)
- warfarin (Coumadin, Jantoven)

Taking alfalfa with these drugs may interfere with the effects of the drug:
- cyproterone and ethinyl estradiol (Diane-35)
- estradiol (Climara, Estrace)
- estradiol and medroxyprogesterone (Lunelle)
- estradiol and norethindrone (Activella, CombiPatch)
- estradiol and testosterone (Climacteron)
- estrogens (conjugated A/synthetic) (Cenestin)
- estrogens (conjugated/equine) (Congest, Premarin)
- estrogens (conjugated/equine) and medroxy-progesterone (Premphase, Prempro)
- estrogens (esterified) (Estratab, Menest)
- estrogens (esterified) and methyltestosterone (Estratest, Estratest H.S.)
- estropipate (Ogen, Ortho-Est)
- ethinyl estradiol (Estinyl)
- ethinyl estradiol and desogestrel (Cyclessa, Ortho-Cept)
- ethinyl estradiol and drospirenone (Yasmin)
- ethinyl estradiol and ethynodiol diacetate (Demulen, Zovia)
- ethinyl estradiol and etonogestrel (NuvaRing)
- ethinyl estradiol and levonorgestrel (Alesse, Triphasil)
- ethinyl estradiol and norelgestromin (Evra, Ortho Evra)
- ethinyl estradiol and norethindrone (Brevicon, Ortho-Novum)
- ethinyl estradiol and norgestimate (Cyclen, Ortho Tri-Cyclen)
- ethinyl estradiol and norgestrel (Cryselle, Ovral)
- levonorgestrel (Mirena, Plan B)
- medroxyprogesterone (Depo-Provera, Provera)
- mestranol and norethindrone (Necon 1/50, Ortho-Novum 1/50)
- norgestrel (Ovrette)
- polyestradiol

Taking alfalfa with these drugs may reduce the drug's immunosuppressive effect:
- azathioprine (Imuran)
- cyclosporine (Neoral, Sandimmune)
- dexamethasone (Decadron, Dexasone)
- methylprednisolone (Depo-Medrol, Medrol)
- prednisone (Apo-Prednisone, Deltasone)

Lab Tests That May Be Altered by Alfalfa
May decrease serum cholesterol levels, particularly in those with type II hyperlipoproteinemia.

Diseases That May Be Worsened or Triggered by Alfalfa
- May reduce blood sugar levels in those with diabetes.
- This herb may have estrogen-like effects and should not be used by women with estrogen-sensitive breast cancer or other hormone-sensitive conditions.
- Latent systemic lupus erythematosus may be reactivated by eating alfalfa seeds.

Foods That May Interact with Alfalfa
None known

Supplements That May Interact with Alfalfa

Increased risk of clotting in people using antico-agulants due to vitamin K content. The saponins in alfalfa may interfere with the absorption or activity of vitamin E.

ALLSPICE

Discovered in the Caribbean by Christopher Columbus (who thought it was pepper), allspice was so named in the seventeenth century because it tastes like a combination of cloves, cinnamon, and nutmeg. A tea made from allspice has been said to be good for couples who are "inharmonious."

Scientific Name

Pimiento officinalis, Eugenia pimento

Allspice Is Also Commonly Known As

Clove pepper, Jamaica pepper, pimenta, pimiento

Medicinal Parts

Fruit

Allspice's Uses

To treat flatulence, indigestion, tooth pain, and muscle pain

Typical Dose

A typical dose of allspice is approximately 2 tsp of powder mixed in 1 cup water, or three drops of essential oil mixed with sugar.

Possible Side Effects

Allspice's side effects include nausea, vomiting, and anorexia.

Drugs That May Interact with Allspice

Taking allspice with these drugs may increase the risk of bleeding or bruising:

- abciximab (ReoPro)
- antithrombin III (Thrombate III)
- argatroban
- aspirin (Bufferin, Ecotrin)
- aspirin and dipyridamole (Aggrenox)
- bivalirudin (Angiomax)
- clopidogrel (Plavix)
- dalteparin (Fragmin)
- danaparoid (Orgaran)
- dipyridamole (Novo-Dipirado, Persantine)
- enoxaparin (Lovenox)
- eptifibatide (Integrillin)
- fondaparinux (Arixtra)
- heparin (Hepalean, Hep-Lock)
- indobufen (Ibustrin)
- lepirudin (Refludan)
- ticlopidine (Alti-Ticlopidine, Ticlid)
- tinzaparin (Innohep)
- tirofiban (Aggrastat)
- warfarin (Coumadin, Jantoven)

Lab Tests That May Be Altered by Allspice

None known

Diseases That May Be Worsened or Triggered by Allspice

None known

Foods That May Interact with Allspice

None known

Supplements That May Interact with Allspice

May interfere with the absorption of iron, zinc, and other minerals from food.

ALOE

> The gel taken from the leaf of the aloe vera plant is an excellent natural moisturizer that soothes skin irritation, sunburn, burns, wounds, and dry skin, and encourages skin regeneration. Aloe also contains acemannan, a compound that appears to boost immunity and, in one study, helped to heal oral ulcers better than standard treatments.

Scientific Name

Aloe barbadensis, Aloe capensis, Aloe vera

Aloe Is Also Commonly Known As

Aloe vera, aloe vera gel

Medicinal Parts

Juice of the leaf

Aloe's Uses

Different forms of aloe have different uses. *Aloe barbadensis* is used to promote bowel movements in cases of hemorrhoids and anal fissures and to treat fungal diseases, stomach tumors, colic, skin diseases, amenorrhea, infections, and worm infestation. *Aloe capensis* is used to soften the stool and to treat eye inflammations, syphilis, and gastrointestinal disorders. *Aloe vera* is used to treat constipation, herpes simplex lesions, psoriasis, sunburn, abrasions, minor burns, and wounds. Germany's Commission E has approved the use of *Aloe barbadensis* and *Aloe capensis* to treat constipation.

Typical Dose

There is no typical dose for external application. Taken internally, a typical dose of aloe is approximately 0.05 gm of *Aloe barbadensis* powder or 0.05 to 0.2 g of *Aloe capensis* powder. Note, however, that due to its potential side effects, aloe is not recommended for internal use.

Possible Side Effects

Taken internally, aloe's side effects include gastrointestinal spasms, diarrhea, red coloring to the urine, and lowered levels of potassium. Applied externally, aloe's side effects include slower healing of deep wounds and contact dermatitis.

Drugs That May Interact with Aloe

Taking aloe internally with these drugs may increase the risk of hypoglycemia (low blood sugar):

- acarbose (Prandase, Precose)
- acetohexamide
- chlorpropamide (Diabinese, Novo-Propamide)
- gliclazide (Diamicron, Novo-Gliclazide)
- glimepiride (Amaryl)
- glipizide (Glucotrol)
- glipizide and metformin (Metaglip)
- gliquidone (Beglynor, Glurenorm)
- glyburide (DiaBeta, Micronase)
- glyburide and metformin (Glucovance)
- insulin (Humulin, Novolin R)
- metformin (Glucophage, Riomet)
- miglitol (Glyset)
- nateglinide (Starlix)
- pioglitazone (Actos)
- repaglinide (GlucoNorm, Prandin)
- rosiglitazone (Avandia)
- rosiglitazone and metformin (Avandamet)
- tolazamide (Tolinase)
- tolbutamide (Apo-Tolbutamide, Tol-Tab)

Taking aloe internally with these drugs may increase drug effects, due to potassium loss:

- acebutolol (Novo-Acebutolol, Sectral)
- adenosine (Adenocard, Adenoscan)
- amiodarone (Cordarone, Pacerone)
- bretylium
- digitalis (Digitek, Lanoxin)
- diltiazem (Cardizem, Tiazac)
- disopyramide (Norpace, Rythmodan)
- dofetilide (Tikosyn)
- esmolol (Brevibloc)
- flecainide (Tambocor)
- ibutilide (Corvert)
- lidocaine (Lidoderm, Xylocaine)
- mexiletine (Mexitil, Novo-Mexiletine)
- moricizine (Ethmozine)
- phenytoin (Dilantin, Phenytek)
- procainamide (Procanbid, Pronestyl-SR)
- propafenone (Gen-Propafenone, Rhythmol)
- propranolol (Inderal, InnoPran XL)
- quinidine (Novo-Quinidin, Quinaglute Dura-Tabs)
- sotalol (Betapace, Sorine)
- tocainide (Tonocard)
- verapamil (Calan, Isoptin SR)

Taking aloe internally with these drugs may increase the risk of hypokalemia (low levels of potassium in the blood):

- azosemide (Diat)
- beclomethasone (Beconase, Vanceril)
- bepridil (Vascor)
- betamethasone (Celestone, Diprolene)
- budesonide (Entocort, Rhinocort)
- budesonide and formoterol (Symbicort)
- bumetanide (Bumex, Burinex)
- chlorothiazide (Diuril)
- cortisone (Cortone)

- deflazacort (Calcort, Dezacor)
- dexamethasone (Decadron, Dexasone)
- ethacrynic acid (Edecrin)
- etozolin (Elkapin)
- flunisolide (AeroBid, Nasarel)
- fluorometholone (Eflone, Flarex)
- fluticasone (Cutivate, Flonase)
- furosemide (Apo-Furosemide, Lasix)
- hydrochlorothiazide (Apo-Hydro, Microzide)
- hydrocortisone (Anusol-HC, Locoid)
- hydroflumethiazide (Diucardin, Saluron)
- insulin (Humulin, Novolin R)
- loteprednol (Alrex, Lotemax)
- medrysone (HMS Liquifilm)
- methyclothiazide (Aquatensen, Enduron)
- methylprednisolone (Depo-Medrol, Medrol)
- olmesartan and hydrochlorothiazide (Benicar HCT)
- polythiazide (Renese)
- prednisolone (Inflamase Forte, Pred Forte)
- prednisone (Apo-Prednisone, Deltasone)
- rimexolone (Vexol)
- sildenafil (Viagra)
- torsemide (Demadex)
- triamcinolone (Aristocort, Trinasal)
- trichlormethiazide (Metatensin, Naqua)
- xipamide (Diurexan, Lumitens)

Taking aloe internally with these drugs may increase the loss of electrolytes and fluids:

- cascara (cascara sagrada)
- docusate and senna (Peri-Colace, Senokot-S)

Lab Tests That May Be Altered by Taking Aloe Internally

- May decrease serum potassium levels with long-term use.
- May decrease blood glucose concentrations.

- May confound results of diagnostic urine tests that rely on a color change by turning urine red.

Diseases That May Be Worsened or Triggered by Taking Aloe Internally
- May worsen ulcerative colitis, Crohn's disease, and other intestinal diseases due to the herb's irritating effects.
- Using large amounts of aloe may trigger or worsen potassium depletion.
- Using large amounts of aloe may cause kidney inflammation.

Foods That May Interact with Aloe
None known

Supplements That May Interact with Aloe When Aloe Is Taken Internally
- Increased action of jimson weed in cases of chronic use or abuse of aloe.
- Increased risk of cardiac glycoside toxicity when used with other herbs that contain cardiac glycosides, such as black hellebore, calotropis, motherwort, and others. (For a list of cardiac glycoside–containing herbs and supplements, see Appendix B.)
- Increased risk of potassium depletion when used in conjunction with horsetail plant or licorice.

ANDROGRAPHIS

Native to India, andrographis has long been used to treat fever; improve cardiovascular, urinary, and digestive health; and fight disease. Some scientific evidence suggests that andrographis may be able to stimulate the immune system, kill bacteria and fungi, reduce pain and fever, and relieve upper respiratory infections.

Scientific Name
Andrographis paniculata

Andrographis Is Also Commonly Known As
Andrographolide, creat, Indian echinacea, kariyat

Medicinal Parts
Leaf, rhizome

Andrographis's Uses
To prevent and treat colds, flu, allergies, constipation, pain, tonsillitis, and sinusitis; as an antiseptic

Typical Dose
A typical daily dose of andrographis may range from 1 to 3 gm.

Possible Side Effects
Andrographis's side effects include gastrointestinal distress, lack of appetite, and hives.

Drugs That May Interact with Andrographis
Taking andrographis with these drugs may increase the risk of bleeding or bruising:
- abciximab (ReoPro)
- antithrombin III (Thrombate III)
- argatroban
- aspirin (Bufferin, Ecotrin)
- aspirin and dipyridamole (Aggrenox)
- bivalirudin (Angiomax)
- clopidogrel (Plavix)
- dalteparin (Fragmin)
- danaparoid (Orgaran)

- dipyridamole (Novo-Dipiradol, Persantine)
- enoxaparin (Lovenox)
- eptifibatide (Integrillin)
- fondaparinux (Arixtra)
- heparin (Hepalean, Hep-Lock)
- indobufen (Ibustrin)
- lepirudin (Refludan)
- ticlopidine (Alti-Ticlopidine, Ticlid)
- tinzaparin (Innohep)
- tirofiban (Aggrastat)
- warfarin (Coumadin, Jantoven)

Taking andrographis with these drugs may increase the risk of hypotension (excessively low blood pressure):

- acebutolol (Novo-Acebutolol, Sectral)
- amlodipine (Norvasc)
- atenolol (Apo-Atenol, Tenormin)
- benazepril (Lotensin)
- betaxolol (Betoptic S, Kerlone)
- bisoprolol (Monocor, Zebeta)
- bumetanide (Bumex, Burinex)
- candesartan (Atacand)
- captopril (Capoten, Novo-Captopril)
- carteolol (Cartrol, Ocupress)
- carvedilol (Coreg)
- chlorothiazide (Diuril)
- chlorthalidone (Apo-Chlorthalidone, Thalitone)
- clonidine (Catapres, Duraclon)
- diazoxide (Hyperstat, Proglycem)
- diltiazem (Cardizem, Tiazac)
- doxazosin (Alti-Doxazosin, Cardura)
- enalapril (Vasotec)
- eplerenone (Inspra)
- eprosartan (Teveten)
- esmolol (Brevibloc)
- felodipine (Plendil, Renedil)
- fenoldopam (Corlopam)
- fosinopril (Monopril)
- furosemide (Apo-Furosemide, Lasix)
- guanabenz (Wytensin)
- guanadrel (Hylorel)
- guanfacine (Tenex)
- hydralazine (Apresoline, Novo-Hylazin)
- hydrochlorothiazide (Apo-Hydro, Microzide)
- hydrochlorothiazide and triamterene (Dyazide, Maxzide)
- indapamide (Lozol, Nu-Indapamide)
- irbesartan (Avapro)
- isradipine (DynaCirc)
- labetalol (Normodyne, Trandate)
- lisinopril (Prinivil, Zestril)
- losartan (Cozaar)
- mefruside (Baycaron)
- mecamylamine (Inversine)
- methyclothiazide (Aquatensen, Enduron)
- methyldopa (Apo-Methyldopa, Nu-Medopa)
- metolazone (Mykrox, Zaroxolyn)
- metoprolol (Betaloc, Lopressor)
- minoxidil (Loniten, Rogaine)
- moexipril (Univasc)
- nadolol (Apo-Nadol, Corgard)
- nicardipine (Cardene)
- nifedipine (Adalat CC, Procardia)
- nisoldipine (Sular)
- nitroglycerin (Minitran, Nitro-Dur)
- nitroprusside (Nipride, Nitropress)
- olmesartan (Benicar)
- oxprenolol (Slow-Trasicor, Trasicor)
- perindopril erbumine (Aceon, Coversyl)
- phenoxybenzamine (Dibenzyline)
- phentolamine (Regitine, Rogitine)
- pindolol (Apo-Pindol, Novo-Pindol)
- polythiazide (Renese)

- prazosin (Minipress, Nu-Prazo)
- propranolol (Inderal, InnoPran XL)
- quinapril (Accupril)
- ramipril (Altace)
- reserpine
- spironolactone (Aldactone, Novo-Spiroton)
- telmisartan (Micardis)
- terazosin (Alti-Terazosin, Hytrin)
- timolol (Betimol, Timoptic)
- torsemide (Demadex)
- trandolapril (Mavik)
- triamterene (Dyrenium)
- trichlormethiazide (Metatensin, Naqua)
- valsartan (Diovan)
- verapamil (Calan, Isoptin SR)

Taking andrographis with these drugs may reduce the drug's ability to suppress the immune system:
- antithymocyte globulin, equine (Atgam)
- antithymocyte globulin, rabbit (Thymoglobulin)
- azathioprine (Imuran)
- basiliximab (Simulect)
- beclomethasone (Beconase, Vanceril)
- betamethasone (Celestone, Diprolene)
- budesonide (Entocort, Rhinocort)
- budesonide and Formoterol (Symbicort)
- cortisone (Cortone)
- cyclosporine (Neoral, Sandimmune)
- daclizumab (Zenapax)
- deflazacort (Calcort, Dezacor)
- dexamethasone (Decadron, Dexasone)
- efalizumab (Raptiva)
- flunisolide (AeroBid, Nasarel)
- fluorometholone (Eflone, Flarex)
- fluticasone (Cutivate, Flonase)
- hydrocortisone (Anusol-HC, Locoid)
- loteprednol (Alrex, Lotemax)

- medrysone (HMS Liquifilm)
- methotrexate (Rheumatrex, Trexall)
- methylprednisolone (DepoMedrol, Medrol)
- muromonab-CD3 (Orthoclone OKT 3)
- mycophenolate (CellCept)
- pimecrolimus (Elidel)
- prednisolone (Inflamase Forte, Pred Forte)
- prednisone (Apo-Prednisone, Deltasone)
- rimexolone (Vexol)
- sirolimus (Rapamune)
- tacrolimus (Prograf, Protopic)
- thalidomide (Thalomid)
- triamcinolone (Aristocort, Trinasal)

Lab Tests That May Be Altered by Andrographis
None known

Diseases That May Be Worsened or Triggered by Andrographis
- May increase the risk of bleeding or bruising in people with bleeding disorders.
- May lower blood pressure too much in people with already low blood pressure.
- May further decrease fertility in men and women with fertility problems.

Foods That May Interact with Andrographis
None known

Supplements That May Interact with Andrographis
- Increased risk of low blood pressure (hypotension) or increased therapeutic effects when used with herbs and supplements that may lower blood pressure, such as black cohosh, danshen, and ginger. (For a list of herbs and supplements with hypotensive activity, see Appendix B.)
- Increased risk of bleeding or bruising when

used with herbs and supplements that might affect platelet aggregation, such as angelica, danshen, garlic, ginger, ginkgo biloba, red clover, turmeric, white willow, and others. (For a list of herbs and supplements that might affect platelet aggregation, see Appendix B.)

ANGEL'S TRUMPET

Angel's trumpet gets its name because its two-inch-long, beautiful white, pink, or yellow flowers are shaped like trumpets. Used during religious ceremonies by South American shamans as a hallucinogen, angel's trumpet has been grown commercially in South America as a source of the alkaloid hyoscine, a drug used to dilate the pupils of the eyes.

Scientific Name
Brugmansia suaveolens

Angel's Trumpet Is Also Commonly Known As
Devil's trumpet

Medicinal Parts
Leaf, flower

Angel's Trumpet's Uses
To treat asthma; to induce euphoria and hallucinations

Typical Dose
There is no typical dose of angel's trumpet.

Possible Side Effects
Angel's trumpet's side effects include delirium, dilated pupils, disorientation, dry skin, fever, hyperexcitability, and visual hallucinations.

Drugs That May Interact with Angel's Trumpet
Taking angel's trumpet with these drugs may enhance the therapeutic and adverse effects of the drug:

- amantadine (Endantadine, Symmetrel)
- amitriptyline (Elavil, Levate)
- amitriptyline and chlordiazepoxide (Limbitrol)
- amitriptyline and perphenazine (Etrafon, Triavil)
- amoxapine (Asendin)
- atropine (Isopto Atropine, Sal-Tropine)
- belladonna and opium (B&O Supprettes)
- belladonna, phenobarbital, and ergotamine (Bellamine S, Bel-Tabs)
- benztropine (Apo-Benztropine, Cogentin)
- chlorpromazine (Largactil, Thorazine)
- clidinium and chlordiazepoxide (Apo-Chlorax, Librax)
- clomipramine (Anafranil, Novo-Clopramine)
- cyclopentolate (Cyclogyl, Cylate)
- desipramine (Alti-Desipramine, Norpramin)
- dicyclomine (Bentyl, Lomine)
- doxepin (Zonalon, Sinequan)
- fluphenazine (Modecate, Prolixin)
- glycopyrrolate (Robinul, Robinul Forte)
- homatropine (Isopto Homatropine)
- hyoscyamine (Hyosine, Levsin)
- hyoscyamine, atropine, scopolamine, and phenobarbital (Donnatal, Donnatal Extentabs)
- imipramine (Apo-Imipramine, Tofranil)
- ipratropium (Atrovent, Nu-Ipratropium)
- lofepramine (Feprapax, Gamanil)
- melitracen (Dixeran)
- mesoridazine (Serentil)
- nortriptyline (Aventyl HCl, Pamelor)

- oxitropium (Oxivent, Tersigat)
- perphenazine (Apo-Perphenazine, Trilafon)
- prifinium (Padrin, Riabel)
- prochlorperazine (Compazine, Compro)
- procyclidine (Kemadrin, Procyclid)
- promethazine (Phenergan)
- propantheline (Propanthel)
- protriptyline (Vivactil)
- scopolamine (Scopace, Transderm Scop)
- thiethylperazine (Torecan)
- thioridazine (Mellaril)
- thiothixene (Navane)
- tiotropium (Spiriva)
- tolterodine (Detrol, Detrol LA)
- trifluoperazine (Novo-Trifluzine, Stelazine)
- trihexyphenidyl (Artane)
- trimethobenzamide (Tigan)
- trimipramine (Apo-Trimip, Surmontil)

Lab Tests That May Be Altered by Angel's Trumpet
None known

Diseases That May Be Worsened or Triggered by Angel's Trumpet
- May cause irregular heartbeat and rapid heartbeat and worsen heart failure due to its constituents hyoscyamine and scopolamine.
- May worsen gastroesophageal reflux disease (GERD), ulcers, constipation, and obstructive gastrointestinal diseases due to its constituents hyoscyamine and scopolamine.
- May worsen urinary retention due to its constituents hyoscyamine and scopolamine.
- May increase the risk of fever due to its constituents hyoscyamine and scopolamine.

Foods That May Interact with Angel's Trumpet
None known

Supplements That May Interact with Angel's Trumpet
None known

ANGELICA

> Known as the "guardian angel herb," angelica was widely used during the mid-1700s to ward off infection, evil spirits, and witches when the Great Plague swept through Europe. Today it's known to have antimicrobial, antispasmodic, and diuretic properties, making it useful in treating colds, bronchitis, painful menstrual periods, headaches, and urinary infections.

Scientific Name
Angelica archangelica

Medicinal Parts
Whole herb, seed, root

Angelica Is Also Commonly Known As
Angel's wort, European angelica, garden angelica

Angelica's Uses
To treat coughs, bronchitis, gastrointestinal cramps, menstrual complaints, poor digestion, liver and biliary duct conditions. Germany's Commission E has approved the use of angelica root to treat dyspeptic complaints such as heartburn and bloating, and loss of appetite.

Typical Dose
A typical dose of angelica is approximately 4.5 gm of the root, 1.5 to 3.0 gm of the liquid extract (1:1), or 10 to 20 drops of the essential oil.

Possible Side Effects

Angelica's side effects include sensitivity of the skin to sunlight.

Drugs That May Interact with Angelica

Taking angelica with these drugs may increase the risk of bleeding or bruising:

- abciximab (ReoPro)
- alteplase (Activase, Cathflo Activase)
- antithrombin III (Thrombate III)
- argatroban
- aspirin (Bufferin, Ecotrin)
- aspirin and dipyridamole (Aggrenox)
- bivalirudin (Angiomax)
- celecoxib (Celebrex)
- clopidogrel (Plavix)
- dalteparin (Fragmin)
- danaparoid (Orgaran)
- dipyridamole (Novo-Dipiradol, Persantine)
- enoxaparin (Lovenox)
- eptifibatide (Integrillin)
- fondaparinux (Arixtra)
- heparin (Hepalean, Hep-Lock)
- indobufen (Ibustrin)
- lepirudin (Refludan)
- meloxicam (MOBIC, Mobicox)
- nadroparin (Fraxiparine)
- naproxen (Aleve, Naprosyn)
- piroxicam (Feldene, Nu-Pirox)
- reteplase (Retavase)
- rofecoxib (Vioxx)
- streptokinase (Streptase)
- tenecteplase (TNKase)
- ticlopidine (Alti-Ticlopidine, Ticlid)
- tinzaparin (Innohep)
- tirofiban (Aggrastat)
- urokinase (Abbokinase)
- warfarin (Coumadin, Jantoven)

Taking angelica with these drugs may interfere with the action of the drug:

- aluminum hydroxide (AlternaGel, Alu-Cap)
- aluminum hydroxide and magnesium carbonate (Gaviscon Extra Strength, Gaviscon Liquid)
- aluminum hydroxide and magnesium hydroxide (Maalox, Rulox)
- aluminum hydroxide and magnesium trisilicate (Gaviscon Tablet)
- aluminum hydroxide, magnesium hydroxide, and simethicone (Maalox, Mylanta Liquid)
- calcium carbonate (Rolaids Extra Strength, Tums)
- calcium carbonate and magnesium hydroxide (Mylanta Gelcaps, Rolaids Extra Strength)
- cimetidine (Nu-Cimet, Tagamet)
- esomeprazole (Nexium)
- famotidine (Apo-Famotidine, Pepcid)
- famotidine, calcium carbonate, and magnesium hydroxide (Pepcid Complete)
- lansoprazole (Prevacid)
- magaldrate and simethicone (Riopan Plus, Riopan Plus Double Strength)
- magnesium hydroxide (Dulcolax Milk of Magnesia, Phillips' Milk of Magnesia)
- magnesium oxide (Mag-Ox 400, Uro-Mag)
- magnesium sulfate (Epsom salts)
- nizatidine (Axid, PMS-Nizatidine)
- omeprazole (Losec, Prilosec)
- pantoprazole (Pantoloc, Protonix)
- rabeprazole (Aciphex, Pariet)
- ranitidine (Alti-Ranitidine, Zantac)
- sodium bicarbonate (Brioschi, Neut)

Taking angelica with these drugs may increase the risk of hyperglycemia (high blood sugar):

- insulin (Humulin, Novolin R)
- metformin (Glucophage, Riomet)
- miglitol (Glyset)

- pioglitazone (Actos)
- repaglinide (GlucoNorm, Prandin)
- rosiglitazone (Avandia)

Taking angelica with these drugs may be harmful: lithium (Eskalith, Carbolith)—may increase effects of lithium, causing lithium toxicity

Lab Tests That May Be Altered by Angelica
May increase plasma partial thromboplastin time (PTT), prothrombin time (PT), and plasma international normalized ratio (INR) in those who are also taking warfarin.

Diseases That May Be Worsened or Triggered by Angelica
None known

Foods That May Interact with Angelica
None known

Supplements That May Interact with Angelica
Increased risk of bleeding or bruising when used with herbs and supplements that might affect platelet aggregation, such as danshen, garlic, ginger, ginkgo biloba, red clover, turmeric, white willow, and others. (For a list of herbs and supplements with anticoagulant/antiplatelet potential, see Appendix B.)

ANISE

Used as a spice and an herbal remedy by the ancient Egyptians, the sweet, licorice-tasting anise seed has long been used in tea form to relieve digestive complaints and ease coughs and colds. It also has been used to increase milk production in nursing mothers and relieve menstrual problems, most likely because it contains phytoestrogens, a plant form of the female hormone estrogen.

Scientific Name
Pimpinella anisum

Anise Is Also Commonly Known As
Aniseed, sweet cumin

Medicinal Parts
Fruit

Anise's Uses
To treat flatulence, digestive disturbances, menstrual complaints, whooping cough, liver disease, the cold, fever, inflammation, and tuberculosis. Germany's Commission E has approved the use of anise to treat the common cold, cough, bronchitis, fevers, inflammation of the mouth and throat, loss of appetite, and dyspeptic complaints such as heartburn and bloating.

Typical Dose
A typical daily dose of anise is approximately 3 gm combined with boiling water, allowed to steep, then strained.

Possible Side Effects
No side effects are known when anise is taken in designated therapeutic doses. Allergic reactions to the herb may occur on rare occasions.

Drugs That May Interact with Anise
Taking anise with these drugs may increase the risk of bleeding or bruising:

- abciximab (ReoPro)
- aspirin (Bufferin, Ecotrin)
- celecoxib (Celebrex)
- enoxaparin (Lovenox)
- etodolac (Lodine, Utradol)
- fondaparinux (Arixtra)
- heparin (Hepalean, Hep-Lock)
- ibuprofen (Advil, Motrin)
- indomethacin (Indocin, Novo-Methacin)
- ketoprofen (Orudis, Rhodis)
- ketorolac (Acular, Toradol)
- meloxicam (MOBIC, Mobicox)
- naproxen (Aleve, Naprosyn)
- piroxicam (Feldene, Nu-Pirox)
- rofecoxib (Vioxx)
- ticlopidine (Alti-Ticlopidine, Ticlid)
- urokinase (Abbokinase)
- warfarin (Coumadin, Jantoven)

Taking anise with these drugs may interfere with contraception and/or hormone replacement therapy:

- cyproterone and ethinyl estradiol (Diane-35)
- estradiol (Climara, Estrace)
- estradiol and medroxyprogesterone (Lunelle)
- estradiol and norethindrone (Activella, Combi-Patch)
- estradiol and testosterone (Climacteron)
- estrogens (conjugated A/synthetic) (Cenestin)
- estrogens (conjugated/equine) (Congest, Premarin)
- estrogens (conjugated/equine) and medroxy-progesterone (Premphase, Prempro)
- estrogens (esterified) (Estratab, Menest)
- estrogens (esterified) and methyltestosterone (Estratest, Estratest H.S.)
- estropipate (Ogen, OrthoEst)

- ethinyl estradiol (Estinyl)
- ethinyl estradiol and desogestrel (Cyclessa, Ortho-Cept)
- ethinyl estradiol and drospirenone (Yasmin)
- ethinyl estradiol and ethynodiol diacetate (Demulen, Zovia)
- ethinyl estradiol and etonogestrel (NuvaRing)
- ethinyl estradiol and levonorgestrel (Alesse, Triphasil)
- ethinyl estradiol and norelgestromin (Ortho Evra, Evra)
- ethinyl estradiol and norethindrone (Brevicon, Ortho-Novum)
- ethinyl estradiol and norgestimate (Cyclen, Ortho Tri-Cyclen)
- ethinyl estradiol and norgestrel (Cryselle, Ovral)
- levonorgestrel (Mirena, Plan B)
- medroxyprogesterone (Depo-Provera, Provera)
- mestranol and norethindrone (Necon 1/50, Ortho-Novum 1/50)
- norgestrel (Ovrette)
- polyestradiol

Taking anise with these drugs may interfere with the action of the drug:

- iproniazid (Marsilid)
- moclobemide (Alti-Moclobemide, Nu-Moclo-bemide)
- phenelzine (Nardil)
- selegiline (Eldepryl)
- tamoxifen (Nolvadex, Tamofen)
- tranylcypromine (Parnate)

Lab Tests That May Be Altered by Anise
May increase blood pressure readings, heart rate, and pulse rate due to the catecholamine activity of its constituent anethole.

Diseases That May Be Worsened or Triggered by Anise

- This herb may have estrogen-like effects and should not be used by women with estrogen-sensitive breast cancer or other hormone-sensitive conditions.
- Various skin conditions may be worsened if anise is applied to the skin.

Foods That May Interact with Anise

None known

Supplements That May Interact with Anise

None known

APPLE CIDER VINEGAR

Vinegar became one of our first medicines around 400 B.C., when Hippocrates, the "Father of Medicine," discovered its antiseptic, soothing qualities. He began prescribing it for conditions ranging from ear infections to skin rashes. Vinegar is made by fermenting the natural sugar contained in its main ingredients, which could be fruit, honey, beer, malt, or grains, into alcohol. Then the alcohol is fermented into acetic acid, which gives vinegar its sharp, sour taste. Apple cider vinegar has long been used as a health aid, and is purported to treat arthritis, high blood pressure, osteoporosis, and obesity, while fighting cancer, infection, and the onset of senility.

Scientific Name

Malus sylvestris

Apple Cider Vinegar Is Also Commonly Known As

Cider vinegar

Medicinal Parts

Fermented juice derived from the fruit of the apple tree

Apple Cider Vinegar's Uses

To treat leg cramps and pain, elevated cholesterol levels, upset stomach, high blood pressure; to encourage weight loss; to rid the body of toxins

Typical Dose

There is no typical dose of apple cider vinegar.

Possible Side Effects

Apple cider vinegar's side effects include lowered potassium levels.

Drugs That May Interact with Apple Cider Vinegar

Taking apple cider vinegar with these drugs may increase the risk of hypokalemia (low levels of potassium in the blood):

- acetazolamide (Apo-Acetazolamide, Diamox Sequels)
- azosemide (Diat)
- bumetanide (Bumex, Burinex)
- chlorothiazide (Diuril)
- chlorthalidone (Apo-Chlorthalidone, Thalitone)
- digitalis (Digitek, Lanoxin)
- ethacrynic acid (Edecrin)
- etozolin (Elkapin)
- furosemide (Apo-Furosemide, Lasix)
- hydrochlorothiazide (Apo-Hydro, Microzide)
- hydroflumethiazide (Diucardin, Saluron)
- indapamide (Lozol, Nu-Indapamide)
- insulin (Humulin, Novolin R)
- mannitol (Osmitrol, Resectisol)
- mefruside (Baycaron)
- methazolamide (Apo-Methazolamide, Neptazane)

- methyclothiazide (Aquatensen, Enduron)
- metolazone (Mykrox, Zaroxolyn)
- olmesartan and hydrochlorothiazide (Benicar HCT)
- polythiazide (Renese)
- torsemide (Demadex)
- trichlormethiazide (Metatensin, Naqua)
- urea (Amino-Cerv, UltraMide)
- xipamide (Diurexan, Lumitens)

Lab Tests That May Be Altered by Apple Cider Vinegar
May decrease serum potassium level and increase urine potassium level when used in high doses or over a long term.

Diseases That May Be Worsened or Triggered by Apple Cider Vinegar
May increase the risk of potassium loss in people using insulin.

Foods That May Interact with Apple Cider Vinegar
None known

Supplements That May Interact with Apple Cider Vinegar
- Increased risk of cardiotoxicity from potassium depletion when taken with cardioactive herbs, such as adonis, digitalis, lily-of-the-valley, and squill. (For a list of cardioactive herbs and supplements, see Appendix B.)
- Increased risk of potassium depletion when used in conjunction with horsetail plant or licorice.

ARECA NUT

Purportedly chewed by over 200 million people worldwide—one-tenth of the world's population—the areca nut (also known as the betel nut) is a mild stimulant used as a recreational drug to impart a feeling of exhilaration, strength, and well-being. The nut, which is a little smaller than a walnut, is sometimes wrapped in betel leaf, with mineral lime added as a catalyst. Then the whole package is placed between the cheek and the gum to let it "soak." Those who use areca nut find that it causes red stains not only to the mouth and lips, but also to the feces.

Scientific Name
Areca catechu

Areca Nut Is Also Commonly Known As
Areca, betel nut, pinag

Medicinal Parts
Nut

Areca Nut's Uses
Areca nut is chewed for its intoxicating qualities but is also used to treat edema, diarrhea, digestive problems, schizophrenia, glaucoma, and chronic hepatitis.

Typical Dose
There is no typical dose of areca nut, although eleven nuts per day is common among frequent users.

Possible Side Effects
Areca nut's side effects include tremors; slowed heart rate; staining of the mouth, lips, and feces; euphoria; and increased salivation. Long-term use can result in cancer of the oral cavity. Taking 8 to 10 gm may be toxic to humans.

Drugs That May Interact with Areca Nut

Taking areca nut with these drugs may enhance the therapeutic and adverse effects of the drug:

- acetylcholine (Miochol-E)
- bethanechol (Duvoid, Urecholine)
- carbachol (Carbastat, Isopto Carbachol)
- cevimeline (Evoxac)
- donepezil (Aricept)
- edrophonium (Enlon, Reversol)
- galantamine (Razadyne)
- methacholine (Provocholine)
- neostigmine (Prostigmin)
- physostigmine (Eserine)
- pilocarpine (Isopto Carpine, Salagen)
- pyridostigmine (Mestinon)
- rivastigmine (Exelon)
- tacrine (Cognex)

Taking areca nut with these drugs may interfere with the actions of the drug:

- atropine (Isopto Atropine, Sal-Tropine)
- benztropine (Apo-Benztropine, Cogentin)
- clidinium and chlordiazepoxide (Apo-Chlorax, Librax)
- cyclopentolate (Cyclogyl, Cylate)
- dicyclomine (Bentyl, Lomine)
- glycopyrrolate (Robinul, Robinul Forte)
- homatropine (Isopto Homatropine)
- hyoscyamine (Hyosine, Levsin)
- hyoscyamine, atropine, scopolamine, and phenobarbital (Donnatal, Donnatal Extentabs)
- ipratropium (Atrovent, Nu-Ipratropium)
- oxitropium (Oxivent, Tersigat)
- prifinium (Padrin, Riabel)
- procyclidine (Kemadrin, Procyclid)
- propantheline (Propanthel)
- scopolamine (Scopace, Transderm Scop)
- tiotropium (Spiriva)
- tolterodine (Detrol, Detrol LA)
- trihexyphenidyl (Artane)
- trimethobenzamide (Tigan)

Lab Tests That May Be Altered by Areca Nut

May interfere with fecal lab tests since chewing areca nuts stains the feces red.

Diseases That May Be Worsened or Triggered by Areca Nut

May worsen asthma.

Foods That May Interact with Areca Nut

None known

Supplements That May Interact with Areca Nut

None known

ARNICA

Sometimes called "mountain tobacco," arnica is used in both herbal and homeopathic forms to treat wounds, bruises, and other types of injuries. The famous eighteenth-century German scholar Goethe claimed that arnica cured him of an otherwise uncontrollable fever that nearly took his life.

Scientific Name

Arnica montana

Arnica Is Also Commonly Known As

Leopard's bane, mountain tobacco, sneezewort, wolf's bane

Medicinal Parts

Flower, leaf, root, rhizome

Arnica's Uses

To treat muscle and joint ailments, inflammation, cough, hair loss, and contusions. Germany's Commission E has approved the use of arnica flower to treat inflammation of the skin, mouth, and throat; cough, bronchitis, the common cold, fever, rheumatism, and blunt injuries.

Typical Dose

A typical dose of arnica has not been established.

Possible Side Effects

When applied topically, arnica's side effects include eczema and skin inflammation. When taken internally, arnica's side effects include dizziness, tremor, stomach pain, or diarrhea. Oral administration of the herb is potentially dangerous, and should be taken only under the supervision of a physician.

Drugs That May Interact with Arnica

Taking arnica with these drugs may increase the risk of bleeding or bruising:

- abciximab (ReoPro)
- alteplase (Activase, Cathflo Activase)
- antithrombin III (Thrombate III)
- argatroban
- aspirin (Bufferin, Ecotrin)
- aspirin and dipyridamole (Aggrenox)
- bivalirudin (Angiomax)
- celecoxib (Celebrex)
- clopidogrel (Plavix)
- dalteparin (Fragmin)
- danaparoid (Orgaran)
- dipyridamole (Persantine, Novo-Dipiradol)
- enoxaparin (Lovenox)
- eptifibatide (Integrillin)
- fondaparinux (Arixtra)
- heparin (Hepalean, Hep-Lock)
- indobufen (Ibustrin)
- lepirudin (Refludan)
- nadroparin (Fraxiparine)
- reteplase (Retavase)
- streptokinase (Streptase)
- tenecteplase (TNKase)
- ticlopidine (Alti-Ticlopidine, Ticlid)
- tinzaparin (Innohep)
- tirofiban (Aggrastat)
- urokinase (Abbokinase)
- warfarin (Coumadin, Jantoven)

Taking arnica with these drugs may interfere with the action of the drug:

- acebutolol (Novo-Acebutolol, Sectral)
- amlodipine (Norvasc)
- atenolol (Apo-Atenol, Tenormin)
- benazepril (Lotensin)
- betaxolol (Betoptic S, Kerlone)
- bisoprolol (Monocor, Zebeta)
- bumetanide (Bumex, Burinex)
- candesartan (Atacand)
- captopril (Capoten, Novo-Captopril)
- carteolol (Cartrol, Ocupress)
- carvedilol (Coreg)
- chlorothiazide (Diuril)
- chlorthalidone (Apo-Chlorthalidone, Thalitone)
- clonidine (Catapres, Duraclon)
- diazoxide (Hyperstat, Proglycem)
- diltiazem (Cardizem, Tiazac)
- doxazosin (Alti-Doxazosin, Cardura)
- enalapril (Vasotec)
- eplerenone (Inspra)

- eprosartan (Teveten)
- esmolol (Brevibloc)
- felodipine (Plendil, Renedil)
- fenoldopam (Corlopam)
- fosinopril (Monopril)
- furosemide (Apo-Furosemide, Lasix)
- guanabenz (Wytensin)
- guanadrel (Hylorel)
- guanfacine (Tenex)
- hydralazine (Apresoline, Novo-Hylazin)
- hydrochlorothiazide (Apo-Hydro, Micro-zide)
- indapamide (Lozol, Nu-Indapamide)
- irbesartan (Avapro)
- isradipine (DynaCirc)
- labetalol (Normodyne, Trandate)
- lisinopril (Prinivil, Zestril)
- losartan (Cozaar)
- mefruside (Baycaron)
- mecamylamine (Inversine)
- methyclothiazide (Aquatensen, Enduron)
- methyldopa (Apo-Methyldopa, Nu-Medopa)
- metolazone (Mykrox, Zaroxolyn)
- metoprolol (Betaloc, Lopressor)
- minoxidil (Loniten, Rogaine)
- moexipril (Univasc)
- nadolol (Apo-Nadol, Corgard)
- nicardipine (Cardene)
- nifedipine (Adalat CC, Procardia)
- nisoldipine (Sular)
- nitroglycerin (Minitran, Nitro-Dur)
- nitroprusside (Nipride, Nitropress)
- olmesartan (Benicar)
- oxprenolol (Slow-Trasicor, Trasicor)
- perindopril erbumine (Aceon, Coversyl)
- phenoxybenzamine (Dibenzyline)
- phentolamine (Regitine, Rogitine)
- pindolol (Apo-Pindol, Novo-Pindol)
- polythiazide (Renese)
- prazosin (Minipress, Nu-Prazo)
- propranolol (Inderal, InnoPran XL)
- quinapril (Accupril)
- ramipril (Altace)
- reserpine
- spironolactone (Aldactone, Novo-Spiroton)
- telmisartan (Micardis)
- terazosin (Alti-Terazosin, Hytrin)
- timolol (Betimol, Timoptic)
- torsemide (Demadex)
- trandolapril (Mavik)
- triamterene (Dyrenium)
- trichlormethiazide (Metatensin, Naqua)
- valsartan (Diovan)
- verapamil (Calan, Isoptin SR)

Lab Tests That May Be Altered by Arnica
May inhibit platelet function.

Diseases That May Be Worsened or Triggered by Arnica
This herb can irritate the gastrointestinal tract and may worsen inflammatory or infectious gastrointestinal ailments.

Foods That May Interact with Arnica
None known

Supplements That May Interact with Arnica
Arnica belongs to the Asteraceae family and is contraindicated in those sensitive to herbs from the Asteraceae family, such as German chamomile, daisy, or dandelion. (For a list of herbs and

supplements from the Asteraceae family, see Appendix B.)

ARTICHOKE

> The artichoke plant contains cynarin and scolymoside, two substances used to stimulate bile secretion and treat sluggish livers and poor digestion. In Europe, artichoke is a popular herbal treatment for arteriosclerosis, as cynarin has been shown to lower both cholesterol and triglyceride levels.

Scientific Name
Cynara scolymus

Artichoke Is Also Commonly Known As
Garden artichoke, globe artichoke

Medicinal Parts
Leaf

Artichoke's Uses
To lower cholesterol and aid digestion; to treat dyspepsia; to prevent the return of gallstones. Germany's Commission E has approved the use of artichoke to treat loss of appetite and liver and gallbladder complaints.

Typical Dose
A typical single dose of artichoke is approximately 500 mg of dry extract; an average daily dose is 6 gm of dry extract or 6 gm of dried herb, divided into three doses.

Possible Side Effects
No side effects are known when artichoke is taken in designated therapeutic doses.

Drugs That May Interact with Artichoke
Taking artichoke with these drugs may increase the drug's diuretic effects:
- bumetanide (Bumex, Burinex)
- furosemide (Apo-Furosemide, Lasix)

Taking artichoke with these drugs may interfere with the absorption of the drug:
- ferric gluconate (Ferrlecit)
- ferrous fumarate (Femiron, Feostat)
- ferrous gluconate (Fergon, Novo-Ferrogluc)
- ferrous sulfate (Feratab, Fer-Iron)
- ferrous sulfate and ascorbic acid (FeroGrad 500, Vitelle Irospan)
- iron-dextran complex (Dexferrum, INFeD)
- polysaccharide-iron complex (Hytinic, Niferex)

Taking artichoke with this drug may increase the risk of hypokalemia (low levels of potassium in the blood):
- hydrochlorothiazide (Apo-Hydro, Microzide)

Lab Tests That May Be Altered by Artichoke
None known

Diseases That May Be Worsened or Triggered by Artichoke
May increase bile flow and exacerbate gallstones or bile duct obstruction.

Foods That May Interact with Artichoke
None known

Supplements That May Interact with Artichoke
None known

ASA FOETIDA

> This odiferous herb, sometimes known as devil's dung or stinking gum, gets its name from the Persian word *asa*, meaning "resin," combined with the Latin word *foetida*, meaning "smelling" or "fetid." Despite its sulfurlike smell, it was used as a folk remedy in the Appalachians for children's colds: a bag of the smelly paste was hung around the child's neck.

Scientific Name
Ferula foetida

Asa Foetida Is Also Commonly Known As
Devil's dung, food of the gods, gum asafoetida

Medicinal Parts
Plant resin

Asa Foetida's Uses
To treat dyspepsia, irritable colon, chronic gastritis, intestinal parasites, asthma, whooping cough, and diseases of the liver and spleen.

Typical Dose
A typical dose of asa foetida is approximately 20 drops of tincture.

Possible Side Effects
No side effects are known when asa foetida is taken in designated therapeutic doses.

Drugs That May Interact with Asa Foetida
Taking asa foetida with these drugs may increase the risk of bleeding or bruising:
- abciximab (ReoPro)
- antithrombin III (Thrombate III)
- argatroban
- aspirin (Bufferin, Ecotrin)
- aspirin and dipyridamole (Aggrenox)
- bivalirudin (Angiomax)
- clopidogrel (Plavix)
- dalteparin (Fragmin)
- danaparoid (Orgaran)
- dipyridamole (Novo-Dipiradol, Persantine)
- enoxaparin (Lovenox)
- eptifibatide (Integrillin)
- fondaparinux (Arixtra)
- heparin (Hepalean, Hep-Lock)
- indobufen (Ibustrin)
- lepirudin (Refludan)
- ticlopidine (Alti-Ticlopidine, Ticlid)
- tinzaparin (Innohep)
- tirofiban (Aggrastat)
- warfarin (Coumadin, Jantoven)

Taking asa foetida with these drugs may increase the risk of hypotension (excessively low blood pressure):
- acebutolol (Novo-Acebutolol, Sectral)
- amlodipine (Norvasc)
- atenolol (Apo-Atenol, Tenormin)
- benazepril (Lotensin)
- betaxolol (Betoptic S, Kerlone)
- bisoprolol (Monocor, Zebeta)
- bumetanide (Bumex, Burinex)
- candesartan (Atacand)
- captopril (Capoten, Novo-Captopril)
- carteolol (Cartrol, Ocupress)
- carvedilol (Coreg)
- chlorothiazide (Diuril)
- chlorthalidone (Apo-Chlorthalidone, Thalitone)
- clonidine (Catapres, Duraclon)
- diazoxide (Hyperstat, Proglycem)

- diltiazem (Cardizem, Tiazac)
- doxazosin (Alti-Doxazosin, Cardura)
- enalapril (Vasotec)
- eplerenone (Inspra)
- eprosartan (Teveten)
- esmolol (Brevibloc)
- felodipine (Plendil, Renedil)
- fenoldopam (Corlopam)
- fosinopril (Monopril)
- furosemide (Apo-Furosemide, Lasix)
- guanabenz (Wytensin)
- guanadrel (Hylorel)
- guanfacine (Tenex)
- hydralazine (Apresoline, Novo-Hylazin)
- hydrochlorothiazide (Apo-Hydro, Microzide)
- hydrochlorothiazide and triamterene (Dyazide, Maxzide)
- indapamide (Lozol, Nu-Indapamide)
- irbesartan (Avapro)
- isradipine (DynaCirc)
- labetalol (Normodyne, Trandate)
- lisinopril (Prinivil, Zestril)
- losartan (Cozaar)
- mecamylamine (Inversine)
- mefruside (Baycaron)
- methyclothiazide (Aquatensen, Enduron)
- methyldopa (Apo-Methyldopa, Nu-Medopa)
- metolazone (Mykrox, Zaroxolyn)
- metoprolol (Betaloc, Lopressor)
- minoxidil (Loniten, Rogaine)
- moexipril (Univasc)
- nadolol (Apo-Nadol, Corgard)
- nicardipine (Cardene)
- nifedipine (Adalat CC, Procardia)
- nisoldipine (Sular)
- nitroglycerin (Minitran, Nitro-Dur)
- nitroprusside (Nipride, Nitropress)
- olmesartan (Benicar)

- oxprenolol (Slow-Trasicor, Trasicor)
- perindopril erbumine (Aceon, Coversyl)
- phenoxybenzamine (Dibenzyline)
- phentolamine (Regitine, Rogitine)
- pindolol (Apo-Pindol, Novo-Pindol)
- polythiazide (Renese)
- prazosin (Minipress, Nu-Prazo)
- propranolol (Inderal, InnoPran XL)
- quinapril (Accupril)
- ramipril (Altace)
- reserpine
- spironolactone (Aldactone, Novo-Spiroton)
- telmisartan (Micardis)
- terazosin (Alti-Terazosin, Hytrin)
- timolol (Betimol, Timoptic)
- torsemide (Demadex)
- trandolapril (Mavik)
- triamterene (Dyrenium)
- trichlormethiazide (Metatensin, Naqua)
- valsartan (Diovan)
- verapamil (Calan, Isoptin SR)

Lab Tests That May Be Altered by Asa Foetida
None known

Diseases That May Be Worsened or Triggered by Asa Foetida

- May increase the risk of bleeding or bruising in those with bleeding diseases.
- May trigger convulsions in those with diseases of the central nervous system.
- May interfere with control of blood pressure.
- This herb can irritate the gastrointestinal tract and may worsen inflammatory or infectious gastrointestinal ailments.

Foods That May Interact with Asa Foetida
None known

Supplements That May Interact with Asa Foetida

None known

ASHWAGANDHA

> Ashwagandha, which in Sanskrit means "that which has the smell of a horse," has been used in Indian medicine for some four thousand years to treat inflammatory diseases and tumors and to promote sexual stimulation and longevity. Some animal and human studies have shown that an extract of the ashwagandha root does have some ability to slow the growth of cancerous tumors and to reduce the inflammation seen in rheumatoid arthritis.

Scientific Name

Withania somnifera

Ashwagandha Is Also Commonly Known As

Asgandh, avarada, Ayurvedic ginseng, winter cherry, withania

Medicinal Parts

Root, berry

Ashwagandha's Uses

To treat anxiety, insomnia, arthritis, tumors, skin ulcers, backache, chronic liver disease, and tuberculosis; to increase resistance to environmental stress

Typical Dose

A typical daily dose of ashwagandha may range from 1 to 6 gm of the whole herb in capsule or tea form.

Possible Side Effects

Ashwagandha's side effects include gastrointestinal upset, vomiting, and diarrhea.

Drugs That May Interact with Ashwagandha

Taking ashwagandha with these drugs may reduce the drug's immunosuppressive effects:

- antithymocyte globulin, equine (Atgam)
- antithymocyte globulin, rabbit (Thymoglobulin)
- azathioprine (Imuran)
- basiliximab (Simulect)
- beclomethasone (Beconase, Vanceril)
- betamethasone (Celestone, Diprolene)
- budesonide (Entocort, Rhinocort)
- budesonide and Formoterol (Symbicort)
- cortisone (Cortone)
- cyclosporine (Neoral, Sandimmune)
- daclizumab (Zenapax)
- deflazacort (Calcort, Dezacor)
- dexamethasone (Decadron, Dexasone)
- efalizumab (Raptiva)
- flunisolide (AeroBid, Nasarel)
- fluorometholone (Eflone, Flarex)
- fluticasone (Cutivate, Flonase)
- hydrocortisone (Anusol-HC, Locoid)
- loteprednol (Alrex, Lotemax)
- medrysone (HMS Liquifilm)
- methotrexate (Rheumatrex, Trexall)
- methylprednisolone (DepoMedrol, Medrol)
- muromonab-CD3 (Orthoclone OKT 3)
- mycophenolate (CellCept)
- pimecrolimus (Elidel)
- prednisolone (Inflamase Forte, Pred Forte)
- prednisone (Apo-Prednisone, Deltasone)
- rimexolone (Vexol)
- sirolimus (Rapamune)
- tacrolimus (Prograf, Protopic)

- thalidomide (Thalomid)
- triamcinolone (Aristocort, Trinasal)

Taking ashwagandha with these drugs may increase both the positive and negative effects of the drug:

- acetaminophen and codeine (Capital and Codeine, Tylenol with Codeine)
- alfentanil (Alfenta)
- alprazolam (Apo-Alpraz, Xanax)
- amobarbital (Amytal)
- amobarbital and secobarbital (Tuinal)
- aspirin and codeine (Coryphen Codeine)
- belladonna and opium (B&O Supprettes)
- bromazepam (Apo-Bromazepam, Gen-Bromazepam)
- brotizolam (Lendorm, Sintonal)
- buprenorphine (Buprenex, Subutex)
- buprenorphine and naloxone (Suboxone)
- butabarbital (Butisol Sodium)
- butalbital, acetaminophen, and caffeine (Esgic, Fioricet)
- butalbital, aspirin, and caffeine (Fiorinal)
- butorphanol (Apo-Butorphanol, Stadol)
- chloral hydrate (Aquachloral Supprettes, Somnote)
- chlordiazepoxide (Apo-Chlordiazepoxide, Librium)
- clobazam (Alti-Clobazam, Frisium)
- clonazepam (Klonopin, Rivotril)
- clorazepate (Tranxene, T-Tab)
- codeine (Codeine Contin)
- dexmedetomidine (Precedex)
- diazepam (Apo-Diazepam, Valium)
- dihydrocodeine, aspirin, and caffeine (Synalgos-DC)
- diphenhydramine (Benadryl Allergy, Nytol)
- estazolam (ProSom)
- fentanyl (Actiq, Duragesic)
- flurazepam (Apo-Flurazepam, Dalmane)
- glutethimide
- haloperidol (Haldol, Novo-Peridol)
- hydrocodone and acetaminophen (Vicodin, Zydone)
- hydrocodone and aspirin (Damason-P)
- hydrocodone and ibuprofen (Vicoprofen)
- hydromorphone (Dilaudid, PMS-Hydromorphone)
- hydroxyzine (Atarax, Vistaril)
- levomethadyl acetate hydrochloride
- levorphanol (LevoDromoran)
- loprazolam (Dormonoct, Havlane)
- lorazepam (Ativan, Nu-Loraz)
- meperidine (Demerol, Meperitab)
- meperidine and promethazine
- mephobarbital (Mebaral)
- methadone (Dolophine, Methadose)
- methohexital (Brevital, Brevital Sodium)
- midazolam (Apo-Midazolam, Versed)
- morphine sulfate (Kadian, MS Contin)
- nalbuphine (Nubain)
- opium tincture
- oxycodone (OxyContin, Roxicodone)
- oxycodone and acetaminophen (Endocet, Percocet)
- oxycodone and aspirin (Endodan, Percodan)
- oxymorphone (Numorphan)
- paregoric
- pentazocine (Talwin)
- pentobarbital (Nembutal)
- phenobarbital (Luminal Sodium, PMS-Phenobarbital)
- phenoperidine
- prazepam
- primidone (Apo-Primidone, Mysoline)
- promethazine (Phenergan)
- propofol (Diprivan)

- propoxyphene (Darvon, Darvon-N)
- propoxyphene and acetaminophen (Darvocet-N 50, Darvocet-N 100)
- propoxyphene, aspirin, and caffeine (Darvon Compound)
- quazepam (Doral)
- remifentanil (Ultiva)
- secobarbital (Seconal)
- sufentanil (Sufenta)
- temazepam (Novo-Temazepam, Restoril)
- tetrazepam (Mobiforton, Musapam)
- thiopental (Pentothal)
- triazolam (Apo-Triazo, Halcion)
- zaleplon (Sonata, Stamoc)
- zolpidem (Ambien)
- zopiclone (Alti-Zopiclone, Gen-Zopiclone)

Lab Tests That May Be Altered by Ashwagandha

May suppress thyroid stimulating hormone (TSH) or increase triiodothyronine (T_3) or thyroxine (T_4) values. May stimulate the synthesis or secretion of thyroid hormone.

Diseases That May Be Worsened or Triggered by Ashwagandha

May worsen peptic ulcer disease by irritating the gastrointestinal tract.

Foods That May Interact with Ashwagandha

None known

Supplements That May Interact with Ashwagandha

May enhance therapeutic and adverse effects of herbs and supplements that have sedative properties, such as 5-HTP, kava kava, St. John's wort, and valerian. (For a list of herbs and supplements that have sedative properties, see Appendix B.)

ASTRAGALUS

One of the premier herbs used in traditional Chinese medicine, astragalus was used as far back as the first century B.C. Some studies have shown that astragalus helps boost the immune system and may also keep malignant cancer cells from spreading to healthy tissue. For these reasons astragalus is used by some cancer patients, especially when undergoing radiation and chemotherapy.

Scientific Name

Astragalus species

Astragalus Is Also Commonly Known As

Beg kei, huang-qi, membranous milk vetch, tragacanth

Medicinal Parts

Root

Astragalus's Uses

To treat depression of the immune system, heart failure, viral infections, respiratory infections, liver disease, and kidney disease

Typical Dose

A typical daily dose of astragalus may range from 2 to 6 gm of dried root or 4 to 12 ml of fluid extract.

Possible Side Effects

Astragalus's more common side effects, as suggested by animal studies, include respiratory depression and allergic reactions.

Drugs That May Interact with Astragalus

Taking astragalus with these drugs may increase the risk of bleeding or bruising:

- abciximab (ReoPro)
- alteplase (Activase, Cathflo Activase)
- antithrombin III (Thrombate III)
- argatroban
- aspirin (Bufferin, Ecotrin)
- aspirin and dipyridamole (Aggrenox)
- bivalirudin (Angiomax)
- clopidogrel (Plavix)
- dalteparin (Fragmin)
- danaparoid (Organ)
- dipyridamole (Novo-Dipiradol, Persantine)
- enoxaparin (Lovenox)
- eptifibatide (Integrillin)
- fondaparinux (Arixtra)
- heparin (Hepalean, Hep-Lock)
- indobufen (Ibustrin)
- lepirudin (Refludan)
- nadroparin (Fraxiparine)
- reteplase (Retavase)
- streptokinase (Streptase)
- tenecteplase (TNKase)
- ticlopidine (Alti-Ticlopidine, Ticlid)
- tinzaparin (Innohep)
- tirofiban (Aggrastat)
- urokinase (Abbokinase)
- warfarin (Coumadin, Jantoven)

Taking astragalus with these drugs may reduce the drug's immunosuppressive effects:
- antithymocyte globulin, equine (Atgam)
- antithymocyte globulin, rabbit (Thymoglobulin)
- azathioprine (Imuran)
- basiliximab (Simulect)
- beclomethasone (Beconase, Vanceril)
- betamethasone (Betatrex, Maxivate)

- budesonide (Entocort, Rhinocort)
- budesonide and formoterol (Symbicort)
- cortisone (Cortone)
- cyclophosphamide (Cytoxan, Neosar)
- cyclosporine (Neoral, Sandimmune)
- daclizumab (Zenapax)
- deflazacort (Calcort, Dezacor)
- dexamethasone (Decadron, Dexasone)
- efalizumab (Raptiva)
- flunisolide (AeroBid, Nasarel)
- fluoromethalone (Eflone, Flarex)
- fluticasone (Cutivate, Flonase)
- hydrocortisone (Cetacort, Locoid)
- loteprednol (Alrex, Lotemax)
- medrysone (HMS Liquifilm)
- methotrexate (Rheumatrex, Trexall)
- methylprednisolone (Depo-Medrol, Medrol)
- muromonab-CD3 (Orthoclone OKT 3)
- mycophenolate (CellCept)
- pimecrolimus (Elidel)
- prednisolone (Inflamase Forte, Pred Forte)
- prednisone (Apo-Prednisone, Deltasone)
- rimexolone (Vexol)
- sirolimus (Rapamune)
- tacrolimus (Prograf, Protopic)
- thalidomide (Thalomid)
- triamcinolone (Aristocort, Trinasal)

Taking astragalus with this drug may increase the drug's tumor cell–killing ability and decrease the drug's side effects:
- aldesleukin (Proleukin)

Lab Tests That May Be Altered by Astragalus
May increase sperm motility in vitro and alter results of semen specimen analysis.

Diseases That May Be Worsened or Triggered by Astragalus

- May worsen autoimmune diseases by increasing the activity of the immune system.
- May interfere with the body's ability to accept transplanted tissues by hampering immunosuppressive medicines.

Foods That May Interact with Astragalus

None known

Supplements That May Interact with Astragalus

None known

AVARAM

> Avaram, an evergreen shrub famous for its beautiful yellow flowers, grows wild in India. Its bark, which contains 18 percent tannin, is often used in the tanning of leather. In Ayurvedic medicine, avaram root is used to treat fevers, diabetes, diseases of the urinary system, and constipation, while the leaves are used as a laxative and the dried flowers are used for polyurea. One study showed that an extract of avaram flowers suppressed elevated blood glucose and lipids in diabetic rats as well as a standard drug.

Scientific Name

Cassia auriculata

Avaram Is Also Commonly Known As

Kalpa herbal tea, ranawara, tanner's cassia

Medicinal Parts

Fruit, flower, leaf, root, bark, seed

Avaram's Uses

To treat diabetes, liver disease, and urinary tract disorders

Typical Dose

A typical daily dose of avaram has not been established.

Possible Side Effects

Serious side effects linked to the use of avaram have not been reported.

Drugs That May Interact with Avaram

Taking avaram with these drugs may increase the risk of hypoglycemia (low blood sugar):

- acarbose (Prandase, Precose)
- acetohexamide
- chlorpropamide (Diabinese, Novo-Propamide)
- gliclazide (Diamicron, Novo-Gliclazide)
- glimepiride (Amaryl)
- glipizide (Glucotrol)
- glipizide and metformin (Metaglip)
- gliquidone (Beglynor, Glurenorm)
- glyburide (DiaBeta, Micronase)
- glyburide and metformin (Glucovance)
- insulin (Humulin, Novolin R)
- metformin (Glucophage, Riomet)
- miglitol (Glyset)
- nateglinide (Starlix)
- pioglitazone (Actos)
- repaglinide (GlucoNorm, Prandin)
- rosiglitazone (Avandia)
- rosiglitazone and metformin (Avandamet)
- tolazamide (Tolinase)
- tolbutamide (Apo-Tolbutamide, Tol-Tab)

Taking avaram with this drug may be harmful:

- Carbamazepine (Tegretol, Carbatrol)— increases drug levels

Lab Tests That May Be Altered by Avaram
None known

Diseases That May Be Worsened or Triggered by Avaram
None known

Foods That May Interact with Avaram
None known

Supplements That May Interact with Avaram
The tannins in avaram may cause substances in certain other herbs to separate and settle, increasing the risk of toxic reactions. (For a list of herbs and other substances high in alkaloids, see Appendix B.)

BALSAM OF PERU

Taken from the bark of the *Myroxolon balsamum* tree, native to El Salvador, balsam of Peru smells like cinnamon and vanilla due to its high amounts of cinnamein (a combination of cinnamic acid, cinnamyl cinnamate, benzyl benzoate, benzoic acid, and vanillin). It also contains essential oils that are much like those found in the peel of citrus fruit. This wonderful-smelling substance is used in perfumes and toiletries. It also has mild antibacterial and antifungal properties and is added to wound-healing ointments.

Scientific Name
Myroxylon balsamum

Balsam of Peru Is Also Commonly Known As
Balsam of Tolu, balsam tree, Peruvian balsam

Medicinal Parts
Bark

Balsam of Peru's Uses
To treat hemorrhoids, coughs, colds, fever, and wounds

Typical Dose
A typical daily dose of balsam of Peru has not been established.

Possible Side Effects
Balsam of Peru's side effects include skin irritation and sun sensitivity.

Drugs That May Interact with Balsam of Peru
Taking balsam of Peru with these drugs may cause or increase kidney damage:

- etodolac (Lodine, Utradol)
- ibuprofen (Advil, Motrin)
- indomethacin (Indocin, Novo-Methacin)
- ketoprofen (Orudis, Rhodis)
- ketorolac (Acular, Toradol)
- metformin (Glucophage, Riomet)

Lab Tests That May Be Altered by Balsam of Peru
None known

Diseases That May Be Worsened or Triggered by Balsam of Peru
None known

Foods That May Interact with Balsam of Peru
None known

Supplements That May Interact with Balsam of Peru

None known

BANABA

Banaba leaves, a popular medicine used in the Philippines to treat diabetes, are high in corosolic acid, a natural plant insulin. In 1999 a study conducted on diabetes patients at the Southwestern Institute of Biomedical Research in Bradenton, Florida, found that corosolic acid universally lowered blood sugar levels in all patients. The more corosolic acid they received, the more their blood sugar levels dropped.

Scientific Name

Lagerstoemia speciosa

Banaba Is Also Commonly Known As

Crape myrtle, crepe myrtle, pride of India, queen's crape myrtle

Medicinal Parts

Leaf

Banaba's Uses

To treat diabetes and aid in weight loss

Typical Dose

A typical daily dose of banaba has not been established.

Possible Side Effects

No serious side effects have been reported when banaba is used properly under a physician's supervision.

Drugs That May Interact with Banaba

Taking banaba with these drugs may increase the risk of hypoglycemia (low blood sugar):

- acarbose (Prandase, Precose)
- acetohexamide
- chlorpropamide (Diabinese, Novo-Propamide)
- gliclazide (Diamicron, Novo-Gliclazide)
- glimepiride (Amaryl)
- glipizide (Glucotrol)
- glipizide and metformin (Metaglip)
- gliquidone (Glurenorm, Beglynor)
- glyburide (DiaBeta, Micronase)
- glyburide and metformin (Glucovance)
- insulin (Humulin, Novolin R)
- metformin (Glucophage, Riomet)
- miglitol (Glyset)
- nateglinide (Starlix)
- pioglitazone (Actos)
- repaglinide (GlucoNorm, Prandin)
- rosiglitazone (Avandia)
- rosiglitazone and metformin (Avandamet)
- tolazamide (Tolinase)
- tolbutamide (Apo-Tolbutamide, Tol-Tab)

Lab Tests That May Be Altered by Banaba

None known

Diseases That May Be Worsened or Triggered by Banaba

May cause blood sugar levels to fall too low in diabetics.

Foods That May Interact with Banaba

None known

Supplements That May Interact with Banaba

May increase blood glucose–lowering effects and risk of hypoglycemia (low blood sugar) when used with herbs and supplements that lower glucose levels, such as alpha-lipoic acid, chromium, devil's claw, Panax ginseng, and psyllium. (For a list of herbs and supplements that lower blood glucose levels, see Appendix B.)

BARLEY

Barley comes in a variety of forms—flour, flakes, pot barley, and pearl barley. Research conducted in Canada, the United States, and Australia has shown that certain components of barley (most notably its soluble and insoluble fiber, tocotrienols, and beta-glucans) play important roles in reducing high cholesterol levels, most likely by inhibiting both the production and the absorption of cholesterol. In addition, some studies have shown that barley has a healing effect and can repair damage to the intestinal tracts of animals.

Scientific Name
Hordeum distichon

Barley Is Also Commonly Known As
Pearl barley, pot barley, Scotch barley

Medicinal Parts
Grain

Barley's Uses
To treat diarrhea, elevated cholesterol, inflammation of the stomach lining, and inflammatory bowel disease

Typical Dose
A typical dose of barley is approximately 450 mg of malt extract in capsule form.

Possible Side Effects
No side effects are known when barley is taken in designated therapeutic doses.

Drugs That May Interact with Barley
Taking barley with these drugs may increase the risk of hypoglycemia (low blood sugar):
- acarbose (Prandase, Precose)
- acetohexamide
- chlorpropamide (Diabinese, Novo-Propamide)
- gliclazide (Diamicron, Novo-Gliclazide)
- glimepiride (Amaryl)
- glipizide (Glucotrol)
- glipizide and metformin (Metaglip)
- gliquidone (Beglynor, Glurenorm)
- glyburide (DiaBeta, Micronase)
- glyburide and metformin (Glucovance)
- insulin (Humulin, Novolin R)
- metformin (Glucophage, Riomet)
- miglitol (Glyset)
- nateglinide (Starlix)
- pioglitazone (Actos)
- repaglinide (GlucoNorm, Prandin)
- rosiglitazone (Avandia)
- rosiglitazone and metformin (Avandamet)
- tolazamide (Tolinase)
- tolbutamide (Apo-Tolbutamide, Tol-Tab)

Taking barley with these drugs may be harmful:
- All oral drugs. The fiber in barley accelerates gastrointestinal transit and may therefore reduce the absorption of some drugs.

Lab Tests That May Be Altered by Barley
May decrease serum total cholesterol, LDL cholesterol, and blood glucose concentrations. May cause false positive test results with ELISA (enzyme-linked immunosorbent assay), RIA

(radioimmunoassay), and TLC (thin-layer chromatography) urine assays for a number of opiate drugs due to its constituent, hordenine.

Diseases That May Be Worsened or Triggered by Barley
May worsen celiac disease due to its gluten content.

Foods That May Interact with Barley
None known

Supplements That May Interact with Barley
May increase blood glucose–lowering effects and risk of hypoglycemia (low blood sugar) when used with herbs and supplements that lower glucose levels, such as alpha-lipoic acid, chromium, devil's claw, Panax ginseng, and psyllium. (For a list of herbs and supplements that lower glucose levels, see Appendix B.)

BASIL

> Today this savory herb is best known as a flavoring in spaghetti sauce, but well into the seventeenth century many believed that if you left a sprig of basil under a pot, in time it would turn into a scorpion. And smelling the herb would cause scorpions to nest in the brain!

Scientific Name
Ocimum basilicum

Basil Is Also Commonly Known As
St. Josephwort

Medicinal Parts
Leaf, oil of the leaf

Basil's Uses
To treat flatulence and a feeling of fullness, earaches, malaria, menstrual problems, and rheumatoid arthritis; to stimulate the appetite and digestion; to help rid the body of excess fluid. Basil oil is used to treat joint pain, wounds, and depression.

Typical Dose
A typical dose of basil is approximately 3 gm of the herb combined with 150 ml hot water.

Possible Side Effects
No side effects are known when basil herb or basil oil is taken in designated therapeutic doses.

Drugs That May Interact with Basil
Taking basil with these drugs may disrupt blood sugar control:
- acarbose (Prandase, Precose)
- acetohexamide
- chlorpropamide (Diabinese, Novo-Propamide)
- gliclazide (Diamicron, Novo-Gliclazide)
- glimepiride (Amaryl)
- glipizide (Glucotrol)
- glipizide and metformin (Metaglip)
- gliquidone (Beglynor, Glurenorm)
- glyburide (DiaBeta, Micronase)
- glyburide and metformin (Glucovance)
- insulin (Humulin, Novolin R)
- metformin (Glucophage, Riomet)
- miglitol (Glyset)
- nateglinide (Starlix)
- pioglitazone (Actos)
- repaglinide (GlucoNorm, Prandin)
- rosiglitazone (Avandia)
- rosiglitazone and metformin (Avandamet)
- tolazamide (Tolinase)
- tolbutamide (Apo-Tolbutamide, Tol-Tab)

Lab Tests That May Be Altered by Basil
None known

Diseases That May Be Worsened or Triggered by Basil
None known

Foods That May Interact with Basil
None known

Supplements That May Interact with Basil
None known

BELLADONNA

Legend has it that belladonna, which means "beautiful woman," sometimes takes the form of a stunningly gorgeous enchantress who is dangerous to behold. Or belladona may be so-named because Italian ladies once used the juice to dilate their pupils, making their eyes more brilliant. Belladonna is a source of atropine, which is used to treat eye diseases and spasms.

Scientific Name
Atropa belladonna

Belladonna Is Also Commonly Known As
Deadly nightshade, devil's herb, great morel, naughty man's cherries

Medicinal Parts
Leaf, root

Belladonna's Uses
To treat spasms and pain in the gastrointestinal tract; to treat gout, meningitis, and tonsillitis, and inflammation of the skin, joints, or gastrointestinal tract. Belladonna root is used to treat irregular heartbeat, pain in the gastrointestinal tract and bile duct, asthma, and bronchitis. Germany's Commission E has approved the use of belladonna leaf and root to treat gallbladder and liver complaints.

Typical Dose
A typical dose of belladonna leaf may range from 50 to 100 mg in powder form, with a maximum daily dose of 600 mg. A typical dose of belladonna root is 50 mg in powder form, with a maximum daily dose of 300 mg.

Possible Side Effects
Belladonna's side effects include dry mouth, dilated pupils, blurred vision, dry skin, tachycardia (rapid heartbeat), and difficulty urinating.

Drugs That May Interact with Belladonna
Taking belladonna with these drugs may enhance the drug's therapeutic and adverse effects:
- acetaminophen, chlorpheniramine, and pseudoephedrine (Children's Tylenol Plus Cold; Sinutab Sinus Allergy Maximum Strength)
- acetaminophen, dextromethorphan, and pseudoephedrine (Alka-Seltzer Plus Flu Liqui-Gels, Sudafed Severe Cold)
- acrivastine and pseudoephedrine (Semprex-D)
- amantadine (Endantadine, Symmetrel)
- amitriptyline (Elavil, Levate)
- amitriptyline and chlordiazepoxide (Limbitrol)
- amitriptyline and perphenazine (Etrafon, Triavil)
- amoxapine (Asendin)
- azatadine (Optimine)
- azatadine and pseudoephedrine (Rynatan Tablet, Trinalin)

- azelastine (Astelin, Optivar)
- brompheniramine and pseudoephedrine (Children's Dimetapp Elixir Cold & Allergy, Lodrane)
- carbinoxamine (Histex CT, Histex PD)
- carbinoxamine and pseudoephedrine (Rondec Drops, Sildec)
- carbinoxamine, pseudoephedrine, and dextromethorphan (Rondec-DM Drops, Tussafed)
- cetirizine (Reactine, Zyrtec)
- chlorpheniramine and acetaminophen (Coricidin HBP Cold and Flu)
- chlorpheniramine and phenylephrine (Histatab Plus, Rynatan)
- chlorpheniramine, ephedrine, phenylephrine, and carbetapentane (Rynatuss, Tynatuss Pediatric)
- chlorpheniramine, phenylephrine, and dextromethorphan (Alka-Seltzer Plus Cold and Cough)
- chlorpheniramine, phenylephrine, and methscopolamine (AH-Chew, Extendryl)
- chlorpheniramine, phenylephrine, and phenyltoloxamine (Comhist, Nalex-A)
- chlorpheniramine, phenylephrine, codeine, and potassium iodide (Pediacof)
- chlorpheniramine, pseudoephedrine, and codeine (Dihistine DH, Ryna-C)
- chlorpheniramine, pseudoephedrine, and dextromethorphan (Robitussin Pediatric Night Relief, Vicks Pediatric 44M)
- chlorpromazine (Thorazine, Largactil)
- cimetidine (Nu-Cimet, Tagamet)
- clemastine (Tavist Allergy)
- clomipramine (Anafranil, Novo-Clopramine)
- cyproheptadine (Periactin)
- deptropine (Deptropine FNA)
- desipramine (Alti-Desipramine, Norpramin)
- desloratadine (Aerius, Clarinex)
- dexbrompheniramine and pseudoephedrine (Drixomed, Drixoral Cold & Allergy)
- dexchlorpheniramine (Polaramine)
- dimethindene (Fenistil)
- diphenhydramine (Benadryl Allergy, Nytol)
- diphenhydramine and pseudoephedrine (Benadryl Allergy/Decongestant, Benadryl Children's Allergy and Sinus)
- doxepin (Sinequan, Zonalon)
- doxylamine and pyridoxine (Diclectin)
- epinastine (Elestat)
- famotidine (Apo-Famotidine, Pepcid)
- fexofenadine (Allegra)
- fexofenadine and pseudoephedrine (Allegra-D)
- fluphenazine (Modecate, Prolixin)
- hydrocodone and chlorpheniramine (Tussionex)
- hydrocodone, carbinoxamine, and pseudoephedrine (Histex HC, Tri-Vent HC)
- hydroxyzine (Atarax, Vistaril)
- imipramine (Apo-Imipramine, Tofranil)
- ketotifen (Novo-Ketotifen, Zaditor)
- levocabastine (Livostin)
- lofepramine (Feprapax, Gamanil)
- loratadine (Alavert, Claritin)
- loratadine and pseudoephedrine (Claritin-D 12 Hour, Claritin-D 24 Hour)
- mebhydrolin (Bexidal, Incidal)
- melitracen (Dixeran)
- mesoridazine (Serentil)
- mizolastine (Elina, Mizollen)
- nizatidine (Axid, PMS-Nizatidine)
- nortriptyline (Aventyl HCl, Pamelor)
- olopatadine (Patanol)
- oxatomide (Cenacert, Tinset)
- perphenazine (Apo-Perphenazine, Trilafon)
- procainamide (Procanbid, Pronestyl-SR)
- prochlorperazine (Compazine, Compro)

- promethazine (Phenergan)
- promethazine and codeine (Phenergan with Codeine)
- promethazine and dextromethorphan (Promatussin DM)
- promethazine and phenylephrine
- promethazine, phenylephrine, and codeine
- protriptyline (Vivactil)
- quinidine (Novo-Quinidin, Quinaglute Dura-Tabs)
- ranitidine (Alti-Ranitidine, Zantac)
- thiethylperazine (Torecan)
- thioridazine (Mellaril)
- thiothixene (Navane)
- trifluoperazine (Novo-Trifluzine, Stelazine)
- trimipramine (Apo-Trimip, Surmontil)
- tripelennamine (PBZ, PBZ-SR)
- triprolidine and pseudoephedrine (Actifed Cold and Allergy, Silafed)
- triprolidine, pseudoephedrine, and codeine (CoActifed, Covan)

Lab Tests That May Be Altered by Belladonna
None known

Diseases That May Be Worsened or Triggered by Belladonna
- May cause tachycardia and exacerbate congestive heart failure.
- May cause constipation.
- May exacerbate gastroesophageal reflux, gastric ulcers, obstructive gastrointestinal tract diseases, and toxic megacolon.
- Increased risk of hyperthermia in patients with fever.
- May suppress gastrointestinal motility.
- May increase ocular tension in those with narrow-angle glaucoma.
- May increase urinary retention.

Foods That May Interact with Belladonna
None known

Supplements That May Interact with Belladonna
None known

BETA-CAROTENE

Part of a large group of health-enhancing substances called carotenes, beta-carotene is found in orange or yellow-orange foods such as carrots, squash, and pumpkin and in dark-green leafy foods such as spinach and broccoli. Beta-carotene is called the "plant form" of vitamin A or provitamin A because it is converted into active vitamin A inside the body.

Beta-carotene's Uses
To treat cardiovascular disease, cataracts, age-related macular degeneration, depression, infertility, psoriasis, and vitiligo

Typical Dose
A typical daily dose of beta-carotene is approximately 25 mg. The Food and Nutrition Board, which sets the RDAs for selected supplements, has not set an RDA or Tolerable Upper Intake Level (UL) for beta-carotene.

Possible Side Effects
Beta-carotene's side effects include yellow skin discoloration, diarrhea, and bruising.

Drugs That May Interfere with the Absorption, Utilization, or Excretion of Beta-carotene
- cholestyramine (Prevalite, Questran)

- clofibrate (Atromid-S, Novo-Fibrate)
- colchicine (ratio-Colchicine)
- colchicine and probenecid (ColBenemid)
- colesevelam (WelChol)
- colestipol (Colestid)
- lansoprazole (Prevacid)
- methotrexate (Folex PFS, Rheumatrex)
- mineral oil (Fleet Mineral Oil Enema, Milkinol)
- neomycin (Myciguent, Neo-Fradin)
- octreotide (Sandostatin)
- omeprazole (Losec, Prilosec)
- orlistat (Xenical)
- pantoprazole (Pantoloc, Protonix)
- rabeprazole (Aciphex, Pariet)
- simvastatin (Apo-Simvastatin, Zocor)

Lab Tests That May Be Altered by Beta-carotene
None known

Diseases That May Be Worsened or Triggered by Beta-carotene
None known

Foods That May Interact with Beta-carotene
The fat substitute Olestra may lower the blood concentrations of beta-carotene absorbed from supplements.

Supplements That May Interact with Beta-carotene
None known

BILBERRY

Used since the sixteenth century as a medicinal herb, the fruit of this ornamental shrub contains flavonoids and anthocyanin, which help strengthen capillaries and thin the blood. Bilberry also stimulates the release of vasodilators, thus reducing the formation of dangerous clots and lowering blood pressure. Studies have shown that bilberry improves night vision and the ability to see again after being exposed to glaring light at night.

Scientific Name
Vaccinium myrtillus

Bilberry Leaf Is Also Commonly Known As
Airelle, bleaberry, dyeberry, huckleberry, trackleberry, whortleberry

Medicinal Parts
Leaf, ripe or dried fruit

Bilberry's Uses
To treat diabetes, arthritis, gout, various problems with the gastrointestinal and urinary tracts, inflammation of the eyes, burns, and various skin diseases. Bilberry fruit is used to treat inflammation of the mouth and throat, diarrhea, vomiting, wounds, and skin ulcers. Germany's Commission E has approved the use of bilberry fruit to treat diarrhea and inflammation of the mouth and throat.

Typical Dose
A typical dose of bilberry leaf has not been established. A typical dose of bilberry fruit may range from 20 to 60 gm of unprocessed fruit.

Possible Side Effects
Bilberry's side effects include digestive complaints (including nausea).

Drugs That May Interact with Bilberry

Taking bilberry with these drugs may increase the risk of bleeding or bruising:

- abciximab (ReoPro)
- alteplase (Activase, Cathflo Activase)
- antithrombin III (Thrombate III)
- argatroban
- aspirin (Bufferin, Ecotrin)
- aspirin and dipyridamole (Aggrenox)
- bivalirudin (Angiomax)
- clopidogrel (Plavix)
- dalteparin (Fragmin)
- danaparoid (Orgaran)
- dipyridamole (Novo-Dipiradol, Persantine)
- enoxaparin (Lovenox)
- eptifibatide (Integrillin)
- fondaparinux (Arixtra)
- heparin (Hepalean, Hep-Lock)
- indobufen (Ibustrin)
- lepirudin (Refludan)
- nadroparin (Fraxiparine)
- reteplase (Retavase)
- streptokinase (Streptase)
- tenecteplase (TNKase)
- ticlopidine (Alti-Ticlopidine, Ticlid)
- tinzaparin (Innohep)
- tirofiban (Aggrastat)
- urokinase (Abbokinase)
- warfarin (Coumadin, Jantoven)

Taking bilberry with these drugs may increase the risk of hypoglycemia (low blood sugar):

- acarbose (Prandase, Precose)
- acetohexamide
- chlorpropamide (Diabinese, Novo-Propamide)
- gliclazide (Diamicron, Novo-Gliclazide)
- glimepiride (Amaryl)
- glipizide (Glucotrol)
- glipizide and metformin (Metaglip)
- gliquidone (Beglynor, Glurenorm)
- glyburide (DiaBeta, Micronase)
- glyburide and metformin (Glucovance)
- insulin (Humulin, Novolin R)
- metformin (Glucophage, Riomet)
- miglitol (Glyset)
- nateglinide (Starlix)
- pioglitazone (Actos)
- repaglinide (GlucoNorm, Prandin)
- rosiglitazone (Avandia)
- rosiglitazone and metformin (Avandamet)
- tolazamide (Tolinase)
- tolbutamide (Apo-Tolbutamide, Tol-Tab)

Taking bilberry with these drugs may interfere with absorption of the drug:

- ferric gluconate (Ferrlecit)
- ferrous fumarate (Femiron, Feostat)
- ferrous gluconate (Fergon, Novo-Ferrogluc)
- ferrous sulfate (Feratab, Fer-Iron)
- ferrous sulfate and ascorbic acid (FeroGrad 500, Vitelle Irospan)
- iron-dextran complex (Dexferrum, INFeD)
- polysaccharide-iron complex (Hytinic, Niferex)

Lab Tests That May Be Altered by Bilberry

Bilberry leaf may lower serum triglycerides.

Diseases That May Be Worsened or Triggered by Bilberry

None known

Foods That May Interact with Bilberry

None known

Supplements That May Interact with Bilberry

- Bilberry leaf may increase blood glucose–lowering effects and risk of hypoglycemia (low blood sugar) when used with herbs and supplements that lower glucose levels, such as alpha-lipoic acid, chromium, devil's claw, Panax ginseng, and psyllium. (For a list of herbs and supplements that lower blood glucose levels, see Appendix B.)
- The tannins in bilberry may cause the alkaloids in certain other herbs to separate and settle, increasing the risk of toxic reactions. (For a list of herbs and other substances high in alkaloids, see Appendix B.)

BIOTIN

Biotin is part of the B-family of vitamins. It helps in the extraction of energy from food and is necessary for a strong immune system, healthy nerves, sex glands, bone marrow, skin, and hair. Should you run short of biotin, you may suffer from nausea, vomiting, exhaustion, skin problems, muscle pain, and liver enlargement.

Biotin's Uses

To treat depression and diabetes and prevent hair loss.

Typical Dose

The Food and Nutrition Board has set the Adequate Intake (AI) for biotin at 30 mcg per day for men and women ages nineteen and over.

Possible Side Effects

When biotin is taken at therapeutic doses, there are no known side effects.

Drugs That May Interfere with the Absorption, Utilization, or Excretion of Biotin

- aikacin (Amikin)
- amoxicillin (Amoxil, Novamoxin)
- ampicillin (Omnipen, Totacillin)
- aithromycin (Zithromax)
- carbenicillin (Geocillin)
- cefaclor (Ceclor)
- cefadroxil (Duricef)
- cefazolin (Ancef, Kefzol)
- cefdinir (Omnicef)
- cefditoren (Spectracef)
- cefepime (Maxipime)
- cefonicid (Monocid)
- cefoperazone (Cefobid)
- cefotaxime (Claforan)
- cefoxitin (Mefoxin)
- cefpodoxime (Vantin)
- cefprozil (Cefzil)
- ceftazidime (Ceptaz, Fortaz)
- ceftibuten (Cedax)
- ceftizoxime (Cefizox)
- ceftriaxone (Rocephin)
- cefuroxime (Ceftin, Kefurox)
- cephalexin (Biocef, Keftab)
- cephalothin (Ceporacin)
- cephapirin (Cefadyl)
- cepharadine (Velosef)
- cinoxacin (Cinobac)
- clarithromycin (Biaxin, Biaxin XL)
- cloxacillin (Cloxapen, Nu-Cloxi)
- dicloxacillin (Dycill, Pathocil)
- dirithromycin (Dynabac)
- ethosuximide (Zarontin)
- gatifloxacin (Tequin, Zymar)
- kanamycin (Kantrex)
- levofloxacin (Levaquin, Quixin)
- linezolid (Zyvox)

- lomefloxacin (Maxaquin)
- loracarbef (Lorabid)
- meclocycline (Meclan Topical)
- nafcillin (Nafcil Injection, Unipen Oral)
- nalidixic acid (NegGram)
- norfloxacin (Chibroxin Ophthalmic, Noroxin Oral)
- penicillin G benzathine (Bicillin L-A, Permapen)
- penicillin G benzathine and penicillin G procaine (Bicillin C-R)
- penicillin G procaine (Pfizerpen-AS, Wycillin)
- penicillin V potassium (Suspen, Truxcillin)
- piperacillin (Pipracil)
- piperacillin and tazobactam sodium (Zosyn)
- sparfloxacin (Zagam)
- sulfadiazine (Microsulfon)
- tulfisoxazole (Gantrisin)
- ticarcillin (Ticar)
- ticarcillin and clavulanate potassium (Timentin)
- tobramycin (Nebcin, Tobrex)
- trimethoprim (Primsol, Trimpex)
- trovafloxacin (Trovan)

Lab Tests That May Be Altered by Biotin
None known

Diseases That May Be Worsened or Triggered by Biotin
None known

Foods That May Interact with Biotin
None known

Supplements That May Interact with Biotin
None known

BIRCH

> Tea made from the birch leaf is a powerful diuretic that can actually dissolve bladder and kidney stones, while killing bacteria in the kidneys and urinary tract and easing fluid retention due to heart or kidney dysfunction.

Scientific Name
Betula species

Birch Is Also Commonly Known As
Common birch, silver birch, white birch

Medicinal Parts
Leaf, bud, wood, and bark

Birch's Uses
Birch leaves are used as a "flushing out" therapy for inflammatory and bacterial ailments of the urinary tract and for kidney gravel; to treat gout and rheumatism; and to purify the blood. Birch tar oil (obtained via the dry distillation of the wood of the white birch) is used to treat gout, rheumatism, and psoriasis and other skin ailments.

Typical Dose
A typical dose of birch leaf is made by steeping 2 to 3 gm of leaf in 150 ml of hot water for fifteen minutes, then straining the leaves and drinking the liquid as a tea. There is no typical dose of birch tar oil.

Possible Side Effects
No side effects are known when birch is taken in designated therapeutic doses. However, birch leaf

should not be used to treat edema if the heart or kidneys are not functioning well.

Drugs That May Interact with Birch
Taking birch with these drugs may reduce the effectiveness of the drug:
- acetazolamide (Apo-Acetazolamide, Diamox Sequels)
- amiloride (Midamor)
- azosemide (Diat)
- bumetanide (Bumex, Burinex)
- chlorthalidone (Apo-Chlorthalidone, Thalitone)
- chlorothiazide (Diuril)
- ethacrynic acid (Edecrin)
- etozolin (Elkapin)
- furosemide (Apo-Furosemide, Lasix)
- hydrochlorothiazide (Apo-Hydro, Microzide)
- hydrochlorothiazide and triamterene (Dyazide, Maxzide)
- hydroflumethiazide (Diucardin, Saluron)
- indapamide (Lozol, Nu-Indapamide)
- mannitol (Osmitrol, Resectisol)
- mefruside (Baycaron)
- methazolamide (Apo-Methazolamide, Neptazane)
- methyclothiazide (Aquatensen, Enduron)
- metolazone (Mykrox, Zaroxolyn)
- olmesartan and hydrochlorothiazide (Benicar HCT)
- polythiazide (Renese)
- spironolactone (Aldactone, Novo-Spiroton)
- torsemide (Demadex)
- triamterene (Dyrenium)
- trichlormethiazide (Metatensin, Naqua)
- urea (Amino-Cerv, UltraMide)
- xipamide (Diurexan, Lumitens)

Lab Tests That May Be Altered by Birch
None known

Diseases That May Be Worsened or Triggered by Birch
May make elevated blood pressure worse by causing the body to retain more sodium and fluid.

Foods That May Interact with Birch
Those allergic to birch may develop an allergy to celery, and vice versa.

Supplements That May Interact with Birch
None known

BIRTHWORT

> Its scientific name, *Aristolochia*, means "excellent birth," and the fresh juice of birthwort was used traditionally to induce labor and remove obstructions after childbirth. Native Americans used this herb, which also is known as snakeroot, to treat snakebites, toothaches, stomach pain, and fevers.

Scientific Name
Aristolochia clematitis

Birthwort Is Also Commonly Known As
Aristolochia, long birthwort, pelican flower, snakeroot, snakeweed

Medicinal Parts
Root, leaf, stem, flower

Birthwort's Uses
To treat gastrointestinal and gallbladder colic caused by allergies, joint pain, stomachache, malaria, and gynecological disorders; to stimulate the immune system

Typical Dose

There is no typical dose of birthwort.

Possible Side Effects

❗ Birthwort is extremely toxic. When taken in low doses over time, its side effects include the development of tumors. Toxic doses lead to vomiting, severe kidney damage, gastroenteritis, and death by kidney failure.

Drugs That May Interact with Birthwort

Taking birthwort with these drugs may interfere with the action of the drug:

- aluminum hydroxide (AlternaGel, Alu-Cap)
- aluminum hydroxide and magnesium carbonate (Gaviscon Extra Strength, Gaviscon Liquid)
- aluminum hydroxide and magnesium hydroxide (Maalox, Rulox)
- aluminum hydroxide and magnesium trisilicate (Gaviscon Tablet)
- aluminum hydroxide, magnesium hydroxide, and simethicone (Maalox, Mylanta Liquid)
- calcium carbonate (Rolaids Extra Strength, Tums)
- calcium carbonate and magnesium hydroxide (Mylanta Gelcaps, Rolaids Extra Strength)
- cimetidine (Nu-Cimet, Tagamet)
- esomeprazole (Nexium)
- famotidine (Apo-Famotidine, Pepcid)
- famotidine, calcium carbonate, and magnesium hydroxide (Pepcid Complete)
- lansoprazole (Prevacid)
- magaldrate and simethicone (Riopan Plus, Riopan Plus Double Strength)
- magnesium hydroxide (Dulcolax Milk of Magnesia, Phillips' Milk of Magnesia)
- magnesium oxide (Mag-Ox 400, Uro-Mag)
- magnesium sulfate (Epsom salts)
- nizatidine (Axid, PMS-Nizatidine)
- omeprazole (Losec, Prilosec)
- pantoprazole (Pantoloc, Protonix)
- rabeprazole (Aciphex, Pariet)
- ranitidine (Alti-Ranitidine, Zantac)
- sodium bicarbonate (Brioschi, Neut)

Lab Tests That May Be Altered by Birthwort

May cause nephropathy and abnormal kidney function test results.

Diseases That May Be Worsened or Triggered by Birthwort

Can irritate the gastrointestinal tract and may worsen inflammatory or infectious gastrointestinal ailments.

Foods That May Interact with Birthwort

None known

Supplements That May Interact with Birthwort

None known

BISHOP'S WEED

The dried, ripe fruit of this native Mediterranean plant eases spasms in the muscles in the walls of blood vessels, bronchial airways, and other tubes and ducts, which explains its use as a treatment for high blood pressure, cough, and bronchitis. It also mildly stimulates the pumping action of the heart and increases blood circulation to the heart muscle.

Scientific Name

Ammi visnaga

Bishop's Weed Is Also Commonly Known As

Greater ammi, khella, khella fruits

Medicinal Parts

Fruit

Bishop's Weed's Uses

To treat angina pectoris, hypertension, asthma, whooping cough, and cramping of the abdomen

Typical Dose

A typical dose of bishop's weed is approximately 0.5 ml of liquid extract.

Possible Side Effects

Bishop's weed's side effects include insomnia, dizziness, nausea, and allergic reactions.

Drugs That May Interact with Bishop's Weed

Taking bishop's weed with these drugs may increase the risk of hypotension (excessively low blood pressure):

- acebutolol (Novo-Acebutolol, Sectral)
- acetazolamide (Apo-Acetazolamide, Diamox Sequels)
- amiloride (Midamor)
- amlodipine (Norvasc)
- atenolol (Apo-Atenol, Tenormin)
- azosemide (Diat)
- benazepril (Lotensin)
- bepridil (Vascor)
- betaxolol (Betoptic S, Kerlone)
- bisoprolol (Monocor, Zebeta)
- bumetanide (Bumex, Burinex)
- candesartan (Atacand)
- captopril (Capoten, Novo-Captopril)
- carteolol (Cartrol, Ocupress)
- carvedilol (Coreg)
- chlorothiazide (Diuril)
- chlorthalidone (Apo-Chlorthalidone, Thalitone)
- clonidine (Catapres, Duraclon)
- diazoxide (Hyperstat, Proglycem)
- diltiazem (Cardizem, Tiazac)
- doxazosin (Alti-Doxazosin, Cardura)
- enalapril (Vasotec)
- eplerenone (Inspra)
- eprosartan (Teveten)
- esmolol (Brevibloc)
- ethacrynic acid (Edecrin)
- etozolin (Elkapin)
- felodipine (Plendil, Renedil)
- fenoldopam (Corlopam)
- fosinopril (Monopril)
- furosemide (Apo-Furosemide, Lasix)
- guanabenz (Wytensin)
- guanadrel (Hylorel)
- guanfacine (Tenex)
- hydralazine (Apresoline, Novo-Hylazin)
- hydrochlorothiazide (Apo-Hydro, Microzide)
- hydrochlorothiazide and triamterene (Dyazide, Maxzide)
- hydroflumethiazide (Diucardin, Saluron)
- indapamide (Lozol, Nu-Indapamide)
- irbesartan (Avapro)
- isradipine (DynaCirc)
- labetalol (Normodyne, Trandate)
- lacidipine (Aponil, Caldine)
- lercanidipine (Cardiovasc, Carmen)
- lisinopril (Prinivil, Zestril)
- losartan (Cozaar)
- manidipine (Calslot, Iperten)
- mannitol (Osmitrol, Resectisol)

- mecamylamine (Inversine)
- mefruside (Baycaron)
- methazolamide (Apo-Methazolamide, Neptazane)
- methyclothiazide (Aquatensen, Enduron)
- methyldopa (Apo-Methyldopa, Nu-Medopa)
- metolazone (Mykrox, Zaroxolyn)
- metoprolol (Betaloc, Lopressor)
- minoxidil (Loniten, Rogaine)
- moexipril (Univasc)
- nadolol (Apo-Nadol, Corgard)
- nicardipine (Cardene)
- nifedipine (Adalat CC, Procardia)
- nilvadipine
- nimodipine (Nimotop)
- nisoldipine (Sular)
- nitrendipine
- nitroglycerin (Minitran, Nitro-Dur)
- nitroprusside (Nitropress, Nipride)
- olmesartan (Benicar)
- olmesartan and hydrochlorothiazide (Benicar HCT)
- oxprenolol (Trasicor, Slow-Trasicor)
- perindopril erbumine (Aceon, Coversyl)
- phenoxybenzamine (Dibenzyline)
- phentolamine (Regitine, Rogitine)
- pinaverium (Dicetel)
- pindolol (Apo-Pindol, Novo-Pindol)
- polythiazide (Renese)
- prazosin (Minipress, Nu-Prazo)
- propranolol (Inderal, InnoPran XL)
- quinapril (Accupril)
- ramipril (Altace)
- reserpine
- spironolactone (Aldactone, Novo-Spiroton)
- telmisartan (Micardis)
- terazosin (Alti-Terazosin, Hytrin)

- timolol (Betimol, Timoptic)
- torsemide (Demadex)
- trandolapril (Mavik)
- triamterene (Dyrenium)
- trichlormethiazide (Metatensin, Naqua)
- urea (Amino-Cerv, UltraMide)
- valsartan (Diovan)
- verapamil (Calan, Isoptin SR)
- xipamide (Diurexan, Lumitens)

Taking bishop's weed with these drugs may increase the risk of bleeding or bruising:

- abciximab (ReoPro)
- antithrombin III (Thrombate III)
- argatroban
- aspirin (Bufferin, Ecotrin)
- aspirin and dipyridamole (Aggrenox)
- bivalirudin (Angiomax)
- clopidogrel (Plavix)
- dalteparin (Fragmin)
- danaparoid (Orgaran)
- dipyridamole (Novo-Dipiradol, Persantine)
- enoxaparin (Lovenox)
- eptifibatide (Integrillin)
- fondaparinux (Arixtra)
- heparin (Hepalean, Hep-Lock)
- indobufen (Ibustrin)
- lepirudin (Refludan)
- ticlopidine (Alti-Ticlopidine, Ticlid)
- tinzaparin (Innohep)
- tirofiban (Aggrastat)
- warfarin (Coumadin, Jantoven)

Lab Tests That May Be Altered by Bishop's Weed
- May increase HDL "good" cholesterol levels.
- May increase the results of certain liver tests (ALT, SGOT, SGPT), giving the impression that the patient may have hepatitis or liver disease.

Diseases That May Be Worsened or Triggered by Bishop's Weed

May worsen liver function in people with liver disease.

Foods That May Interact with Bishop's Weed

None known

Supplements That May Interact with Bishop's Weed

- May increase the risk of liver damage when combined with herbs and supplements that can cause hepatotoxicity (destructive effects on the liver), such as borage, chaparral, uva ursi, and others. (For a list of herbs and supplements that can cause hepatotoxicity, see Appendix B.)
- Increased risk of bleeding when used with herbs and supplements that might affect platelet aggregation, such as angelica, danshen, garlic, ginger, ginkgo biloba, red clover, turmeric, white willow, and others. (For a list of herbs and supplements with anticoagulant/antiplatelet potential, see Appendix B.)
- May have additive effects when used with herbs and supplements that increase photosensitivity, such as St. John's wort. (For a list of herbs and supplements that increase photosensitivity, see Appendix B.)

BITTER ALMOND

> Bitter almond differs from the sweet almond that we commonly eat in that it contains a compound called amygdalin, from which the alternative cancer drug laetrile is made. For the most part, it has been found that amygdalin has no significant activity against tumor cells and can be lethal if taken in excessive amounts.

Scientific Name

Prunus dulcis

Bitter Almond Is Also Commonly Known As

Amygdala amara, badama, vatadha, volatile almond oil

Medicinal Parts

Fruit

Bitter Almond's Uses

To treat cough and itching; as a local anesthetic

Typical Dose

There is no typical dose of bitter almond.

Possible Side Effects

Bitter almond's side effects include depression of the central nervous system.

Drugs That May Interact with Bitter Almond

Taking bitter almond with these drugs may cause excessive sedation and mental depression and impairment:

- acetaminophen and codeine (Capital and Codeine, Tylenol with Codeine)
- alfentanil (Alfenta)
- alprazolam (Apo-Alpraz, Xanax)
- amobarbital (Amytal)
- amobarbital and secobarbital (Tuinal)
- aspirin and codeine (Coryphen Codeine)
- belladonna and opium (B&O Supprettes)
- bromazepam (Apo-Bromazepam, Gen-Bromazepam)
- brotizolam (Lendorm, Sintonal)
- buprenorphine (Buprenex, Subutex)
- buprenorphine and naloxone (Suboxone)
- butabarbital (Butisol Sodium)

- butalbital, acetaminophen, and caffeine (Esgic, Fioricet)
- butalbital, aspirin, and caffeine (Fiorinal)
- butorphanol (Apo-Butorphanol, Stadol)
- chloral hydrate (Aquachloral Supprettes, Somnote)
- chlordiazepoxide (Apo-Chlordiazepoxide, Librium)
- clobazam (Alti-Clobazam, Frisium)
- clonazepam (Klonopin, Rivotril)
- clorazepate (Tranxene, T-Tab)
- codeine (Codeine Contin)
- dexmedetomidine (Precedex)
- diazepam (Apo-Diazepam, Valium)
- dihydrocodeine, aspirin, and caffeine (Synalgos-DC)
- diphenhydramine (Benadryl Allergy, Nytol)
- estazolam (ProSom)
- fentanyl (Actiq, Duragesic)
- flurazepam (Apo-Flurazepam, Dalmane)
- glutethimide
- haloperidol (Haldol, Novo-Peridol)
- hydrocodone and acetaminophen (Vicodin, Zydone)
- hydrocodone and aspirin (Damason-P)
- hydrocodone and ibuprofen (Vicoprofen)
- hydromorphone (Dilaudid, PMS-Hydromorphone)
- hydroxyzine (Atarax, Vistaril)
- levomethadyl acetate hydrochloride
- levorphanol (LevoDromoran)
- loprazolam (Dormonoct, Havlane)
- lorazepam (Ativan, Nu-Loraz)
- meperidine (Demerol, Meperitab)
- meperidine and promethazine
- mephobarbital (Mebaral)
- methadone (Dolophine, Methadose)
- methohexital (Brevital, Brevital Sodium)
- midazolam (Apo-Midazolam, Versed)
- morphine sulfate (Kadian, MS Contin)
- nalbuphine (Nubain)
- opium tincture
- oxycodone (OxyContin, Roxicodone)
- oxycodone and acetaminophen (Endocet, Percocet)
- oxycodone and aspirin (Endodan, Percodan)
- oxymorphone (Numorphan)
- paregoric
- pentazocine (Talwin)
- pentobarbital (Nembutal)
- phenobarbital (Luminal Sodium, PMS-Phenobarbital)
- phenoperidine
- prazepam
- primidone (Apo-Primidone, Mysoline)
- promethazine (Phenergan)
- propofol (Diprivan)
- propoxyphene (Darvon, Darvon-N)
- propoxyphene and acetaminophen (Darvocet-N 50, Darvocet-N 100)
- propoxyphene, aspirin, and caffeine (Darvon Compound)
- quazepam (Doral)
- remifentanil (Ultiva)
- secobarbital (Seconal)
- sufentanil (Sufenta)
- temazepam (Novo-Temazepam, Restoril)
- tetrazepam (Mobiforton, Musapam)
- thiopental (Pentothal)
- triazolam (Apo-Triazo, Halcion)
- zaleplon (Sonata, Stamoc)
- zolpidem (Ambien)
- zopiclone (Alti-Zopiclone, Gen-Zopiclone)

Lab Tests That May Be Altered by Bitter Almond
None known

Diseases That May Be Worsened or Triggered by Bitter Almond

None known

Foods That May Interact with Bitter Almond

None known

Supplements That May Interact with Bitter Almond

None known

BITTER MELON

Found in many Asian grocery stores, the juice of this extremely bitter fruit has been used traditionally to treat diabetes, cancer, and infections. A study on one hundred people showed that bitter melon can reduce both fasting and after-meal blood glucose levels in people with non–insulin-dependent diabetes.

Scientific Name

Momordica charantia

Bitter Melon Is Also Commonly Known As

Balsam apple, balsam pear, bitter apple, carilla gourd

Medicinal Parts

Fruit, leaf, seed

Bitter Melon's Uses

To treat diabetes, gastrointestinal upset, colitis, ulcers, constipation, intestinal worms, fever, kidney stones, and psoriasis

Typical Dose

A typical daily dose of bitter melon is approximately 15 gm of aqueous extract or 2 oz of juice.

Possible Side Effects

Bitter melon's side effects include nausea, vomiting, and anorexia.

Drugs That May Interact with Bitter Melon

Taking bitter melon with these drugs may cause or increase liver damage:

- abacavir (Ziagen)
- acarbose (Prandase, Precose)
- acetaminophen (Genapap, Tylenol)
- allopurinol (Aloprim, Zyloprim)
- atorvastatin (Lipitor)
- celecoxib (Celebrex)
- cidofovir (Vistide)
- cyclosporine (Neoral, Sandimmune)
- meloxicam (MOBIC, Mobicox)
- methotrexate (Rheumatrex, Trexall)
- methyldopa (Apo-Methyldopa, Nu-Medopa)
- modafinil (Alertec, Provigil)
- morphine hydrochloride
- morphine sulfate (Kadian, MS Contin)
- naproxen (Aleve, Naprosyn)
- nelfinavir (Viracept)
- nevirapine (Viramune)
- nitrofurantoin (Furadantin, Macrobid)
- ondansetron (Zofran)
- paclitaxel (Onxol, Taxol)
- pantoprazole (Pantoloc, Protonix)
- phenytoin (Dilantin, Phenytek)
- pioglitazone (Actos)
- piroxicam (Feldene, Nu-Pirox)
- pravastatin (Novo-Pravastatin, Pravachol)
- prochlorperazine (Compazine, Compro)
- propoxyphene (Darvon, Darvon-N)
- repaglinide (GlucoNorm, Prandin)
- rifampin (Rifadin, Rimactane)
- rifapentine (Priftin)
- ritonavir (Norvir)

- rofecoxib (Vioxx)
- rosiglitazone (Avandia)
- saquinavir (Fortovase, Invirase)
- simvastatin (Apo-Simvastatin, Zocor)
- stavudine (Zerit)
- tamoxifen (Nolvadex, Tamofen)
- tramadol (Ultram)
- zidovudine (Novo-AZT, Retrovir)

Taking bitter melon with these drugs may increase the risk of hypoglycemia (low blood sugar):

- acarbose (Prandase, Precose)
- acetohexamide
- chlorpropamide (Diabinese, Novo-Propamide)
- gliclazide (Diamicron, Novo-Gliclazide)
- glimepiride (Amaryl)
- glipizide (Glucotrol)
- glipizide and metformin (Metaglip)
- gliquidone (Beglynor, Glurenorm)
- glyburide (DiaBeta, Micronase)
- glyburide and metformin (Glucovance)
- insulin (Humulin, Novolin R)
- metformin (Glucophage, Riomet)
- miglitol (Glyset)
- nateglinide (Starlix)
- pioglitazone (Actos)
- repaglinide (GlucoNorm, Prandin)
- rosiglitazone (Avandia)
- rosiglitazone and metformin (Avandamet)
- tolazamide (Tolinase)
- tolbutamide (Apo-Tolbutamide, Tol-Tab)

Lab Tests That May Be Altered by Bitter Melon

- May decrease blood glucose test values if taken with chlorpropamide.
- May lower blood glucose in those with type 2 diabetes.

- May lower glycosylated hemoglobin (HbA1c) in type 2 diabetes patients after seven weeks of treatment.

Diseases That May Be Worsened or Triggered by Bitter Melon

May lower blood sugar levels and trigger hypoglycemia (low blood sugar) in people with diabetes.

Foods That May Interact with Bitter Melon

None known

Supplements That May Interact with Bitter Melon

May increase blood glucose–lowering effects and risk of hypoglycemia (low blood sugar) when used with herbs and supplements that lower glucose levels, such as alpha-lipoic acid, chromium, devil's claw, Panax ginseng, and psyllium. (For a list of herbs and supplements that lower blood glucose levels, see Appendix B.)

BITTER ORANGE

> Bitter orange is native to tropical Asia. Its peel is used to stimulate the appetite and ease indigestion. Bitter orange is also frequently found in modern weight-loss formulas because it contains synephrine and octopamine—chemicals similar to the ephedrine found in ma-huang. However, when taken in very large doses, bitter orange may be just as dangerous as ma-huang because these chemicals can cause high blood pressure and irregular heartbeat, which can lead to heart attack, stroke, and even death.

Scientific Name

Citrus aurantium

Bitter Orange Is Also Commonly Known As

Neroli, bigarade orange

Medicinal Parts

Fruit peel, flower, flower oil, seed

Bitter Orange's Uses

To treat loss of appetite, coughs, colds, apathy, uterine and anal prolapse, heartburn, bloating, and nausea. Germany's Commission E has approved the use of bitter orange peel to treat loss of appetite and dyspeptic complaints such as heartburn, bloating, and nausea.

Typical Dose

A typical dose of bitter orange peel is 1 tsp cut and coarsely powdered drug added to 150 ml of hot water, steeped for 10 minutes, then strained and taken as tea approximately 30 minutes before meals. There are no standard doses of bitter orange flower or flower oil.

Possible Side Effects

No side effects are known when bitter orange is taken in designated therapeutic doses, although there may be an increase in photosensitivity in light-skinned individuals.

Drugs That May Interact with Bitter Orange

Taking bitter orange with these drugs may increase drug levels in the body and risk of side effects:

- dextromethorphan (found in various formulations of Alka-Seltzer, Contac, PediaCare, Robitussin, Sudafed, Triaminic, and other over-the counter medications)
- felodipine (Plendil, Renedil)
- iproniazid (Marsilid)
- midazolam (Apo-Midazolam, Versed)
- moclobemide (Alti-Moclobemide, Nu-Moclobemide)
- phenelzine (Nardil)
- selegiline (Eldepryl)
- tranylcypromine (Parnate)

Lab Tests That May Be Altered by Bitter Orange

None known

Diseases That May Be Worsened or Triggered by Bitter Orange

The synephrine and doctopamine in bitter orange may cause cluster or migraine headaches, or exacerbate elevated blood pressure, narrow-angle glaucoma, or an overly rapid heart rate.

Foods That May Interact with Bitter Orange

Increased risk of hypertension and adverse cardiovascular effects when used in conjunction with large amounts of caffeine.

Supplements That May Interact with Bitter Orange

Increased risk of hypertension and adverse cardiovascular effects when used with herbs and supplements that have stimulant properties (for example, caffeine, coffee, cola, ma-huang, and others).

BLACK COHOSH

A member of the buttercup family, black cohosh has long been used by Native Americans to treat menstrual discomfort and the pains of childbirth. Western civilizations have used it to treat menopausal symptoms since the 1700s due to its estrogen-like effects on the body.

Scientific Name

Cimicifuga racemosa

Black Cohosh Is Also Commonly Known As

Black snakeroot, bugwort, cimicifuga, rattleweed

Medicinal Parts

Root, rhizome

Black Cohosh's Uses

To treat rheumatism, bronchitis, sore throats, fever, snakebite, and lumbago; to calm involuntary muscle motions; as a sedative. Germany's Commission E has approved the use of black cohosh to treat premenstrual syndrome (PMS) and symptoms of menopause.

Typical Dose

A typical dose of black cohosh may range from 40 to 200 mg of powdered rhizome daily; alcoholic-aqueous extracts corresponding to 40 mg of the drug; or 0.4 to 2 ml of tincture (1:10 in 60 percent alcohol).

Possible Side Effects

Black cohosh's side effects include nausea, vomiting, and diarrhea.

Drugs That May Interact with Black Cohosh

Taking black cohosh with these drugs may increase the risk of hypotension (excessively low blood pressure):

- acebutolol (Sectral)
- amlodipine (Norvasc)
- atenolol (Apo-Atenol, Tenormin)
- benazepril (Lotensin)
- betaxolol (Betoptic S, Kerlone)
- bisoprolol (Monocor, Zebeta)
- bumetanide (Bumex, Burinex)
- candesartan (Atacand)
- captopril (Capoten, Novo-Captopril)
- carteolol (Cartrol, Ocupress)
- carvedilol (Coreg)
- chlorothiazide (Diuril)
- chlorthalidone (Apo-Chlorthalidone, Thalitone)
- clonidine (Catapres, Duraclon)
- diazoxide (Hyperstat, Proglycem)
- diltiazem (Cardizem, Tiazac)
- doxazosin (Alti-Doxazosin, Cardura)
- enalapril (Vasotec)
- eplerenone (Inspra)
- eprosartan (Teveten)
- esmolol (Brevibloc)
- felodipine (Plendil, Renedil)
- fenoldopam (Corlopam)
- fosinopril (Monopril)
- furosemide (Apo-Furosemide, Lasix)
- guanabenz (Wytensin)
- guanadrel (Hylorel)
- guanfacine (Tenex)
- hydralazine (Apresoline, Novo-Hylazin)
- hydrochlorothiazide (Apo-Hydro, Microzide)
- hydrochlorothiazide and triamterene (Dyazide, Maxzide)
- indapamide (Lozol, Nu-Indapamide)
- irbesartan (Avapro)
- isradipine (DynaCirc)
- labetalol (Normodyne, Trandate)
- lisinopril (Prinivil, Zestril)
- losartan (Cozaar)
- mecamylamine (Inversine)
- mefruside (Baycaron)
- methyclothiazide (Aquatensen, Enduron)
- methyldopa (Apo-Methyldopa, Nu-Medopa)
- metolazone (Mykrox, Zaroxolyn)
- metoprolol (Betaloc, Lopressor)
- minoxidil (Loniten, Rogaine)
- moexipril (Univasc)

- nadolol (Apo-Nadol, Corgard)
- nicardipine (Cardene)
- nifedipine (Adalat CC, Procardia)
- nisoldipine (Sular)
- nitroglycerin (Minitran, Nitro-Dur)
- nitroprusside (Nipride, Nitropress)
- olmesartan (Benicar)
- oxprenolol (Slow-Trasicor, Trasicor)
- perindopril erbumine (Aceon, Coversyl)
- phenoxybenzamine (Dibenzyline)
- phentolamine (Regitine, Rogitine)
- pindolol (Apo-Pindol, Novo-Pindol)
- polythiazide (Renese)
- prazosin (Minipress, Nu-Prazo)
- propranolol (Inderal, InnoPran XL)
- quinapril (Accupril)
- ramipril (Altace)
- reserpine
- sildenafil (Viagra)
- sotalol (Betapace, Sorine)
- spironolactone (Aldactone, Novo-Spiroton)
- telmisartan (Micardis)
- terazosin (Alti-Terazosin, Hytrin)
- timolol (Betimol, Timoptic)
- torsemide (Demadex)
- trandolapril (Mavik)
- triamterene (Dyrenium)
- trichlormethiazide (Metatensin, Naqua)
- valsartan (Diovan)
- verapamil (Calan, Isoptin SR)

Taking black cohosh with these drugs may alter/interfere with the action of the drug and is best avoided by those with estrogen-dependent tumors:
- anastrozole (Arimidex)
- carbocysteine (Mucopront, Rhinatiol)
- cisplatin (Platinol-AQ)

- cyclophosphamide (Cytoxan, Neosar)
- cyproterone and ethinyl estradiol (Diane-35)
- doxorubicin (Adriamycin, Rubex)
- epirubicin (Ellence, Pharmorubicin)
- estradiol (Climara, Estrace)
- estrogens (conjugated A/synthetic) (Cenestin)
- estrogens (conjugated/equine) (Cenestin, Premarin)
- estrogens (esterified) (Estratab, Menest)
- estropipate (Ogen, Ortho-Est)
- ethinyl estradiol (Estinyl)
- ethinyl estradiol and ethynodiol diacetate (Demulen, Zovia)
- ethinyl estradiol and etonogestrel (NuvaRing)
- ethinyl estradiol and levonorgestrel (Alesse, Triphasil)
- ethinyl estradiol and norenthindrone (Brevicon, Ortho-Novum)
- ethinyl estradiol and norgestimate (Cyclen, Ortho Tri-Cyclen)
- ethinyl estradiol and norgestrel (Cryselle, Ovral)
- exemestane (Aromasin)
- fluorouracil (Adrucil, Efudex)
- megestrol (Lin-Megestrol, Megace)
- mitomycin (Mutamycin)
- mitoxantrone (Novantrone)
- norgestrel (Ovrette)
- paclitaxel (Onxol, Taxol)
- tamoxifen (Nolvadex, Tamofen)
- thiotepa (Thioplex)
- vinblastine (Velban)

Taking black cohosh with these drugs may reduce or prevent drug absorption:
- ferric gluconate (Ferrlecit)
- ferrous fumarate (Femiron, Feostat)

- ferrous gluconate (Fergon, Novo-Ferrogluc)
- ferrous sulfate (Feratab, Fer-Iron)
- ferrous sulfate and ascorbic acid (Fero-Grad 500, Vitelle Irospan)
- iron-dextran complex (Dexferrum, INFeD)
- polysaccharide-iron complex (Hytinic, Niferex)

Lab Tests That May Be Altered by Black Cohosh
None known

Diseases That May Be Worsened or Triggered by Black Cohosh
May increase the risk of breast cancer metastasis.

Foods That May Interact with Black Cohosh
None known

Supplements That May Interact with Black Cohosh
May adversely affect the liver and increase the risk of liver damage when combined with herbs and supplements that can cause hepatotoxicity (destructive effects on the liver), such as bishop's weed, borage, chaparral, uva ursi, and others. (For a list of herbs and supplements that can cause hepatotoxicity, see Appendix B.)

BLACK HELLEBORE

Black hellebore, which takes its name from the Greek *elein*, meaning "injure," and *bora*, meaning "food," is a very poisonous plant that has been used in the treatment of edema, amenorrhoea, nervous disorders, and hysteria. Because it is so toxic and its medicinal value has not been proven, it is not recommended for use.

Scientific Name
Helleborus niger

Black Hellebore Is Also Commonly Known As
Christe herbe, Christmas rose

Medicinal Parts
Dried rhizome, root

Black Hellebore's Uses
To treat nausea, worm infestation, constipation, irregular menstruation, and head colds

Typical Dose
A typical dose of black hellebore may range from 0.2 to 1.0 gm per day.

Possible Side Effects
❶ Black hellebore's side effects include poisoning, symptoms of which include a scratchy feeling in the mouth and throat, shortness of breath, nausea, vomiting, possible spasm, and asphyxiation. Black hellebore contains cardiac glycosides, which can help control irregular heartbeat, reduce the backup of blood and fluid in the body, and increase blood flow through the kidneys, helping to excrete sodium and relieve swelling in body tissues. However, a buildup of cardiac glycosides can occur, especially when the herb is combined with certain medications or other herbs that contain cardiac glycosides, causing arrhythmias, abnormally slow heartbeat, heart failure, and even death.

Drugs That May Interact with Black Hellebore
Taking black hellebore with this drug may increase the risk of cardiac glycoside toxicity:
- digitalis (Digitek, Lanoxin)

Lab Tests That May Be Altered by Black Hellebore
None known

Diseases That May Be Worsened or Triggered by Black Hellebore
Can worsen gastrointestinal inflammation.

Foods That May Interact with Black Hellebore
None known

Supplements That May Interact with Black Hellebore
- May cause hypokalemia (low levels of potassium in the blood) when combined with buckthorn or cascara sagrada.
- Increased risk of cardiac glycoside toxicity when used with other herbs that contain cardiac glycosides, such as calotropis, digitalis leaf, hedge mustard, motherwort, and others. (For a list of cardiac glycoside–containing herbs and supplements, see Appendix B.)

BLACK MUSTARD

> Mixing the powdered seeds of the black mustard plant with water causes the release of a volatile compound called allylisothiocyanate that is so potent it can actually blister the skin. Historically, mustard has been used to treat snakebites, treat epilepsy, ease arthritis, and increase circulation.

Scientific Name
Brassica nigra

Black Mustard Is Also Commonly Known As
Brown mustard, red mustard, mustard seed

Medicinal Parts
Seed, oil

Black Mustard's Uses
To treat sciatica, bronchial pneumonia, sinusitis, the common cold, rheumatism, and arthritis; in footbaths to treat aching feet

Typical Dose
There is no typical dose of black mustard.

Possible Side Effects
Black mustard can cause diarrhea, vomiting, stomach pain, difficulty breathing, and coma. Applied topically, black mustard's side effects include blistering of the skin and skin allergies.

Drugs That May Interact with Black Mustard
Taking black mustard with these drugs may interfere with the action of the drug:
- aluminum hydroxide (AlternaGel, Alu-Cap)
- aluminum hydroxide and magnesium carbonate (Gaviscon Extra Strength, Gaviscon Liquid)
- aluminum hydroxide and magnesium hydroxide (Maalox, Rulox)
- aluminum hydroxide and magnesium trisilicate (Gaviscon Tablet)
- aluminum hydroxide, magnesium hydroxide, and simethicone (Maalox, Mylanta Liquid)
- calcium carbonate (Rolaids Extra Strength, Tums)
- calcium carbonate and magnesium hydroxide (Mylanta Gelcaps, Rolaids Extra Strength)
- cimetidine (Nu-Cimet, Tagamet)
- esomeprazole (Nexium)
- famotidine (Apo-Famotidine, Pepcid)
- famotidine, calcium carbonate, and magnesium hydroxide (Pepcid Complete)

- lansoprazole (Prevacid)
- magaldrate and simethicone (Riopan Plus, Riopan Plus Double Strength)
- magnesium hydroxide (Dulcolax Milk of Magnesia, Phillips' Milk of Magnesia)
- magnesium sulfate (Epsom salts)
- nizatidine (Axid, PMS-Nizatidine)
- omeprazole (Losec, Prilosec)
- pantoprazole (Pantoloc, Protonix)
- rabeprazole (Aciphex, Pariet)
- ranitidine (Alti-Ranitidine, Zantac)
- sodium bicarbonate (Brioschi, Neut)
- sucralfate (Carafate, Sulcrate)

Lab Tests That May Be Altered by Black Mustard
None known

Diseases That May Be Worsened or Triggered by Black Mustard
May worsen ulcers in the stomach or small intestines by irritating the lining of the stomach or small intestine.

Foods That May Interact with Black Mustard
None known

Supplements That May Interact with Black Mustard
None known

BLACK PEPPER

Legend has it that Attila the Hun demanded three thousand pounds of pepper, among other items, as ransom for the city of Rome. Black pepper was a highly sought after spice during the Middle Ages that was available only to the wealthy, although to-day it is in virtually every home. Studies with laboratory animals dating back to the 1980s suggest that black pepper may protect against cancer of the colon by reducing the amount of toxins in the body.

Scientific Name
Piper nigrum

Black Pepper Is Also Commonly Known As
Pepper bark, peppercorn, pimenta, piper, vellaja, white pepper

Medicinal Parts
Berry

Black Pepper's Uses
To treat digestive problems, scabies, nerve pain, arthritis, asthma, cough, and hemorrhoids

Typical Dose
A typical dose of black pepper may range from 0.3 to 0.6 gm, totaling 1.5 gm daily.

Possible Side Effects
No side effects are known when black pepper is taken in designated therapeutic doses.

Drugs That May Interact with Black Pepper
Taking black pepper with these drugs may increase absorption and blood levels of the drug:
- phenytoin (Dilantin, Phenytek)
- propranolol (Inderal, InnoPran XL)
- theophylline (Elixophyllin, Theochron)

Lab Tests That May Be Altered by Black Pepper
May increase phenytoin, propranolol, and theophylline serum concentrations.

Diseases That May Be Worsened or Triggered by Black Pepper
None known

Foods That May Interact with Black Pepper
None known

Supplements That May Interact with Black Pepper
When taken with Scotch broom, black pepper may increase the activity of sparteine, the principal alkaloid in Scotch broom, which can be toxic in large doses.

BLACK ROOT

> Native to the eastern United States, the root and below-ground parts of this plant are used medicinally to stimulate bowel movements, the flow of bile from the gallbladder, the release of intestinal gas, and perspiration. The fresh root has a much more potent effect than the dried root.

Scientific Name
Leptandra virginica

Black Root Is Also Commonly Known As
Bowman's root, physic root, tall Veronica, whorlywort

Medicinal Parts
Rhizome, root

Black Root's Uses
To treat diarrhea, chronic constipation, disorders of the liver and gallbladder

Typical Dose
A typical homeopathic dose of black root may be 1 tablet, 5 drops, or 10 globules one or more times a day, depending on whether the problem is acute or chronic.

Possible Side Effects
No side effects are known when black root is taken in designated therapeutic doses.

Drugs That May Interact with Black Root
Taking black root with these drugs increases the risk of hypokalemia (low levels of potassium in the blood):

- acetazolamide (Apo-Acetazolamide, Diamox Sequels)
- azosemide (Diat)
- bumetanide (Bumex, Burinex)
- chlorothiazide (Diuril)
- chlorthalidone (Apo-Chlorthalidone, Thalitone)
- ethacrynic acid (Edecrin)
- etozolin (Elkapin)
- furosemide (Apo-Furosemide, Lasix)
- hydrochlorothiazide (Apo-Hydro, Microzide)
- hydroflumethiazide (Diucardin, Saluron)
- indapamide (Lozol, Nu-Indapamide)
- mannitol (Osmitrol, Resectisol)
- mefruside (Baycaron)
- methazolamide (Apo-Methazolamide, Neptazane)
- methyclothiazide (Aquatensen, Enduron)
- metolazone (Mykrox, Zaroxolyn)
- olmesartan and hydrochlorothiazide (Benicar HCT)
- polythiazide (Renese)
- torsemide (Demadex)
- trichlormethiazide (Metatensin, Naqua)
- urea (Amino-Cerv, UltraMide)
- xipamide (Diurexan, Lumitens)

Taking black root with these drugs decreases drug absorption:

- atropine (Isopto Atropine, Sal-Tropine)
- digitalis (Digitek, Lanoxin)
- scopolamine (Scopace, Transderm Scop)

Lab Tests That May Be Altered by Black Root
None known

Diseases That May Be Worsened or Triggered by Black Root
May worsen cases of inflammatory disease of the gastrointestinal tract.

Foods That May Interact with Black Root
None known

Supplements That May Interact with Black Root
- May increase the risk of cardiac toxicity due to potassium depletion when taken with horsetail plant or licorice.
- Increased risk of potassium depletion when used with other stimulant laxative herbs (such as cascara sagrada, castor oil, and senna). (For a list of stimulant laxative herbs and supplements, see Appendix B.)

BLACK TEA

> Black tea, like green tea, comes from the leaves of the *Camellia sinensis* bush, but unlike green tea, its leaves are fermented during processing. This produces health-enhancing substances called thearubigens and theaflavins, which are strong antioxidants that may help lower the risk of death due to heart disease.

Scientific Name
Camellia sinensis

Black Tea Is Also Commonly Known As
Black leaf tea, English tea, tea

Medicinal Parts
Leaf, stem

Black Tea's Uses
To treat kidney stones, cardiovascular disease, Parkinson's disease, and headaches; to increase mental alertness; to reduce the risk of atherosclerosis

Typical Dose
A typical dose of black tea may range from one to several cups per day.

Possible Side Effects
Black tea's side effects include nervousness, restlessness, insomnia, and gastric irritation.

Drugs That May Interact with Black Tea
Taking black tea with these drugs may interfere with the absorption of the drug:

- amitriptyline (Elavil, Levate)
- amitriptyline and chlordiazepoxide (Limbitrol)
- amitriptyline and perphenazine (Etrafon, Triavil)
- amoxapine (Asendin)
- chlorpromazine (Thorazine, Largactil)
- clomipramine (Anafranil, Novo-Clopramine)
- desipramine (Alti-Desipramine, Norpramin)
- doxepin (Sinequan, Zonalon)
- fluphenazine (Modecate, Prolixin)
- imipramine (Apo-Imipramine, Tofranil)
- lofepramine (Feprapax, Gamanil)
- melitracen (Dixeran)

- mesoridazine (Serentil)
- nortriptyline (Aventyl HCl, Pamelor)
- perphenazine (Apo-Perphenazine, Trilafon)
- prochlorperazine (Compazine, Compro)
- promethazine (Phenergan)
- protriptyline (Vivactil)
- thiethylperazine (Torecan)
- thioridazine (Mellaril)
- thiothixene (Navane)
- trifluoperazine (Novo-Trifluzine, Stelazine)
- trimipramine (Apo-Trimip, Surmontil)

Black tea contains caffeine, so see Caffeine and Caffeine-Containing Herbs on p. 111 for an additional list of drugs that may interact with this herb.

Lab Tests That May Be Altered by Black Tea

See Caffeine and Caffeine-Containing Herbs on p. 112 for a list of lab tests that may interact with the caffeine in this herb.

Diseases That May Be Worsened or Triggered by Black Tea

Increased risk of microcytic anemia in infants who are given tea.

See Caffeine and Caffeine-Containing Herbs on p. 113 for a list of diseases that may be worsened or triggered by the caffeine in this herb.

Foods That May Interact with Black Tea

- May increase therapeutic and adverse effects of caffeine when taken together with caffeine-containing foods and drinks. (For a list of caffeine-containing herbs, foods, and supplements, see Appendix B.)
- May interfere with the absorption of nonheme iron (iron from sources other than meat) in the diet.

- Milk can bind the antioxidants in black tea and decrease their beneficial effects.
- Increased excretion of both calcium and magnesium when black tea is taken in large amounts.

Supplements That May Interact with Black Tea

See Caffeine and Caffeine-Containing Herbs on p. 113 for a list of supplements that may interact with the caffeine in this herb.

BLACK WALNUT

> Black walnut gets its scientific name from the Latin words *Juglans*, meaning "acorn" or "Jupiter," and *nigra*, meaning "black," which is the color of the bark of the tree. The reference to Jupiter comes from the idea that the gods who lived on earth were able to subsist on walnuts. Asians and certain Native American tribes have used the bark of the black walnut tree to treat various kinds of intestinal worms.

Scientific Name

Juglans nigra

Black Walnut Is Also Commonly Known As

Nogal Americano, schwarze walnuss

Medicinal Parts

Hull of nut

Black Walnut's Uses

To treat worms, leukemia, diphtheria, and syphilis; as a gargle for mouth sores or sore throats

Typical Dose

There is no typical dose of black walnut.

Possible Side Effects

There are no adverse side effects reported with the use of black walnut.

Drugs That May Interact with Black Walnut

Taking black walnut with these drugs may interfere with absorption of the drug:

- all drugs taken by mouth

Lab Tests That May Be Altered by Black Walnut

None known

Diseases That May Be Worsened or Triggered by Black Walnut

None known

Foods That May Interact with Black Walnut

None known

Supplements That May Interact with Black Walnut

The tannins in black walnut may cause the alkaloids in certain other herbs to separate and settle, increasing the risk of toxic reactions. (For a list of herbs high in alkaloids, see Appendix B.)

BLADDERWRACK

A type of brown seaweed, bladderwrack has a reputation for being a weight-loss aid. If it does help speed weight loss, it's probably because bladderwrack contains high amounts of iodine, which can stimulate an underactive thyroid gland.

Scientific Name

Fucus vesiculosus

Bladderwrack Is Also Commonly Known As

Black-tang, cutweed, fucus, kelpware, seawrack

Medicinal Parts

Thallus (plant body)

Bladderwrack's Uses

To treat obesity, arteriosclerosis, digestive disorders, diseases of the thyroid, and sprains

Typical Dose

A typical dose of bladderwrack may range from 5 to 10 gm in the form of an infusion, taken three times daily, or 4 to 8 ml of extract, taken three times daily.

Possible Side Effects

Bladderwrack's more common side effects include acne, allergic reactions, and triggering or worsening hyperthyroidism.

Drugs That May Interact with Bladderwrack

Taking bladderwrack with these drugs may increase the risk of bleeding or bruising:

- abciximab (ReoPro)
- alteplase (Activase, Cathflo Activase)
- antithrombin III (Thrombate III)
- argatroban
- aspirin (Bufferin, Ecotrin)
- aspirin and dipyridamole (Aggrenox)
- bivalirudin (Angiomax)
- clopidogrel (Plavix)
- dalteparin (Fragmin)
- danaparoid (Orgaran)
- dipyridamole (Novo-Dipiradol, Persantine)
- enoxaparin (Lovenox)
- eptifibatide (Integrillin)

- fondaparinux (Arixtra)
- heparin (Hepalean, Hep-Lock)
- indobufen (Ibustrin)
- lepirudin (Refludan)
- nadroparin (Fraxiparine)
- reteplase (Retavase)
- streptokinase (Streptase)
- tenecteplase (TNKase)
- ticlopidine (Alti-Ticlopidine, Ticlid)
- tinzaparin (Innohep)
- tirofiban (Aggrastat)
- urokinase (Abbokinase)
- warfarin (Coumadin, Jantoven)

Taking bladderwrack with these drugs may reduce the effectiveness of the drug:

- acetazolamide (Apo-Acetazolamide, Diamox Sequels)
- amiloride (Midamor)
- azosemide (Diat)
- bumetanide (Bumex, Burinex)
- chlorothiazide (Diuril)
- chlorthalidone (Apo-Chlorthalidone, Thalitone)
- ethacrynic acid (Edecrin)
- etozolin (Elkapin)
- furosemide (Apo-Furosemide, Lasix)
- hydrochlorothiazide (Apo-Hydro, Microzide)
- hydrochlorothiazide and triamterene (Dyazide, Maxzide)
- hydroflumethiazide (Diucardin, Saluron)
- indapamide (Lozol, Nu-Indapamide)
- levothyroxine (Synthroid, Levothroid)
- liothyronine (Cytomel, Triostat)
- liotrix (Thyrolar)
- mannitol (Osmitrol, Resectisol)
- mefruside (Baycaron)
- methazolamide (Apo-Methazolamide, Neptazane)

- methyclothiazide (Aquatensen, Enduron)
- metolazone (Mykrox, Zaroxolyn)
- olmesartan and hydrochlorothiazide (Benicar HCT)
- polythiazide (Renese)
- spironolactone (Aldactone, Novo-Spiroton)
- thyroid (Nature-Throid NT, Westhroid)
- torsemide (Demadex)
- triamterene (Dyrenium)
- trichlormethiazide (Metatensin, Naqua)
- urea (Amino-Cerv, UltraMide)
- xipamide (Diurexan, Lumitens)

Taking bladderwrack with these drugs may increase the risk of hypoglycemia (low blood sugar):
- acarbose (Prandase, Precose)
- acetohexamide
- chlorpropamide (Diabinese, Novo-Propamide)
- gliclazide (Diamicron, Novo-Gliclazide)
- glimepiride (Amaryl)
- glipizide (Glucotrol)
- glipizide and metformin (Metaglip)
- gliquidone (Beglynor, Glurenorm)
- glyburide (DiaBeta, Glynase)
- glyburide and metformin (Glucovance)
- insulin (Humulin, Novolin R)
- metformin (Glucophage, Riomet)
- miglitol (Glyset)
- nateglinide (Starlix)
- pioglitazone (Actos)
- repaglinide (GlucoNorm, Prandin)
- rosiglitazone (Avandia)
- rosiglitazone and metformin (Avandamet)
- tolazamide (Tolinase)
- tolbutamide (Apo-Tolbutamide, Tol-Tab)

Lab Tests That May Be Altered by Bladderwrack
None known

Diseases That May Be Worsened or Triggered by Bladderwrack

- May worsen cases of acne.
- May worsen hyperthyroidism.
- May worsen iron deficiency by hindering the body's ability to absorb iron.

Foods That May Interact with Bladderwrack

None known

Supplements That May Interact with Bladderwrack

None known

BLESSED THISTLE

Cultivated in Europe as long ago as the sixteenth century, this herb, which was often grown in monastery gardens, was named blessed thistle because of its reputation as a cure-all and one of the most effective remedies for the plague. Blessed thistle is also one of the earliest folk remedies for amenorrhea (the absence of the menstrual cycle) and is still used today for menstrual problems.

Scientific Name

Cnicus benedictus

Blessed Thistle Is Also Commonly Known As

Holy thistle, spotted thistle, St. Benedict's thistle

Medicinal Parts

Leaf, upper stems, seed

Blessed Thistle's Uses

To treat fevers, colds, digestive problems, ulcers, and wounds; as a diuretic. Germany's Commission E has approved the use of blessed thistle to treat loss of appetite and dyspeptic complaints such as heartburn and bloating.

Typical Dose

A typical daily dose of blessed thistle may range from 4 to 6 gm of the herb. Tea is prepared by pouring 150 ml of boiling water over 1.5 to 2 gm of herb, steeping for five to ten minutes, then drinking the tea thirty minutes before a meal.

Possible Side Effects

Blessed thistle's side effects include stomach irritation and vomiting.

Drugs That May Interact with Blessed Thistle

Taking blessed thistle with these drugs may interfere with the action of the drug:

- aluminum hydroxide (AlternaGel, Alu-Cap)
- aluminum hydroxide and magnesium carbonate (Gaviscon Extra Strength, Gaviscon Liquid)
- aluminum hydroxide and magnesium hydroxide (Maalox, Rulox)
- aluminum hydroxide and magnesium trisilicate (Gaviscon Tablet)
- aluminum hydroxide, magnesium hydroxide, and simethicone (Maalox, Mylanta Liquid)
- calcium carbonate (Rolaids Extra Strength, Tums)
- calcium carbonate and magnesium hydroxide (Mylanta Gelcaps, Rolaids Extra Strength)
- cimetidine (Nu-Cimet, Tagamet)
- esomeprazole (Nexium)
- famotidine (Apo-Famotidine, Pepcid)
- famotidine, calcium carbonate, and magnesium hydroxide (Pepcid Complete)
- lansoprazole (Prevacid)
- magaldrate and simethicone (Riopan Plus, Riopan Plus Double Strength)

- magnesium hydroxide (Dulcolax Milk of Magnesia, Phillips' Milk of Magnesia)
- magnesium oxide (Mag-Ox 400, Uro-Mag)
- magnesium sulfate (Epsom salts)
- nizatidine (Axid, PMS-Nizatidine)
- omeprazole (Losec, Prilosec)
- pantoprazole (Pantoloc, Protonix)
- rabeprazole (Aciphex, Pariet)
- ranitidine (Alti-Ranitidine, Zantac)
- sodium bicarbonate (Brioschi, Neut)
- sucralfate (Carafate, Sulcrate)

Lab Tests That May Be Altered by Blessed Thistle
None known

Diseases That May Be Worsened or Triggered by Blessed Thistle
May worsen inflammatory or infectious gastrointestinal ailments by irritating the gastrointestinal tract.

Foods That May Interact with Blessed Thistle
None known

Supplements That May Interact with Blessed Thistle
May cause an allergic reaction in those sensitive to herbs from the Asteraceae family, such as German chamomile, daisy, or dandelion. (For a list of herbs and supplements from the Asteraceae family, see Appendix B.)

BLUE COHOSH

> The flowers of the blue cohosh plant (which is not related to the black cohosh plant) were used by Native Americans to induce labor and menstruation.

> Today the herb's ability to stimulate uterine contractions is thought to stem from a substance it contains called caulosaponin. Blue cohosh has also been used traditionally to treat painful periods, kidney infections, arthritis, and other ailments.

Scientific Name
Caulophyllum thalictroides

Blue Cohosh Is Also Commonly Known As
Beechdrops, blue ginseng, blueberry root, squawroot

Medicinal Parts
Rhizome, root

Blue Cohosh's Uses
To treat menstrual difficulties, lack of menstruation, impending miscarriage, and rheumatic symptoms

Typical Dose
A typical dose of blue cohosh may range from 0.3 to 1.0 gm of herb or 0.5 to 1.0 ml of liquid extract per day.

Possible Side Effects
Blue cohosh's side effects include nausea, vomiting, abdominal pain, diarrhea, inflammation of the skin, excessive sweating, and weakness.

Drugs That May Interact with Blue Cohosh
Taking blue cohosh with these drugs may alter the effects of the drug:
- acarbose (Prandase, Precose)
- acebutolol (Novo-Acebutolol, Sectral)
- acetohexamide
- amlodipine (Norvasc)

- atenolol (Apo-Atenol, Tenormin)
- benazepril (Lotensin)
- betaxolol (Betoptic S, Kerlone)
- bisoprolol (Monocor, Zebeta)
- bumetanide (Bumex, Burinex)
- candesartan (Atacand)
- captopril (Capoten, Novo-Captopril)
- carteolol (Cartrol, Ocupress)
- carvedilol (Coreg)
- chlorothiazide (Diuril)
- chlorpropamide (Diabinese, Novo-Propamide)
- chlorthalidone (Apo-Chlorthalidone, Thalitone)
- clonidine (Catapres, Duraclon)
- diazoxide (Hyperstat, Proglycem)
- diltiazem (Cardizem, Tiazac)
- doxazosin (Alti-Doxazosin, Cardura)
- enalapril (Vasotec)
- eplerenone (Inspra)
- eprosartan (Teveten)
- esmolol (Brevibloc)
- felodipine (Plendil, Renedil)
- fenoldopam (Corlopam)
- fosinopril (Monopril)
- furosemide (Apo-Furosemide, Lasix)
- gliclazide (Diamicron, Novo-Gliclazide)
- glimepiride (Amaryl)
- glipizide (Glucotrol)
- glipizide and metformin (Metaglip)
- gliquidone (Beglynor, Glurenorm)
- glyburide (DiaBeta, Micronase)
- glyburide and metformin (Glucovance)
- guanabenz (Wytensin)
- guanadrel (Hylorel)
- guanfacine (Tenex)
- hydralazine (Apresoline, Novo-Hylazin)
- hydrochlorothiazide (Apo-Hydro, Microzide)
- hydrochlorothiazide and triamterene (Dyazide, Maxzide)
- indapamide (Lozol, Nu-Indapamide)
- insulin (Humulin, Novolin R)
- irbesartan (Avapro)
- isradipine (DynaCirc)
- labetalol (Normodyne, Trandate)
- lisinopril (Prinivil, Zestril)
- losartan (Cozaar)
- mecamylamine (Inversine)
- mefruside (Baycaron)
- metformin (Glucophage, Riomet)
- methyclothiazide (Aquatensen, Enduron)
- methyldopa (Apo-Methyldopa, Nu-Medopa)
- metolazone (Mykrox, Zaroxolyn)
- metoprolol (Betaloc, Lopressor)
- miglitol (Glyset)
- minoxidil (Loniten, Rogaine)
- moexipril (Univasc)
- nadolol (Apo-Nadol, Corgard)
- nateglinide (Starlix)
- nicardipine (Cardene)
- nifedipine (Adalat CC, Procardia)
- nisoldipine (Sular)
- nitroglycerin (Minitran, Nitro-Dur)
- nitroprusside (Nipride, Nitropress)
- olmesartan (Benicar)
- oxprenolol (Slow-Trasicor, Trasicor)
- perindopril erbumine (Aceon, Coversyl)
- phenoxybenzamine (Dibenzyline)
- phentolamine (Regitine, Rogitine)
- pindolol (Apo-Pindol, Novo-Pindol)
- pioglitazone (Actos)
- polythiazide (Renese)
- prazosin (Minipress, Nu-Prazo)
- propranolol (Inderal, InnoPran XL)
- quinapril (Accupril)
- ramipril (Altace)

- repaglinide (GlucoNorm, Prandin)
- reserpine
- rosiglitazone (Avandia)
- rosiglitazone and metformin (Avandamet)
- spironolactone (Aldactone, Novo-Spiroton)
- telmisartan (Micardis)
- terazosin (Alti-Terazosin, Hytrin)
- timolol (Betimol, Timoptic)
- tolazamide (Tolinase)
- tolbutamide (Apo-Tolbutamide, Tol-Tab)
- torsemide (Demadex)
- trandolapril (Mavik)
- triamterene (Dyrenium)
- trichlormethiazide (Metatensin, Naqua)
- valsartan (Diovan)
- verapamil (Calan, Isoptin SR)

Lab Tests That May Be Altered by Blue Cohosh
None known

Diseases That May Be Worsened or Triggered by Blue Cohosh

- May worsen elevated blood pressure, angina, and other cardiovascular ailments by increasing blood pressure.
- May worsen diarrhea by encouraging the movement of feces through the bowels.
- May worsen diabetes by raising blood sugar levels.
- This herb may have estrogen-like effects and should not be used by women with estrogen-sensitive breast cancer or other hormone-sensitive conditions.

Foods That May Interact with Blue Cohosh
None known

Supplements That May Interact with Blue Cohosh
None known

BLUE FLAG

A common Native American remedy, blue flag was traditionally used as an immunity enhancer, blood purifier, and intestinal detoxifier. Some herbalists treat impetigo (a bacterial skin infection often seen in children) by applying fresh slices of the blue flag rhizome to the infected wounds.

Scientific Name
Iris versicolor

Blue Flag Is Also Commonly Known As
Dragonflower, fleur-de-lis, snake lily, wild iris

Medicinal Parts
Rhizome and root

Blue Flag's Uses
To treat constipation, infections, sores, bites, and skin eruptions; as a diuretic

Typical Dose
A typical dose of blue flag as a laxative may range from 650 to 1300 mg of powdered root or 2.5 to 15 ml of tincture.

Possible Side Effects
When taken internally, blue flag's side effects include nausea, vomiting, irritation of the throat, and headache. When used externally, there may be skin irritation or eye inflammation.

Drugs That May Interact with Blue Flag
Taking blue flag with these drugs may increase the risk of hypokalemia (low levels of potassium in the blood):

- acetazolamide (Apo-Acetazolamide, Diamox Sequels)
- azosemide (Diat)
- bumetanide (Bumex, Burinex)
- chlorothiazide (Diuril)
- chlorthalidone (Apo-Chlorthalidone, Thalitone)
- digitalis (Digitek, Lanoxin)
- ethacrynic acid (Edecrin)
- etozolin (Elkapin)
- furosemide (Apo-Furosemide, Lasix)
- hydrochlorothiazide (Apo-Hydro, Microzide)
- hydroflumethiazide (Diucardin, Saluron)
- indapamide (Lozol, Nu-Indapamide)
- mannitol (Osmitrol, Resectisol)
- mefruside (Baycaron)
- methazolamide (Apo-Methazolamide, Neptazane)
- methyclothiazide (Aquatensen, Enduron)
- metolazone (Mykrox, Zaroxolyn)
- olmesartan and hydrochlorothiazide (Benicar HCT)
- polythiazide (Renese)
- torsemide (Demadex)
- trichlormethiazide (Metatensin, Naqua)
- urea (Amino-Cerv, UltraMide)
- xipamide (Diurexan, Lumitens)

Lab Tests That May Be Altered by Blue Flag
None known

Diseases That May Be Worsened or Triggered by Blue Flag
This herb can irritate the gastrointestinal tract and may worsen inflammatory or infectious gastrointestinal ailments.

Foods That May Interact with Blue Flag
None known

Supplements That May Interact with Blue Flag
- Increased risk of potassium depletion when used in conjunction with horsetail plant or licorice.
- Increased risk of potassium depletion when used with other stimulant laxative herbs (such as black root, cascara sagrada, castor oil, and senna). (For a list of stimulant laxative herbs and supplements, see Appendix B.)

BOG BEAN

Bog bean, a small aquatic plant with leaves similar to those seen on bean plants, grows well in a bog, a standing body of water that has no underground spring of fresh water to feed it. Found throughout the Northern Hemisphere, bog bean is used to treat appetite loss and indigestion because its strong, bitter taste stimulates the production of saliva and gastric juices.

Scientific Name
Menyanthes trifoliata

Bog Bean Is Also Commonly Known As
Bog myrtle, buck bean, marsh clover, water shamrock

Medicinal Parts
Leaf

Bog Bean's Uses
To treat diseases of digestive system, fever, insomnia, headache, and lack of menstruation. Germany's Commission E has approved the use of bog bean to treat loss of appetite and dyspeptic complaints such as heartburn, bloating, and nausea.

Typical Dose

A typical daily dose of bog bean may range from 1.5 to 3.0 gm of the herb. Tea is prepared by pouring boiling water over 0.5 to 1.0 gm of herb, steeping for five to ten minutes, then drinking before meals.

Possible Side Effects

No side effects are known when bog bean is taken in designated therapeutic doses.

Drugs That May Interact with Bog Bean

Taking bog bean with these drugs may increase the risk of bleeding or bruising:

- abciximab (ReoPro)
- acemetacin (Acemetacin Heumann, Acemetacin Sandoz)
- antithrombin III (Thrombate III)
- argatroban
- aspirin (Bufferin, Ecotrin)
- aspirin and dipyridamole (Aggrenox)
- bivalirudin (Angiomax)
- celecoxib (Celebrex)
- choline magnesium trisalicylate (Trilisate)
- choline salicylate (Teejel)
- clopidogrel (Plavix)
- dalteparin (Fragmin)
- danaparoid (Orgaran)
- diclofenac (Cataflam, Voltaren)
- diflunisal (Apo-Diflunisal, Dolobid)
- dipyridamole (Novo-Dipiradol, Persantine)
- dipyrone (Analgina, Dinador)
- enoxaparin (Lovenox)
- eptifibatide (Integrillin)
- etodolac (Lodine, Utradol)
- etoricoxib (Arcoxia)
- fenoprofen (Nalfon)
- flurbiprofen (Ansaid, Ocufen)
- fondaparinux (Arixtra)
- heparin (Hepalean, Hep-Lock)
- ibuprofen (Advil, Motrin)
- indobufen (Ibustrin)
- indomethacin (Indocin, Novo-Methacin)
- ketoprofen (Orudis, Rhodis)
- ketorolac (Acular, Toradol)
- lepirudin (Refludan)
- magnesium salicylate (Doan's, Mobidin)
- meclofenamate (Meclomen)
- mefenamic acid (Ponstan, Ponstel)
- meloxicam (MOBIC, Mobicox)
- nabumetone (Apo-Nabumetone, Relafen)
- naproxen (Aleve, Naprosyn)
- niflumic acid (Niflam, Nifluril)
- nimesulide (Areuma, Aulin)
- oxaprozin (Apo-Oxaprozin, Daypro)
- piroxicam (Feldene, Nu-Pirox)
- rofecoxib (Vioxx)
- salsalate (Amgesic, Salflex)
- sulindac (Clinoril, Nu-Sundac)
- tenoxicam (Dolmen, Mobiflex)
- tiaprofenic acid (Dom Tiaprofenic, Surgam)
- ticlopidine (Alti-Ticlopidine, Ticlid)
- tinzaparin (Innohep)
- tirofiban (Aggrastat)
- tolmetin (Tolectin)
- valdecoxib (Bextra)
- warfarin (Coumadin, Jantoven)

Taking bog bean with these drugs may interfere with the action of the drug:

- cimetidine (Nu-Cimet, Tagamet)
- famotidine (Apo-Famotidine, Pepcid)
- famotidine, calcium carbonate, and magnesium hydroxide (Pepcid Complete)
- lansoprazole (Prevacid)

- omeprazole (Losec, Prilosec)
- pantoprazole (Pantoloc, Protonix)
- ranitidine (Alti-Ranitidine, Zantac)
- sucralfate (Carafate, Sulcrate)

Lab Tests That May Be Altered by Bog Bean
None known

Diseases That May Be Worsened or Triggered by Bog Bean
May increase risk of bleeding in those with bleeding disorders.

Foods That May Interact with Bog Bean
None known

Supplements That May Interact with Bog Bean
None known

BOLDO

Native to Chile, boldo has long been used in South America as a liver tonic, treatment for gallstones, and cure for gonorrhea. Its major alkaloid, boldine, is thought to be responsible for its bile-stimulating and diuretic actions.

Scientific Name
Peumus boldo

Boldo Is Also Commonly Known As
Boldu, boldus

Medicinal Parts
Leaf

Boldo's Uses
To treat gallstones, liver disease, gonorrhea; as a diuretic and sedative

Typical Dose
A typical daily dose of boldo is approximately 60 to 200 mg of dried leaves, taken as a tea.

Possible Side Effects
Boldo's side effects include skin irritation and convulsions.

Drugs That May Interact with Boldo
Taking boldo with these drugs may increase the risk of bleeding or bruising:

- abciximab (ReoPro)
- antithrombin III (Thrombate III)
- argatroban
- aspirin (Bufferin, Ecotrin)
- aspirin and dipyridamole (Aggrenox)
- bivalirudin (Angiomax)
- clopidogrel (Plavix)
- dalteparin (Fragmin)
- danaparoid (Orgaran)
- dipyridamole (Novo-Dipiradol, Persantine)
- enoxaparin (Lovenox)
- eptifibatide (Integrillin)
- fondaparinux (Arixtra)
- heparin (Hepalean, Hep-Lock)
- indobufen (Ibustrin)
- lepirudin (Refludan)
- ticlopidine (Alti-Ticlopidine, Ticlid)
- tinzaparin (Innohep)
- tirofiban (Aggrastat)
- warfarin (Coumadin, Jantoven)

Lab Tests That May Be Altered by Boldo
None known

Diseases That May Be Worsened or Triggered by Boldo

Boldo may worsen cases of gallstones, liver or kidney disease, and bile duct obstruction.

Foods That May Interact with Boldo

None known

Supplements That May Interact with Boldo

None known

BONESET

> Theories abound as to the origins of this herb's interesting name. It may be because of its use in treating "breakbone fever," a particularly virulent form of the flu, or because its leaves join together like the ends of a broken bone. Another theory is that it's called boneset because taking a tea made from the herb twice a day was believed to help broken bones heal.

Scientific Name

Eupatorium perfoliatum

Boneset Is Also Commonly Known As

Agueweed, crosswort, feverwort, Indian sage, teasel

Medicinal Parts

Whole herb, leaf, flower

Boneset's Uses

To treat the flu and other diseases involving fever

Typical Dose

A typical dose of boneset has not been established.

Possible Side Effects

Boneset's side effects include loss of appetite, diarrhea, nausea, and vomiting.

Drugs That May Interact with Boneset

Taking boneset with these drugs may cause or increase liver damage:

- abacavir (Ziagen)
- acarbose (Prandase, Precose)
- acetaminophen (Genapap, Tylenol)
- allopurinol (Aloprim, Zyloprim)
- atorvastatin (Lipitor)
- celecoxib (Celebrex)
- cidofovir (Vistide)
- cyclosporine (Neoral, Sandimmune)
- docetaxel (Taxotere)
- dofetilide (Tikosyn)
- erythromycin (Erythrocin, Staticin)
- etodolac (Lodine, Utradol)
- fluconazole (Apo-Fluconazole, Diflucan)
- fluphenazine (Modecate, Prolixin)
- fluvastatin (Lescol)
- foscarnet (Foscavir)
- ganciclovir (Cytovene, Vitrasert)
- gemfibrozil (Apo-Gemfibrozil, Lopid)
- gentamicin (Alcomicin, Gentacidin)
- ibuprofen (Advil, Motrin)
- indinavir (Crixivan)
- isoniazid (Isotamine, Nydrazid)
- ketoconazole (Apo-Ketoconazole, Nizoral)
- ketoprofen (Orudis, Rhodis)
- ketorolac (Acular, Toradol)
- lamivudine (Epivir, Heptovir)
- levodopa-carbidopa (Nu-Levocarb, Sinemet)
- lovastatin (Altocor, Mevacor)
- meloxicam (MOBIC, Mobicox)
- methotrexate (Rheumatrex, Trexall)
- methyldopa (Apo-Methyldopa, Nu-Medopa)

- morphine hydrochloride
- morphine sulfate (Kadian, MS Contin)
- naproxen (Aleve, Naprosyn)
- nelfinavir (Viracept)
- nevirapine (Viramune)
- nitrofurantoin (Furadantin, Macrobid)
- ondansetron (Zofran)
- paclitaxel (Onxol, Taxol)
- pantoprazole (Pantoloc, Protonix)
- phenytoin (Dilantin, Phenytek)
- pioglitazone (Actos)
- piroxicam (Feldene, Nu-Pirox)
- pravastatin (Novo-Pravastatin, Pravachol)
- prochlorperazine (Compazine, Compro)
- propoxyphene (Darvon, Darvon-N)
- repaglinide (GlucoNorm, Prandin)
- rifampin (Rifadin, Rimactane)
- rifapentine (Priftin)
- ritonavir (Norvir)
- rofecoxib (Vioxx)
- rosiglitazone (Avandia)
- saquinavir (Fortovase, Invirase)
- simvastatin (Apo-Simvastatin, Zocor)
- stavudine (Zerit)
- tamoxifen (Nolvadex, Tamofen)
- tramadol (Ultram)
- zidovudine (Novo-AZT, Retrovir)

Lab Tests That May Be Altered by Boneset
None known

Diseases That May Be Worsened or Triggered by Boneset
None known

Foods That May Interact with Boneset
None known

Supplements That May Interact with Boneset
None known

BORAGE (*See also* Borage Seed Oil)

> The ability of borage to counteract melancholia has been known for centuries. In the 1600s, diarist John Evelyn wrote that borage could "revive the hypochondriac and cheer the hard student," possibly by supporting the adrenal glands.

Scientific Name
Borago officinalis

Borage Is Also Commonly Known As
Bugloss, burrage

Medicinal Parts
Flower, leaf, stem

Borage's Uses
To treat coughs, various throat and bronchial conditions, rheumatism, menopausal complaints, and pain; to reduce inflammation; to purify the blood

Typical Dose
There is no typical dose of borage.

Possible Side Effects
Borage's side effects include gastrointestinal distress.

Drugs That May Interact with Borage
Taking borage with these drugs may increase the risk of bleeding or bruising:
- abciximab (ReoPro)

- alteplase (Activase, Cathflo Activase)
- antithrombin III (Thrombate III)
- argatroban
- aspirin (Bufferin, Ecotrin)
- aspirin and dipyridamole (Aggrenox)
- bivalirudin (Angiomax)
- clopidogrel (Plavix)
- dalteparin (Fragmin)
- danaparoid (Orgaran)
- dipyridamole (Novo-Dipiradol, Persantine)
- enoxaparin (Lovenox)
- eptifibatide (Integrillin)
- fondaparinux (Arixtra)
- heparin (Hepalean, Hep-Lock)
- indobufen (Ibustrin)
- lepirudin (Refludan)
- nadroparin (Fraxiparine)
- reteplase (Retavase)
- streptokinase (Streptase)
- tenecteplase (TNKase)
- ticlopidine (Alti-Ticlopidine, Ticlid)
- tinzaparin (Innohep)
- tirofiban (Aggrastat)
- urokinase (Abbokinase)
- warfarin (Coumadin, Jantoven)

Taking borage with these drugs may reduce or prevent drug absorption:
- ferric gluconate (Ferrlecit)
- ferrous fumarate (Femiron, Feostat)
- ferrous gluconate (Fergon, Novo-Ferrogluc)
- ferrous sulfate (Feratab, Fer-Iron)
- ferrous sulfate and ascorbic acid (Fero-Grad 500, Vitelle Irospan)
- iron-dextran complex (Dexferrum, INFeD)
- polysaccharide-iron complex (Hytinic, Niferex)

Lab Tests That May Be Altered by Borage
None known

Diseases That May Be Worsened or Triggered by Borage
May worsen cases of liver disease.

Foods That May Interact with Borage
None known

Supplements That May Interact with Borage
- Increased risk of unsaturated pyrrolizidine alkaloid (UPA) toxicity when used with eucalyptus.
- Increased risk of additive toxicity when used with herbs and supplements containing unsaturated pyrrolizidine alkaloids (UPAs), such as butterbur, comfrey, and colt's foot. (For a list of herbs and supplements containing unsaturated pyrrolizidine alkaloids, see Appendix B.)

BORAGE SEED OIL (*See also* Borage)

Perhaps the best source of gamma-linolenic acid (outdoing even black currant oil and evening primrose oil), borage seed oil has anti-inflammatory properties and may also act as a blood thinner and blood vessel dilator. Several studies have shown that borage seed oil is helpful in reducing joint inflammation and other symptoms of rheumatoid arthritis.

Scientific Name
Borago officinalis

Borage Seed Oil Is Also Commonly Known As
Borage oil, bugloss, burrage, starflower

Medicinal Parts

Oil of the seed

Borage Seed Oil's Uses

To treat premenstrual syndrome, rheumatoid arthritis, diabetes, stress, and eczema; to prevent stroke and heart disease

Typical Dose

A typical dose of borage seed oil for eczema may range from 2 to 3 gm daily in divided doses; for rheumatoid arthritis the range is 6 to 7 gm daily in divided doses after meals.

Possible Side Effects

Borage seed oil's side effects include diarrhea, bloating, and belching.

Drugs That May Interact with Borage Seed Oil

Taking borage seed oil with these drugs may increase the risk of bleeding or bruising:

- abciximab (ReoPro)
- antithrombin III (Thrombate III)
- argatroban
- aspirin (Bufferin, Ecotrin)
- aspirin and dipyridamole (Aggrenox)
- bivalirudin (Angiomax)
- clopidogrel (Plavix)
- dalteparin (Fragmin)
- danaparoid (Orgaran)
- dipyridamole (Novo-Dipiradol, Persantine)
- enoxaparin (Lovenox)
- eptifibatide (Integrillin)
- fondaparinux (Arixtra)
- heparin (Hepalean, Hep-Lock)
- indobufen (Ibustrin)
- lepirudin (Refludan)
- rofecoxib (Vioxx)
- ticlopidine (Alti-Ticlopidine, Ticlid)
- tinzaparin (Innohep)
- tirofiban (Aggrastat)
- urokinase (Abbokinase)
- warfarin (Coumadin, Jantoven)

Lab Tests That May Be Altered by Borage Seed Oil

- May increase bleeding time.
- May lower plasma triglycerides and increase HDL "good" cholesterol.

Diseases That May Be Worsened or Triggered by Borage Seed Oil

May worsen bleeding disorders and liver disease.

Foods That May Interact with Borage Seed Oil

None known

Supplements That May Interact with Borage Seed Oil

- Increased risk of additive toxicity when used with herbs and supplements containing unsaturated pyrrolizidine alkaloids (UPAs), such as butterbur, comfrey, and colt's foot. (For a list of herbs and supplements containing unsaturated pyrrolizidine alkaloids, see Appendix B.)
- Increased risk of bleeding when used with herbs and supplements that might affect platelet aggregation, such as angelica, danshen, garlic, ginger, ginkgo biloba, red clover, turmeric, white willow, and others. (For a list of herbs and supplements with anticoagulant/antiplatelet potential, see Appendix B.)

BREWER'S YEAST

The dried, ground-up cells of a kind of fungus called *Saccharomyces cerevisiae*, a by-product of the beer-brewing process, brewer's yeast is an excellent source of vitamins, minerals, and amino acids. Specifically, it contains all the major B vitamins (except B_{12}), all of the essential amino acids, and at least fourteen minerals. Brewer's yeast is also the best source of a biologically active form of chromium known as glucose tolerance factor (GTF). In several studies, brewer's yeast has been shown to lower blood sugar levels.

Scientific Name
Saccharomyces cerevisiae

Brewer's Yeast Is Also Commonly Known As
Baker's yeast, medicinal yeast

Medicinal Parts
Yeast developed during the beer-brewing process

Brewer's Yeast's Uses
To treat constipation and itching skin diseases. Germany's Commission E has approved the use of brewer's yeast to treat acne, eczema, skin infections known as furuncles, loss of appetite, and dyspeptic complaints such as heartburn and bloating.

Typical Dose
A typical dose of brewer's yeast is approximately 6 gm in powder or tablet form per day.

Possible Side Effects
Side effects are not typically seen in those taking brewer's yeast in recommended doses. However, when taken in large doses, brewer's yeast has side effects that include intestinal gas, allergic reactions such as itching and hives, or migraine headaches in susceptible people.

Drugs That May Interact with Brewer's Yeast
Taking brewer's yeast with these drugs may increase the risk of hypertension (high blood pressure):
- iproniazid (Marsilid)
- moclobemide (Alti-Moclobemide, Nu-Moclobemide)
- phenelzine (Nardil)
- selegiline (Eldepryl)
- tranylcypromine (Parnate)

Lab Tests That May Be Altered by Brewer's Yeast
May alter results of antimicrobial tests.

Diseases That May Be Worsened or Triggered by Brewer's Yeast
May worsen cases of Crohn's disease.

Foods That May Interact with Brewer's Yeast
None known

Supplements That May Interact with Brewer's Yeast
None known

BROMELAIN

Derived from the pineapple, bromelain is a proteolytic enzyme, which means it's capable of breaking down protein. This explains why it is found in certain digestive aids. Its main function, however,

continued

is as an anti-inflammatory used to treat burns, sprains, strains, and muscle injuries and to relieve the accompanying pain and swelling. Bromelain is also used to clean away debris from wounds.

Scientific Name
Ananas comosus

Bromelain Is Also Commonly Known As
Bromelin, pineapple enzyme, plant protease concentrate

Medicinal Parts
Extract of enzymes from pineapple stem

Bromelain's Uses
To treat inflammation, burns, and swelling; to inhibit platelet aggregation. Germany's Commission E has approved the use of bromelain to treat burns and wounds.

Typical Dose
A typical dose of bromelain may range from 200 to 400 mg daily.

Possible Side Effects
Bromelain's side effects include gastrointestinal upset.

Drugs That May Interact with Bromelain
Taking bromelain with these drugs may increase the risk of bleeding and bruising:
- abciximab (ReoPro)
- antithrombin III (Thrombate III)
- argatroban
- aspirin (Bufferin, Ecotrin)
- aspirin and dipyridamole (Aggrenox)
- bivalirudin (Angiomax)
- celecoxib (Celebrex)
- clopidogrel (Plavix)
- dalteparin (Fragmin)
- danaparoid (Orgaran)
- dipyridamole (Novo-Dipiradol, Persantine)
- enoxaparin (Lovenox)
- eptifibatide (Integrillin)
- etodolac (Lodine, Utradol)
- fondaparinux (Arixtra)
- heparin (Hepalean, Hep-Lock)
- ibuprofen (Advil, Motrin)
- indobufen (Ibustrin)
- indomethacin (Indocin, Novo-Methacin)
- ketoprofen (Orudis, Rhodis)
- ketorolac (Acular, Toradol)
- lepirudin (Refludan)
- ticlopidine (Alti-Ticlopidine, Ticlid)
- tinzaparin (Innohep)
- tirofiban (Aggrastat)
- warfarin (Coumadin, Jantoven)

Taking bromelain with these drugs can increase drug concentrations in plasma and urine:
- demeclocycline (Declomycin)
- doxycycline (Apo-Doxy, Vibramycin)
- minocycline (Dynacin, Minocin)
- oxytetracycline (Terramycin, Terramycin IM)
- tetracycline (Novo-Tetra, Sumycin)

Lab Tests That May Be Altered by Bromelain
None known

Diseases That May Be Worsened or Triggered by Bromelain
Pineapple allergy may be triggered by taking bromelain.

Foods That May Interact with Bromelain

Potato protein and soybean can inhibit bromelain activity.

Supplements That May Interact with Bromelain

- Increased risk of bleeding when used with herbs and supplements that might affect platelet aggregation, such as angelica, danshen, garlic, ginger, ginkgo biloba, red clover, turmeric, white willow, and others. (For a list of herbs and supplements with anticoagulant/antiplatelet potential, see Appendix B.)
- Bromelain activity may be inhibited by zinc, which oxidizes bromelain.

Buchu

The leaves of the buchu, a low, stubby shrub from the Cape region of South Africa, have been used traditionally to treat urinary tract inflammation and infections as well as inflammation of the prostate gland. Buchu's ability to treat infections is thought to be due to its volatile oils, especially disophenol, which may have antibacterial action.

Scientific Name

Agathosma betulina

Buchu Is Also Commonly Known As

Bookoo, bucco, diosma, short buchu

Medicinal Parts

Leaf

Buchu's Uses

To treat venereal disease, infections of the prostate, kidneys, and other parts of the urinary tract

Typical Dose

A typical dose of buchu is 3 to 6 gm of dried leaves per day, taken as tea in divided doses; or 2 to 4 ml of fluid extract per day (1:2 dilution); or 5 to 10 ml of tincture per day (1:5 dilution).

Possible Side Effects

Buchu's side effects include loss of appetite, diarrhea, nausea, and increased menstrual flow.

Drugs That May Interact with Buchu

Taking buchu with these drugs can increase the risk of bleeding or bruising:

- abciximab (ReoPro)
- antithrombin III (Thrombate III)
- argatroban
- aspirin (Bufferin, Ecotrin)
- aspirin and dipyridamole (Aggrenox)
- bivalirudin (Angiomax)
- clopidogrel (Plavix)
- dalteparin (Fragmin)
- danaparoid (Orgaran)
- dipyridamole (Novo-Dipiradol, Persantine)
- enoxaparin (Lovenox)
- eptifibatide (Integrillin)
- fondaparinux (Arixtra)
- heparin (Hepalean, Hep-Lock)
- indobufen (Ibustrin)
- lepirudin (Refludan)
- ticlopidine (Alti-Ticlopidine, Ticlid)
- tinzaparin (Innohep)
- tirofiban (Aggrastat)
- warfarin (Coumadin, Jantoven)

Taking buchu with these drugs can increase the risk of hyperglycemia (high blood sugar):

- acarbose (Prandase, Precose)
- acetohexamide
- chlorpropamide (Diabinese, Novo-Propamide)
- gliclazide (Diamicron, Novo-Gliclazide)
- glimepiride (Amaryl)
- glipizide (Glucotrol)
- glipizide and metformin (Metaglip)
- gliquidone (Beglynor, Glurenorm)
- glyburide (DiaBeta, Micronase)
- glyburide and metformin (Glucovance)
- insulin (Humulin, Novolin R)
- metformin (Glucophage, Riomet)
- miglitol (Glyset)
- nateglinide (Starlix)
- pioglitazone (Actos)
- repaglinide (GlucoNorm, Prandin)
- rosiglitazone (Avandia)
- rosiglitazone and metformin (Avandamet)
- tolazamide (Tolinase)
- tolbutamide (Apo-Tolbutamide, Tol-Tab)

Taking buchu with these drugs can be harmful:
- lithium (Carbolith, Eskalith)—may increase the action of the drug and cause lithium toxicity.

Lab Tests That May Be Altered by Buchu
None known

Diseases That May Be Worsened or Triggered by Buchu
May worsen cases of kidney infection or urinary tract inflammation.

Foods That May Interact with Buchu
None known

Supplements That May Interact with Buchu
None known

BUCKTHORN

This laxative herb is so strong that it's usually used only as a last resort. Chemicals in buckthorn called anthraquinones stimulate the muscles of the intestinal tract, greatly increasing the urge to defecate and sometimes causing diarrhea and abdominal pain.

Scientific Name
Rhamnus catharticus

Buckthorn Is Also Commonly Known As
Hartsthorn, highwaythorn, ramsthorn, waythorn

Medicinal Parts
Fruit, bark

Buckthorn's Uses
To treat constipation and poor digestion; as a diuretic in "blood-purifying" remedies. Germany's Commission E has approved the use of buckthorn to treat constipation.

Typical Dose
A typical dose of buckthorn may range from 2 to 5 gm per day.

Possible Side Effects
Buckthorn's side effects include nausea, vomiting, loss of appetite, abdominal cramps, and nervousness. Long-term use leads to dehydration and loss of electrolytes, especially potassium.

Drugs That May Interact with Buckthorn
Taking buckthorn with these drugs may reduce or prevent drug absorption:
- all drugs taken orally (due to herb's laxative effect)

Taking buckthorn with these drugs may interfere with the action of the drug:

- acebutolol (Novo-Acebutolol, Sectral)
- adenosine (Adenocard, Adenoscan)
- amiodarone (Cordarone, Pacerone)
- bretylium
- digoxin (Digitek, Lanoxin)
- diltiazem (Cardizem, Tiazac)
- disopyramide (Norpace, Rhythmodan)
- dofetilide (Tikosyn)
- esmolol (Brevibloc)
- flecainide (Tambocor)
- ibutilide (Corvert)
- lidocaine (Lidoderm, Xylocaine)
- mexiletine (Mexitil, Novo-Mexiletine)
- moricizine (Ethmozine)
- phenytoin (Dilantin, Phenytek)
- procainamide (Procanbid, Pronestyl-SR)
- propafenone (Gen-Propafenone, Rhythmol)
- propranolol (Inderal, InnoPran XL)
- quinidine (Novo-Quinidin, Quinaglute Dura-Tabs)
- sotalol (Betapace, Sorine)
- tocainide (Tonocard)
- verapamil (Calan, Isoptin SR)

Taking buckthorn with these drugs may increase the risk of hypokalemia (low levels of potassium in the blood):

- acetazolamide (Apo-Acetazolamide, Diamox Sequels)
- azosemide (Diat)
- beclomethasone (Beconase, Vanceril)
- betamethasone (Celestone, Diprolene)
- budesonide (Entocort, Rhinocort)
- budesonide and formoterol (Symbicort)
- bumetanide (Bumex, Burinex)
- chlorothiazide (Diuril)
- chlorthalidone (Apo-Chlorthalidone, Thalitone)

- cortisone (Cortone)
- deflazacort (Calcort, Dezacor)
- dexamethasone (Decadron, Dexasone)
- ethacrynic acid (Edecrin)
- etozolin (Elkapin)
- flunisolide (AeroBid, Nasarel)
- fluorometholone (Eflone, Flarex)
- fluticasone (Cutivate, Flonase)
- furosemide (Apo-Furosemide, Lasix)
- hydrochlorothiazide (Apo-Hydro, Microzide)
- hydrocortisone (Anusol-HC, Locoid)
- hydroflumethiazide (Diucardin, Saluron)
- indapamide (Lozol, Nu-Indapamide)
- loteprednol (Alrex, Lotemax)
- mannitol (Osmitrol, Resectisol)
- medrysone (HMS Liquifilm)
- mefruside (Baycaron)—used for elevated blood pressure
- methazolamide (Apo-Methazolamide, Neptazane)
- methyclothiazide (Aquatensen, Enduron)
- methylprednisolone (Depo-Medrol, Medrol)
- metolazone (Mykrox, Zaroxolyn)
- olmesartan and hydrochlorothiazide (Benicar HCT)
- polythiazide (Renese)
- prednisolone (Inflamase Forte, Pred Forte)
- prednisone (Apo-Prednisone, Deltasone)
- rimexolone (Vexol)
- torsemide (Demadex)
- triamcinolone (Aristocort, Trinasal)
- trichlormethiazide (Metatensin, Naqua)
- urea (Amino-Cerv, UltraMide)
- xipamide (Diurexan, Lumitens)

Taking buckthorn with these drugs may interfere with the action of the herb:

- aluminum hydroxide (AlternaGel, AluCap)
- aluminum hydroxide and magnesium

carbonate (Gaviscon Extra Strength, Gaviscon Liquid)
- aluminum hydroxide and magnesium hydroxide (Maalox, Rulox)
- aluminum hydroxide and magnesium trisilicate (Gaviscon Tablet)
- aluminum hydroxide, magnesium hydroxide, and simethicone (Maalox, Mylanta Liquid)
- calcium carbonate (Rolaids Extra Strength, Tums)
- calcium carbonate and magnesium hydroxide (Mylanta Gelcaps, Rolaids Extra Strength)
- famotidine, calcium carbonate, and magnesium hydroxide (Pepcid Complete)
- magaldrate and simethicone (Riopan Plus, Riopan Plus Double Strength)
- magnesium hydroxide (Dulcolax Milk of Magnesia, Phillips' Milk of Magnesia)
- magnesium oxide (Mag-Ox 400, Uro-Mag)
- magnesium sulfate (Epsom salts)
- sodium bicarbonate (Brioschi, Neut)

Lab Tests That May Be Altered by Buckthorn

May confound results of diagnostic urine tests that rely on a color change by turning urine different colors.

Diseases That May Be Worsened or Triggered by Buckthorn

May worsen cases of Crohn's disease, irritable bowel syndrome, ulcerative colitis, or other gastrointestinal diseases.

Foods That May Interact with Buckthorn

The action of buckthorn may be inhibited by milk.

Supplements That May Interact with Buckthorn

- May cause increased action of jimson weed in cases of chronic abuse of buckthorn.
- Increased risk of hypokalemia (low blood levels of potassium) when used with adonis, black or green hellebore, licorice, lily-of-the-valley, or strophanthus.
- Increased risk of potassium deficiency when used with licorice.

BUGLEWEED

Traditionally, bugleweed was used to treat coughs, but it's used in modern times primarily to reduce the activity of an overactive thyroid. Bugleweed contains lithospermic acid and other organic acids that appear to decrease the levels of several hormones in the body, particularly thyroid-stimulating hormone and the thyroid hormone thyroxine.

Scientific Name

Lycopus virginicus

Bugleweed Is Also Commonly Known As

Gypsywort, sweet bugle, Virginia water horehound, water bugle

Medicinal Parts

Leaf, flower, stem, and root

Bugleweed's Uses

To treat mild thyroid hyperfunction, liver and kidney disease, tension, PMS, and pain in the breast (mastodynia). Germany's Commission E has approved the use of bugleweed to treat premenstrual syndrome, insomnia, and nervousness.

Typical Dose

A typical dose of bugleweed may range from 1 to 3 gm of dried herb taken three times a day.

Possible Side Effects

No side effects are known when bugleweed is taken in designated therapeutic dosages.

Drugs That May Interact with Bugleweed

Taking bugleweed with these drugs may increase the risk of hypertension (high blood pressure):

- ephedrine (Pretz-D)
- ergotamine (Cafergor, Cafergot)
- rizatriptan benzoate (Maxalt)
- zolmitriptan (Zomig)

Taking bugleweed with these drugs may increase the risk of hypoglycemia (low blood sugar):

- acarbose (Prandase, Precose)
- acetohexamide
- chlorpropamide (Diabinese, Novo-Propamide)
- gliclazide (Diamicron, Novo-Gliclazide)
- glimepiride (Amaryl)
- glipizide (Glucotrol)
- glipizide and metformin (Metaglip)
- gliquidone (Beglynor, Glurenorm)
- glyburide (DiaBeta, Micronase)
- glyburide and metformin (Glucovance)
- insulin (Humulin, Novolin R)
- metformin (Glucophage, Riomet)
- miglitol (Glyset)
- nateglinide (Starlix)
- pioglitazone (Actos)
- repaglinide (GlucoNorm, Prandin)
- rosiglitazone (Avandia)
- rosiglitazone and metformin (Avandamet)
- tolazamide (Tolinase)
- tolbutamide (Apo-Tolbutamide, Tol-Tab)

Taking bugleweed with these drugs may interfere with diagnostic procedures related to thyroid deficiency:

- levothyroxine (Levothroid, Synthroid)
- liothyronine (Cytomel, Triostat)
- liotrix (Thyrolar)
- thyroid (Nature-Throid NT, Westhroid)

Lab Tests That May Be Altered by Bugleweed

- May interfere with diagnostic procedures using radioactive isoptopes, such as positron emission tomography (PET scans).
- May improve thyroid function in those with mild hyperthyroidism.

Diseases That May Be Worsened or Triggered by Bugleweed

- May trigger hypoglycemia (low blood sugar) in people with diabetes.
- May interfere with thyroid treatments.

Foods That May Interact with Bugleweed

None known

Supplements That May Interact with Bugleweed

May alter effects of herbs and supplements that have thyroid activity, such as balm leaf and wild thyme. (For a list of herbs that can affect thyroid function, see Appendix B.)

Burdock

> Burdock has antimicrobial action, earning it a reputation as an effective treatment for skin eruptions, cystitis, sore throats, colds, and flu. A lotion made from the leaves or root of burdock is purported to be good for thinning hair.

Scientific Name

Arctium lappa

Burdock Is Also Commonly Known As

Bardana, burr seed, cockle buttons, cocklebur, hardock, lappa

Medicinal Parts

Leaf, root, seed

Burdock's Uses

To treat various gastrointestinal problems, psoriasis, seborrhea of the scalp, and ichthyosis (dry, scaly skin); as a diuretic; and to help purify the blood

Typical Dose

A typical dose of burdock is approximately 2.5 gm (1 tsp) of the drug steeped in 150 ml of boiling water, then strained and taken as tea.

Possible Side Effects

No side effects are known when burdock is taken in designated therapeutic dosages.

Drugs That May Interact with Burdock

Taking burdock with these drugs may increase the risk of hypoglycemia (low blood sugar):

- acarbose (Prandase, Precose)
- acetohexamide
- chlorpropamide (Diabinese, Novo-Propamide)
- gliclazide (Diamicron, Novo-Gliclazide)
- glimepiride (Amaryl)
- glipizide (Glucotrol)
- glipizide and metformin (Metaglip)
- gliquidone (Beglynor, Glurenorm)
- glyburide (DiaBeta, Micronase)
- glyburide and metformin (Glucovance)
- insulin (Humulin, Novolin R)
- metformin (Glucophage, Riomet)
- miglitol (Glyset)
- nateglinide (Starlix)
- pioglitazone (Actos)
- repaglinide (GlucoNorm, Prandin)
- rosiglitazone (Avandia)
- rosiglitazone and metformin (Avandamet)
- tolazamide (Tolinase)
- tolbutamide (Apo-Tolbutamide, Tol-Tab)

Lab Tests That May Be Altered by Burdock

None known

Diseases That May Be Worsened or Triggered by Burdock

May trigger hypoglycemia (low blood sugar) in people with diabetes.

Foods That May Interact with Burdock

None known

Supplements That May Interact with Burdock

None known

BUTCHER'S BROOM

Chemicals in butcher's broom known as ruscogenins and flavonoids tighten weak, stretched-out blood vessels, such as those seen in hemorrhoids or varicose veins, and help keep blood circulating throughout the body. Some studies have suggested that butcher's broom may be helpful in treating varicose veins. One study involving forty people found that a combination of butcher's broom, vitamin C, and hesperidin led to a rapid improvement in the appearance of varicose veins.

Scientific Name

Ruscus aculeatus

Butcher's Broom Is Also Commonly Known As
Knee holly, Jew's myrtle, sweet broom

Medicinal Parts
Leaf, rhizome

Butcher's Broom's Uses
To treat hemorrhoids, and pain and other symptoms of poor circulation in the legs. Germany's Commission E has approved the use of butcher's broom to treat hemorrhoids and vein ailments.

Typical Dose
There is no typical dose of butcher's broom.

Possible Side Effects
Loss of appetite, nausea, vomiting

Drugs That May Interact with Butcher's Broom
Taking butcher's broom with this drug may interfere with the actions of the drug:
- prazosin (Minipress, Nu-Prazo)

Taking butcher's broom with these drugs may increase the risk of a hypertensive crisis (a rapid and severe increase in blood pressure that can trigger a heart attack, stroke, and other problems):
- iproniazid (Marsilid)
- moclobemide (Alti-Moclobemide, Nu-Moclobemide)
- phenelzine (Nardil)
- selegiline (Eldepryl)
- tranylcypromine (Parnate)

Lab Tests That May Be Altered by Butcher's Broom
None known

Diseases That May Be Worsened or Triggered by Butcher's Broom
None known

Foods That May Interact with Butcher's Broom
None known

Supplements That May Interact with Butcher's Broom
- May have additive effects when combined with herbs with alpha-agonist properties. (For a list of herbs with alpha-agonist properties, see Appendix B.)
- May decrease effects of herbs with alpha-antagonist properties. (For a list of herbs and supplements with alpha-antagonist properties, see Appendix B.)

BUTTERBUR

Butterbur, taken from a shrub found in Europe, North America, and Asia, was used during the Middle Ages to treat fever and the plague. Later it became known as a remedy for ulcers, asthma, migraine headaches, anxiety, coughs, and wounds, probably due to its ability to calm inflammation and relax smooth muscle spasms.

Scientific Name
Petasites hybridus

Butterbur Is Also Commonly Known As
Blatterdock, bog rhubarb, European pestroot, flapperdock, sweet colt's foot

Medicinal Parts
Flower, leaf, stem, root

Butterbur's Uses

To treat asthma, whooping cough, migraine headaches, allergic rhinitis (hay fever), irritable bowel syndrome, and anxiety; to stimulate the appetite

Typical Dose

A typical dose of butterbur for allergic rhinitis is approximately 50 mg of whole butterbur root extract taken twice daily.

Possible Side Effects

Butterbur's side effects include asthma, stomach upset, fatigue, and headache.

Drugs That May Interact with Butterbur

Taking butterbur with these drugs may cause or increase liver damage:

- abacavir (Ziagen)
- acarbose (Prandase, Precose)
- allopurinol (Aloprim, Zyloprim)
- atorvastatin (Lipitor)
- celecoxib (Celebrex)
- cidofovir (Vistide)
- cyclosporine (Neoral, Sandimmune)
- docetaxel (Taxotere)
- dofetilide (Tikosyn)
- erythromycin (Erythrocin, Staticin)
- etodolac (Lodine, Utradol)
- fluconazole (Apo-Fluconazole, Diflucan)
- fluphenazine (Modecate, Prolixin)
- fluvastatin (Lescol)
- foscarnet (Foscavir)
- ganciclovir (Cytovene, Vitrasert)
- gemfibrozil (Apo-Gemfibrozil, Lopid)
- gentamicin (Alcomicin, Gentacidin)
- ibuprofen (Advil, Motrin)
- indinavir (Crixivan)
- isoniazid (Isotamine, Nydrazid)
- ketoconazole (Apo-Ketoconazole, Nizoral)
- ketoprofen (Orudis, Rhodis)
- ketorolac (Acular, Toradol)
- lamivudine (Epivir, Heptovir)
- levodopa-carbidopa (Nu-Levocarb, Sinemet)
- lovastatin (Altocor, Mevacor)
- meloxicam (MOBIC, Mobicox)
- methotrexate (Rheumatrex, Trexall)
- methyldopa (Apo-Methyldopa, Nu-Medopa)
- morphine hydrochloride
- morphine sulfate (Kadian, MS Contin)
- naproxen (Aleve, Naprosyn)
- nelfinavir (Viracept)
- nevirapine (Viramune)
- nitrofurantoin (Furadantin, Macrobid)
- ondansetron (Zofran)
- paclitaxel (Onxol, Taxol)
- pantoprazole (Pantoloc, Protonix)
- phenytoin (Dilantin, Phenytek)
- pioglitazone (Actos)
- piroxicam (Feldene, Nu-Pirox)
- pravastatin (Novo-Pravastatin, Pravachol)
- prochlorperazine (Compazine, Compro)
- propoxyphene (Darvon, Darvon-N)
- repaglinide (GlucoNorm, Prandin)
- rifampin (Rifadin, Rimactane)
- rifapentine (Priftin)
- ritonavir (Norvir)
- rofecoxib (Vioxx)
- rosiglitazone (Avandia)
- saquinavir (Fortovase, Invirase)
- simvastatin (Apo-Simvastatin, Zocor)
- tamoxifen (Nolvadex, Tamofen)
- tramadol (Ultram)
- zidovudine (Novo-AZT, Retrovir)

Taking butterbur with these drugs may enhance the drug's therapeutic and adverse effects:

- acebutolol (Novo-Acebutolol, Sectral)
- atenolol (Apo-Atenol, Tenormin)
- atropine (Isopto Atropine, Sal-Tropine)
- befunolol (Bentos, Betaclar)
- benztropine (Apo-Benztropine, Cogentin)
- betaxolol (Betoptic S, Kerlone)
- bisoprolol (Monocor, Zebeta)
- carteolol (Cartrol, Ocupress)
- carvedilol (Coreg)
- celiprolol
- clidinium and chlordiazepoxide (Apo-Chlorax, Librax)
- cyclopentolate (Cylate, Cyclogyl)
- dicyclomine (Bentyl, Lomine)
- esmolol (Brevibloc)
- glycopyrrolate (Robinul, Robinul Forte)
- homatropine (Isopto Homatropine)
- hyoscyamine (Hyosine, Levsin)
- hyoscyamine, atropine, scopolamine, and phenobarbital (Donnatal, Donnatal Extentabs)
- ipratropium (Atrovent, Nu-Ipratropium)
- labetalol (Normodyne, Trandate)
- levobetaxolol (Betaxon)
- levobunolol (Betagan, Novo-Levobunolol)
- metipranolol (OptiPranolol)
- metoprolol (Betaloc, Lopressor)
- nadolol (Apo-Nadol, Corgard)
- oxitropium (Oxivent, Tersigat)
- oxprenolol (Slow-Trasicor, Trasicor)
- pindolol (Apo-Pindol, Novo-Pindol)
- prifinium (Padrin, Riabel)
- procyclidine (Kemadrin, Procyclid)
- propantheline (Propanthel)
- propranolol (Inderal, InnoPran XL)
- scopolamine (Scopace, Transderm Scop)
- sotalol (Betapace, Sorine)
- timolol (Betimol, Timoptic)
- tiotropium (Spiriva)
- tolterodine (Detrol, Detrol LA)
- trihexyphenidyl (Artane)
- trimethobenzamide (Tigan)

Taking butterbur with these drugs may increase the drug's adverse effects:

- amitriptyline (Elavil, Levate)
- cyclobenzaprine (Flexeril, Novo-Cycloprine)
- desipramine (Alti-Desipramine, Norpramin)
- diphenhydramine (Benadryl Allergy, Nytol)
- doxepin (Sinequan, Zonalon)
- fluphenazine (Modecate, Prolixin)
- haloperidol (Haldol, Novo-Peridol)
- imipramine (Apo-Imipramine, Tofranil)
- loratadine (Alavert, Claritin)
- prochlorperazine (Compazine, Compro)

Lab Tests That May Be Altered by Butterbur

May cause increases in liver enzyme activity, changing the results of liver function tests (LFTs)

Diseases That May Be Worsened or Triggered by Butterbur

None known

Foods That May Interact with Butterbur

None known

Supplements That May Interact with Butterbur

Increased risk of toxicity when used with herbs and supplements containing unsaturated pyrrolizidine alkaloids (UPAs), such as comfrey and colt's foot. (For a list of herbs containing unsaturated pyrrolizidine alkaloids, see Appendix B.)

BUTTERNUT

Butternut gets its name because Native Americans took kernels from the nut of the *Juglans cinerea* tree, boiled them to extract the oil, and then used the oil like butter. The inner rind of the bark of the root is used as a gentle laxative for chronic constipation. Butternut is also used to expel, rather than kill, intestinal worms and is an old-fashioned remedy for sluggish liver, hemmorrhoids, and fevers.

Scientific Name
Juglans cinerea

Butternut Is Also Commonly Known As
Black walnut, lemon walnut, oil nut, white walnut

Medicinal Parts
Bark, root

Butternut's Uses
To treat hemorrhoids and skin and gallbladder diseases. Germany's Commission E has approved the use of butternut to treat skin inflammations and excessive perspiration of the hands and feet.

Typical Dose
There is no typical dose of butternut.

Possible Side Effects
Diarrhea and gastrointestinal irritation

Drugs That May Interact with Butternut
Taking butternut with these drugs may increase the risk of hypokalemia (low levels of potassium in the blood):

- acetazolamide (Apo-Acetazolamide, Diamox Sequels)
- azosemide (Diat)
- beclomethasone (Beconase, Vanceril)
- betamethasone (Celestone, Diprolene)
- budesonide (Entocort, Rhinocort)
- budesonide and formoterol (Symbicort)
- bumetanide (Bumex, Burinex)
- chlorothiazide (Diuril)
- chlorthalidone (Apo-Chlorthalidone, Thalitone)
- cortisone (Cortone)
- deflazacort (Calcort, Dezacor)
- dexamethasone (Decadron, Dexasone)
- ethacrynic acid (Edecrin)
- etozolin (Elkapin)
- flunisolide (AeroBid, Nasarel)
- fluorometholone (Eflone, Flarex)
- fluticasone (Cutivate, Flonase)
- furosemide (Apo-Furosemide, Lasix)
- hydrochlorothiazide (Apo-Hydro, Microzide)
- hydrocortisone (Anusol-HC, Locoid)
- hydroflumethiazide (Diucardin, Saluron)
- indapamide (Lozol, Nu-Indapamide)
- loteprednol (Alrex, Lotemax)
- mannitol (Osmitrol, Resectisol)
- medrysone (HMS Liquifilm)
- mefruside (Baycaron)
- methazolamide (Apo-Methazolamide, Neptazane)
- methyclothiazide (Aquatensen, Enduron)
- methylprednisolone (DepoMedrol, Medrol)
- metolazone (Mykrox, Zaroxolyn)
- olmesartan and hydrochlorothiazide (Benicar HCT)
- polythiazide (Renese)
- prednisolone (Inflamase Forte, Pred Forte)
- prednisone (Apo-Prednisone, Deltasone)
- rimexolone (Vexol)

- torsemide (Demadex)
- triamcinolone (Aristocort, Trinasal)
- trichlormethiazide (Metatensin, Naqua)
- urea (Amino-Cerv, UltraMide)
- xipamide (Diurexan, Lumitens)

Taking butternut with these drugs may increase the loss of electrolytes and fluids:
- cascara (cascara sagrada)
- docusate and senna (Peri-Colace, Senokot-S)

Taking butternut with these drugs may increase the adverse effects of the drug:
- digitalis (Digitek, Lanoxin)

Taking butternut with these drugs may reduce or prevent drug absorption:
- ferric gluconate (Ferrlecit)
- ferrous fumarate (Femiron, Feostat)
- ferrous gluconate (Fergon, Novo-Ferrogluc)
- ferrous sulfate (Feratab, Fer-Iron)
- ferrous sulfate and ascorbic acid (Fero-Grad 500, Vitelle Irospan)
- iron-dextran complex (Dexferrum, INFeD)
- polysaccharide-iron complex (Hytinic, Niferex)

Taking butternut with these drugs may be harmful:
- All drugs. Butternut reduces gastrointestinal transit time and may therefore reduce the absorption of some drugs.

Lab Tests That May Be Altered by Butternut
None known

Diseases That May Be Worsened or Triggered by Butternut
None known

Foods That May Interact with Butternut
None known

Supplements That May Interact with Butternut
- Increased risk of cardiac glycoside toxicity when used with other herbs that contain cardiac glycosides, such as black hellebore, calotropis, motherwort, and others. (For a list of cardiac glycoside–containing herbs and supplements, see Appendix B.)
- Increased risk of potassium depletion when used in conjunction with horsetail plant or licorice.
- Increased risk of potassium depletion when used with other stimulant laxative herbs (such as black root, cascara sagrada, castor oil, and senna). (For a list of stimulant laxative herbs and supplements, see Appendix B.)

CABBAGE

The ancient Romans used cabbage to treat cancer, colic, paralysis, wounds, and drunkenness. Today we know that cabbage, a member of the cruciferous family of vegetables, contains many health-enhancing substances, including indoles, sulforaphane, beta-carotene, vitamin C, and fiber. It may have antibacterial and antiviral properties, help reduce the risk of cancer, and even be useful in treating ulcers.

Scientific Name
Brassica oleracea

Cabbage Is Also Commonly Known As
Colewort

Medicinal Parts

Cabbage head, juice from fresh leaves

Cabbage's Uses

To treat ulcers, thyroid disorders, itching, asthma, gout, and hemorrhoids

Typical Dose

A typical dose of cabbage is approximately 1 liter of juice per day, taken for at least three weeks in conjunction with a bland diet.

Possible Side Effects

No side effects or health hazards are known when cabbage is taken in designated therapeutic dosages.

Drugs That May Interact with Cabbage

Taking cabbage with these drugs may increase drug metabolism and reduce drug levels in body:

- acetaminophen (Genapap, Tylenol)
- oxazepam (Novoxapam, Serax)
- clozapine (Clozaril, Gen-Clozapine)
- cyclobenzaprine (Flexeril, Novo-Cycloprine)
- fluvoxamine (Alti-Fluvoxamine, Luvox)
- haloperidol (Haldol, Novo-Peridol)
- imipramine (Apo-Imipramine, Tofranil)
- mexiletine (Mextil, Novo-Mexiletine)
- olanzapine (Zydis, Zyprexa)
- pentazocine (Talwin)
- propranolol (Inderal, InnoPran XL)
- tacrine (Cognex)
- theophylline (Elixophyllin, Theochron)
- zileuton (Zyflo)
- zolmitriptan (Zomig)

Taking cabbage with this drug may be harmful:

- warfarin (Coumadin, Jantoven)—cabbage may interfere with the action of the drug

Lab Tests That May Be Altered by Cabbage

May decrease the results of coagulation tests, such as international normalized ratio (INR)/ prothrombin time (PT), because of herb's high vitamin K content.

Diseases That May Be Worsened or Triggered by Cabbage

May exacerbate hypothyroidism.

Foods That May Interact with Cabbage

None known

Supplements That May Interact with Cabbage

None known

Caffeine and Caffeine-Containing Herbs*

Caffeine, although classified as a drug, is also a natural constituent of many plant parts, including cocoa beans, coffee beans, cola nuts, guarana seeds, maté leaves, and tea leaves. On the positive side, it has been found to enhance physical performance, ease certain kinds of headaches, and improve alertness, concentration, and mental stamina. On the negative side, it can contribute to insomnia, anxiety, nervousness, and the depletion of B vitamins, and may play a role in recurring depression.

Scientific Name

1,3,7-trimethylxanthine

Caffeine Is Also Commonly Known As

Anhydrous caffeine, caffeine citrate, methylxanthine

*See separate listings for black tea, cocoa, coffee, cola nut, green tea, guarana, and maté.

Caffeine's Uses

To treat headaches, attention-deficit hyperactivity disorder (ADHD), and asthma; to increase mental alertness; to reduce the risk of Parkinson's disease

Typical Dose

A typical daily dose of caffeine may range from 150 to 600 mg.

Possible Side Effects

Caffeine's side effects include insomnia, restlessness, nervousness, gastric irritation, vomiting, and increased urination (diuresis).

Drugs That May Interact with Caffeine

Taking caffeine with these drugs may have an unpredictable effect on blood sugar levels:

- acarbose (Prandase, Precose)
- acetohexamide
- chlorpropamide (Diabinese, Novo-Propamide)
- gliclazide (Diamicron, Novo-Gliclazide)
- glimepiride (Amaryl)
- glipizide (Glucotrol)
- glipizide and metformin (Metaglip)
- gliquidone (Beglynor, Glurenorm)
- glyburide (DiaBeta, Micronase)
- glyburide and metformin (Glucovance)
- insulin (Humulin, Novolin R)
- metformin (Glucophage, Riomet)
- miglitol (Glyset)
- nateglinide (Starlix)
- pioglitazone (Actos)
- repaglinide (GlucoNorm, Prandin)
- rosiglitazone (Avandia)
- rosiglitazone and metformin (Avandamet)
- tolazamide (Tolinase)
- tolbutamide (Apo-Tolbutamide, Tol-Tab)

Taking caffeine with these drugs may increase the risk of side effects due to a buildup of caffeine in the body:

- cimetidine (Nu-Cimet, Tagamet)
- cinoxacin (Cinobac)
- ciprofloxacin (Ciloxan, Cipro)
- disulfiram (Antabuse)
- ephedrine (Pretz-D)
- ergotamine (Cafergor, Cafergot)
- estrogens (conjugated A/synthetic) (Cenestin)
- estrogens (conjugated/equine) (Congest, Premarin)
- estrogens (conjugated/equine) and medroxyprogesterone (Premphase, Prempro)
- estrogens (esterified) (Estratab, Menest)
- estrogens (esterified) and methyltestosterone (Estratest, Estratest H.S.)
- ethinyl estradiol and desogestrel (Cyclessa, Ortho-Cept)
- ethinyl estradiol and ethynodiol diacetate (Demulen, Zovia)
- ethinyl estradiol and etonogestrel (NuvaRing)
- ethinyl estradiol and levonorgestrel (Alesse, Triphasil)
- ethinyl estradiol and norelgestromin (Evra, Ortho Evra)
- ethinyl estradiol and norethindrone (Brevicon, Ortho-Novum)
- ethinyl estradiol and norgestimate (Cyclen, Ortho Tri-Cyclen)
- ethinyl estradiol and norgestrel (Cryselle, Ovral)
- fluconazole (Apo-Fluconazole, Diflucan)
- fluvoxamine (Alti-Fluvoxamine, Luvox)
- gatifloxacin (Tequin, Zymar)
- gemifloxacin (Factive)
- levofloxacin (Levaquin, Quixin)
- lomefloxacin (Maxaquin)
- mestranol and norethindrone (Necon 1/50, Ortho-Novum 1/50)

- mexiletine (Mextil, Novo-Mexiletine)
- moxifloxacin (Avelox, Vigamox)
- nalidixic acid (NegGram)
- norfloxacin (Apo-Norflox, Noroxin)
- ofloxacin (Floxin, Ocuflox)
- pefloxacin (Peflacine, Perflox)
- riluzole (Rilutek)
- sparfloxacin (Zagam)
- terbinafine (Lamisil, Lamisil AT)
- trovafloxacin
- verapamil (Calan, Isoptin SR)

Taking large amounts of caffeine with these drugs may increase the risk of hypertension (high blood pressure):

- ephedrine (Pretz-D)
- iproniazid (Marsilid)
- moclobemide (Alti-Moclobemide, Nu-Moclobemide)
- phenelzine (Nardil)
- selegiline (Eldepryl)
- tranylcypromine (Parnate)

Taking caffeine with these drugs may increase central nervous system stimulation:

- albuterol (Proventil, Ventolin)
- clobenzorex (Asenlix)
- diethylpropion (Tenuate)
- epinephrine (Adrenalin, EpiPen)
- fenoterol (Berotec)
- modafinil (Alertec, Provigil)
- phentermine (Adipex-P, Ionamin)
- pseudoephedrine (Dimetapp Decongestant, Sudafed)

Taking caffeine with these drugs may cause or increase gastrointestinal irritation:

- celecoxib (Celebrex)
- ibuprofen (Advil, Motrin)
- indomethacin (Indocin, Novo-Methacin)
- ketoprofen (Orudis, Rhodis)
- ketorolac (Acular, Toradol)
- naproxen (Aleve, Naprosyn)
- piroxicam (Feldene, Nu-Pirox)
- rofecoxib (Vioxx)

Taking caffeine with these drugs may be harmful:

- alendronate (Fosamax, Novo-Alendronate)—may reduce drug effectiveness
- clozapine (Clozaril, Gen-Clozapine)—may cause increased psychotic symptoms
- dipyridamole (Novo-Dipiradol, Persantine)—may reduce drug effectiveness
- ergotamine (Cafergor, Cafergot)—may increase drug absorption
- etodolac (Lodine, Utradol)—may increase risk of liver damage
- lithium (Carbolith, Eskalith)—may cause drug levels in the body to rise, heightening "lithium tremor," when high amounts of caffeine are taken over time and suddenly stopped
- riluzole (Rilutek)—increases risk of drug side effects
- selegiline (Eldepryl)—may increase risk of arrhythmia (irregular heartbeat)
- theophylline (Elixophyllin, Theochron)—may increase toxic effects of the drug

Lab Tests That May Be Altered by Caffeine
- May increase urine 5-hydroxyindoleacetic acid concentrations.
- May increase urine catecholamine concentrations.
- May increase bleeding time due to antiplatelet activity.

- May increase plasma catecholamine levels.
- May increase urine creatine levels.
- May alter test results with dipyridamole thallium imaging studies.
- May increase or decrease blood glucose levels.
- May increase blood lactate levels when combined with ephedrine (a constituent of ma-huang).
- May cause a false positive diagnosis of neuroblastoma, when diagnosis is based on tests of urine vanillylmandelic acid (VMA) or catecholamine concentrations, because caffeine can increase both of these.
- May cause a false positive diagnosis of pheochromocytoma, when diagnosis is based on tests of urine vanillylmandelic acid (VMA) or catecholamine concentrations, because caffeine can increase both of these.
- May alter results of pulmonary function tests, including forced expiratory volume at one minute (FEV1) and midexpiratory flow rates.
- May increase serum urate test results determined by the Bittner method.
- May increase urinary calcium levels.
- May increase urine vanillylmandelic acid (VMA) concentrations.
- May increase two-hour postprandial glucose test if caffeine is ingested during test.

Diseases That May Be Worsened or Triggered by Caffeine

- May worsen anxiety disorders.
- May worsen bleeding disorders.
- May trigger irregular heartbeat.
- May worsen gastroesophageal reflux disease (GERD), irritable bowel syndrome, and ulcers.
- May contribute to insulin resistance and raise blood sugar following a meal.

- May play a role in glaucoma by increasing the intraocular pressure ("eye pressure").
- May raise blood pressure in those with hypertension.
- May contribute to osteoporosis by encouraging the body to excrete calcium.

Foods That May Interact with Caffeine

None known

Supplements That May Interact with Caffeine

- May increase therapeutic and adverse effects of caffeine when taken with herbs and supplements containing caffeine, such as cola nut, guarana, and maté. (For a list of caffeine-containing herbs, foods, and supplements, see Appendix B.)
- May increase urinary calcium excretion.
- Increased risk of serious life-threatening or debilitating effects, such as low blood pressure (hypotension), heart attack (myocardial infarction), stroke, seizures, and death when used with ma-huang.
- Increased risk of ischemic stroke when combined with ma-huang and creatine.
- Possible decreased beneficial effects of creatine on athletic performance due to inhibition of phosphocreatine resynthesis.

CALABAR BEAN

This very poisonous plant, native to Africa, earned the name "ordeal bean" when natives forced prisoners accused of witchcraft to eat its seeds. If the prisoner vomited within half an hour, he was considered innocent; if he died, he was found guilty. Used primarily to treat glaucoma, calabar bean contains physostigmine, which relieves pressure within the eyeball.

Scientific Name
Physostigma venenosum

Calabar Bean Is Also Commonly Known As
Chop nut, ordeal bean

Medicinal Parts
Seed

Calabar Bean's Uses
To treat glaucoma; to stimulate the peristaltic movements that move food through the digestive tract; as an antidote to poison

Typical Dose
A typical dose of calabar bean in the form of physostigmine eye drops may range from 1 to 2 drops taken three times daily.

Possible Side Effects
❶ Calabar bean is very poisonous, and can even be poisonous as eye drops when they are inappropriately administered. Symptoms of poisoning may include nausea, diarrhea, vomiting, salivation, exhaustion, chills, dizziness, and muscle paralysis.

Drugs That May Interact with Calabar Bean
Taking calabar bean with these drugs may interfere with the action of the drug:
- atropine (Isopto Atropine, Sal-Tropine)
- benztropine (Apo-Benztropine, Cogentin)
- clidinium and chlordiazepoxide (Apo-Chlorax, Librax)
- cyclopentolate (Cyclogyl, Cylate)
- dicyclomine (Bentyl, Lomine)
- glycopyrrolate (Robinul, Robinul Forte)
- homatropine (Isopto Homatropine)
- hyoscyamine (Hyosine, Levsin)
- hyoscyamine, atropine, scopolamine, and phenobarbital (Donnatal, Donnatal Extentabs)
- ipratropium (Atrovent, Nu-Ipratropium)
- oxitropium (Oxivent, Tersigat)
- prifinium (Padrin, Riabel)
- procyclidine (Kemadrin, Procyclid)
- propantheline (Propanthel)
- scopolamine (Scopace, Transderm Scop)
- tiotropium (Spiriva)
- tolterodine (Detrol, Detrol LA)
- trihexyphenidyl (Artane)
- trimethobenzamide (Tigan)

Lab Tests That May Be Altered by Calabar Bean
None known

Diseases That May Be Worsened or Triggered by Calabar Bean
May exacerbate or interfere with the treatment of asthma, diabetes, cardiovascular disease, Parkinson's disease, gangrene, slow heart rate, and intestinal obstructions.

Foods That May Interact with Calabar Bean
None known

Supplements That May Interact with Calabar Bean
None known

CALAMUS

Calamus is a tall, reedy wetland plant whose long, scented aromatic rhizomes are used for medicinal purposes and as a psychotropic drug. It has been said that 5 cm of dried calamus rhizome, either chewed or chopped and prepared as tea, is "stimulating and evokes a cheerful mood," while 25 cm can lead to hallucinations. Calamus is also reputed to be an aphrodisiac, especially when added to bathwater.

Scientific Name
Acorus calamus

Calamus Is Also Commonly Known As
Cinnamon sedge, myrtle flag, sweet cane, sweet flag, sweet myrtle

Medicinal Parts
Rhizome

Calamus's Uses
To treat ulcers, rheumatism, toothache, pain syndrome, gastrointestinal disorders, gum disease, tonsillitis, and fungal infections

Typical Dose
There is no typical dose of calamus.

Possible Side Effects
No side effects or health hazards are known when calamus is taken in designated therapeutic dosages. However, rats receiving calamus oil over an extended period of time developed malignant tumors; therefore, long-term use of calamus should probably be avoided.

Drugs That May Interact with Calamus
Taking calamus with these drugs may interfere with the action of the drug:
- aluminum hydroxide (AlternaGel, Alu-Cap)
- aluminum hydroxide and magnesium carbonate (Gaviscon Extra Strength, Gaviscon Liquid)
- aluminum hydroxide and magnesium hydroxide (Maalox, Rulox)
- aluminum hydroxide and magnesium trisilicate (Gaviscon Tablet)
- aluminum hydroxide, magnesium hydroxide, and simethicone (Maalox, Mylanta Liquid)
- calcium carbonate (Rolaids Extra Strength, Tums)
- calcium carbonate and magnesium hydroxide (Mylanta Gelcaps, Rolaids Extra Strength)
- cimetidine (Nu-Cimet, Tagamet)
- esomeprazole (Nexium)
- famotidine (Apo-Famotidine, Pepcid)
- famotidine, calcium carbonate, and magnesium hydroxide (Pepcid Complete)
- lansoprazole (Prevacid)
- magaldrate and simethicone (Riopan Plus, Riopan Plus Double Strength)
- magnesium hydroxide (Dulcolax Milk of Magnesia, Phillips' Milk of Magnesia)
- magnesium oxide (Mag-Ox 400, Uro-Mag)
- magnesium sulfate (Epsom salts)
- nizatidine (Axid, PMS-Nizatidine)
- omeprazole (Losec, Prilosec)
- pantoprazole (Pantoloc, Protonix)
- rabeprazole (Aciphex, Pariet)
- ranitidine (Alti-Ranitidine, Zantac)
- sodium bicarbonate (Brioschi, Neut)

Taking calamus with these drugs may increase the drug's therapeutic and adverse effects:
- iproniazid (Marsilid)
- moclobemide (Alti-Moclobemide, Nu-Moclobemide)
- phenelzine (Nardil)
- selegiline (Eldepryl)
- tranylcypromine (Parnate)

Lab Tests That May Be Altered by Calamus
None known

Diseases That May Be Worsened or Triggered by Calamus

None known

Foods That May Interact with Calamus

None known

Supplements That May Interact with Calamus

May enhance therapeutic and adverse effects of herbs and supplements that have sedative properties, such as 5-HTP, kava kava, St. John's wort, and valerian. (For a list of herbs and supplements that have sedative properties, see Appendix B.)

CALCIUM

> Besides its well-known prowess as the mineral that builds strong bones, calcium assists in wound healing, blood clotting, cellular metabolism, and muscle contraction. Taking in too little dietary calcium can cause spastic muscle contractions and a thinning of the bones that leads to osteoporosis.

Calcium's Uses

Calcium, most of which resides in your bones, has many duties in the body, including helping to control blood pressure, promote blood clotting and wound healing, induce muscle contraction and relaxation, send signals through the nervous system, and keep the heart beating properly.

Typical Dose

The Food and Nutrition Board has set the Adequate Intake (AI) for calcium at 1,000 mg per day for men and women ages nineteen to fifty and 1,200 per day for men and women fifty-one years old and up.

Possible Side Effects

Excessive amounts of calcium can cause kidney damage.

Drugs That May Interact with Calcium

Taking calcium with these drugs may interfere with the action of the drug:

- amlodipine (Norvasc)
- aspirin (Bufferin, Ecotrin)
- aspirin and codeine (Coryphen Codeine)
- aspirin and dipyridamole (Aggrenox)
- bepridil (Vascor)
- bismuth subcitrate (DE-NOL)
- cefpodoxime (Vantin)
- cinoxacin (Cinobac)
- ciprofloxacin (Ciloxan, Cipro)
- demeclocycline (Declomycin)
- diltiazem (Cardizem, Tiazac)
- doxycycline (Apo-Doxy, Vibramycin)
- felodipine (Plendil, Renedil)
- gatifloxacin (Tequin, Zymar)
- gemifloxacin (Factive)
- isradipine (DynaCirc)
- itraconazole (Sporanox)
- ketoconazole (Apo-Ketoconazole, Nizoral)
- lacidipine (Aponil, Caldine)
- lercanidipine (Cardiovasc, Carmen)
- levofloxacin (Levaquin, Quixin)
- lomefloxacin (Maxaquin)
- manidipine (Calslot, Iperten)
- minocycline (Dynacin, Minocin)
- moxifloxacin (Avelox, Vigamox)
- nalidixic acid (NegGram)
- nicardipine (Cardene)
- nifedipine (Adalat CC, Procardia)

- nilvadipine
- nimodipine (Nimotop)
- nisoldipine (Sular)
- nitrendipine
- norfloxacin (Apo-Norflox, Noroxin)
- ofloxacin (Floxin, Ocuflox)
- oxytetracycline (Terramycin, Terramycin IM)
- pefloxacin (Peflacine, Perflox)
- pinaverium (Dicetel)
- sparfloxacin (Zagam)
- sucralfate (Carafate, Sulcrate)
- tetracycline (Novo-Tetra, Sumycin)
- ticlopidine (Alti-Ticlopidine, Ticlid)
- trovafloxacin
- verapamil (Calan, Isoptin SR)

Taking calcium with these drugs may reduce or prevent absorption of the drug:
- alendronate (Fosamax, Novo-Alendronate)
- atenolol (Apo-Atenol, Tenormin)
- clodronate (Bonefos, Ostac)
- etidronate (Didronel)
- hyoscyamine (Hyosine, Levsin)
- ibandronic acid (Bondronat)
- levothyroxine (Levothroid, Synthroid)
- methscopolamine (an ingredient in AH-Chew, Extendryl)
- pamidronate (Aredia)
- risedronate (Actonel)
- sulfasalazine (Azulfidine, Azulfidine EN-tabs)
- tiludronate (Skelid)
- zoledronic acid (Zometa)

Taking calcium with these drugs may cause elevated calcium levels, possibly leading to kidney damage and other problems:
- chlorothiazide (Diuril)
- hydrochlorothiazide (Apo-Hydro, Microzide)

- hydrochlorothiazide and triamterene (Dyazide, Maxzide)
- hydroflumethiazide (Diucardin, Saluron)
- methyclothiazide (Aquatensen, Enduron)
- olmesartan and hydrochlorothiazide (Benicar HCT)
- polythiazide (Renese)
- trichlormethiazide (Metatensin, Naqua)
- xipamide (Diurexan, Lumitens)

Taking calcium with these drugs may increase calcium absorption in postmenopausal women:
- cyproterone and ethinyl estradiol (Diane-35)
- estradiol (Climara, Estrace)
- estradiol and norethindrone (Activella, CombiPatch)
- estradiol and testosterone (Climacteron)
- estrogens (conjugated A/synthetic) (Cenestin)
- estrogens (conjugated/equine) (Congest, Premarin)
- estrogens (conjugated/equine) and medroxy-progesterone (Premprase, Prempro)
- estrogens (esterified) (Estratab, Menest)
- estrogens (esterified) and methyltestosterone (Estratest, Estratest H.S.)
- estropipate (Ogen, Ortho-Est)
- ethinyl estradiol (Estinyl)
- ethinyl estradiol and desogestrel (Cyclessa, Ortho-Cept)
- ethinyl estradiol and ethynodiol diacetate (Demulen, Zovia)
- ethinyl estradiol and etonogestrel (NuvaRing)
- ethinyl estradiol and levonorgestrel (Alesse, Triphasil)
- ethinyl estradiol and norelgestromin (Evra, Ortho Evra)
- ethinyl estradiol and norethindrone (Brevicon, Ortho-Novum)

- ethinyl estradiol and norgestimate (Cyclen, Ortho Tri-Cyclen)
- ethinyl estradiol and norgestrel (Cryselle, Ovral)
- mestranol and norethindrone (Necon 1/50, Ortho-Novum 1/50)
- polyestradiol

Taking calcium with these drugs may be harmful:
- digitalis (Digitek, Lanoxin)—taking calcium and digitalis simultaneously can lead to increased digitalis levels
- gentamicin (Alcomicin, Gentacidin)—increases the risk of kidney failure

Drugs That May Interfere with the Absorption, Utilization, or Excretion of Calcium

- alendronate (Fosamax, Novo-Alendronate)
- aluminum hydroxide (AlternaGel, Alu-Cap)
- aluminum hydroxide and magnesium carbonate (Gaviscon Liquid)
- aluminum hydroxide and magnesium hydroxide (Maalox, Mylanta)
- aluminum hydroxide and magnesium hydroxide and simethicone (Mylanta Liquid)
- aluminum hydroxide and magnesium trisilicate (Gaviscon Tablet)
- amifostine (Ethyol)
- amikacin (Amikin)
- amiloride (Midamor)
- amphotericin B (Amphocin, Fungizone)
- arsenic trioxide (Trisenox)
- basiliximab (Simulect)
- beclomethasone (Beconase, Vanceril)
- betamethasone (Betatrex, Maxivate)
- bisacodyl (Carter's Little Pills, Dulcolax)
- budesonide (Entocort, Rhinocort)
- bumetanide (Bumex, Burinex)
- butabarbital (Butisol Sodium)
- butalbital and acetaminophen and caffeine (Esgic, Fioricet)
- butalbital and aspirin and caffeine (Fiorinal)
- carbamazepine (Carbatrol, Tegretol)
- carboplatin (Paraplatin, Paraplatin-AQ)
- cascara (cascara sagrada)
- cholestyramine (Prevalite, Questran)
- cidofovir (Vistide)
- cimetidine (Nu-Cimet, Tagamet)
- cisplatin (Platinol, Platinol-AQ)
- colchicine (ratio-Colchicine)
- colestipol (Colestid)
- cortisone (Cortone)
- dactinomycin (Cosmegen)
- deferoxamine (Desferal)
- demeclocycline (Declomycin)
- denileukin diftitox (Ontak)
- dexamethasone (Decadron, Dexasone)
- diflorasone (Florone, Maxiflor)
- digitalis (Digitek, Lanoxin)
- doxycycline (Apo-Doxy, Vibramycin)
- ethacrynic acid (Edecrin)
- ethosuximide (Zarontin)
- etidronate (Didronel)
- famotidine (Apo-Famotidine, Pepcid)
- flucytosine (Ancobon)
- flunisolide (AeroBid-M, Nasarel)
- fluticasone (Cutivate, Flonase)
- foscarnet (Foscavir)
- fosphenytoin (Cerebyx)
- frovatriptan (Frova)
- furosemide (Apo-Furosemide, Lasix)
- gentamicin (Alcomicin, Gentacidin)
- halobetasol (Ultravate)
- heparin (Hepalean, Hep-Lock)
- hydrochlorothiazide (Apo-Hydro, Microzide)

- hydrochlorothiazide and triamterene (Dyazide, Maxzide)
- hydrocortisone (Cetacort, Locoid)
- interferon Alfa-2a (Roferon-A)
- interferon Alfa-2b (Intron A)
- isoniazid (Laniazid Oral, PMS-Isoniazid)
- kanamycin (Kantrex)
- magnesium hydroxide (Dulcolax Milk of Magnesia, Phillips' Milk of Magnesia)
- magnesium oxide (Mag-Ox 400, Uro-Mag)
- magnesium sulfate (Epsom salts)
- meclocycline (Meclan Topical)
- methotrexate (Folex PFS, Rheumatrex)
- methsuximide (Celontin)
- methylprednisolone (Depoject Injection, Medrol Oral)
- mineral oil (Fleet Mineral Oil Enema, Milkinol)
- minocycline (Dynacin, Minocin)
- mometasone furoate (Elocom, Nasonex)
- mycophenolate (CellCept)
- neomycin (Myciguent, Neo-Fradin)
- nizatidine (Apo-Nizatidine, Axid)
- oxcarbazepine (Trileptal)
- pamidronate (Aredia)
- pentamidine (NebuPent, Pentacarinat)
- phenobarbital (Luminal Sodium, PMS-Pheno-barbital)
- phenytoin (Dilantin, Phenytek)
- plicamycin (Mithracin)
- potassium and sodium phosphate (K-Phos Neutral, Uro-KP-Neutral)
- prednisolone (Inflamase Forte, Pred Forte)
- prednisone (Apo-Prednisone, Deltasone)
- primidone (Mysoline, Sertan)
- ranitidine (Alti-Ranitidine, Zantac)
- rifampin (Rifadin, Rimactane)
- rifampin and isoniazid (Rifamate)
- sodium bicarbonate (Brioschi, Neut)
- sodium phosphate (Fleet Enema, Fleet Phospho-Soda)
- sodium polystyrene sulfonate (Kayexalate)
- streptomycin
- sucralfate (Carafate, Sulcrate)
- tacrolimus (Prograf, Protopic)
- tetracycline (Novo-Tetra, Sumycin)
- tiludronate (Skelid)
- tobramycin (Nebcin, Tobrex)
- torsemide (Demadex)
- trandolapril (Mavik)
- trandolapril and verapamil (Tarka)
- triamcinolone (Aristocort, Trinasal)
- triamterene (Dyrenium)
- zalcitabine (Hivid)
- zoledronic acid (Zometa)
- zonisamide (Zonegran)

Lab Tests That May Be Altered by Calcium

- Increased plasma 11-hydroxycorticosteroid concentrations when calcium gluconate is given intravenously.
- Decreased urinary 17-hyrdroxycorticosteroid concentrations due to ingestion of calcium gluconate.
- Decreased rate of bone mineral loss as reflected in bone mineral density (BMD) tests due to ingestion of supplemental calcium.
- Increased serum gastrin concentrations within thirty to seventy-five minutes due to ingestion of calcium carbonate.
- Decreased serum glucose concentrations in newborns due to calcium gluconate.
- Decreased serum uptake of I-131 due to calcium gluconate.

- Decreased test results when measuring serum lipase concentrations greater than 5 mmol/l using the Teitz method.
- Decreased test results for serum magnesium and urine magnesium when measured by titan yellow, due to calcium gluconate.

Diseases That May Be Worsened or Triggered by Calcium

- May increase problems associated with hyperphosphatemia or hypophosphatemia (elevated or lowered phosphate levels in the blood).
- Calcium in the form of calcium carbonate (for example, Tums) may reduce effectiveness of the drug levothyroxine used for underactive thyroid gland (hypothyroidism).
- May trigger elevated levels of calcium in those with the chronic disease called sarcoidosis.

Foods That May Interact with Calcium

- Increased urinary calcium excretion when caffeine intake is high.
- Increased urinary calcium excretion when sodium intake is high.
- Decreased absorption of calcium when ingested with certain constituents of dietary fiber, such as oxalic acid, phytic acid, and uronic acid.
- Calcium supplements may decrease absorption of dietary iron, magnesium, and zinc.

Supplements That May Interact with Calcium

Increased active absorption of calcium in the small intestine when taken with vitamin D

CALIFORNIA POPPY

The beautiful bright-orange California poppy was prized by California Indians as a source of both food and oil. They also used its mildly narcotic juice to treat toothaches. A sedative, hypnotic, and antispasmodic, California poppy has a reputation for being a less powerful, nonaddictive alternative to opium poppy.

Scientific Name

Eschscholtzia californica

California Poppy Is Also Commonly Known As

Poppy California

Medicinal Parts

Leaf, stem, flower

California Poppy's Uses

To treat insomnia, nervous agitation, bedwetting in children, depression, and mood swings

Typical Dose

A typical dose of California poppy is approximately 2 gm of the herb mixed with 150 ml of boiling water, taken as a tea up to four times daily. A single dose of the liquid extract ranges from 1 to 2 ml.

Possible Side Effects

No side effects have been recorded when California poppy is taken in recommended therapeutic doses.

Drugs That May Interact with California Poppy

Taking California poppy with these drugs may increase the drug's therapeutic and adverse effects:

- acetaminophen and codeine (Capital and Codeine, Tylenol with Codeine)
- alfentanil (Alfenta)
- alprazolam (Apo-Alpraz, Xanax)
- amobarbital (Amytal)
- amobarbital and secobarbital (Tuinal)
- aspirin and codeine (Coryphen Codeine)
- belladonna and opium (B&O Supprettes)
- bromazepam (Apo-Bromazepam, Gen-Bromazepam)
- brotizolam (Lendorm, Sintonal)
- buprenorphine (Buprenex, Subutex)
- buprenorphine and naloxone (Suboxone)
- butabarbital (Butisol Sodium)
- butalbital, acetaminophen, and caffeine (Esgic, Fioricet)
- butalbital, aspirin, and caffeine (Fiorinal)
- butorphanol (Apo-Butorphanol, Stadol)
- chloral hydrate (Aquachloral Supprettes, Somnote)
- chlordiazepoxide (Apo-Chlordiazepoxide, Librium)
- clobazam (Alti-Clobazam, Frisium)
- clonazepam (Klonopin, Rivotril)
- clorazepate (Tranxene, T-Tab)
- codeine (Codeine Contin)
- dexmedetomidine (Precedex)
- diazepam (Apo-Diazepam, Valium)
- dihydrocodeine, aspirin, and caffeine (Synalgos-DC)
- diphenhydramine (Benadryl Allergy, Nytol)
- estazolam (ProSom)
- fentanyl (Actiq, Duragesic)
- flurazepam (Apo-Flurazepam, Dalmane)
- glutethimide
- haloperidol (Haldol, Novo-Peridol)
- hydrocodone and acetaminophen (Vicodin, Zydone)
- hydrocodone and aspirin (Damason-P)
- hydrocodone and ibuprofen (Vicoprofen)
- hydromorphone (Dilaudid, PMS-Hydromorphone)
- hydroxyzine (Atarax, Vistaril)
- levomethadyl acetate hydrochloride
- levorphanol (LevoDromoran)
- loprazolam (Dormonoct, Havlane)
- lorazepam (Ativan, Nu-Loraz)
- meperidine (Demerol, Meperitab)
- meperidine and promethazine
- mephobarbital (Mebaral)
- methadone (Dolophine, Methadose)
- methohexital (Brevital, Brevital Sodium)
- midazolam (Apo-Midazolam, Versed)
- morphine sulfate (Kadian, MS Contin)
- nalbuphine (Nubain)
- opium tincture
- oxycodone (OxyContin, Roxicodone)
- oxycodone and acetaminophen (Endocet, Percocet)
- oxycodone and aspirin (Endodan, Percodan)
- oxymorphone (Numorphan)
- paregoric
- pentazocine (Talwin)
- pentobarbital (Nembutal)
- phenobarbital (Luminal Sodium, PMS-Phenobarbital)
- phenoperidine
- prazepam
- primidone (Apo-Primidone, Mysoline)
- promethazine (Phenergan)
- propofol (Diprivan)
- propoxyphene (Darvon, DarvonN)
- propoxyphene and acetaminophen (Darvocet-N 50, Darvocet-N 100)
- propoxyphene, aspirin, and caffeine (Darvon Compound)
- quazepam (Doral)
- remifentanil (Ultiva)

- secobarbital (Seconal)
- sodium oxybate (Xyrem)
- sufentanil (Sufenta)
- temazepam (Novo-Temazepam, Restoril)
- tetrazepam (Mobiforton, Musapam)
- thiopental (Pentothal)
- triazolam (Apo-Triazo, Halcion)
- zaleplon (Sonata, Stamoc)
- zolpidem (Ambien)
- zopiclone (Alti-Zopiclone, Gen-Zopiclone)

Lab Tests That May Be Altered by California Poppy
None known

Diseases That May Be Worsened or Triggered by California Poppy
None known

Foods That May Interact with California Poppy
Increased risk of drowsiness and impaired motor skills when combined with alcohol.

Supplements That May Interact with California Poppy
May enhance therapeutic and adverse effects of herbs and supplements that have sedative properties, such as 5-HTP, kava kava, St. John's wort, and valerian. (For a list of herbs and supplements that have sedative properties, see Appendix B.)

CALOTROPIS

This giant milkweed species grows in tropical regions of Asia, Africa, and India. It produces a milk-like liquid used in traditional Indian medicine to treat skin diseases, rheumatism, and aches. When taken orally, calotropis reportedly has potent anti-inflammatory, antifever, and antipain effects, although it can also be quite toxic.

Scientific Name
Calotropis procera

Calotropis Is Also Commonly Known As
Mudar bark, mudar yercum

Medicinal Parts
Root, root bark

Calotropis's Uses
To treat dysentery, cancer, leprosy, worms, fever, epilepsy, and snakebite

Typical Dose
A typical dose of calotropis may range from 200 to 600 mg.

Possible Side Effects
Calotropis contains cardiac glycosides, which can help control irregular heartbeat, reduce the backup of blood and fluid in the body, and increase blood flow through the kidneys, helping to excrete sodium and relieve swelling in body tissues. However, a buildup of cardiac glycosides can occur, especially when the herb is combined with certain medications or other herbs that contain cardiac glycosides, causing arrhythmias, abnormally slow heartbeat, heart failure, and even death.

Drugs That May Interact with Calotropis
Taking calotropis with these drugs may increase the toxic effects of the drug:

- acetazolamide (Apo-Acetazolamide, Diamox Sequels)
- azosemide (Diat)
- bumetanide (Bumex, Burinex)
- cascara (cascara sagrada)
- chlorothiazide (Diuril)
- chlorthalidone (Apo-Chlorthalidone, Thalitone)
- digitalis (Digitek, Lanoxin)
- docusate and senna (Peri-Colace, Senokot-S)
- ethacrynic acid (Edecrin)
- etozolin (Elkapin)
- furosemide (Apo-Furosemide, Lasix)
- hydrochlorothiazide (Apo-Hydro, Microzide)
- hydroflumethiazide (Diucardin, Saluron)
- indapamide (Lozol, Nu-Indapamide)
- mannitol (Osmitrol, Resectisol)
- mefruside (Baycaron)
- methazolamide (Apo-Methazolamide, Neptazane)
- methyclothiazide (Aquatensen, Enduron)
- metolazone (Mykrox, Zaroxolyn)
- olmesartan and hydrochlorothiazide (Benicar HCT)
- polythiazide (Renese)
- torsemide (Demadex)
- trichlormethiazide (Metatensin, Naqua)
- urea (Amino-Cerv, UltraMide)
- xipamide (Diurexan, Lumitens)

Lab Tests That May Be Altered by Calotropis
None known

Diseases That May Be Worsened or Triggered by Calotropis
None known

Foods That May Interact with Calotropis
None known

Supplements That May Interact with Calotropis

- Increased risk of cardiac glycoside toxicity when used with other herbs that contain cardiac glycosides, such as black hellebore, motherwort, and others. (For a list of cardiac glycoside–containing herbs and supplements, see Appendix B.)
- Increased risk of cardiotoxicity due to potassium depletion when taken with cardioactive herbs, such as adonis, digitalis, lily-of-the-valley, and squill. (For a list of cardioactive herbs and supplements, see Appendix B.)
- Increased risk of potassium depletion when used in conjunction with horsetail plant or licorice.
- Increased risk of potassium depletion when used with other stimulant laxative herbs, such as black root, cascara sagrada, castor oil, and senna. (For a list of stimulant laxative herbs and supplements, see Appendix B.)

CARRAGEEN

Also known as Irish moss, carrageen is an edible North Atlantic seaweed that produces a moist, sticky substance used medicinally and in the preparation of jellies and puddings. Carrageen, which contains iodine, calcium, magnesium, sodium, and potassium, as well as various antiviral and antimicrobial agents, has long been a favorite of the Irish and the Scots as a treatment for colds, flu, and other respiratory ailments.

Scientific Name
Chondrus crispus

Carrageen Is Also Commonly Known As
Carrageenan, chondrus, Irish moss

Medicinal Parts
Thallus

Carrageen's Uses
To treat constipation, diarrhea, colds, flu, and symptoms of bronchitis and tuberculosis

Typical Dose
There is no typical dose of carrageen.

Possible Side Effects
Carrageen's side effects include lowered blood pressure, nausea, and abdominal pain.

Drugs That May Interact with Carrageen
Taking carrageen with these drugs may reduce absorption of the drug:
- all drugs taken orally

Taking carrageen with these drugs may increase the risk of bleeding or bruising:
- abciximab (ReoPro)
- antithrombin III (Thrombate III)
- argatroban
- aspirin (Bufferin, Ecotrin)
- aspirin and dipyridamole (Aggrenox)
- bivalirudin (Angiomax)
- clopidogrel (Plavix)
- dalteparin (Fragmin)
- danaparoid (Orgaran)
- dipyridamole (Novo-Dipiradol, Persantine)
- enoxaparin (Lovenox)
- eptifibatide (Integrillin)
- fondaparinux (Arixtra)
- heparin (Hepalean, Hep-Lock)
- indobufen (Ibustrin)
- lepirudin (Refludan)
- ticlopidine (Alti-Ticlopidine, Ticlid)
- tinzaparin (Innohep)
- tirofiban (Aggrastat)
- warfarin (Coumadin, Jantoven)

Taking carrageen with these drugs may increase drug effects:
- acebutolol (Novo-Acebutolol, Sectral)
- amlodipine (Norvasc)
- atenolol (Apo-Atenol, Tenormin)
- benazepril (Lotensin)
- betaxolol (Betoptic S, Kerlone)
- bisoprolol (Monocor, Zebeta)
- bumetanide (Bumex, Burinex)
- candesartan (Atacand)
- captopril (Capoten, Novo-Captopril)
- carteolol (Cartrol, Ocupress)
- carvedilol (Coreg)
- chlorothiazide (Diuril)
- chlorthalidone (Apo-Chlorthalidone, Thalitone)
- clonidine (Catapres, Duraclon)
- diazoxide (Hyperstat, Proglycem)
- diltiazem (Cardizem, Tiazac)
- doxazosin (Alti-Doxazosin, Cardura)
- enalapril (Vasotec)
- eplerenone (Inspra)
- eprosartan (Teveten)
- esmolol (Brevibloc)
- felodipine (Plendil, Renedil)
- fenoldopam (Corlopam)
- fosinopril (Monopril)
- furosemide (Apo-Furosemide, Lasix)
- guanabenz (Wytensin)
- guanadrel (Hylorel)
- guanfacine (Tenex)
- hydralazine (Apresoline, Novo-Hylazin)
- hydrochlorothiazide (Apo-Hydro, Microzide)
- hydrochlorothiazide and triamterene (Dyazide, Maxzide)

- indapamide (Lozol, Nu-Indapamide)
- irbesartan (Avapro)
- isradipine (DynaCirc)
- labetalol (Normodyne, Trandate)
- lisinopril (Prinivil, Zestril)
- losartan (Cozaar)
- mecamylamine (Inversine)
- mefruside (Baycaron)
- methyclothiazide (Aquatensen, Enduron)
- methyldopa (Apo-Methyldopa, Nu-Medopa)
- metolazone (Mykrox, Zaroxolyn)
- metoprolol (Betaloc, Lopressor)
- minoxidil (Loniten, Rogaine)
- moexipril (Univasc)
- nadolol (Apo-Nadol, Corgard)
- nicardipine (Cardene)
- nifedipine (Adalat CC, Procardia)
- nisoldipine (Sular)
- nitroglycerin (Minitran, Nitro-Dur)
- nitroprusside (Nipride, Nitropress)
- olmesartan (Benicar)
- oxprenolol (Slow-Trasicor, Trasicor)
- perindopril erbumine (Aceon, Coversyl)
- phenoxybenzamine (Dibenzyline)
- phentolamine (Regitine, Rogitine)
- pindolol (Apo-Pindol, Novo-Pindol)
- polythiazide (Renese)
- prazosin (Minipress, Nu-Prazo)
- propranolol (Inderal, InnoPran XL)
- quinapril (Accupril)
- ramipril (Altace)
- reserpine
- spironolactone (Aldactone, Novo-Spiroton)
- telmisartan (Micardis)
- terazosin (Alti-Terazosin, Hytrin)
- timolol (Betimol, Timoptic)
- torsemide (Demadex)
- trandolapril (Mavik)
- triamterene (Dyrenium)
- trichlormethiazide (Metatensin, Naqua)
- valsartan (Diovan)
- verapamil (Calan, Isoptin SR)

Lab Tests That May Be Altered by Carrageen
None known

Diseases That May Be Worsened or Triggered by Carrageen
None known

Foods That May Interact with Carrageen
None known

Supplements That May Interact with Carrageen
None known

CASCARA SAGRADA

Cascara sagrada, which means "sacred bark," got its name from seventeenth-century Spanish missionaries who noticed its excellent effects on constipation and upset stomach among Native Americans. One of the safest natural laxatives available, cascara sagrada helps restore tone to the colon and overcome laxative dependence in the elderly.

Scientific Name
Rhamnus purshiana

Cascara Sagrada Is Also Commonly Known As
Bitter bark, California buckthorn, dogwood bark, sagrada bark, yellow bark

Medicinal Parts
Bark

Cascara Sagrada's Uses

To treat hemorrhoids, constipation, rheumatism, and poor digestion; as a tonic; for cleaning wounds. Germany's Commission E has approved the use of cascara sagrada to treat constipation.

Typical Dose

A typical daily dose of cascara sagrada may range from 20 to 30 mg of the active ingredient (hydroxyanthracene derivatives).

Possible Side Effects

Cascara sagrada's side effects include abdominal discomfort, colic, and cramps.

Drugs That May Interact with Cascara Sagrada

Taking cascara sagrada with these drugs may reduce absorption of the drug:

- all oral medicines
- ferric gluconate (Ferrlecit)
- ferrous fumarate (Femiron, Feostat)
- ferrous gluconate (Fergon, Novo-Ferrogluc)
- ferrous sulfate (Feratab, Fer-Iron)
- ferrous sulfate and ascorbic acid (Fero-Grad 500, Vitelle Irospan)
- iron-dextran complex (Dexferrum, INFeD)
- polysaccharide-iron complex (Hytinic, Niferex)

Taking cascara sagrada with these drugs may increase the risk of arrhythmia (irregular heartbeat):

- acebutolol (Novo-Acebutolol, Sectral)
- adenosine (Adenocard, Adenoscan)
- amiodarone (Cordarone, Pacerone)
- bepridil (Vascor)
- bretylium
- digitalis (Digitek, Lanoxin)
- diltiazem (Cardizem, Tiazac)

- disopyramide (Norpace, Rhythmodan)
- dofetilide (Tikosyn)
- esmolol (Brevibloc)
- flecainide (Tambocor)
- ibutilide (Corvert)
- insulin (Humulin, Novolin R)
- lidocaine (Lidoderm, Xylocaine)
- mexiletine (Mexitil, Novo-Mexiletine)
- moricizine (Ethmozine)
- phenytoin (Dilantin, Phenytek)
- procainamide (Procanbid, Pronestyl-SR)
- propafenone (Gen-Propafenone, Rhythmol)
- propranolol (Inderal, InnoPran XL)
- quinidine (Novo-Quinidin, Quinaglute Dura-Tabs)
- sildenafil (Viagra)
- sotalol (Betapace, Sorine)
- tocainide (Tonocard)
- verapamil (Calan, Isoptin SR)

Taking cascara sagrada with these drugs may increase the risk of hypokalemia (low levels of potassium in the blood):

- acetazolamide (Apo-Acetazolamide, Diamox Sequels)
- azosemide (Diat)
- beclomethasone (Beconase, Vanceril)
- betamethasone (Celestone, Diprolene)
- budesonide (Entocort, Rhinocort)
- budesonide and formoterol (Symbicort)
- bumetanide (Bumex, Burinex)
- chlorothiazide (Diuril)
- chlorthalidone (Apo-Chlorthalidone, Thalitone)
- cortisone (Cortone)
- deflazacort (Calcort, Dezacor)
- dexamethasone (Decadron, Dexasone)
- digitalis (Digitek, Lanoxin)

- ethacrynic acid (Edecrin)
- etozolin (Elkapin)
- flunisolide (AeroBid, Nasarel)
- fluorometholone (Eflone, Flarex)
- fluticasone (Cutivate, Flonase)
- furosemide (Apo-Furosemide, Lasix)
- hydrochlorothiazide (Apo-Hydro, Microzide)
- hydrocortisone (Cetacort, Locoid)
- hydroflumethiazide (Diucardin, Saluron)
- indapamide (Lozol, Nu-Indapamide)
- loteprednol (Alrex, Lotemax)
- mannitol (Osmitrol, Resectisol)
- medrysone (HMS Liquifilm)
- mefruside (Baycaron)
- methazolamide (Apo-Methazolamide, Neptazane)
- methyclothiazide (Aquatensen, Enduron)
- methylprednisolone (Depo-Medrol, Medrol)
- metolazone (Mykrox, Zaroxolyn)
- olmesartan and hydrochlorothiazide (Benicar HCT)
- polythiazide (Renese)
- prednisolone (Inflamase Forte, Pred Forte)
- prednisone (Apo-Prednisone, Deltasone)
- rimexolone (Vexol)
- torsemide (Demadex)
- triamcinolone (Aristocort, Trinasal)
- trichlormethiazide (Metatensin, Naqua)
- urea (Amino-Cerv, UltraMide)
- xipamide (Diurexan, Lumitens)

Taking cascara sagrada with these drugs may increase the loss of electrolytes and fluids:
- docusate and senna (Peri-Colace, Senokot-S)

Taking cascara sagrada with these drugs may be harmful:

- indomethacin (Indocin, Novo-Methacin)—may interefere with the action of the drug

Lab Tests That May Be Altered by Cascara Sagrada

- Increased or decreased test values of serum and 24-hour urine estrogens.
- May confound results of diagnostic urine tests that rely on a color change by discoloring urine.
- May decrease serum potassium concentrations and cause potassium depletion.

Diseases That May Be Worsened or Triggered by Cascara Sagrada

May worsen Crohn's disease, ulcerative colitis, and other gastrointestinal disesases.

Foods That May Interact with Cascara Sagrada

Decreased action of cascara sagrada when taken with milk.

Supplements That May Interact with Cascara Sagrada

- Increased risk of hypokalemia (low levels of potassium in the blood) when used with potassium-depleting herbs, such as horsetail plant, licorice root, and strophanthus. (For a list of herbs that can deplete potassium stores, see Appendix B.)
- Increased action of jimson weed in cases of chronic use of cascara sagrada.
- Increased risk of cardiotoxicity from potassium depletion especially when cascara sagrada is overused or taken with cardioactive herbs, such as adonis, digitalis, lily-of-the-valley, and squill. (For a list of cardioactive herbs and supplements, see Appendix B.)
- Increased risk of potassium depletion when used in conjunction with horsetail plant or licorice.

- Increased risk of potassium depletion when used with other stimulant laxative herbs, such as black root, castor oil, and senna. (For a list of stimulant laxative herbs and supplements, see Appendix B.)

Castor Oil Plant

> Ancient Egyptians apparently valued the laxative effects of the castor oil plant highly, as its seeds have been found in their tombs. Castor oil's laxative action comes from its ability to draw fluid into the colon and encourage peristalsis, the rhythmic movements of the bowel muscles that push the stool through the system.

Scientific Name
Ricinus communis

Castor Oil Is Also Commonly Known As
Castor bean, Mexico seed, palma Christi, wonder tree, wunderbaum

Medicinal Parts
Seed, oil, and fat taken from seed

Castor Oil's Uses
To treat constipation, intestinal worms, sore throat, ulcers, joint pain, diarrhea, inflammation of the skin and intestines

Typical Dose
A typical dose of castor oil to treat constipation is approximately 15 ml.

Possible Side Effects
Castor oil's side effects include abdominal discomfort, cramps, faintness, and nausea.

Drugs That May Interact with Castor Oil
Taking castor oil with these drugs may increase the risk of hypokalemia (low levels of potassium in the blood):

- acetazolamide (Apo-Acetazolamide, Diamox Sequels)
- azosemide (Diat)
- beclomethasone (Beconase, Vanceril)
- betamethasone (Celestone, Diprolene)
- budesonide (Entocort, Rhinocort)
- budesonide and formoterol (Symbicort)
- bumetanide (Bumex, Burinex)
- chlorothiazide (Diuril)
- chlorthalidone (Apo-Chlorthalidone, Thalitone)
- cortisone (Cortone)
- deflazacort (Calcort, Dezacor)
- dexamethasone (Decadron, Dexasone)
- digitalis (Digitek, Lanoxin)
- ethacrynic acid (Edecrin)
- etozolin (Elkapin)
- flunisolide (AeroBid, Nasarel)
- fluorometholone (Eflone, Flarex)
- fluticasone (Cutivate, Flonase)
- furosemide (Apo-Furosemide, Lasix)
- hydrochlorothiazide (Apo-Hydro, Microzide)
- hydrocortisone (Anusol-HC, Locoid)
- hydroflumethiazide (Diucardin, Saluron)
- indapamide (Lozol, Nu-Indapamide)
- loteprednol (Alrex, Lotemax)
- mannitol (Osmitrol, Resectisol)
- medrysone (HMS Liquifilm)
- mefruside (Baycaron)
- methazolamide (Apo-Methazolamide, Neptazane)
- methyclothiazide (Aquatensen, Enduron)
- methylprednisolone (Depo-Medrol, Medrol)
- metolazone (Mykrox, Zaroxolyn)
- olmesartan and hydrochlorothiazide (Benicar HCT)

- polythiazide (Renese)
- prednisolone (Inflamase Forte, Pred Forte)
- prednisone (Apo-Prednisone, Deltasone)
- rimexolone (Vexol)
- torsemide (Demadex)
- triamcinolone (Aristocort, Trinasal)
- trichlormethiazide (Metatensin, Naqua)
- urea (Amino-Cerv, UltraMide)
- xipamide (Diurexan, Lumitens)

Taking castor oil with these drugs may reduce absorption of the drug:
- all drugs taken orally

Taking castor oil with these drugs may increase the loss of electrolytes and fluids:
- cascara
- docusate and senna (Peri-Colace, Senokot-S)

Lab Tests That May Be Altered by Castor Oil
None known

Diseases That May Be Worsened or Triggered by Castor Oil
May worsen cases of Crohn's disease, irritable bowel syndrome, or other gastrointestinal ailments.

Foods That May Interact with Castor Oil
Absorption of castor oil may be decreased if taken within one hour of drinking milk.

Supplements That May Interact with Castor Oil
- Increased risk of cardiac glycoside toxicity when used with other herbs that contain cardiac glycosides, such as black hellebore, calotropis, motherwort, and others. (For a list of cardiac glycoside–containing herbs and supplements, see Appendix B.)

- Increased risk of potassium depletion when used in conjunction with horsetail plant or licorice.
- Increased risk of potassium depletion when used with other stimulant laxative herbs, such as black root, cascara sagrada, and senna. (For a list of stimulant laxative herbs and supplements, see Appendix B.)
- Enhanced absorption of castor oil when taken with oil-soluble anthelmintic herbs, such as male fern.
- May decrease toxicity and efficacy of wormseed oil when taken concurrently with castor oil.

CAT'S CLAW

Cat's claw is a woody vine originating in the Peruvian rain forest. It gets its name from two curved thorns resembling the claws of a cat that sit at the base of each leaf. In studies, cat's claw has been shown to enhance the ability of immune-system cells to engulf and destroy invading cells and cellular debris. It may also improve the body's ability to repair damaged DNA.

Scientific Name
Uncaria tomentosa

Cat's Claw Is Also Commonly Known As
Garbato, toron, una de gato

Medicinal Parts
Root, bark

Cat's Claw's Uses
To treat rheumatism, diarrhea, wounds, asthma, and menstrual irregularity; as a contraceptive

Typical Dose

A typical daily dose of cat's claw may range from 250 to 5,000 mg in capsule form.

Possible Side Effects

Cat's claw's side effects include decreased serum estradiol and progesterone levels with long-term use.

Drugs That May Interact with Cat's Claw

Taking cat's claw with these drugs may increase the risk of bleeding or bruising:

- abciximab (ReoPro)
- alteplase (Activase, Cathflo Activase)
- antithrombin III (Thrombate III)
- argatroban
- aspirin (Bufferin, Ecotrin)
- aspirin and dipyridamole (Aggrenox)
- bivalirudin (Angiomax)
- choline magnesium trysalicylate (Trilisate)
- clopidogrel (Plavix)
- dalteparin (Fragmin)
- danaparoid (Orgaran)
- diclofenac (Cataflam, Voltaren)
- diflunisal (Apo-Diflunisal, Dolobid)
- dipyridamole (Novo-Dipiradol, Persantine)
- drotrecogin alfa (Xigris)
- eptifibatide (Integrillin)
- etodolac (Lodine, Utradol)
- fenoprofen (Nalfon)
- flurbiprofen (Ansaid, Ocufen)
- fondaparinux (Arixtra)
- heparin (Hepalean, Hep-Lock)
- hydrocodone and aspirin (Damason-P)
- hydrocodone and ibuprofen (Vicoprofen)
- ibritumomab (Zevalin)
- ibuprofen (Advil, Motrin)
- indobufen (Ibustrin)
- indomethacin (Indocin, Novo-Methacin)

- ketorolac (Acular, Toradol)
- lepirudin (Refludan)
- nabumetone (Apo-Nabumetone, Relefan)
- nadroparin (Fraxiparine)
- naproxen (Aleve, Naprosyn)
- oxaprozin (Apo-Oxaprozin, Daypro)
- piroxicam (Feldene, Nu-Pirox)
- reteplase (Retavase)
- salsalate (Amgesic, Salflex)
- streptokinase (Streptase)
- sulindac (Clinoril, Nu-Sundac)
- tenecteplase (TNKase)
- tiaprofenic acid (Dom-Tiaprofenic, Surgam)
- ticlopidine (Alti-Ticlopidine, Ticlid)
- tinzaparin (Innohep)
- tirofiban (Aggrastat)
- tolmetin (Tolectin)
- urokinase (Abbokinase)
- valdecoxib (Bextra)
- warfarin (Coumadin, Jantoven)

Taking cat's claw with these drugs may increase the drug's effects on the pain and feeling of suffocation characteristic of angina:

- bepridil (Vascor)
- diltiazem (Cardizem, Tiazac)
- nifedipine (Adalat CC, Procardia)
- verapamil (Calan, Isoptin SR)

Taking cat's claw with these drugs may increase the risk of hypotension (excessively low blood pressure):

- acebutolol (Novo-Acebutolol, Sectral)
- amlodipine (Norvasc)
- atenolol (Apo-Atenol, Tenormin)
- benazepril (Lotensin)
- betaxolol (Betoptic S, Kerlone)
- bisoprolol (Monocor, Zebeta)
- bumetanide (Bumex, Burinex)

- candesartan (Atacand)
- captopril (Capoten, Novo-Captopril)
- carteolol (Cartrol, Ocupress)
- carvedilol (Coreg)
- chlorothiazide (Diuril)
- chlorthalidone (Apo-Chlorthalidone, Thalitone)
- clonidine (Catapres, Duraclon)
- diazoxide (Hyperstat, Proglycem)
- diltiazem (Cardizem, Tiazac)
- doxazosin (Alti-Doxazosin, Cardura)
- enalapril (Vasotec)
- eplerenone (Inspra)
- eprosartan (Teveten)
- esmolol (Brevibloc)
- felodipine (Plendil, Renedil)
- fenoldopam (Corlopam)
- fosinopril (Monopril)
- furosemide (Apo-Furosemide, Lasix)
- guanabenz (Wytensin)
- guanadrel (Hylorel)
- guanfacine (Tenex)
- hydralazine (Apresoline, Novo-Hylazin)
- hydrochlorothiazide (Apo-Hydro, Microzide)
- hydrochlorothiazide and triamterene (Dyazide, Maxzide)
- indapamide (Lozol, Nu-Indapamide)
- irbesartan (Avapro)
- isradipine (DynaCirc)
- labetalol (Normodyne, Trandate)
- lisinopril (Prinivil, Zestril)
- losartan (Cozaar)
- mecamylamine (Inversine)
- mefruside (Baycaron)
- methyclothiazide (Aquatensen, Enduron)
- methyldopa (Apo-Methyldopa, Nu-Medopa)
- metolazone (Mykrox, Zaroxolyn)
- metoprolol (Betaloc, Lopressor)
- minoxidil (Loniten, Rogaine)
- moexipril (Univasc)
- nadolol (Apo-Nadol, Corgard)
- nicardipine (Cardene)
- nifedipine (Adalat CC, Procardia)
- nisoldipine (Sular)
- nitroglycerin (Minitran, Nitro-Dur)
- nitroprusside (Nipride, Nitropress)
- olmesartan (Benicar)
- oxprenolol (Slow-Trasicor, Trasicor)
- perindopril erbumine (Aceon, Coversyl)
- phenoxybenzamine (Dibenzyline)
- phentolamine (Regitine, Rogitine)
- pindolol (Apo-Pindol, Novo-Pindol)
- polythiazide (Renese)
- prazosin (Minipress, Nu-Prazo)
- propranolol (Inderal, InnoPran XL)
- quinapril (Accupril)
- ramipril (Altace)
- reserpine
- spironolactone (Aldactone, Novo-Spiroton)
- telmisartan (Micardis)
- terazosin (Alti-Terazosin, Hytrin)
- timolol (Betimol, Timoptic)
- torsemide (Demadex)
- trandolapril (Mavik)
- triamterene (Dyrenium)
- trichlormethiazide (Metatensin, Naqua)
- valsartan (Diovan)
- verapamil (Calan, Isoptin SR)

Taking cat's claw with these drugs may interfere with the immunosuppressant action of the drug:
- antithymocyte globulin, equine (Atgam)
- antithymocyte globulin, rabbit (Thymoglobulin)
- azathioprine (Imuran)
- basiliximab (Simulect)
- betamethasone (Betatrex, Maxivate)

- cyclosporine (Neoral, Sandimmune)
- daclizumab (Zenapax)
- dexamethasone (Decadron, Dexasone)
- efalizumab (Raptiva)
- hydrocortisone (Cetacort, Locoid)
- methotrexate (Rheumatrex, Trexall)
- methylprednisolone (Depo-Medrol, Medrol)
- muromonab-CD3 (Orthoclone OKT 3)
- mycophenolate (CellCept)
- pimecrolimus (Elidel)
- prednisolone (Inflamase Forte, Pred Forte)
- prednisone (Apo-Prednisone, Deltasone)
- sirolimus (Rapamune)
- tacrolimus (Prograf, Protopic)
- thalidomide (Thalomid)
- triamcinolone (Aristocort, Trinasal)

Lab Tests That May Be Altered by Cat's Claw
None known

Diseases That May Be Worsened or Triggered by Cat's Claw
May worsen autoimmune diseases, such as systemic lupus erythematosus or multiple sclerosis.

Foods That May Interact with Cat's Claw
None known

Supplements That May Interact with Cat's Claw
None known

CATECHU

Catechu is an extract made from the rust-colored inner wood of the *Acacia catechu* tree, which is native to India. It has strong astringent properties and is traditionally used to ease respiratory congestion, coughs, and sore throats. One of its constituents, taxifolin, has anti-inflammatory, antibacterial, antifungal, and antioxidant properties.

Scientific Name
Acacia catechu

Catechu Is Also Commonly Known As
Black catechu, catechu wood extract, cutch

Medicinal Parts
Heartwood

Catechu's Uses
To treat diabetes, hypertension, diarrhea, and mouth ulcers; as a contraceptive

Typical Dose
A typical dose of catechu may range from 0.3 to 2 gm of dried extract.

Possible Side Effects
Catechu's side effects include low blood pressure, low blood sugar, and constipation.

Drugs That May Interact with Catechu
Taking catechu with these drugs may increase the risk of hypotension (excessively low blood pressure):

- acebutolol (Novo-Acebutolol, Sectral)
- amlodipine (Norvasc)
- atenolol (Apo-Atenol, Tenormin)
- benazepril (Lotensin)
- betaxolol (Betoptic S, Kerlone)
- bisoprolol (Monocor, Zebeta)

- bumetanide (Bumex, Burinex)
- candesartan (Atacand)
- captopril (Capoten, Novo-Captopril)
- carteolol (Cartrol, Ocupress)
- carvedilol (Coreg)
- chlorothiazide (Diuril)
- chlorthalidone (Apo-Chlorthalidone, Thalitone)
- clonidine (Catapres, Duraclon)
- diazoxide (Hyperstat, Proglycem)
- diltiazem (Cardizem, Tiazac)
- doxazosin (Alti-Doxazosin, Cardura)
- enalapril (Vasotec)
- eplerenone (Inspra)
- eprosartan (Teveten)
- esmolol (Brevibloc)
- felodipine (Plendil, Renedil)
- fenoldopam (Corlopam)
- fosinopril (Monopril)
- furosemide (Apo-Furosemide, Lasix)
- guanabenz (Wytensin)
- guanadrel (Hylorel)
- guanfacine (Tenex)
- hydralazine (Apresoline, Novo-Hylazin)
- hydrochlorothiazide (Apo-Hydro, Microzide)
- hydrochlorothiazide and triamterene (Dyazide, Maxzide)
- indapamide (Lozol, Nu-Indapamide)
- irbesartan (Avapro)
- isradipine (DynaCirc)
- labetalol (Normodyne, Trandate)
- lisinopril (Prinivil, Zestril)
- losartan (Cozaar)
- mecamylamine (Inversine)
- mefruside (Baycaron)
- methyclothiazide (Aquatensen, Enduron)
- methyldopa (Apo-Methyldopa, Nu-Medopa)
- metolazone (Mykrox, Zaroxolyn)
- metoprolol (Betaloc, Lopressor)
- minoxidil (Loniten, Rogaine)
- moexipril (Univasc)
- nadolol (Apo-Nadol, Corgard)
- nicardipine (Cardene)
- nifedipine (Adalat CC, Procardia)
- nisoldipine (Sular)
- nitroglycerin (Minitran, Nitro-Dur)
- nitroprusside (Nipride, Nitropress)
- olmesartan (Benicar)
- oxprenolol (Slow-Trasicor, Trasicor)
- perindopril erbumine (Aceon, Coversyl)
- phenoxybenzamine (Dibenzyline)
- phentolamine (Regitine, Rogitine)
- pindolol (Apo-Pindol, Novo-Pindol)
- polythiazide (Renese)
- prazosin (Minipress, Nu-Prazo)
- propranolol (Inderal, InnoPran XL)
- quinapril (Accupril)
- ramipril (Altace)
- reserpine
- spironolactone (Aldactone, Novo-Spiroton)
- telmisartan (Micardis)
- terazosin (Alti-Terazosin, Hytrin)
- timolol (Betimol, Timoptic)
- torsemide (Demadex)
- trandolapril (Mavik)
- triamterene (Dyrenium)
- trichlormethiazide (Metatensin, Naqua)
- valsartan (Diovan)
- verapamil (Calan, Isoptin SR)

Taking catechu with these drugs may reduce the absorption of the drug:
- ferric gluconate (Ferrlecit)
- ferrous fumarate (Femiron, Feostat)

- ferrous gluconate (Fergon, Novo-Ferrogluc)
- ferrous sulfate (Feratab, Fer-Iron)
- ferrous sulfate and ascorbic acid (Fero-Grad 500, Vitelle Irospan)
- iron-dextran complex (Dexferrum, INFeD)
- polysaccharide-iron complex (Hytinic, Niferex)

Taking catechu with these drugs may increase the risk of constipation:
- atropine (Isopto Atropine, Sal-Tropine)
- benztropine (Apo-Benztropine, Cogentin)
- clidinium and chlordiazepoxide (Apo-Chlorax, Librax)
- cyclopentolate (Cyclogyl, Cylate)
- dicyclomine (Bentyl, Lomine)
- glycopyrrolate (Robinul, Robinul Forte)
- homatropine (Isopto Homatropine)
- hyoscyamine (Hyosine, Levsin)
- hyoscyamine, atropine, scopolamine, and phenobarbital (Donnatal, Donnatal Extentabs)
- ipratropium (Atrovent, Nu-Ipratropium)
- oxitropium (Oxivent, Tersigat)
- prifinium (Padrin, Riabel)
- procyclidine (Kemadrin, Procyclid)
- propantheline (Propanthel)
- scopolamine (Scopace, Transderm Scop)
- tiotropium (Spiriva)
- tolterodine (Detrol, Detrol LA)
- trihexyphenidyl (Artane)
- trimethobenzamide (Tigan)

Lab Tests That May Be Altered by Catechu
None known

Diseases That May Be Worsened or Triggered by Catechu
None known

Foods That May Interact with Catechu
None known

Supplements That May Interact with Catechu
None known

Catnip

> Catnip, best known for the euphoric effect it has on cats, acts as a mild sedative in humans, making it useful for soothing the nervous system and easing cramps. It also helps to calm an upset stomach and ease diarrhea and colic. In the form of a hot infusion, catnip promotes sweating, which can help ease colds and flu.

Scientific Name
Nepeta cataria

Catnip Is Also Commonly Known As
Catmint, catswort, field balm

Medicinal Parts
Leaf, stem, flower

Catnip's Uses
To treat colds, fever, colic, migraine headaches, gynecological disorders, and nervous disorders

Typical Dose
A typical dose of catnip is two 380 mg capsules three times daily at meals.

Possible Side Effects
Catnip's side effects include vomiting and headache.

Drugs That May Interact with Catnip

Taking catnip with these drugs may cause excessive sedation and mental depression and impairment:

- alprazolam (Apo-Alpraz, Xanax)
- amitriptyline (Elavil, Levate)
- amoxapine (Asendin)
- bupropion (Wellbutrin, Zyban)
- buspirone (BuSpar, Nu-Buspirone)
- clonazepam (Klonopin, Rivotril)
- cyclobenzaprine (Flexeril, Novo-Cycloprine)
- desipramine (Alti-Desipramine, Norpramin)
- diazepam (Apo-Diazepam, Valium)
- diphenhydramine (Benadryl Allergy, Nytol)
- doxepin (Sinequan, Zonalon)
- fluoxetine (Prozac, Sarafem)
- fluphenazine (Modecate, Prolixin)
- flurazepam (Apo-Flurazepam, Dalmane)
- imipramine (Apo-Imipramine, Tofranil)
- lorazepam (Ativan, Nu-Loraz)
- metoclopramide (Apo-Metoclop, Reglan)
- midazolam (Apo-Midazolam, Versed)
- morphine hydrochloride
- morphine sulfate (Kadian, MS Contin)
- nefazodone (Serzone)
- nortriptyline (Aventyl HCl, Pamelor)
- olanzapine (Zydis, Zyprexa)
- oxazepam (Novoxapam, Serax)
- oxcarbazepine (Trileptal)
- prochlorperazine (Compazine, Compro)
- propoxyphene (Darvon, Darvon-N)
- quetiapine (Seroquel)
- risperidone (Risperdal)
- temazepam (Restoril, Novo-Temazepam)
- tramadol (Ultram)
- triazolam (Apo-Triazo, Halcion)
- zolpidem (Ambien)

Lab Tests That May Be Altered by Catnip

None known

Diseases That May Be Worsened or Triggered by Catnip

May worsen cases of pelvic inflammatory disease and extra-heavy menstrual bleeding.

Foods That May Interact with Catnip

None known

Supplements That May Interact with Catnip

May enhance therapeutic and adverse effects of herbs and supplements that have sedative properties, such as 5-HTP, kava kava, St. John's wort, and valerian. (For a list of herbs and supplements that have sedative properties, see Appendix B.)

CAYENNE

The cayenne plant, a close cousin of bell peppers, jalapeños, paprika, and other peppers, contains a chemical called capsaicin that relieves pain and itching. It does this by temporarily stimulating the release of various neurotransmitters from the affected nerves, leading to depletion of these neurotransmitters. Without them, pain messages can no longer be delivered. Although the capsaicin in cayenne was once thought to trigger cancer, studies have indicated that it may actually interfere with certain biochemical processes needed to activate cancer cells.

Scientific Name

Capsicum species

Cayenne Is Also Commonly Known As

Capsicum chili pepper, goat's pod, Hungarian pepper, paprika, red pepper, Zanzibar pepper

Medicinal Parts

Fruit

Cayenne's Uses

To treat frostbite, sore throats, "clogged arteries," muscle spasms, and seasickness. Topically, in the form of capsaicin cream, it is used to ease joint pain. Germany's Commission E has approved the use of cayenne to treat muscular tension and rheumatism.

Typical Dose

A typical dose of cayenne used internally is approximately 400 to 500 mg in capsule form taken three times a day. Topically a 0.025 to 0.075 percent capsaicin concentration may be applied to the affected area up to four times a day.

Possible Side Effects

When cayenne is taken internally, its side effects include gastrointestinal irritation and flushing of the head and neck. When used topically, cayenne may cause burning and inflammation of the skin.

Drugs That May Interact with Cayenne

Taking cayenne internally with these drugs may increase the risk of bleeding and bruising:

- abciximab (ReoPro)
- alteplase (Activase, Cathflo Activase)
- antithrombin III (Thrombate III)
- argatroban
- aspirin (Bufferin, Ecotrin)
- aspirin and dipyridamole (Aggrenox)
- bivalirudin (Angiomax)
- clopidogrel (Plavix)
- dalteparin (Fragmin)
- danaparoid (Orgaran)
- dipyridamole (Novo-Dipiradol, Persantine)
- enoxaparin (Lovenox)
- eptifibatide (Integrillin)
- fondaparinux (Arixtra)
- heparin (Hepalean, Hep-Lock)
- indobufen (Ibustrin)
- lepirudin (Refludan)
- nadroparin (Fraxiparine)
- reteplase (Retavase)
- streptokinase (Streptase)
- tenecteplase (TNKase)
- ticlopidine (Alti-Ticlopidine, Ticlid)
- tinzaparin (Innohep)
- tirofiban (Aggrastat)
- urokinase (Abbokinase)
- warfarin (Coumadin, Jantoven)

Taking cayenne internally with these drugs may trigger a cough:

- benazepril (Lotensin)
- captopril (Capoten, Novo-Captopril)
- cilazapril (Inhibace)
- delapril (Adecut, Delakete)
- enalapril (Vasotec)
- fosinopril (Monopril)
- imidapril (Novarok, Tanatril)
- lisinopril (Prinivil, Zestril)
- moexipril (Univasc)
- perindopril erbumine (Aceon, Coversyl)
- quinapril (Accupril)
- ramipril (Altace)
- spirapril
- trandolapril (Mavik)

Taking cayenne internally with these drugs may reduce absorption of the drug:

- aminosalicylic acid (Nemasol Sodium, Paser)
- aspirin (Bufferin, Ecotrin)
- choline magnesium trisalicylate (Trilisate)
- choline salicylate (Teejel)
- salsalate (Amgesic, Salflex)

Taking cayenne internally with these drugs may trigger a hypertensive crisis (a rapid and severe increase in blood pressure that can trigger a heart attack, stroke, and other problems):

- iproniazid (Marsilid)
- moclobemide (Alti-Moclobemide, Nu-Moclobemide)
- phenelzine (Nardil)
- selegiline (Eldepryl)
- tranylcypromine (Parnate)

Taking cayenne internally with these drugs may be harmful:

- sucralfate (Carafate, Sulcrate)—interferes with action of the drug
- theophylline (Elixophyllin, Theochron)—may trigger theophylline toxicity

Lab Tests That May Be Altered by Cayenne
None known

Diseases That May Be Worsened or Triggered by Cayenne
May worsen gastrointestinal ailments involving inflammation or infection.

Foods That May Interact with Cayenne
None known

Supplements That May Interact with Cayenne
None known

CEDAR LEAF

> Cedar leaf's scientific name, *Thuja*, comes from the Greek *thuo*, which means "to sacrifice" and alludes to the Greek practice of burning the fragrant cedar wood when making sacrifices. The aromatic cedar leaf oil has been used for respiratory, menstrual, and urinary problems; rheumatism; psoriasis; and wart removal. It has also been used as an antifungal agent for ringworm and thrush. Cedar leaf's major constituent, thujone, is toxic in large doses, so long-term use should be avoided.

Scientific Name
Thuja occidentalis

Cedar Leaf Is Also Commonly Known As
American arborvitae, eastern white cedar, swamp cedar, thuja, tree of life

Medicinal Parts
Leaf, oil of the leaf

Cedar Leaf's Uses
To treat respiratory tract infections, arthritis, bacterial skin infections, and herpes simplex

Typical Dose
A typical dose of cedar leaf may range from 2 to 4 ml of liquid extract (no specified concentration).

Possible Side Effects
Cedar leaf's side effects include asthma, seizures, nausea, and painful diarrhea.

Drugs That May Interact with Cedar Leaf
Taking cedar leaf with these drugs may increase the risk of seizures:

- acetazolamide (Apo-Acetazolamide, Diamox Sequels)
- amobarbital (Amytal)
- barbexaclone (Maliasin)
- arbamazepine (Carbatrol, Tegretol)
- clonazepam (Klonopin, Rivotril)
- clorazepate (Tranxene, T-Tab)
- diazepam (Apo-Diazepam, Valium)
- ethosuximide (Zarontin)
- felbamate (Felbatol)
- fosphenytoin (Cerebyx)
- gabapentin (Neurontin, Nu-Gabapentin)
- lamotrigine (Lamictal)
- levetiracetam (Keppra)
- lorazepam (Ativan, Nu-Loraz)
- mephobarbital (Mebaral)
- methsuximide (Celontin)
- oxazepam (Novoxapam, Serax)
- oxcarbazepine (Trileptal)
- pentobarbital (Nembutal)
- phenobarbital (Luminal Sodium, PMS-Phenobarbital)
- phenytoin (Dilantin, Phenytek)
- primidone (Apo-Primidone, Mysoline)
- thiopental (Pentothal)
- tiagabine (Gabitril)
- topiramate (Topamax)
- valproic acid (Depacon, Depakote ER)
- vigabatrin (Sabril)
- zonisamide (Zonegran)

Lab Tests That May Be Altered by Cedar Leaf
None known

Diseases That May Be Worsened or Triggered by Cedar Leaf
May irrigate the gastrointestinal tract and worsen gastrointestinal ailments.

Foods That May Interact with Cedar Leaf
None known

Supplements That May Interact with Cedar Leaf
Increased risk of thujone toxicity when taken with herbs containing thujone, such as oak moss, oriental arborvitae, sage, tansy, tree moss, and wormwood.

CEDARWOOD OIL

Cedarwood oil is extracted from the red cedar, a coniferous tree native to North America whose wood is often used to make pencils. Cedarwood oil has astringent, antiseptic, and sedative properties, and when applied to the skin, it is good for relieving itching and repelling insects.

Scientific Name
Juniperus virginiana

Cedarwood Oil Is Also Commonly Known As
Ashe juniper, cedar, red cedar, red juniper, Texas cedarwood

Medicinal Parts
Oil distilled from the wood of the tree

Cedarwood Oil's Uses
To treat baldness, rheumatism, skin rash, and cough

Typical Dose
There is no typical dose of cedarwood oil.

Possible Side Effects
Cedarwood oil's side effects include allergic reactions.

Drugs That May Interact with Cedarwood Oil

Taking cedarwood oil with these drugs may reduce the effectiveness of the drug:

- amobarbital (Amytal)
- amobarbital and secobarbital (Tuinal)
- butabarbital (Butisol Sodium)
- butalbital, acetaminophen, and caffeine (Esgic, Fioricet)
- butalbital, aspirin, and caffeine (Fiorinal)
- mephobarbital (Mebaral)
- methohexital (Brevital, Brevital Sodium)
- pentobarbital (Nembutal)
- phenobarbital (Luminal Sodium, PMS-Phenobarbital)
- primidone (Apo-Primidone, Mysoline)
- secobarbital (Seconal)
- thiopental (Pentothal)

Lab Tests That May Be Altered by Cedarwood Oil

None known

Diseases That May Be Worsened or Triggered by Cedarwood Oil

None known

Foods That May Interact with Cedarwood Oil

None known

Supplements That May Interact with Cedarwood Oil

Increased risk of toxicity when taken with herbs containing thujone, such as oak moss, oriental arborvitae, sage, tansy, tree moss, and wormwood.

CELERY

Celery, a member of the carrot family, was used in ancient Egypt to treat impotence and during the Middle Ages as a remedy for gallstones and animal bites. Madame Pompadour, mistress to France's King Louis XV, used celery as an aphrodisiac for her royal lover. Animal studies have indicated that substances in celery can reduce the levels of dopamine and other hormones in the body, which may in turn reduce blood pressure.

Scientific Name

Apium graveolens

Celery Is Also Commonly Known As

Apium, celery seed, marsh parsley, smallage

Medicinal Parts

Whole plant, seed

Celery's Uses

To treat loss of appetite, exhaustion, gout, kidney stones, gallstones, nervous agitation, rheumatism; to regulate the bowels; as a diuretic

Typical Dose

A typical dose of celery may range from 1 to 4 gm of seeds per day.

Possible Side Effects

No side effects have been recorded when celery is taken in recommended therapeutic doses.

Drugs That May Interact with Celery

Taking celery with these drugs may increase skin sensitivity to sunlight:

- bumetanide (Bumex, Burinex)
- ciprofloxacin (Ciloxan, Cipro)
- doxycycline (Apo-Doxy, Vibramycin)
- enalapril (Vasotec)
- etodolac (Lodine, Utradol)
- fluphenazine (Modecate, Prolixin)
- fosinopril (Monopril)
- furosemide (Apo-Furosemide, Lasix)
- gatifloxacin (Tequin, Zymar)
- hydrochlorothiazide (Apo-Hydro, Microzide)
- ibuprofen (Advil, Motrin)
- indomethacin (Indocin, Novo-Methacin)
- ketoprofen (Orudis, Rhodis)
- ketorolac (Acular, Toradol)
- lansoprazole (Prevacid)
- levofloxacin (Levaquin, Quixin)
- lisinopril (Prinivil, Zestril)
- loratadine (Alavert, Claritin)
- methotrexate (Rheumatrex, Trexall)
- naproxen (Aleve, Naprosyn)
- nortriptyline (Aventyl HCl, Pamelor)
- ofloxacin (Floxin, Ocuflox)
- omeprazole (Losec, Prilosec)
- phenytoin (Dilantin, Phenytek)
- piroxicam (Feldene, Nu-Pirox)
- prochlorperazine (Compazine, Compro)
- quinapril (Accupril)
- risperidone (Risperdal)
- rofecoxib (Vioxx)
- tetracycline (Novo-Tetra, Sumycin)

Taking celery with these drugs may be harmful:
- fondaparinux (Arixtra)—may increase risk of bleeding or bruising
- levothyroxine (Levothroid, Synthroid)—may reduce effectiveness of the drug

Lab Tests That May Be Altered by Celery
Celery seed may decrease thyroxine (T-4) serum levels.

Diseases That May Be Worsened or Triggered by Celery
May worsen kidney ailments by triggering inflammation.

Foods That May Interact with Celery
None known

Supplements That May Interact with Celery
None known

CEREUS

Cereus is a long, spindly cactus that grows like a vine on hillsides. A tincture made from its sliced, fresh stems has been used to treat a host of conditions ranging from tinnitus to emphysema. It primarily affects the muscle fibers of the heart and arterioles, and herbalists use it most often to treat cardiac weakness, congestive heart failure, and the chest pain known as angina.

Scientific Name
Selenicereus grandiflorus

Cereus Is Also Commonly Known As
Night-blooming cereus, sweet-scented cactus

Medicinal Parts
Flower, stem

Cereus's Uses

To treat angina pectoris, urinary ailments, menstrual problems, tinnitus, emphysema, and rheumatism; to stimulate the heart

Typical Dose

A typical dose of cereus is approximately 0.6 ml of a 1:1 fluid extract, taken one to ten times daily.

Possible Side Effects

When cereus is taken as a fresh juice, its side effects include nausea, vomiting, diarrhea, and burning of the mouth.

Drugs That May Interact with Cereus

Taking cereus with this drug may be harmful:

- digitalis (Digitek, Lanoxin)—may increase effects of the drug

Lab Tests That May Be Altered by Cereus

None known

Diseases That May Be Worsened or Triggered by Cereus

May worsen heart ailments or interfere with treatment.

Foods That May Interact with Cereus

None known

Supplements That May Interact with Cereus

None known

CHANCA PIEDRA

"Chanca piedra" literally means "break stone," and an extract taken from this small shrublike plant native to the Amazon rain forest is used to break up and expel kidney stones and gallstones. Chanca piedra is also used to treat edema, gout, asthma, and fever, and it appears to have antispasmodic, antiviral, and hypoglycemic activity.

Scientific Name

Phyllanthus niruri

Chanca Piedra Is Also Commonly Known As

Derriere dos, dukong anak, niruri, rami buah, seed on the leaf

Medicinal Parts

Entire plant

Chanca Piedra's Uses

To treat urinary tract infections, poor appetite, constipation, the flu, and pain

Typical Dose

There is no standard dose of chanca piedra.

Possible Side Effects

Chanca piedra has no reported side effects when used properly under a physician's supervision.

Drugs That May Interact with Chanca Piedra

Taking chanca piedra with these drugs may increase the risk of hypoglycemia (low blood sugar):

- acarbose (Prandase, Precose)
- acetohexamide

- chlorpropamide (Diabinese, Novo-Propamide)
- gliclazide (Diamicron, Novo-Gliclazide)
- glimepiride (Amaryl)
- glipizide (Glucotrol)
- glipizide and metformin (Metaglip)
- gliquidone (Beglynor, Glurenorm)
- glyburide (DiaBeta, Micronase)
- glyburide and metformin (Glucovance)
- insulin (Humulin, Novolin R)
- metformin (Glucophage, Riomet)
- miglitol (Glyset)
- nateglinide (Starlix)
- pioglitazone (Actos)
- repaglinide (GlucoNorm, Prandin)
- rosiglitazone (Avandia)
- rosiglitazone and metformin (Avandamet)
- tolazamide (Tolinase)
- tolbutamide (Apo-Tolbutamide, Tol-Tab)

Lab Tests That May Be Altered by Chanca Piedra
None known

Diseases That May Be Worsened or Triggered by Chanca Piedra
None known

Foods That May Interact with Chanca Piedra
None known

Supplements That May Interact with Chanca Piedra
None known

CHAPARRAL

A tea made from the leaves and twigs of the chaparral, an evergreen desert shrub, is an old Native American remedy for cancer that has also been used to treat arthritis, venereal disease, and colds. Chaparral may also contain substances that have anti-HIV and antitumor actions, and at least one study has shown that it can lower blood sugar. However, because chapparal tea can cause severe liver toxicity, its use is not recommended.

Scientific Name
Larrea divaricata, Larrea tridentata

Chaparral Is Also Commonly Known As
Creosote bush, greasewood, hediondilla

Medicinal Parts
Leaf, twig

Chaparral's Uses
To treat bronchitis, fever, diabetes, joint pain, and colds; as a "blood purifier" for infections of the genitourinary and respiratory tracts

Typical Dose
A typical dose of chaparral may range from 1 to 3 ml of a 1:5 dilution of tincture three times a day.

Possible Side Effects
❶ Chaparral's side effects include liver damage and, when used externally, contact dermatitis.

Drugs That May Interact with Chaparral
Taking chaparral internally with these drugs may cause or increase liver damage:

- abacavir (Ziagen)
- acarbose (Prandase, Precose)
- acetaminophen (Genapap, Tylenol)
- allopurinol (Aloprim, Zyloprim)
- atorvastatin (Lipitor)
- celecoxib (Celebrex)
- cidofovir (Vistide)
- cyclosporine (Neoral, Sandimmune)
- docetaxel (Taxotere)
- dofetilide (Tikosyn)
- erythromycin (Erythrocin, Staticin)
- etodolac (Lodine, Utradol)
- fluconazole (Apo-Fluconazole, Diflucan)
- fluphenazine (Modecate, Prolixin)
- fluvastatin (Lescol)
- foscarnet (Foscavir)
- ganciclovir (Cytovene, Vitrasert)
- gemfibrozil (Apo-Gemfibrozil, Lopid)
- gentamicin (Alcomicin, Gentacidin)
- ibuprofen (Advil, Motrin)
- indinavir (Crixivan)
- isoniazid (Isotamine, Nydrazid)
- ketoconazole (Apo-Ketoconazole, Nizoral)
- ketoprofen (Orudis, Rhodis)
- ketorolac (Acular, Toradol)
- lamivudine (Epivir, Heptovir)
- levodopa-carbidopa (Nu-Levocarb, Sinemet)
- lovastatin (Altocor, Mevacor)
- meloxicam (MOBIC, Mobicox)
- methotrexate (Rheumatrex, Trexall)
- methyldopa (Apo-Methyldopa, Nu-Medopa)
- morphine hydrochloride
- morphine sulfate (Kadian, MS Contin)
- naproxen (Aleve, Naprosyn)
- nelfinavir (Viracept)
- nevirapine (Viramune)
- nitrofurantoin (Furadantin, Macrobid)
- ondansetron (Zofran)
- paclitaxel (Onxol, Taxol)
- pantoprazole (Pantoloc, Protonix)
- phenytoin (Dilantin, Phenytek)
- pioglitazone (Actos)
- piroxicam (Feldene, Nu-Pirox)
- pravastatin (Novo-Pravastatin, Pravachol)
- prochlorperazine (Compazine, Compro)
- propoxyphene (Darvon, Darvon-N)
- repaglinide (GlucoNorm, Prandin)
- rifampin (Rifadin, Rimactane)
- rifapentine (Priftin)
- ritonavir (Norvir)
- rofecoxib (Vioxx)
- rosiglitazone (Avandia)
- saquinavir (Fortovase, Invirase)
- simvastatin (Apo-Simvastatin, Zocor)
- stavudine (Zerit)
- tamoxifen (Nolvadex, Tamofen)
- tramadol (Ultram)
- zidovudine (Novo-AZT, Retrovir)

Lab Tests That May Be Altered by Chaparral

May increase results of liver function tests including alkaline phosphatase, aspartic acid transaminase (AST, SGOT), alanine aminotransferase (ALT, SGPT), total bilirubin, urine bilirubin, gamma-glutamyltransferase, and lactate dehydrogenase.

Diseases That May Be Worsened or Triggered by Chaparral

May worsen liver disease.

Foods That May Interact with Chaparral

None known

Supplements That May Interact with Chaparral

May increase the risk of liver damage when combined with herbs and supplements that can cause hepatotoxicity (destructive effects on the liver), such as bishop's weed, borage, uva ursi, and others. (For a list of herbs and supplements that can cause hepatotoxicity, see Appendix B.)

CHASTE TREE BERRY

The Greek physician Hippocrates prescribed the berry of the chaste tree, a shrub native to the Mediterranean area, for menstrual difficulties. Medieval monks took the berry to help reduce their sex drive (thus its name, the "chaste" berry). Some experts believe that the chaste tree berry can relieve female hormonal imbalances by boosting progesterone levels, which may ease the symptoms of premenstrual syndrome (PMS) and other menstrual problems.

Scientific Name

Vitex agnus-castus

Chaste Tree Berry Is Also Commonly Known As

Chasteberry, monk's pepper, vitex

Medicinal Parts

Fruit, leaf

Chaste Tree Berry's Uses

To treat impotence; to increase lactation, suppress appetite, and induce sleep. Germany's Commission E has approved the use of chaste tree berry to treat premenstrual syndrome, menstrual cycle irregularities, and breast pain.

Typical Dose

A typical dose of chaste tree berry may range from 250 to 500 mg of dry powdered extract (4:1 dilution) taken three times daily.

Possible Side Effects

Chaste tree berry's side effects include rash, depression, diarrhea, and loss of appetite.

Drugs That May Interact with Chaste Tree Berry

Taking chaste tree berry with these drugs may increase the risk of dopaminergic side effects (such as nausea, vomiting, headache, and dizziness):

- amantadine (Endantadine, Symmetrel)
- bromocriptine (Apo-Bromocriptine, Parlodel)
- carbidopa (Lodsoyn)
- levodopa (Dopar, Larodopa)
- levodopa-carbidopa (Nu-Levocarb, Sinemet)
- pergolide (Permax)
- pramipexole (Mirapex)
- ropinirole (Requip)

Taking chaste tree berry with these drugs may interfere with the action of the drug:

- ethinyl estradiol and desogestrel (Cyclessa, Ortho- Cept)
- ethinyl estradiol and drospirenone (Yasmin)
- ethinyl estradiol and ethynodiol diacetate (Demulen, Zovia)
- ethinyl estradiol and levonorgestrel (Alesse, Triphasil)
- ethinyl estradiol and norethindrone (Brevicon, Ortho-Novum)
- ethinyl estradiol and norgestimate (Cyclen, Ortho Tri-Cyclen)
- ethinyl estradiol and norgestrel (Cryselle, Ovral)

- mestranol and norethindrone (Necon 1/50, Ortho-Novum 1/50)
- norgestrel (Ovrette)

Lab Tests That May Be Altered by Chaste Tree Berry
Decreased serum prolactin

Diseases That May Be Worsened or Triggered by Chaste Tree Berry
- This herb may have hormonal effects and should not be used by women with estrogen-sensitive breast cancer or other hormone-sensitive conditions.
- May interfere with in vitro fertilization.

Foods That May Interact with Chaste Tree Berry
None known

Supplements That May Interact with Chaste Tree Berry
None known

CHEROKEE ROSEHIP

The earliest written record of this herb, which is also known as Chinese rosehip and was an important Chinese food and medicine, dates back fifteen hundred years. Traditionally used to treat male sexual problems, replenish the "vital essence" of the kidneys, and stimulate ovulation, Cherokee rosehip contains high amounts of vitamin C and other antioxidants that are known health-enhancers.

Scientific Name
Rosa laevigata

Cherokee Rosehip Is Also Commonly Known As
Chinese rosehip, fructus rosae laevigatae, jinyingzi

Medicinal Parts
Fruit

Cherokee Rosehip's Uses
To treat male sexual dysfunction, uterine bleeding, night sweats, bedwetting, chronic cough, and hypertension

Typical Dose
There is no typical dose of Cherokee rosehip.

Possible Side Effects
Cherokee rosehip's side effects include nausea, abdominal cramps, insomnia, fatigue, and diarrhea.

Drugs That May Interact with Cherokee Rosehip
Taking Cherokee rosehip with these drugs may increase drug absorption and effects:
- estrogens (conjugated A/synthetic) (Cenestin)
- estrogens (conjugated/equine) (Premarin, Congest)
- estrogens (conjugated/equine) and medroxy-progesterone (Prempro, Premprase)
- estrogens (esterified) (Estratab, Menest)
- estrogens (esterified) and methyltestosterone (Estratest, Estratest H.S.)
- ethinyl estradiol and desogestrel (Cyclessa, Ortho-Cept)
- ethinyl estradiol and ethynodiol diacetate (Demulen, Zovia)
- ethinyl estradiol and etonogestrel (NuvaRing)
- ethinyl estradiol and levonogestrel (Alesse, Triphasil)
- ethinyl estradiol and norelgestromin (Evra, Ortho Evra)

- ethinyl estradiol and norethindrone (Brevicon, Ortho-Novum)
- ethinyl estradiol and norgestimate (Cyclen, Ortho Tri-Cyclen)
- ethinyl estradiol and norgestrel (Cryselle, Ovral)
- mestranol and norethindrone (Necon 1/50, Ortho-Novum 1/50)

Taking Cherokee rosehip with these drugs may be harmful:
- aspirin (Bufferin, Ecotrin)—may reduce the body's ability to excrete the drug
- fluphenazine (Modecate, Prolixin)—may reduce blood levels of the drug
- warfarin (Coumadin, Jantoven)—may reduce effectiveness of the drug

Lab Tests That May Be Altered by Cherokee Rosehip
- May cause false negative results in stool occult blood tests if large amounts of Cherokee rosehip are ingested forty-eight to seventy-two hours before the test.
- May cause false readings in urine glucose tests: increases in results of glucose oxidase tests (such as Clinistix) and decreases in results of cupric sulfate tests (such as Clinitest) when large amounts of vitamin C (more than 500 mg) are ingested. This may be a problem as Cherokee rosehip contains large amounts of vitamin C.

Diseases That May Be Worsened or Triggered by Cherokee Rosehip
May interfere with therapy to control blood sugar in diabetics.

Foods That May Interact with Cherokee Rosehip
May increase gastrointestinal absorption of iron from food (ferric) but not iron from supplements (ferrous), due to vitamin C content.

Supplements That May Interact with Cherokee Rosehip
Increased risk of the adverse effects that are seen with large dosages of vitamin C (such as nausea, gastrointestinal upset, heartburn, and diarrhea) when Cherokee rosehip is used with other products containing vitamin C.

CHICORY

Also known as the "friend of the liver," chicory helps increase the flow of bile. According to the Roman scholar Pliny, those who mix chicory juice with oil and apply it to their bodies will "become more popular and obtain their requests more easily."

Scientific Name
Cichorium intybus

Chicory Is Also Commonly Known As
Blue sailors, garden endive, hendibeh, succory, wild chicory

Medicinal Parts
Leaf, root

Chicory's Uses
To treat digestive problems, headaches, skin allergies, and diarrhea; as a laxative. Germany's Commission E has approved the use of chicory to treat dyspeptic complaints (such as fullness, heartburn, and bloating) and loss of appetite.

Typical Dose
A typical daily dose of chicory may range from 3 to 5 gm of the root per day.

Possible Side Effects

Chicory's side effects include allergic reactions in those who are sensitive to the Asteraceae (daisy) family (chrysanthemums, daisies, marigolds, ragweed, etc.).

Drugs That May Interact with Chicory

Taking chicory with these drugs may increase the drug's antianginal effects:

- bepridil (Vascor)
- diltiazem (Cardizem, Tiazac)
- nifedipine (Adalat CC, Procardia)
- verapamil (Calan, Isoptin SR)

Lab Tests That May Be Altered by Chicory

None known

Diseases That May Be Worsened or Triggered by Chicory

None known

Foods That May Interact with Chicory

None known

Supplements That May Interact with Chicory

None known

CHINESE CLUB MOSS

Used for centuries to treat inflammation and fever, Chinese club moss is known for its mild diuretic action. The herb also contains a chemical called huperzine A. Several studies of memory-impaired animals and humans have shown that taking huperzine A may help to relieve dementia, most likely by temporarily blocking the breakdown of an important neurotransmitter called acetylcholine. A small study of normal teenagers also showed that general mental functioning appeared to be enhanced when huperzine A was taken consistently for as little as one month.

Scientific Name

Huperzia serrata

Chinese Club Moss Is Also Commonly Known As

Huperazon, qian ceng ta

Medicinal Parts

Entire plant

Chinese Club Moss's Uses

To treat memory disorders, Alzheimer's disease, fever, inflammation, irregular menstruation, and blood loss; as a diuretic

Typical Dose

There is no typical dose of Chinese club moss. However, a typical dose of its active ingredient, huperzine A, may range from 50 to 200 mcg twice daily for Alzheimer's disease.

Possible Side Effects

There are no known side effects due to the administration of Chinese club moss. However, its active ingredient, huperzine A, can cause nausea, blurred vision, sweating, and dizziness.

Drugs That May Interact with Chinese Club Moss

Taking Chinese club moss with these drugs may increase the effects of the drug:

- acetylcholine (Miochol-E)
- bethanechol (Duvoid, Urecholine)
- carbachol (Carbastat, Isopto Carbachol)

- cevimeline (Evoxac)
- donepezil (Aricept)
- edrophonium (Enlon, Reversol)
- galantamine (Razadyne)
- methacholine (Provocholine)
- neostigmine (Prostigmin)
- physostigmine (Eserine)
- pilocarpine (Isopto Carpine, Salagen)
- pyridostigmine (Mestinon)
- rivastigmine (Exelon)
- tacrine (Cognex)

Taking Chinese club moss with these drugs may reduce the effects of the herb or the drug:
- atropine (Isopto Atropine, Sal-Tropine)
- benztropine (Apo-Benztropine, Cogentin)
- clidinium and chlordiazepoxide (Apo-Chlorax, Librax)
- cyclopentolate (Cyclogyl, Cylate)
- dicyclomine (Bentyl, Lomine)
- glycopyrrolate (Robinul, Robinul Forte)
- homatropine (Isopto Homatropine)
- hyoscyamine (Hyosine, Levsin)
- hyoscyamine, atropine, scopolamine, and phenobarbital (Donnatal, Donnatal Extentabs)
- ipratropium (Atrovent, Nu-Ipratropium)
- oxitropium (Oxivent, Tersigat)
- prifinium (Padrin, Riabel)
- procyclidine (Kemadrin, Procyclid)
- propantheline (Propanthel)
- scopolamine (Scopace, Transderm Scop)
- tiotropium (Spiriva)
- tolterodine (Detrol, Detrol LA)
- trihexyphenidyl (Artane)
- trimethobenzamide (Tigan)

Lab Tests That May Be Altered by Chinese Club Moss
None known

Diseases That May Be Worsened or Triggered by Chinese Club Moss
May worsen cases of chronic obstructive pulmonary disease, asthma, cardiovascular disease, ulcers, seizures, intestinal obstructions, or urogenital obstructions.

Foods That May Interact with Chinese Club Moss
None known

Supplements That May Interact with Chinese Club Moss
None known

CHINESE CUCUMBER ROOT

Chinese cucumber root has been used to treat breast abscesses and breast cancer since the Ming Dynasty. A protein fraction taken from the root, called trichosanthin, was originally developed for clinical use in inducing abortion. Today it is used to treat some cancers and has been shown to have anti-HIV action.

Scientific Name
Trichosanthes kirilowii

Chinese Cucumber Root Is Also Commonly Known As
Chinese snake gourd, Compound Q, tian hua fen

Medicinal Parts
Root

Chinese Cucumber Root's Uses
To treat coughs, fever, tumors, HIV infection, and diabetes

Typical Dose

A typical oral dose of Chinese cucumber root may range from 9 to 15 gm of the root.

Possible Side Effects

❗ Chinese cucumber root's side effects include fever, seizures, abortion, allergic reactions, heart damage, and death. Extracts of Chinese cucumber can be very toxic.

Drugs That May Interact with Chinese Cucumber Root

Taking Chinese cucumber root with these drugs may increase the drug's therapeutic and/or adverse effects:

- acarbose (Prandase, Precose)
- acetohexamide
- chlorpropamide (Diabinese, Novo-Propamide)
- gliclazide (Diamicron, Novo-Gliclazide)
- glimepiride (Amaryl)
- glipizide (Glucotrol)
- glipizide and metformin (Metaglip)
- gliquidone (Beglynor, Glurenorm)
- glyburide (DiaBeta, Micronase)
- glyburide and metformin (Glucovance)
- insulin (Humulin, Novolin R)
- metformin (Glucophage, Riomet)
- miglitol (Glyset)
- nateglinide (Starlix)
- pioglitazone (Actos)
- repaglinide (GlucoNorm, Prandin)
- rosiglitazone (Avandia)
- rosiglitazone and metformin (Avandamet)
- tolazamide (Tolinase)
- tolbutamide (Apo-Tolbutamide, Tol-Tab)

Lab Tests That May Be Altered by Chinese Cucumber Root

May decrease blood glucose test values.

Diseases That May Be Worsened or Triggered by Chinese Cucumber Root

May hamper effects to control blood sugar in diabetes.

Foods That May Interact with Chinese Cucumber Root

None known

Supplements That May Interact with Chinese Cucumber Root

May increase blood glucose–lowering effects and risk of hypoglycemia (low blood sugar) when used with herbs and supplements that lower glucose levels, such as alpha-lipoic acid, chromium, devil's claw, Panax ginseng, and psyllium. (For a list of herbs and supplements that lower blood glucose levels, see Appendix B.)

CHINESE RHUBARB

Numerous studies show that Chinese rhubarb is an effective laxative. It works by irritating the colon and encouraging the body to push the stool through the system more rapidly. It may also help protect the kidneys. In one study, when the herb was combined with standard medicines, the combination of herb plus medicine was more effective at slowing kidney failure than standard drugs alone.

Scientific Name

Rheum palmatum

Chinese Rhubarb Is Also Commonly Known As

Da-huang, Indian rhubarb, rhubarb, Russian rhubarb

Medicinal Parts

Root, root bark

Chinese Rhubarb's Uses

To treat constipation, delirium, abdominal pain, lack of menstruation, teething, burns, and various skin conditions. Approved by Germany's Commission E to treat constipation.

Typical Dose

A typical dose of Chinese rhubarb may range from 1 to 2 gm of coarse powdered herb.

Possible Side Effects

Chinese rhubarb's side effects include irregular heartbeat, potassium deficiency, and nerve damage.

Drugs That May Interact with Chinese Rhubarb

Taking Chinese rhubarb with these drugs may increase the risk of hypokalemia (low levels of potassium in the blood):

- bepridil (Vascor)
- digitalis (Digitek, Lanoxin)
- diltiazem (Cardizem, Tiazac)
- dofetilide (Tikosyn)
- flecainide (Tambocor)
- insulin (Humulin, Novolin R)
- quinidine (Novo-Quinidin, Quinaglute Dura-Tabs)
- sildenafil (Viagra)
- sotalol (Betapace, Sorine)
- verapamil (Calan, Isoptin SR)

Lab Tests That May Be Altered by Chinese Rhubarb

- May cause potassium depletion when overused.
- May confound results of diagnostic urine tests that rely on a color change by discoloring urine (pink, red, purple, or orange).

Diseases That May Be Worsened or Triggered by Chinese Rhubarb

- May worsen diarrhea or constipation.
- May worsen inflammatory or obstructive conditions of the gastrointestinal tract.

Foods That May Interact with Chinese Rhubarb

Taking milk concurrently may decrease effectiveness of Chinese rhubarb.

Supplements That May Interact with Chinese Rhubarb

- May increase action of jimson weed in cases of chronic use or abuse of Chinese rhubarb.
- May decrease mineral absorption when taken with calcium, iron, or zinc supplements.
- May increase risk of cardiac toxicity when used with herbs that contain cardiac glycosides, such as black hellebore, calotropis, motherwort, and others. (For a list of cardiac glycoside–containing herbs and supplements, see Appendix B.)
- Overuse of Chinese rhubarb might cause potassium depletion, increasing the risk of cardioactive herb toxicity. Avoid concomitant use with cardioactive herbs, such as colt's foot, devil's claw, English hawthorn, European mistletoe, and others, because of increased risk of cardiotoxicity due to potassium depletion. (For a list of cardioactive herbs and supplements, see Appendix B.)
- May increase risk of potassium depletion when used in conjunction with horsetail plant or licorice.

- May increase risk of potassium depletion when used with other stimulant laxative herbs, such as black root, cascara sagrada, castor oil, and senna. (For a list of stimulant laxative herbs and supplements, see Appendix B.)

CHLORELLA

A single-celled green algae high in chlorophyll, chlorella gets its name from the Greek word *chloros*, meaning "green," and the Latin *ella*, meaning "small." Because it is high in protein, chlorella has been researched as a potential food substitute. It is also believed to have antitumor activity, to stimulate immune system function, and to rid the body of harmful toxins and heavy metals.

Scientific Name
Chlorella pyrenoidosa

Chlorella Is Also Commonly Known As
Bulgarian green algae, freshwater seaweed, green algae

Medicinal Parts
Whole plant

Chlorella's Uses
To strengthen the immune system, counteract the effects of aging, and protect against the harmful effects of lead and other toxic minerals

Typical Dose
A typical daily dose of chlorella is approximately 10 gms.

Possible Side Effects
Chlorella's side effects include nausea, abdominal cramping, and fatigue.

Drugs That May Interact with Chlorella
Taking chlorella with this drug may be harmful:
- warfarin (Coumadin, Jantoven)—may interfere with the action of the drug

Lab Tests That May Be Altered by Chlorella
None known

Diseases That May Be Worsened or Triggered by Chlorella
May encourage infections in those with weakened immune systems.

Foods That May Interact with Chlorella
None known

Supplements That May Interact with Chlorella
None known

CINNAMON

Used for embalming in ancient Egypt and highly sought after by fifteenth- and sixteenth-century explorers for its sweet and spicy fragrance, cinnamon has a long history of use as a medicinal herb. It has antibacterial properties, helps regulate blood sugar, is a strong immune system booster, and may even help prevent cancer. Used in China as early as 2700 B.C., cinnamon is still highly recommended there as a treatment for nausea, menstrual problems, fever, and diarrhea.

Scientific Name

Cinnamomum verum

Cinnamon Is Also Commonly Known As

Cassia, cassia lignea, Ceylon cinnamon, padang cassia, Saigon cassia

Medicinal Parts

Bark

Cinnamon's Uses

To treat exhaustion, flatulence, nausea, vomiting, and toothache. Germany's Commission E has approved the use of cinnamon to treat loss of appetite as well as dyspeptic complaints, such as heartburn and bloating.

Typical Dose

A typical dose of cinnamon may range from 0.5 to 1 gm cinnamon bark mixed with 150 ml of boiling water, steeped for ten minutes and strained. This dosage of the tea/infusion may be taken two to three times daily at mealtimes.

Possible Side Effects

No side effects have been recorded when cinnamon is taken in recommended therapeutic doses.

Drugs That May Interact with Cinnamon

Taking cinnamon with these drugs may increase the risk of hypoglycemia (low blood sugar):

- acarbose (Prandase, Precose)
- acetohexamide
- chlorpropamide (Diabinese, Novo-Propamide)
- gliclazide (Diamicron, Novo-Gliclazide)
- glimepiride (Amaryl)
- glipizide (Glucotrol)
- glipizide and metformin (Metaglip)
- gliquidone (Beglynor, Glurenorm)
- glyburide (DiaBeta, Micronase)
- glyburide and metformin (Glucovance)
- insulin (Humulin, Novolin R)
- metformin (Glucophage, Riomet)
- miglitol (Glyset)
- nateglinide (Starlix)
- pioglitazone (Actos)
- repaglinide (GlucoNorm, Prandin)
- rosiglitazone (Avandia)
- rosiglitazone and metformin (Avandamet)
- tolazamide (Tolinase)
- tolbutamide (Apo-Tolbutamide, Tol-Tab)

Lab Tests That May Be Altered by Cinnamon

May decrease blood glucose test values.

Diseases That May Be Worsened or Triggered by Cinnamon

None known

Foods That May Interact with Cinnamon

May interfere with diabetic therapy by lowering blood sugar levels.

Supplements That May Interact with Cinnamon

May increase blood glucose–lowering effects and risk of hypoglycemia (low blood sugar) when used with herbs and supplements that lower glucose levels, such as alpha-lipoic acid, chromium, devil's claw, Panax ginseng, and psyllium. (For a list of herbs and supplements that lower blood glucose levels, see Appendix B.)

CLOVE

The clove, the sweet, spicy flower bud of the clove tree, has been used for some 2,400 years in China, when courtiers began tucking it inside their cheeks to avoid offending the emperor with their bad breath. When applied directly to an aching tooth, clove oil is a strong antiseptic that can bring immediate relief. Clove is also used to treat indigestion, dyspepsia, and nausea.

Scientific Name
Syzygium aromaticum

Clove Is Also Commonly Known As
Caryophylli, lavanga, clove flower, clous de girolfe

Medicinal Parts
Flower bud

Clove's Uses
To treat headaches, colds, stomach ulcers, eye disease, toothaches, colic, inflammation, and flatulence. Germany's Commission E has approved the use of clove to treat inflammation of the mouth and throat and as a dental analgesic.

Typical Dose
A typical dose of clove may range from 1 to 5 percent essential oil in an aqueous solution as a mouthwash; 5 to 30 drops (1:3 dilution) of a tincture; or 1 to 5 drops of essential oil applied topically.

Possible Side Effects
Irritation of the throat or skin, spasms of the bronchial tubes

Drugs That May Interact with Clove
Taking clove internally with these drugs may increase the risk of bleeding and bruising:

- abciximab (ReoPro)
- alteplase (Activase, Cathflo Activase)
- antithrombin III (Thrombate III)
- argatroban
- aspirin (Bufferin, Ecotrin)
- aspirin and dipyridamole (Aggrenox)
- bivalirudin (Angiomax)
- celecoxib (Celebrex)
- clopidogrel (Plavix)
- dalteparin (Fragmin)
- danaparoid (Orgaran)
- dipyridamole (Novo-Dipiradol, Persantine)
- enoxaparin (Lovenox)
- eptifibatide (Integrillin)
- etodolac (Lodine, Utradol)
- fondaparinux (Arixtra)
- heparin (Hepalean, Hep-Lock)
- ibuprofen (Advil, Motrin)
- indobufen (Ibustrin)
- indomethacin (Indocin, Novo-Methacin)
- ketoprofen (Orudis, Rhodis)
- ketorolac (Acular, Toradol)
- lepirudin (Refludan)
- nadroparin (Fraxiparine)
- reteplase (Retavase)
- streptokinase (Streptase)
- tenecteplase (TNKase)
- ticlopidine (Alti-Ticlopidine, Ticlid)
- tinzaparin (Innohep)
- tirofiban (Aggrastat)
- urokinase (Abbokinase)
- warfarin (Coumadin, Jantoven)

Lab Tests That May Be Altered by Clove
May cause false increase in phenytoin levels.

Diseases That May Be Worsened or Triggered by Clove

Clove oil may worsen cases of platelet abnormalities.

Foods That May Interact with Clove

None known

Supplements That May Interact with Clove

Increased risk of bleeding when used with herbs and supplements that might affect platelet aggregation, such as angelica, danshen, garlic, ginger, ginkgo biloba, red clover, turmeric, white willow, and others. (For a list of herbs and supplements with anticoagulant/antiplatelet potential, see Appendix B.)

Cocoa

Cocoa is the dried and partially fermented fatty seed of the cacao tree, native to South America. It was brought to Central America by the seventh century A.D., where it became a favorite of the Aztecs, Mayans, and Toltecs. Its scientific name, *Theobroma cacao*, means "food of the gods," and it was so revered by the Aztecs that their emperor, Moctezuma II, insisted on having a beverage made out of crushed cocoa beans, which he ate with a golden spoon out of a golden goblet, with every meal.

Scientific Name

Theobroma cacao

Cocoa Is Also Commonly Known As

Cacao, chocolate tree

Medicinal Parts

Seed

Cocoa's Uses

To treat infectious intestinal diseases, diarrhea, diabetes, liver and kidney disease; as a mild stimulant; to regulate the thyroid

Typical Dose

There is no typical dose of cocoa.

Possible Side Effects

Cocoa's side effects include nausea, gastrointestinal discomfort, allergic skin reactions, and migraine headaches.

Drugs That May Interact with Cocoa

Cocoa contains caffeine, so see Caffeine and Caffeine-Containing Herbs on p. 111 for a list of drugs that may interact with this herb.

Lab Tests That May Be Altered by Cocoa

See Caffeine and Caffeine-Containing Herbs on p. 112 for a list of lab tests that may interact with the caffeine in this herb.

Diseases That May Be Worsened or Triggered by Cocoa

See Caffeine and Caffeine-Containing Herbs on p. 113 for a list of diseases that may be worsened or triggered by the caffeine in this herb.

Foods That May Interact with Cocoa

May increase therapeutic and adverse effects of caffeine when taken together with caffeine-containing foods and drinks. (For a list of herbs, foods, and supplements that contain caffeine, see Appendix B.)

Supplements That May Interact with Cocoa

See Caffeine and Caffeine-Containing Herbs on p. 113 for a list of supplements that may interact with the caffeine in this herb.

COFFEE

Known for its ability to clear the mind and perk up the energy, coffee has some surprising health benefits. According to a study done at the University of Scranton, in Pennsylvania, it provides more healthful antioxidants than any other food or beverage in the American diet. Researchers at the Harvard School of Public Health found that drinking more than six cups of coffee a day may reduce the risk of diabetes. And a team of Japanese researchers reported that people who drank coffee daily, or nearly every day, had half the liver cancer risk of those who never drank it.

Scientific Name

Coffea arabica

Coffee Is Also Commonly Known As

Arabica coffee, Arabian coffee, caffea, java, mocha

Medicinal Parts

Seed (bean)

Coffee's Uses

To treat hepatitis, inflammation, migraines, fever, and diarrhea. Germany's Commission E has approved the use of coffee to treat diarrhea and inflammation of the mouth and throat.

Typical Dose

A typical dose of coffee for treating headaches is approximately 2 cups of the infusion, containing a total of 250 mg caffeine.

Possible Side Effects

Coffee's side effects include tremors, gastro-esophageal reflux disease (GERD), insomnia, and irritability.

Drugs That May Interact with Coffee

Taking coffee with these drugs may interfere with the absorption of the drug:

- alendronate (Novo-Alendronate, Fosamax)
- amitriptyline (Elavil, Levate)
- amitriptyline and chlordiazepoxide (Limbitrol)
- amitriptyline and perphenazine (Etrafon, Triavil)
- amoxapine (Asendin)
- chlorpromazine (Largactil, Thorazine)
- clomipramine (Anafranil, Novo-Clopramine)
- desipramine (Alti-Desipramine, Norpramin)
- doxepin (Sinequan, Zonalon)
- fluphenazine (Modecate, Prolixin)
- imipramine (Apo-Imipramine, Tofranil)
- lofepramine (Feprapax, Gamanil)
- melitracen (Dixeran)
- mesoridazine (Serentil)
- nortriptyline (Aventyl HCl, Pamelor)
- perphenazine (Apo-Perphenazine, Trilafon)
- prochlorperazine (Compazine, Compro)
- promethazine (Phenergan)
- protriptyline (Vivactil)
- thiethylperazine (Torecan)
- thioridazine (Mellaril)
- thiothixene (Navane)
- trifluoperazine (Novo-Trifluzine, Stelazine)

• trimipramine (Apo-Trimip, Surmontil) Coffee contains caffeine, so see Caffeine and Caffeine-Containing Herbs on p. 111 for an additional list of drugs that may interact with coffee.

Lab Tests That May Interact with Coffee

See Caffeine and Caffeine-Containing Herbs on p. 112 for a list of lab tests that may interact with the caffeine in this herb.

Diseases That May Be Worsened or Triggered by Coffee

See Caffeine and Caffeine-Containing Herbs on p. 113 for a list of diseases that may be worsened or triggered by the caffeine in this herb.

Foods That May Interact with Coffee

May increase therapeutic and adverse effects of caffeine when taken together with caffeine-containing foods and drinks. (For a list of herbs, foods, and supplements that contain caffeine, see Appendix B.)

Supplements That May Interact with Coffee

See Caffeine and Caffeine-Containing Herbs on p. 113 for a list of supplements that may interact with the caffeine in this herb.

COLA NUT

Grown in western Africa, the West Indies, Brazil, and Java, cola nuts are high in caffeine and traditionally are chewed or used in ground or extract form to fight fatigue and enhance mental alertness. Cola nuts have also been used as an aphrodisiac, an appetite suppressant, and a treatment for migraines, morning sickness, and indigestion. In 1898 North Carolina pharmacist Caleb D. Bradham created a beverage made of cola nut extract, carbonated water, sugar, vanilla, oils, and pepsin, and called it Brad's Drink, later changing its name to Pepsi-Cola and securing the trademark.

Scientific Name

Cola acuminata

Cola Nut Is Also Commonly Known As

Bissy nut, guru nut, kola nut, kola tree

Medicinal Parts

Seed

Cola Nut's Uses

To treat inflammation and wounds; to suppress hunger; to reduce physical and mental fatigue; to prevent migraine and morning sickness. Germany's Commission E has approved the use of cola nut to treat lack of stamina.

Typical Dose

A typical dose of cola nut may range from 2 to 6 gm per day.

Possible Side Effects

Cola nut's side effects include insomnia, nervousness, restlessness, gastric irritation, and nausea.

Drugs That May Interact with Cola Nut

Cola nut contains caffeine, so see Caffeine and Caffeine-Containing Herbs on p. 111 for a list of drugs that may interact with this herb.

Lab Tests That May Interact with Cola Nut

See Caffeine and Caffeine-Containing Herbs on p. 112 for a list of lab tests that may interact with the caffeine in this herb.

Diseases That May Be Worsened or Triggered by Cola Nut

See Caffeine and Caffeine-Containing Herbs on p. 113 for a list of diseases that may be worsened or triggered by the caffeine in this herb.

Foods That May Interact with Cola Nut

May increase therapeutic and adverse effects of caffeine when taken together with caffeine-containing foods and drinks. (For a list of herbs, foods, and supplements that contain caffeine, see Appendix B.)

Supplements That May Interact with Cola Nut

See Caffeine and Caffeine-Containing Herbs on p. 113 for a list of supplements that may interact with the caffeine in this herb.

COLCHICUM

Although known since ancient times, colchicum, the highly toxic autumn crocus plant, was not used medicinally until the eighteenth century, when it was first discovered to be an effective treatment for gout. Colchicum is the source of the alkaloid colchicine, which is a modern medication for gout, cancer, and certain types of liver disease. Its use is usually confined to the short term, however, as side effects occur with long-term usage.

Scientific Name

Colchicum autumnale

Colchicum Is Also Commonly Known As

Autumn crocus, crocus, meadow saffron, upstart

Medicinal Parts

Flower, seed, tuber (fleshy, rounded stem or root)

Colchicum's Uses

To treat psoriasis, gout, Mediterranean fever, gastrointestinal inflammation, asthma, and lice. Germany's Commission E has approved the use of colchicum bulbs, seeds, and flowers to treat Mediterranean fever and gout.

Typical Dose

There is no typical dose of colchicum. The herb is considered toxic and is rarely used.

Possible Side Effects

Colchicum's side effects include thirst, burning of the mouth and throat, nausea, vomiting, and diarrhea.

Drugs That May Interact with Colchicum

Taking colchicum with this drug may be harmful:

- colchicine (ratio-Colchicine)—may enhance drug's therapeutic and adverse effects

Lab Tests That May Be Altered by Colchicum

May decrease serum uric acid concentrations.

Diseases That May Be Worsened or Triggered by Colchicum

None known

Foods That May Interact with Colchicum

None known

Supplements That May Interact with Colchicum

None known

Colocynth

Cultivated since the time of the ancient Assyrians and related to the watermelon, the yellow-green, spongy, and extremely bitter colocynth is traditionally used as a strong laxative and antidiabetic agent. One study found that extracts of the seed of the colocynth promote the release of insulin, which could at least partially account for the fruit's antidiabetic action.

Scientific Name

Citrullus colocynthis

Colocynth Is Also Commonly Known As

Bitter apple, colocynth pulp, vine-of-Sodom, wild gourd

Medicinal Parts

Fruit, seed

Colocynth's Uses

To treat constipation and liver and gallbladder ailments

Typical Dose

There is no typical dose of colocynth.

Possible Side Effects

Colocynth's side effects include severe irritation of gastric mucosa, bloody diarrhea, acute toxic colitis, and kidney damage.

Drugs That May Interact with Colocynth

Taking colocynth with these drugs may increase the risk of hypokalemia (low levels of potassium in the blood):

- acetazolamide (Apo-Acetazolamide, Diamox Sequels)
- azosemide (Diat)
- bumetanide (Bumex, Burinex)
- chlorothiazide (Diuril)
- chlorthalidone (Apo-Chlorthalidone, Thalitone)
- ethacrynic acid (Edecrin)
- etozolin (Elkapin)
- furosemide (Apo-Furosemide, Lasix)
- hydrochlorothiazide (Apo-Hydro, Microzide)
- hydroflumethiazide (Diucardin, Saluron)
- indapamide (Lozol, Nu-Indapamide)
- mannitol (Osmitrol, Resectisol)
- mefruside (Baycaron)
- methazolamide (Apo-Methazolamide, Neptazane)
- methyclothiazide (Aquatensen, Enduron)
- metolazone (Mykrox, Zaroxolyn)
- olmesartan and hydrochlorothiazide (Benicar HCT)
- polythiazide (Renese)
- torsemide (Demadex)
- trichlormethiazide (Metatensin, Naqua)
- urea (Amino-Cerv, UltraMide)
- xipamide (Diurexan, Lumitens)

Taking colocynth with these drugs may be harmful:
- digitalis (Digitek, Lanoxin)—may increase adverse effects of the drug

Lab Tests That May Be Altered by Colocynth

- Excessive use may deplete potassium stores, reducing serum potassium levels.

- Excessive use may cause anuria (cessation of urine output).

Diseases That May Be Worsened or Triggered by Colocynth

May irritate the gastrointestinal tract and worsen gastrointestinal ailments.

Foods That May Interact with Colocynth

None known

Supplements That May Interact with Colocynth

- Increased risk of potassium depletion when used in conjunction with horsetail plant or licorice.
- Increased risk of potassium depletion when used with other stimulant laxative herbs, such as black root, cascara sagrada, castor oil, and senna. (For a list of stimulant laxative herbs and supplements, see Appendix B.)

COLOMBO

Colombo was first recorded in herbal medicine in 1671, when Portuguese traders brought it back to Europe from Africa. A gentle but very effective digestive bitter, colombo is commonly cultivated as a medicinal plant in Brazil, where herbalists use the root to treat poor digestion, loss of appetite, low stomach acid, diarrhea, and flatulence.

Scientific Name

Jateorhiza palmata

Colombo Is Also Commonly Known As

Calomba root, calumba

Medicinal Parts

Root

Colombo's Uses

To treat diarrhea, gastritis, dyspepsia, and colitis

Typical Dose

A typical dose of colombo is approximately 2 tsp of boiled root strained and taken as a tea every hour.

Possible Side Effects

Colombo's side effects include vomiting and stomach pain.

Drugs That May Interact with Colombo

Taking colombo with these drugs may interfere with the action of the drug:

- aluminum hydroxide (AlternaGel, Alu-Cap)
- aluminum hydroxide and magnesium carbonate (Gaviscon Extra Strength, Gaviscon Liquid)
- aluminum hydroxide and magnesium hydroxide (Maalox, Rulox)
- aluminum hydroxide and magnesium trisilicate (Gaviscon Tablet)
- aluminum hydroxide, magnesium hydroxide, and simethicone (Maalox, Mylanta Liquid)
- calcium carbonate (Rolaids Extra Strength, Tums)
- calcium carbonate and magnesium hydroxide (Mylanta Gelcaps, Rolaids Extra Strength)
- cimetidine (Nu-Cimet, Tagamet)
- esomeprazole (Nexium)
- famotidine (Apo-Famotidine, Pepcid)
- famotidine, calcium carbonate, and magnesium hydroxide (Pepcid Complete)
- lansoprazole (Prevacid)
- magaldrate and simethicone (Riopan Plus, Riopan Plus Double Strength)

- magnesium hydroxide (Dulcolax Milk of Magnesia, Phillips' Milk of Magnesia)
- magnesium oxide (Mag-Ox 400, Uro-Mag)
- magnesium sulfate (Epsom salts)
- nizatidine (Axid, PMS-Nizatidine)
- omeprazole (Losec, Prilosec)
- pantoprazole (Pantoloc, Protonix)
- rabeprazole (Aciphex, Pariet)
- ranitidine (Alti-Ranitidine, Zantac)
- sodium bicarbonate (Brioschi, Neut)

Lab Tests That May Be Altered by Colombo
None known

Diseases That May Be Worsened or Triggered by Colombo
None known

Foods That May Interact with Colombo
None known

Supplements That May Interact with Colombo
None known

Colt's Foot

Colt's foot takes its name from the shape of its leaves, which resemble a horse's hoof. The ancient Greeks and Romans believed that smoking colt's foot leaves was an effective treatment for coughs and colds—a practice that continued for some fifteen hundred years. Today colt's foot is still used for respiratory problems, but instead of being smoked, it's taken in the form of a tincture, juice, or infusion.

Scientific Name
Tussilago farfara

Colt's Foot Is Also Commonly Known As
British tobacco, bullsfoot, foalswort, horsehoof

Medicinal Parts
Leaf, flower, root

Colt's Foot's Uses
To treat asthma, cough, and bronchitis. Germany's Commission E has approved the use of colt's foot to treat cough, bronchitis, and inflammation of the mouth and throat.

Typical Dose
A typical daily dose of colt's foot may range from 0.6–2 mL fluid extract three times a day.

Possible Side Effects
Colt's foot's side effects include elevated blood pressure, fever, diarrhea, and nausea.

Drugs That May Interact with Colt's Foot
Taking colt's foot with these drugs may cause or increase liver damage:
- abacavir (Ziagen)
- acarbose (Prandase, Precose)
- acetaminophen (Genapap, Tylenol)
- allopurinol (Aloprim, Zyloprim)
- atorvastatin (Lipitor)
- celecoxib (Celebrex)
- cidofovir (Vistide)
- cyclosporine (Neoral, Sandimmune)
- docetaxel (Taxotere)
- dofetilide (Tikosyn)
- erythromycin (Erythrocin, Staticin)

- etodolac (Lodine, Utradol)
- fluconazole (Apo-Fluconazole, Diflucan)
- fluphenazine (Modecate, Prolixin)
- fluvastatin (Lescol)
- foscarnet (Foscavir)
- ganciclovir (Cytovene, Vitrasert)
- gemfibrozil (Apo-Gemfibrozil, Lopid)
- gentamicin (Alcomicin, Gentacidin)
- ibuprofen (Advil, Motrin)
- indinavir (Crixivan)
- isoniazid (Isotamine, Nydrazid)
- ketoconazole (Apo-Ketoconazole, Nizoral)
- ketoprofen (Orudis, Rhodis)
- ketorolac (Acular, Toradol)
- lamivudine (Epivir, Heptovir)
- levodopa-carbidopa (Nu-Levocarb, Sinemet)
- lovastatin (Altocor, Mevacor)
- meloxicam (MOBIC, Mobicox)
- methotrexate (Rheumatrex, Trexall)
- methyldopa (Apo-Methyldopa, Nu-Medopa)
- morphine hydrochloride
- morphine sulfate (Kadian, MS Contin)
- naproxen (Aleve, Naprosyn)
- nelfinavir (Viracept)
- nevirapine (Viramune)
- nitrofurantoin (Furadantin, Macrobid)
- ondansetron (Zofran)
- paclitaxel (Onxol, Taxol)
- pantoprazole (Pantoloc, Protonix)
- phenytoin (Dilantin, Phenytek)
- pioglitazone (Actos)
- piroxicam (Feldene, Nu-Pirox)
- pravastatin (Novo-Pravastatin, Pravachol)
- prochlorperazine (Compazine, Compro)
- propoxyphene (Darvon, Darvon-N)
- repaglinide (GlucoNorm, Prandin)
- rifampin (Rifadin, Rimactane)
- rifapentine (Priftin)
- ritonavir (Norvir)
- rofecoxib (Vioxx)
- rosiglitazone (Avandia)
- saquinavir (Fortovase, Invirase)
- simvastatin (Apo-Simvastatin, Zocor)
- stavudine (Zerit)
- tamoxifen (Nolvadex, Tamofen)
- tramadol (Ultram)
- zidovudine (Novo-AZT, Retrovir)

Lab Tests That May Be Altered by Colt's Foot
None known

Diseases That May Be Worsened or Triggered by Colt's Foot
- May interfere with treatment for elevated blood pressure or cardiovascular disease, if taken in large amounts.
- May worsen liver disease.

Foods That May Interact with Colt's Foot
None known

Supplements That May Interact with Colt's Foot
- Increased risk of unsaturated pyrrolizidine alkaloid (UPA) toxicity when used with eucalyptus.
- Increased risk of additive toxicity when used with herbs and supplements containing unsaturated pyrrolizidine alkaloids (UPAs), such as butterbur and comfrey. (For a list of herbs and supplements containing unsaturated pyrrolizidine alkaloids, see Appendix B.)

Comfrey

> Applied in cream form or as a poultice, comfey, also known as bruisewort, has long been used to heal bruises and other tissue damage, as it contains allantoin, a substance that stimulates the growth of new cells. However, it also contains pyrrolizidine alkaloids that, when ingested over a period of time, may cause liver cancer, so internal use is not recommended.

Scientific Name
Symphytum officinale

Comfrey Is Also Commonly Known As
Black root, bruisewort, slippery root, wallwort

Medicinal Parts
Leaf, root

Comfrey's Uses
To treat gum disease, strep throat, inflammation of the throat, stomach ulcers, bruises, sprains, and pulled ligaments and muscles; to promote bone healing. Germany's Commission E has approved the use of comfrey to treat blunt injuries.

Typical Dose
Internal use is no longer recommended because of the potential for liver damage. For external use, topical products containing comfrey (5 to 20 percent of dried herb present in product) may be used as needed, but not for longer than four weeks and only on unbroken skin.

Possible Side Effects
Comfrey's side effects include allergic reactions (from oral or topical use) and nausea, vomiting, abdominal pain, liver damage, and liver cancer (from oral use).

Drugs That May Interact with Comfrey
Taking comfrey internally with these drugs may cause or increase liver damage:
- abacavir (Ziagen)
- acarbose (Prandase, Precose)
- acetaminophen (Genapap, Tylenol)
- allopurinol (Aloprim, Zyloprim)
- atorvastatin (Lipitor)
- celecoxib (Celebrex)
- cidofovir (Vistide)
- cyclosporine (Neoral, Sandimmune)
- docetaxel (Taxotere)
- dofetilide (Tikosyn)
- erythromycin (Erythrocin, Staticin)
- etodolac (Lodine, Utradol)
- fluconazole (Apo-Fluconazole, Diflucan)
- fluphenazine (Modecate, Prolixin)
- fluvastatin (Lescol)
- foscarnet (Foscavir)
- ganciclovir (Cytovene, Vitrasert)
- gemfibrozil (Apo-Gemfibrozil, Lopid)
- gentamicin (Alcomicin, Gentacidin)
- ibuprofen (Advil, Motrin)
- indinavir (Crixivan)
- isoniazid (Isotamine, Nydrazid)
- ketoconazole (Apo-Ketoconazole, Nizoral)
- ketoprofen (Orudis, Rhodis)
- ketorolac (Acular, Toradol)
- lamivudine (Epivir, Heptovir)
- levodopa-carbidopa (Nu-Levocarb, Sinemet)
- lovastatin (Altocor, Mevacor)
- meloxicam (MOBIC, Mobicox)
- methotrexate (Rheumatrex, Trexall)
- methyldopa (Apo-Methyldopa, Nu-Medopa)
- morphine hydrochloride

- morphine sulfate (Kadian, MS Contin)
- naproxen (Aleve, Naprosyn)
- nelfinavir (Viracept)
- nevirapine (Viramune)
- nitrofurantoin (Macrobid, Furadantin)
- ondansetron (Zofran)
- paclitaxel (Onxol, Taxol)
- pantoprazole (Pantoloc, Protonix)
- phenytoin (Dilantin, Phenytek)
- pioglitazone (Actos)
- piroxicam (Feldene, Nu-Pirox)
- pravastatin (Novo-Pravastatin, Pravachol)
- prochlorperazine (Compazine, Compro)
- propoxyphene (Darvon, Darvon-N)
- repaglinide (GlucoNorm, Prandin)
- rifampin (Rifadin, Rimactane)
- rifapentine (Priftin)
- ritonavir (Norvir)
- rofecoxib (Vioxx)
- rosiglitazone (Avandia)
- saquinavir (Fortovase, Invirase)
- simvastatin (Apo-Simvastatin, Zocor)
- stavudine (Zerit)
- tamoxifen (Nolvadex, Tamofen)
- tramadol (Ultram)
- zidovudine (Novo-AZT, Retrovir)

Lab Tests That May Be Altered by Comfrey

May increase values on liver function tests, including aspartic acid transaminase (AST), alanine aminotransferase (ALT), total bilirubin, and urine bilirubin.

Diseases That May Be Worsened or Triggered by Comfrey

May worsen liver disease.

Foods That May Interact with Comfrey

None known

Supplements That May Interact with Comfrey

- May increase the risk of liver damage when combined with herbs and supplements that can cause hepatotoxicity (destructive effects on the liver), such as bishop's weed, borage, chaparral, uva ursi, and others. (For a list of herbs and supplements that can cause hepatotoxicity, see Appendix B.)
- Enhanced toxicity when taken with herbs and supplements that induce Cytochrome P450 3A4, such as garlic and St. John's wort.
- Increased risk of additive toxicity when used with herbs and supplements containing unsaturated pyrrolizidine alkaloids (UPAs), such as butterbur and colt's foot. (For a list of herbs and supplements containing unsaturated pyrrolizidine alkaloids, see Appendix B.)

CORDYCEPS

Cordyceps, also known as caterpillar fungus or winter worm summer grass, is a fungus that begins its life cycle by growing in the backs of caterpillars and later becomes a tiny grasslike mushroom. Some fifteen hundred years ago, Tibetan shepherds noticed that when their sheep and yaks grazed on this little mushroom, they had much more energy and endurance. During the Ming Dynasty, Chinese royalty ate cordyceps cooked inside the stomach of a duck to increase energy and ward off illnesses. Long used in traditional Chinese medicine to restore energy, promote longevity, stimulate the immune system, and improve the quality of life, cordyceps was virtually unheard of in the western world until 1993, when the Chinese women's track team broke records in the world track and field championships. Their secret, they claimed, was none other than good old caterpillar fungus.

Scientific Name
Cordyceps sinensis

Cordyceps Is Also Commonly Known As
Caterpillar fungus, dong chong xia cao, vegetable caterpillar, winter worm summer grass

Medicinal Parts
Mycellium (main body of the fungus)

Cordyceps's Uses
To improve athletic performance, strengthen the immune system, reduce effects of aging, and promote longevity

Typical Dose
A typical daily dose of cordyceps is approximately 3 gm of fermented *cordyceps sinensis*.

Possible Side Effects
There is little scientific information about cordyceps's potential side effects.

Drugs That May Interact with Cordyceps
Taking cordyceps with these drugs may interfere with the action of the drug:
- cyclophosphamide (Cytoxan, Neosar)
- prednisolone (Inflamase Forte, Pred Forte)

Taking cordyceps with this drug may be harmful:
- fondaparinux (Arixtra)—may increase the risk of bleeding or bruising

Lab Tests That May Be Altered by Cordyceps
Improved liver function in those with chronic hepatitis B.

Diseases That May Be Worsened or Triggered by Cordyceps
None known

Foods That May Interact with Cordyceps
None known

Supplements That May Interact with Cordyceps
None known

CORIANDER

> Pliny, the famous Roman scholar and encyclopedist, named this cousin of the parsley plant *coriandrum*, taken from *coris*, which means "bug," possibly because the coriander seed resembles a European bedbug. Coriander seed is used as an aromatic stimulant, a remedy for flatulence and poor appetite, and to improve digestion, while the seed oil is strongly antibacterial. In studies with laboratory animals, coriander lowered total cholesterol, LDL "bad" cholesterol, and blood fats, while increasing HDL "good" cholesterol.

Scientific Name
Coriandrum sativum

Coriander Is Also Commonly Known As
Chinese parsley, cilantro

Medicinal Parts
Leaf, fruit, seed, oil of seed

Coriander's Uses
To treat digestive complaints, headaches, halitosis, and postpartum complications. Germany's Com-

mission E has approved the use of coriander to treat loss of appetite and dyspeptic complaints, such as heartburn and bloating.

Typical Dose

A typical daily dose of coriander is 3.0 gm of the crushed and powdered herb in divided doses.

Possible Side Effects

Coriander's side effects include nausea, vomiting, anorexia, and allergic reactions such as hay fever, dermatitis, or allergic asthma.

Drugs That May Interact with Coriander

Taking coriander with these drugs may increase skin sensitivity to sunlight:
- bumetanide (Bumex, Burinex)
- celecoxib (Celebrex)
- ciprofloxacin (Ciloxan, Cipro)
- doxycycline (Apo-Doxy, Vibramycin)
- enalapril (Vasotec)
- etodolac (Lodine, Utradol)
- fluphenazine (Modecate, Prolixin)
- fosinopril (Monopril)
- furosemide (Apo-Furosemide, Lasix)
- gatifloxacin (Tequin, Zymar)
- hydrochlorothiazide (Apo-Hydro, Microzide)
- ibuprofen (Advil, Motrin)
- indomethacin (Indocin, Novo-Methacin)
- ketoprofen (Orudis, Rhodis)
- ketorolac (Acular, Toradol)
- lansoprazole (Prevacid)
- levofloxacin (Levaquin, Quixin)
- lisinopril (Prinivil, Zestril)
- loratadine (Alavert, Claritin)
- methotrexate (Rheumatrex, Trexall)
- naproxen (Aleve, Naprosyn)
- nortriptyline (Aventyl HCl, Pamelor)
- ofloxacin (Floxin, Ocuflox)
- omeprazole (Losec, Prilosec)
- phenytoin (Dilantin, Phenytek)
- piroxicam (Feldene, Nu-Pirox)
- prochlorperazine (Compazine, Compro)
- quinapril (Accupril)
- risperidone (Risperdal)
- rofecoxib (Vioxx)
- tetracycline (Novo-Tetra, Sumycin)

Taking coriander may increase the risk of hypoglycemia (low blood sugar):
- acarbose (Prandase, Precose)
- acetohexamide
- chlorpropamide (Diabinese, Novo-Propamide)
- gliclazide (Diamicron, Novo-Gliclazide)
- glimepiride (Amaryl)
- glipizide (Glucotrol)
- glipizide and metformin (Metaglip)
- gliquidone (Beglynor, Glurenorm)
- glyburide (DiaBeta, Micronase)
- glyburide and metformin (Glucovance)
- metformin (Glucophage, Riomet)
- miglitol (Glyset)
- nateglinide (Starlix)
- pioglitazone (Actos)
- repaglinide (GlucoNorm, Prandin)
- rosiglitazone (Avandia)
- rosiglitazone and metformin (Avandamet)
- tolazamide (Tolinase)
- tolbutamide (Apo-Tolbutamide, Tol-Tab)

Lab Tests That May Be Altered by Coriander
None known

Diseases That May Be Worsened or Triggered by Coriander
None known

Foods That May Interact with Coriander
None known

Supplements That May Interact with Coriander
None known

CORKWOOD

The small Australian corkwood tree grows on the margins of rain forests and is named for its soft, corky, yellow-gray bark. Its leaves contain an alkaloid called duboisine, which is very similar to the drug hyoscyamine, used to treat bladder spasms, pancreatitis, and disorders of the gastrointestinal tract, and to control the symptoms of Parkinson's disease.

Scientific Name
Duboisia myoporoides

Corkwood Is Also Commonly Known As
Pituri

Medicinal Parts
Leaf, stem, root

Corkwood's Uses
To ease hunger, pain, and fatigue; to prevent nausea and vomiting due to motion sickness; to decrease gastrointestinal spasms

Typical Dose
There is no typical dose of corkwood.

Possible Side Effects
Corkwood's side effects include confusion, anxiety, restlessness, and dizziness.

Drugs That May Interact with Corkwood
Taking corkwood with these drugs may enhance the drug's therapeutic and/or adverse effects:

- acetaminophen and codeine (Capital and Codeine, Tylenol with Codeine)
- acetaminophen, chlorpheniramine, and pseudoephedrine (Children's Tylenol Plus Cold, Sinutab Sinus Allergy Maximum Strength)
- acetaminophen, dextromethorphan, and pseudoephedrine (Alka-Seltzer Plus Flu Liqui-Gels, Sudafed Severe Cold)
- acrivastine and pseudoephedrine (Semprex-D)
- alfentanil (Alfenta)
- amitriptyline (Elavil, Levate)
- amitriptyline and chlordiazepoxide (Limbitrol)
- amitriptyline and perphenazine (Etrafon, Triavil)
- amoxapine (Asendin)
- aspirin and codeine (Coryphen Codeine)
- azatadine (Optimine)
- azatadine and pseudoephedrine (Rynatan Tablet, Trinalin)
- azelastine (Astelin, Optivar)
- belladonna and opium (B&O Supprettes)
- brompheniramine and pseudoephedrine (Children's Dimetapp Elixir Cold & Allergy, Lodrane)
- buprenorphine (Buprenex, Subutex)
- buprenorphine and naloxone (Suboxone)
- butorphanol (Apo-Butorphanol, Stadol)
- carbinoxamine (Histex CT, Histex PD)
- carbinoxamine and pseudoephedrine (Rondec Drops, Sildec)
- carbinoxamine, pseudoephedrine, and dextromethorphan (Rondec-DM Drops, Tussafed)
- cetirizine (Reactine, Zyrtec)
- chlorpheniramine and acetaminophen (Coricidin HBP Cold and Flu)
- chlorpheniramine and phenylephrine (Histatab Plus, Rynatan)

- chlorpheniramine, ephedrine, phenylephrine, and carbetapentane (Rynatuss, Tynatuss Pediatric)
- chlorpheniramine, phenylephrine, and dextromethorphan (Alka-Seltzer Plus Cold and Cough)
- chlorpheniramine, phenylephrine, and methscopolamine (AH-Chew, Extendryl)
- chlorpheniramine, phenylephrine, and phenyltoloxamine (Comhist, Nalex-A)
- chlorpheniramine, phenylephrine, codeine, and potassium iodide (Pediacof)
- chlorpheniramine, pseudoephedrine, and codeine (Dihistine DH, Ryna-C)
- chlorpheniramine, pseudoephedrine, and dextromethorphan (Robitussin Pediatric Night Relief, Vicks Pediatric 44M)
- chlorpromazine (Largactil, Thorazine)
- cimetidine (Nu-Cimet, Tagamet)
- clemastine (Tavist Allergy)
- clomipramine (Anafranil, Novo-Clopramine)
- codeine (Codeine Contin)
- cyclobenzaprine (Flexeril, Novo-Cycloprine)
- cyproheptadine (Periactin)
- deptropine (Deptropine FNA)
- desipramine (Alti-Desipramine, Norpramin)
- desloratadine (Aerius, Clarinex)
- dexbrompheniramine and pseudoephedrine (Drixomed, Drixoral Cold & Allergy)
- dexchlorpheniramine (Polaramine)
- dihydrocodeine, aspirin, and caffeine (Synalgos-DC)
- dimethindene (Fenistil)
- diphenhydramine (Benadryl Allergy, Nytol)
- diphenhydramine and pseudoephedrine (Benadryl Allergy/Decongestant, Benadryl Children's Allergy and Sinus)
- doxepin (Sinequan, Zonalon)
- epinastine (Elestat)
- famotidine (Apo-Famotidine, Pepcid)
- fentanyl (Actiq, Duragesic)
- fexofenadine (Allegra)
- fexofenadine and pseudoephedrine (Allegra-D)
- fluphenazine (Modecate, Prolixin)
- haloperidol (Haldol, Novo-Peridol)
- hydrocodone and acetaminophen (Zydone, Vicodin)
- hydrocodone and aspirin (Damason-P)
- hydrocodone and chlorpheniramine (Tussionex)
- hydrocodone and ibuprofen (Vicoprofen)
- hydrocodone, carbinoxamine, and pseudoephedrine (Histex HC, Tri-Vent HC)
- hydromorphone (Dilaudid, PMS-Hydromorphone)
- hydroxyzine (Atarax, Vistaril)
- imipramine (Apo-Imipramine, Tofranil)
- ketotifen (Novo-Ketotifen, Zaditor)
- levocabastine (Livostin)
- levomethadyl acetate hydrochloride
- levorphanol (LevoDromoran)
- lofepramine (Feprapax, Gamanil)
- loratadine (Alavert, Claritin)
- loratadine and pseudoephedrine (Claritin-D 12 Hour, Claritin-D 24 Hour)
- mebhydrolin (Bexidal, Incidal)
- melitracen (Dixeran)
- meperidine (Demerol, Meperitab)
- meperidine and promethazine
- mesoridazine (Serentil)
- methadone (Dolophine, Methadose)
- mizolastine (Elina, Mizollen)
- morphine sulfate (Kadian, MS Contin)
- nalbuphine (Nubain)
- nizatidine (Axid, PMS-Nizatidine)
- nortriptyline (Aventyl HCl, Pamelor)
- olopatadine (Patanol)
- opium tincture

- oxatomide (Cenacert, Tinset)
- oxycodone (OxyContin, Roxicodone)
- oxycodone and acetaminophen (Endocet, Percocet)
- oxycodone and aspirin (Endodan, Percodan)
- oxymorphone (Numorphan)
- paregoric
- pentazocine (Talwin)
- perphenazine (Apo-Perphenazine, Trilafon)
- phenoperidine
- prochlorperazine (Compazine, Compro)
- promethazine (Phenergan)
- promethazine and codeine (Phenergan with Codeine)
- promethazine and dextromethorphan (Promatussin DM)
- promethazine and phenylephrine
- promethazine, phenylephrine, and codeine
- propoxyphene (Darvon, Darvon N)
- propoxyphene and acetaminophen (Darvocet-N 50, Darvocet-N 100)
- propoxyphene, aspirin, and caffeine (Darvon Compound)
- protriptyline (Vivactil)
- ranitidine (Alti-Ranitidine, Zantac)
- remifentanil (Ultiva)
- sufentanil (Sufenta)
- thiethylperazine (Torecan)
- thioridazine (Mellaril)
- thiothixene (Navane)
- trifluoperazine (Novo-Trifluzine, Stelazine)
- trimipramine (Apo-Trimip, Surmontil)
- tripelennamine (PBZ, PBZ-SR)
- triprolidine and pseudoephedrine (Actifed Cold and Allergy, Silafed)
- triprolidine, pseudoephedrine, and codeine (CoActifed, Covan)

Lab Tests That May Be Altered by Corkwood
None known

Diseases That May Be Worsened or Triggered by Corkwood
None known

Foods That May Interact with Corkwood
None known

Supplements That May Interact with Corkwood
None known

CORN SILK

Corn silk, the long, silky, yellow threads that grow between the leaves and ears of corn, gets its scientific name from the Greek word *zea*, which means "to live," and the Spanish word *maiz*, the name used for corn in Haiti, where corn is believed to have originated. The corn silk threads, which are the female portion of the corn plant, are gathered once the plant sheds its pollen and used in the form of tea or powder to treat urinary problems.

Scientific Name
Zea mays

Corn Silk Is Also Commonly Known As
Indian corn, maize silk, stigmata maydis

Medicinal Parts
Flower stigma

Corn Silk's Uses
To treat disorders of the liver and urinary tract

Typical Dose

A typical daily dose of corn silk may range from 4 to 8 gm of dried stigma.

Possible Side Effects

Corn silk's side effects include lowered levels of potassium in the blood.

Drugs That May Interact with Corn Silk

Taking corn silk with these drugs may increase the risk of hypokalemia (low levels of potassium in the blood):

- acetazolamide (Apo-Acetazolamide, Diamox Sequels)
- azosemide (Diat)
- bumetanide (Bumex, Burinex)
- chlorothiazide (Diuril)
- chlorthalidone (Apo-Chlorthalidone, Thalitone)
- ethacrynic acid (Edecrin)
- etozolin (Elkapin)
- furosemide (Apo-Furosemide, Lasix)
- hydrochlorothiazide (Apo-Hydro, Microzide)
- hydroflumethiazide (Diucardin, Saluron)
- indapamide (Lozol, Nu-Indapamide)
- mannitol (Osmitrol, Resectisol)
- mefruside (Baycaron)
- methazolamide (Apo-Methazolamide, Neptazane)
- methyclothiazide (Aquatensen, Enduron)
- metolazone (Mykrox, Zaroxolyn)
- olmesartan and hydrochlorothiazide (Benicar HCT)
- polythiazide (Renese)
- torsemide (Demadex)
- trichlormethiazide (Metatensin, Naqua)
- urea (Amino-Cerv, UltraMide)
- xipamide (Diurexan, Lumitens)

Taking corn silk with this drug may be harmful:

- warfarin (Coumadin, Jantoven)—may increase risk of bleeding or bruising

Lab Tests That May Be Altered by Corn Silk

None known

Diseases That May Be Worsened or Triggered by Corn Silk

- May interfere with control of blood sugar in diabetes.
- May interfere with control of blood pressure in those with elevated or lowered blood pressure.
- May worsen cases of potassium loss.

Foods That May Interact with Corn Silk

None known

Supplements That May Interact with Corn Silk

None known

COUNTRY MALLOW

Used for two thousand years in India to treat asthma, colds, flu, headache, and joint aches, this common weed is found throughout India and Sri Lanka. Country mallow contains ephedrine alkaloids like those found in ma-huang, but in smaller quantities, making it a popular alternative to ma-huang for the treatment of asthma, fatigue, and obesity.

Scientific Name

Sida cordifolia

Country Mallow Is Also Commonly Known As
Bala, heartleaf, vatya

Medicinal Parts
Root, leaf, seed

Country Mallow's Uses
To treat asthma, colds, and flu; to strengthen the skeletal system; to aid in weight loss and fat burning; to increase energy

Typical Dose
A typical dose of country mallow may range from 0.5 to 1.0 gm of the powdered root, leaves, and/or seeds two times daily, or 15 to 30 ml of fresh juice two times daily.

Possible Side Effects
Country mallow's side effects include dizziness, irritability, insomnia, and heart palpitations.

Drugs That May Interact with Country Mallow
Taking country mallow with these drugs may increase the risk of hypoglycemia (low blood sugar):
- acarbose (Prandase, Precose)
- acetohexamide
- chlorpropamide (Diabinese, Novo-Propamide)
- gliclazide (Diamicron, Novo-Gliclazide)
- glimepiride (Amaryl)
- glipizide (Glucotrol)
- glipizide and metformin (Metaglip)
- gliquidone (Beglynor, Glurenorm)
- glyburide (DiaBeta, Micronase)
- glyburide and metformin (Glucovance)
- insulin (Humulin, Novolin R)
- metformin (Glucophage, Riomet)
- miglitol (Glyset)
- nateglinide (Starlix)
- pioglitazone (Actos)
- repaglinide (GlucoNorm, Prandin)
- rosiglitazone (Avandia)
- rosiglitazone and metformin (Avandamet)
- tolazamide (Tolinase)
- tolbutamide (Apo-Tolbutamide, Tol-Tab)

Taking country mallow with these drugs may increase the risk of hypertension (high blood pressure):
- belladonna, phenobarbital, and ergotamine (Bellamine S, Bel-Tabs)
- bromocriptine (Apo-Bromocriptine, Parlodel)
- cabergoline (Dostinex)
- dihydroergotamine (Migranal)
- ergoloid mesylates (Hydergine)
- ergonovine
- ergotamine (Cafergor, Cafergot)
- iproniazid (Marsilid)
- methylergonovine (Methergine)
- methysergide (Sansert)
- moclobemide (Alti-Moclobemide, Nu-Moclobemide)
- pergolide (Permax)
- phenelzine (Nardil)
- selegiline (Eldepryl)
- tranylcypromine (Parnate)

Taking country mallow with these drugs may increase the risk of adverse effects:
- pentoxifylline (Pentoxil, Trental)
- theophylline (Elixophyllin, Theochron)
- theophylline and guaifenesin (Elixophyllin-GC, Quibron)

Taking country mallow with this drug may be harmful:
- dexamethasone (Decadron, Dexasone)—may reduce the drug's effectiveness

Lab Tests That May Be Altered by Country Mallow

- May increase or decrease blood glucose levels.
- Positive urine tests for ephedrine (a constituent of country mallow), which is typically banned by athletic organizations.

Diseases That May Be Worsened or Triggered by Country Mallow

- May encourage the formation of kidney stones.
- May increase anxiety.
- May worsen anorexia by diminishing the appetite.
- May worsen cases of benign prostatic hypertrophy (BPH) by causing the bladder to retain urine.
- May worsen cases of cardiovascular disease by causing the heart to beat rapidly or irregularly, by raising blood pressure, or by triggering angina.
- May worsen cases of essential tremor.
- May worsen cases of hyperthyroid by stimulating the thyroid gland.
- May worsen cases of poor blood flow to the brain by constricting blood vessels.
- May worsen cases of narrow-angle glaucoma.
- May worsen diabetes by interfering with control of blood sugar.

Foods That May Interact with Country Mallow

Increased stimulatory and adverse effects of caffeine and ephedrine when taken with caffeine-containing beverages, due to ephedrine content of country mallow. (For a list of herbs, foods, and supplements that contain caffeine, see Appendix B.)

Supplements That May Interact with Country Mallow

- Increased risk of hypertension and adverse cardiovascular effects when used with herbs and supplements that have stimulant properties, such as caffeine, coffee, cola nut, ma-huang, and others. (For a list of herbs and supplements that have stimulant properties, see Appendix B.)
- Increased risk of cardiac arrhythmias when used with digitalis.
- Increased risk of hypertension (elevated blood pressure) when used with secale alkaloid derivatives (ergot).

COWHAGE

The cowhage plant is found in Asia, South America, Africa, and the Fiji Islands, and has crooked seed pods covered with stinging hairs that stick to the fingers and cause intense itching. But when these hairs are mixed with syrup, molasses, or honey and taken internally, they pierce the bodies of worms, which detach themselves from intestinal walls and can be whisked alive out of the body with a cathartic. Not surprisingly, inflammation of the small intestine sometimes follows its use.

Scientific Name

Mucuna pruriens

Cowhage Is Also Commonly Known As

Couhage, cowitch, kiwach

Medicinal Parts

Hairs from the pod and seed

Cowhage's Uses

To treat worm infestation, muscle pain, and rheumatism

Typical Dose

A typical dose of cowhage has not been determined.

Possible Side Effects

Cowhage's side effects include itching, burning, headache, and sweating.

Drugs That May Interact with Cowhage

Taking cowhage with these drugs may reduce the effectiveness of the drug:

- acetophenazine
- aniracetam (Ampamet, Draganon)
- aripiprazole (Abilify)
- benperidol (Anquil, Glianimon)
- bromperidol (Impromen, Tesoprel)
- chlorpromazine (Largactil, Thorazine)
- clozapine (Clozaril, Gen-Clozapine)
- droperidol (Inapsine)
- flupenthixol (Fluanxol)
- fluphenazine (Modecate, Prolixin)
- haloperidol (Haldol, Novo-Peridol)
- loxapine (Loxitane, Nu-Loxapine)
- mesoridazine (Serentil)
- molindone (Moban)
- olanzapine (Zydis, Zyprexa)
- perphenazine (Apo-Perphenazine, Trilafon)
- pimozide (Orap)
- pipamperone (Dipiperon, Piperonil)
- piracetam (Geram, Piracetam Verla)
- prochlorperazine (Compazine, Compro)
- quetiapine (Seroquel)
- risperidone (Risperdal)
- thioridazine (Mellaril)
- thiothixene (Navane)
- trifluoperazine (Novo-Trifluzine, Stelazine)
- ziprasidone (Geodon)—used for schizophrenia
- zuclopenthixol (Clopixol)

Taking cowhage with this drug may increase the risk of a hypertensive crisis (excessively high blood pressure):

- phenelzine (Nardil)
- tranylcypromine (Parnate)

Lab Tests That May Be Altered by Cowhage

- May cause false decrease in glucose oxidase test (e.g., Clinistix).
- May cause false increases in cupric sulfate test (e.g., Clinitest).

Diseases That May Be Worsened or Triggered by Cowhage

- May worsen cardiovascular disease because the herb contains L-dopa, which can cause irregular heartbeat and other problems.
- May push blood sugar too low in diabetes or hypoglycemia (low blood sugar).
- May worsen psychiatric diseases due to its L-dopa content.

Foods That May Interact with Cowhage

None known

Supplements That May Interact with Cowhage

- May increase blood glucose–lowering effects and risk of hypoglycemia (low blood sugar) when used with herbs and supplements that lower glucose levels, such as alpha-lipoic acid, chromium, devil's claw, Panax ginseng, and psyllium. (For a list of herbs and supplements that lower blood glucose levels, see Appendix B.)
- Kava kava and vitamin B_6 may reduce cowhage's effects by counteracting the L-dopa in cowhage.

COWSLIP

In ancient times, the shape of the cowslip, a relative of the primrose, was thought to resemble a bunch of keys. The flower was dedicated to the Virgin Mary, thus its various common names: our lady's keys, key of heaven, and key flower. Used traditionally to treat respiratory conditions, cowslip has been shown in some studies to relieve symptoms of bronchitis just as well as standard medications.

Scientific Name
Primula veris

Cowslip Is Also Commonly Known As
Butter rose, key flower, key of heaven, mayflower, our lady's keys, oxlip

Medicinal Parts
Flower, root

Cowslip's Uses
Cowslip flower is used to treat insomnia, dizziness, headaches, bronchitis, and anxiety. Cowslip root is used to treat whooping cough, gout, bladder and kidney disease, rheumatoid arthritis, stomach cramps, and headaches. Germany's Commission E has approved the use of cowslip flower and cowslip root to treat cough and bronchitis.

Typical Dose
A typical dose of cowslip flower is 1 to 2 ml of liquid extract, taken three times a day.

Possible Side Effects
No side effects are known when cowslip is taken in recommended therapeutic dosages. However, allergic reactions are possible.

Drugs That May Interact with Cowslip
Taking cowslip with these drugs may increase the drug's effects:

- acetazolamide (Apo-Acetazolamide, Diamox Sequels)
- alprazolam (Apo-Alpraz, Xanax)
- amiloride (Midamor)
- amobarbital (Amytal)
- aspirin and meprobamate (Equagesic, 292 MEP)
- azosemide (Diat)
- bumetanide (Bumex, Burinex)
- buspirone (BuSpar, Nu-Buspirone)
- butabarbital (Butisol Sodium)
- carpipramine (Defecton, Prazinil)
- chloral hydrate (Aquachloral Supprettes, Somnote)
- chlordiazepoxide (Apo-Chlordiazepoxide, Librium)
- chlorothiazide (Diuril)
- chlorthalidone (Apo-Chlorthalidone, Thalitone)
- clorazepate (Tranxene, T-Tab)
- dexmedetomidine (Precedex)
- diazepam (Apo-Diazepam, Valium)
- diphenhydramine (Benadryl Allergy, Nytol)
- doxepin (Sinequan, Zonalon)
- estazolam (ProSom)
- ethacrynic acid (Edecrin)
- etozolin (Elkapin)
- flurazepam (Apo-Flurazepam, Dalmane)
- furosemide (Apo-Furosemide, Lasix)
- glutethimide
- haloperidol (Haldol, Novo-Peridol)
- hydrochlorothiazide (Apo-Hydro, Microzide)
- hydrochlorothiazide and triamterene (Dyazide, Maxzide)
- hydroflumethiazide (Diucardin, Saluron)
- hydroxyzine (Atarax, Vistaril)
- indapamide (Lozol, Nu-Indapamide)

- lorazepam (Ativan, Nu-Loraz)
- mannitol (Osmitrol, Resectisol)
- mefruside (Baycaron)
- mephobarbital (Mebaral)
- meprobamate (Miltown, Novo-Mepro)
- methazolamide (Apo-Methazolamide, Neptazane)
- methyclothiazide (Aquatensen, Enduron)
- metolazone (Mykrox, Zaroxolyn)
- midazolam (Apo-Midazolam, Versed)
- olmesartan and hydrochlorothiazide (Benicar HCT)
- oxazepam (Novoxapam, Serax)
- pentazocine (Talwin)
- pentobarbital (Nembutal)
- phenobarbital (Luminal Sodium, PMS-Phenobarbital)
- polythiazide (Renese)
- promethazine (Phenergan)
- propofol (Diprivan)
- quazepam (Doral)
- secobarbital (Seconal)
- spironolactone (Aldactone, Novo-Spiroton)
- temazepam (Novo-Temazepam, Restoril)
- thiopental (Pentothal)
- torsemide (Demadex)
- triamterene (Dyrenium)
- triazolam (Apo-Triazo, Halcion)
- trichlormethiazide (Metatensin, Naqua)
- trifluoperazine (Novo-Trifluzine, Stelazine)
- urea (Amino-Cerv, UltraMide)
- xipamide (Diurexan, Lumitens)
- zaleplon (Sonata, Stamoc)
- zolpidem (Ambien)
- zopiclone (Alti-Zopiclone, Gen-Zopiclone)

Lab Tests That May Be Altered by Cowslip
None known

Diseases That May Be Worsened or Triggered by Cowslip
None known

Foods That May Interact with Cowslip
None known

Supplements That May Interact with Cowslip
None known

CUBEB

A shrubby vine that originated in Indonesia, cubeb produces peppery berries that are used medically or in perfumes and are sometimes smoked in cigarettes. Because it has a stimulating effect on the mucous membranes of the urinary and respiratory tracts, cubeb has often been used in the treatment of bronchitis, gonorrhea, urethritis, and prostate infections. Traditionally, cubeb is believed to be an aphrodisiac and is sometimes used in love spells.

Scientific Name
Piper cubeba

Cubeb Is Also Commonly Known As
Java pepper, tailed cubebs, tailed pepper

Medicinal Parts
Fruit

Cubeb's Uses
To treat gastrointestinal complaints, flatulence, diseases of the urinary tract, chronic bronchitis, and poor memory

Typical Dose

A typical daily dose of cubeb may range from 2 to 4 gm of powder, or 2 to 4 ml of 1:1 extract.

Possible Side Effects

No side effects are known when cubeb is taken in recommended therapeutic dosages.

Drugs That May Interact with Cubeb

Taking cubeb with these drugs may reduce the effectiveness of the drug:

- aluminum hydroxide (AlternaGel, Alu-Cap)
- aluminum hydroxide and magnesium carbonate (Gaviscon Extra Strength, Gaviscon Liquid) aluminum hydroxide and magnesium hydroxide (Maalox, Rulox)
- aluminum hydroxide and magnesium trisilicate (Gaviscon Tablet)
- aluminum hydroxide, magnesium hydroxide, and simethicone (Maalox, Mylanta Liquid)
- calcium carbonate (Rolaids Extra Strength, Tums)
- calcium carbonate and magnesium hydroxide (Mylanta Gelcaps, Rolaids Extra Strength)
- cimetidine (Nu-Cimet, Tagamet)
- esomeprazole (Nexium)
- famotidine (Apo-Famotidine, Pepcid)
- famotidine, calcium carbonate, and magnesium hydroxide (Pepcid Complete)
- lansoprazole (Prevacid)
- magaldrate and simethicone (Riopan Plus, Riopan Plus Double Strength)
- magnesium hydroxide (Dulcolax Milk of Magnesia, Phillips' Milk of Magnesia)
- magnesium oxide (Mag-Ox 400, Uro-Mag)
- magnesium sulfate (Epsom salts)
- nizatidine (Axid, PMS-Nizatidine)
- omeprazole (Losec, Prilosec)
- pantoprazole (Pantoloc, Protonix)
- rabeprazole (Aciphex, Pariet)
- ranitidine (Alti-Ranitidine, Zantac)
- sodium bicarbonate (Brioschi, Neut)

Lab Tests That May Be Altered by Cubeb

None known

Diseases That May Be Worsened or Triggered by Cubeb

May worsen gastrointestinal ailments by irritating the gastrointestinal tract.

Foods That May Interact with Cubeb

None known

Supplements That May Interact with Cubeb

None known

CUCUMBER

The watery, mild-tasting cucumber is one of the oldest foods around, having been gathered and possibly cultivated as long ago as 9750 B.C. in Southeast Asia. Yet Englishmen in the seventeenth century were convinced that eating cucumbers would be fatal, although lying on a bed of the same was one of their cures for fever.

Scientific Name

Cucumis sativus

Cucumber Is Also Commonly Known As

Wild cucumber

Medicinal Parts

Fruit, seed

Cucumber's Uses

To treat hypotension and hypertension; as a diuretic

Typical Dose

A typical dose of cucumber may range from 1 to 2 oz of ground seeds steeped in 150 ml of hot water, strained and taken as a decoction.

Possible Side Effects

Cucumber's side effects include belching and heartburn.

Drugs That May Interact with Cucumber

Taking cucumber with these drugs may increase the drug's diuretic effects:

- acetazolamide (Apo-Acetazolamide, Diamox Sequels)
- amiloride (Midamor)
- azosemide (Diat)
- bumetanide (Bumex, Burinex)
- chlorothiazide (Diuril)
- chlorthalidone (Apo-Chlorthalidone, Thalitone)
- ethacrynic acid (Edecrin)
- etozolin (Elkapin)
- furosemide (Apo-Furosemide, Lasix)
- hydrochlorothiazide (Apo-Hydro, Microzide)
- hydrochlorothiazide and triamterene (Dyazide, Maxzide)
- hydroflumethiazide (Diucardin, Saluron)
- indapamide (Lozol, Nu-Indapamide)
- mannitol (Osmitrol, Resectisol)
- mefruside (Baycaron)
- methazolamide (Apo-Methazolamide, Neptazane)
- methyclothiazide (Aquatensen, Enduron)
- metolazone (Mykrox, Zaroxolyn)
- olmesartan and hydrochlorothiazide (Benicar HCT)
- polythiazide (Renese)
- spironolactone (Aldactone, Novo-Spiroton)
- torsemide (Demadex)
- triamterene (Dyrenium)
- trichlormethiazide (Metatensin, Naqua)
- urea (Amino-Cerv, UltraMide)
- xipamide (Diurexan, Lumitens)

Taking cucumber with this drug may be harmful:

- digitalis (Digitek, Lanoxin)—may increase risk of drug toxicity

Lab Tests That May Be Altered by Cucumber

None known

Diseases That May Be Worsened or Triggered by Cucumber

None known

Foods That May Interact with Cucumber

None known

Supplements That May Interact with Cucumber

None known

CUMIN

Originating in Iran and the Mediterranean region, cumin, the dried seed of a member of the parsley family, plays a major role in the flavoring of Mexican, Indian, and Thai cuisines. The ancient Greeks kept a jar of cumin at the dining table, much like the modern salt shaker. In the Middle Ages, it was believed that cumin would keep chickens and lovers from slipping away and that carrying the seed on your wedding day would ensure a happy married life.

Scientific Name
Cuminum cyminum

Cumin Is Also Commonly Known As
Cummin, jeeraka, zira

Medicinal Parts
Fruit

Cumin's Uses
To treat diarrhea, colic, leprosy, and kidney and bladder stones; to induce abortions

Typical Dose
A typical dose of cumin may range from 300 to 600 mg of the herb.

Possible Side Effects
No side effects are known when cumin is taken in recommended therapeutic dosages.

Drugs That May Interact with Cumin
Taking cumin with these drugs may increase the risk of hypoglycemia (low blood sugar):
- acarbose (Prandase, Precose)
- acetohexamide
- chloropropamide (Diabinese, Novo-Propamide)
- gliclazide (Diamicron, Novo-Gliclazide)
- glimepiride (Amaryl)
- glipizide (Glucotrol)
- glipizide and metformin (Metaglip)
- gliquidone (Beglynor, Glurenorm)
- glyburide (DiaBeta, Micronase)
- glyburide and metformin (Glucovance)
- insulin (Humulin, Novolin R)
- metformin (Glucophage, Riomet)
- miglitol (Glyset)
- nateglinide (Starlix)
- pioglitazone (Actos)
- repaglinide (GlucoNorm, Prandin)
- rosiglitazone (Avandia)
- rosiglitazone and metformin (Avandamet)
- tolazamide (Tolinase)
- tolbutamide (Apo-Tolbutamide, Tol-Tab)

Lab Tests That May Be Altered by Cumin
None known

Diseases That May Be Worsened or Triggered by Cumin
May interfere with blood sugar control in diabetes.

Foods That May Interact with Cumin
None known

Supplements That May Interact with Cumin
None known

DAMIANA

The leaves of the damiana shrub, which grows in the Caribbean, southern Africa, and the Gulf of Mexico, are said to have antidepressant and aphrodisiac properties, although researchers have not identified any real physiological effects in humans. However,

> when damiana extract was given to impotent and/or sexually "sluggish" male rats, it increased their sexual activity and ability to complete the sexual act, while reducing the amount of time required before the animals could engage in sex again.

Scientific Name
Turnera diffusa

Damiana Is Also Commonly Known As
Herba de la pastora, mizibcoc, old woman's broom

Medicinal Parts
Leaf

Damiana's Uses
To treat bladder inflammation, diabetes, kidney ailments, and depression; as an aphrodisiac; to get a mild "high" when smoked and inhaled

Typical Dose
A typical dose of damiana may range from 2 to 4 gm of dried leaf taken three times daily.

Possible Side Effects
There are no known adverse side effects when damiana is taken in recommended therapeutic doses. High doses have been associated with convulsions similar to those caused by tetanus.

Drugs That May Interact with Damiana
Taking damiana with these drugs may increase the risk of hypoglycemia (low blood sugar):

- acarbose (Prandase, Precose)
- acetohexamide
- chlorpropamide (Diabinese, Novo-Propamide)
- gliclazide (Diamicron, Novo-Gliclazide)
- glimepiride (Amaryl)
- glipizide (Glucotrol)
- glipizide and metformin (Metaglip)
- gliquidone (Beglynor, Glurenorm)
- glyburide (DiaBeta, Micronase)
- glyburide and metformin (Glucovance)
- insulin (Humulin, Novolin R)
- metformin (Glucophage, Riomet)
- miglitol (Glyset)
- nateglinide (Starlix)
- pioglitazone (Actos)
- repaglinide (GlucoNorm, Prandin)
- rosiglitazone (Avandia)
- rosiglitazone and metformin (Avandamet)
- tolazamide (Tolinase)
- tolbutamide (Apo-Tolbutamide, Tol-Tab)

Lab Tests That May Be Altered by Damiana
None known

Diseases That May Be Worsened or Triggered by Damiana
May interfere with control of blood sugar in diabetes.

Foods That May Interact with Damiana
None known

Supplements That May Interact with Damiana
None known

DANDELION

> A humble weed that grows uninvited in many gardens, dandelion is a medicine that can play several roles: liver and gallbladder stimulant; mild laxative; blood cleanser; wart remover; and powerful diuretic that has earned the English name of "pee in the bed."

Scientific Name
Taraxacum officinale

Dandelion Is Also Commonly Known As
Blowball, Irish daisy, priest's crown, wild endive

Medicinal Parts
Whole herb

Dandelion's Uses
To treat hemorrhoids, gout, liver and gallbladder problems, rheumatic ailments, eczema, heartburn, bloating, constipation, and elevated blood pressure. Germany's Commission E has approved the use of dandelion to treat loss of appetite, dyspeptic problems such as heartburn, liver and gallbladder complaints, and urinary tract infections.

Typical Dose
A typical dose of dandelion may range from 4 to 10 gm of the whole herb, taken three times a day.

Possible Side Effects
Dandelion's side effects include nausea, loss of appetite, and inflammation of the gallbladder. The herb may trigger allergic reactions in those who are sensitive to herbs from the Asteraceae (daisy) family, such as German chamomile or daisy. (For a list of herbs from the Asteraceae family, see Appendix B.)

Drugs That May Interact with Dandelion
Taking dandelion with these drugs may interfere with the action of the drug:
- aluminum hydroxide (AlternaGel, AluCap)
- aluminum hydroxide and magnesium carbonate (Gaviscon Extra Strength, Gaviscon Liquid)
- aluminum hydroxide and magnesium hydroxide (Maalox, Rulox)
- aluminum hydroxide and magnesium trisilicate (Gaviscon Tablet)
- aluminum hydroxide, magnesium hydroxide, and simethicone (Maalox, Mylanta Liquid)
- benazepril (Lotensin)
- calcium carbonate (Rolaids Extra Strength, Tums)
- calcium carbonate and magnesium hydroxide (Mylanta Gelcaps, Rolaids Extra Strength)
- cimetidine (Nu-Cimet, Tagamet)
- esomeprazole (Nexium)
- famotidine (Apo-Famotidine, Pepcid)
- famotidine, calcium carbonate, and magnesium hydroxide (Pepcid Complete)
- lansoprazole (Prevacid)
- magaldrate and simethicone (Riopan Plus, Riopan Plus Double Strength)
- magnesium hydroxide (Dulcolax Milk of Magnesia, Phillips' Milk of Magnesia)
- magnesium oxide (Mag-Ox 400, Uro-Mag)
- magnesium sulfate (Epsom salts)
- nizatidine (Axid, PMS-Nizatidine)
- omeprazole (Losec, Prilosec)
- pantoprazole (Pantoloc, Protonix)
- rabeprazole (Aciphex, Pariet)

- ranitidine (Alti-Ranitidine, Zantac)
- sodium bicarbonate (Brioschi, Neut)

Taking dandelion with these drugs may increase the risk of hyperkalemia (high blood levels of potassium):
- amiloride (Midamor)
- hydrochlorothiazide and triamterene (Dyazide, Maxzide)
- spironolactone (Aldactone, Novo-Spiroton)
- triamterene (Dyrenium)

Taking dandelion with these drugs may increase the drug's diuretic effects:
- acetazolamide (Apo-Acetazolamide, Diamox Sequels)
- amiloride (Midamor)
- azosemide (Diat)
- bumetanide (Bumex, Burinex)
- chlorothiazide (Diuril)
- chlorthalidone (Apo-Chlorthalidone, Thalitone)
- ethacrynic acid (Edecrin)
- etozolin (Elkapin)
- furosemide (Apo-Furosemide, Lasix)
- hydrochlorothiazide (Apo-Hydro, Microzide)
- hydrochlorothiazide and triamterene (Dyazide, Maxzide)
- hydroflumethiazide (Diucardin, Saluron)
- indapamide (Lozol, Nu-Indapamide)
- mannitol (Osmitrol, Resectisol)
- mefruside (Baycaron)
- methazolamide (Apo-Methazolamide, Neptazane)
- methyclothiazide (Aquatense, Enduron)
- metolazone (Mykrox, Zaroxolyn)
- olmesartan and hydrochlorothiazide (Benicar HCT)
- polythiazide (Renese)

- spironolactone (Aldactone, Novo-Spiroton)
- torsemide (Demadex)
- triamterene (Dyrenium)
- trichlormethiazide (Metatensin, Naqua)
- urea (Amino-Cerv, UltraMide)
- xipamide (Diurexan, Lumitens)

Taking dandelion with these drugs may increase the risk of hypoglycemia (low blood sugar):
- acarbose (Prandase, Precose)
- acetohexamide
- chlorpropamide (Diabinese, Novo-Propamide)
- gliclazide (Diamicron, Novo-Gliclazide)
- glimepiride (Amaryl)
- glipizide (Glucotrol)
- glipizide and metformin (Metaglip)
- gliquidone (Beglynor, Glurenorm)
- glyburide (DiaBeta, Micronase)
- glyburide and metformin (Glucovance)
- insulin (Humulin, Novolin R)
- metformin (Glucophage, Riomet)
- miglitol (Glyset)
- nateglinide (Starlix)
- pioglitazone (Actos)
- repaglinide (GlucoNorm, Prandin)
- rosiglitazone (Avandia)
- rosiglitazone and metformin (Avandamet)
- tolazamide (Tolinase)
- tolbutamide (Apo-Tolbutamide, Tol-Tab)

Taking dandelion with these drugs may be harmful because:
- lithium (Eskalith, Carbolith)—may increase the effects of the drug and cause lithium toxicity

Lab Tests That May Be Altered by Dandelion
None known

Diseases That May Be Worsened or Triggered by Dandelion

- May lower blood sugar in diabetes.
- May worsen cases of gallstones, gallbladder inflammation, or intestinal or bile duct blockages.

Foods That May Interact with Dandelion

None known

Supplements That May Interact with Dandelion

- May enhance the effects of herbs and supplements that have diuretic properties, such as agrimony, celery, shepherd's purse, and yarrow. (For a list of herbs that have diuretic properties, see Appendix B.)
- May increase blood glucose–lowering effects and risk of hypoglycemia (low blood sugar) when used with herbs and supplements that lower glucose levels, such as alpha-lipoic acid, chromium, devil's claw, Panax ginseng, and psyllium. (For a list of herbs and supplements that lower blood glucose levels, see Appendix B.)

DANSHEN

> Widely used in traditional Chinese medicine, danshen is given to improve the circulation of the blood by limiting the stickiness of the platelets. Certain chemicals in danshen may also help relax and widen blood vessels, especially those in the area of the heart. In addition, results from some recent laboratory studies have shown that danshen may have anticancer and anti-HIV activity.

Scientific Name

Salvia bowleyana, Salvia miltiorrhiza

Danshen Is Also Commonly Known As

Dan-shen, huang ken, red sage, salvia root

Medicinal Parts

Root

Danshen's Uses

To treat angina pectoris (chest pain due to low blood flow to the heart muscle), ischemic stroke (a stroke caused by lack of blood flow to a portion of the brain), menstrual problems, circulatory ailments, hepatitis, and psoriasis; to help wounds heal

Typical Dose

There is no typical dose of danshen.

Possible Side Effects

Danshen's side effects include decreased appetite, stomach upset, and itching.

Drugs That May Interact with Danshen

Taking danshen with these drugs may increase the risk of bleeding or bruising:

- abciximab (ReoPro)
- antithrombin III (Thrombate III)
- argatroban
- aspirin (Bufferin, Ecotrin)
- aspirin and dipyridamole (Aggrenox)
- bivalirudin (Angiomax)
- celecoxib (Celebrex)
- clopidogrel (Plavix)
- dalteparin (Fragmin)
- danaparoid (Orgaran)
- dipyridamole (Novo-Dipiradol, Persantine)
- enoxaparin (Lovenox)
- eptifibatide (Integrillin)

- etodolac (Lodine, Utradol)
- fondaparinux (Arixtra)
- heparin (Hepalean, Hep-Lock)
- ibuprofen (Advil, Motrin)
- indobufen (Ibustrin)
- indomethacin (Indocin, Novo-Methacin)
- ketoprofen (Orudis, Rhodis)
- ketorolac (Acular, Toradol)
- lepirudin (Refludan)
- meloxicam (MOBIC, Mobicox)
- naproxen (Aleve, Naprosyn)
- piroxicam (Feldene, Nu-Pirox)
- rofecoxib (Vioxx)
- ticlopidine (Alti-Ticlopidine, Ticlid)
- tinzaparin (Innohep)
- tirofiban (Aggrastat)
- urokinase (Abbokinase)
- warfarin (Coumadin, Jantoven)

Taking danshen with these drugs may be harmful:
- alprazolam (Apo-Alpraz, Xanax)—may increase depression of the central nervous system (sedation, mental depression and impairment)
- digitalis (Digitek, Lanoxin)—may increase the risk of arrhythmia (irregular heartbeat)

Lab Tests That May Be Altered by Danshen

- False increase in serum digoxin concentrations with fluorescence polarization immunoassay (FPIA).
- False decrease in serum digoxin with microparticle enzyme immunoassay (MEIA).

Diseases That May Be Worsened or Triggered by Danshen

May worsen cases of bleeding disorders.

Foods That May Interact with Danshen

None known

Supplements That May Interact with Danshen

- Increased risk of cardiac glycoside toxicity when used with other herbs that contain cardiac glycosides, such as black hellebore, calotropis, motherwort, and others. (For a list of cardiac glycoside–containing herbs and supplements, see Appendix B.)
- Increased risk of bleeding when used with herbs and supplements that might affect platelet aggregation, such as angelica, garlic, ginger, ginkgo biloba, turmeric, and others. (For a list of herbs and supplements with anticoagulant/antiplatelet effects, see Appendix B.)

DEER'S TONGUE

The leaves of this native of the southeastern United States smell like vanilla and are often used to flavor tobacco. Deer's tongue also contains coumarin, a well-known blood thinner.

Scientific Name

Trilisa odoratissima

Deer's Tongue Is Also Commonly Known As

Carolina vanilla, deertongue, hound's tongue, vanilla plant, wild vanilla

Medicinal Parts

Leaf

Deer's Tongue's Uses

To treat malaria

Typical Dose

There is no typical dose of deer's tongue.

Possible Side Effects

Deer's tongue's side effects include allergic reactions in those sensitive to herbs from the *Asteraceae* (daisy) family, such as German chamomile, daisy, or dandelion. (For a list of herbs from the *Asteraceae* family, see Appendix B.) Unexplained bleeding and liver damage are also possible.

Drugs That May Interact with Deer's Tongue

Taking deer's tongue with these drugs may increase the risk of bleeding or bruising:

- abciximab (ReoPro)
- antithrombin III (Thrombate III)
- argatroban
- aspirin (Bufferin, Ecotrin)
- aspirin and dipyridamole (Aggrenox)
- bivalirudin (Angiomax)
- clopidogrel (Plavix)
- dalteparin (Fragmin)
- danaparoid (Orgaran)
- dipyridamole (Novo-Dipiradol, Persantine)
- enoxaparin (Lovenox)
- eptifibatide (Integrillin)
- fondaparinux (Arixtra)
- heparin (Hepalean, Hep-Lock)
- indobufen (Ibustrin)
- lepirudin (Refludan)
- ticlopidine (Alti-Ticlopidine, Ticlid)
- tinzaparin (Innohep)
- tirofiban (Aggrastat)
- warfarin (Coumadin, Jantoven)

Lab Tests That May Be Altered by Deer's Tongue

None known

Diseases That May Be Worsened or Triggered by Deer's Tongue

None known

Foods That May Interact with Deer's Tongue

None known

Supplements That May Interact with Deer's Tongue

Increased risk of bleeding when used with herbs and supplements that might affect platelet aggregation. (For a list of herbs and supplements with anticoagulant/antiplatelet effects, see Appendix B.)

DEVIL'S CLAW

An old folk remedy for arthritis, rheumatism, and gout, devil's claw, a desert plant from southern and eastern Africa, contains a substance that exerts a powerful anti-inflammatory effect on the joints. German researchers tested the effects of devil's claw in seventy-five people with arthritis of the knee or hip and found that the herb reduced joint pain and stiffness while improving overall physical functioning of the affected joint.

Scientific Name

Harpagophytum procumbens

Devil's Claw Is Also Commonly Known As

Grapple pant, wood spider

Medicinal Parts

Root, tuber (fleshy rounded stem or root)

Devil's Claw's Uses

To treat skin ailments and injuries, allergies, metabolic disturbances, and problems with digestion, the kidney, bladder, liver, and gallbladder; to relieve pain. Germany's Commission E has approved the use of devil's claw to treat loss of appetite, dyspeptic complaints such as bloating and heartburn, and rheumatism.

Typical Dose

A typical daily dose of devil's claw may range from 1 to 2 gm of dried powdered root taken three times a day.

Possible Side Effects

Devil's claw's side effects include nausea and vomiting.

Drugs That May Interact with Devil's Claw

Taking devil's claw with these drugs may increase the risk of bleeding or bruising:

- abciximab (ReoPro)
- aspirin (Bufferin, Ecotrin)
- celecoxib (Celebrex)
- enoxaparin (Lovenox)
- etodolac (Lodine, Utradol)
- heparin (Hepalean, Hep-Lock)
- ibuprofen (Advil, Motrin)
- indomethacin (Indocin, Novo-Methacin)
- ketoprofen (Orudis, Rhodis)
- ketorolac (Acular, Toradol)
- meloxicam (MOBIC, Mobicox)
- naproxen (Aleve, Naprosyn)
- piroxicam (Feldene, Nu-Pirox)
- rofecoxib (Vioxx)
- ticlopidine (Alti-Ticlopidine, Ticlid)
- urokinase (Abbokinase)
- warfarin (Coumadin, Jantoven)

Taking devil's claw with these drugs may interfere with the action of the drug:

- aluminum hydroxide (AlternaGel, AluCap)
- aluminum hydroxide and magnesium carbonate (Gaviscon Extra Strength, Gaviscon Liquid)
- aluminum hydroxide and magnesium hydroxide (Maalox, Rulox)
- aluminum hydroxide and magnesium trisilicate (Gaviscon Tablet)
- aluminum hydroxide, magnesium hydroxide, and simethicone (Maalox, Mylanta Liquid)
- calcium carbonate (Rolaids Extra Strength, Tums)
- calcium carbonate and magnesium hydroxide (Mylanta Gelcaps, Rolaids Extra Strength)
- cimetidine (Nu-Cimet, Tagamet)
- esomeprazole (Nexium)
- famotidine (Apo-Famotidine, Pepcid)
- famotidine, calcium carbonate, and magnesium hydroxide (Pepcid Complete)
- lansoprazole (Prevacid)
- magaldrate and simethicone (Riopan Plus, Riopan Plus Double Strength)
- magnesium hydroxide (Dulcolax Milk of Magnesia, Phillips' Milk of Magnesia)
- magnesium oxide (Mag-Ox 400, Uro-Mag)
- magnesium sulfate (Epsom salts)
- nizatidine (Axid, PMS-Nizatidine)
- omeprazole (Losec, Prilosec)
- pantoprazole (Pantoloc, Protonix)
- rabeprazole (Aciphex, Pariet)
- ranitidine (Alti-Ranitidine, Zantac)
- sodium bicarbonate (Brioschi, Neut)

Taking devil's claw with these drugs may increase the risk of hypoglycemia (low blood sugar):

- acarbose (Prandase, Precose)
- acetohexamide
- chlorpropamide (Diabinese, Novo-Propamide)
- gliclazide (Diamicron, Novo-Gliclazide)

- glimepiride (Amaryl)
- glipizide (Glucotrol)
- glipizide and metformin (Metaglip)
- gliquidone (Beglynor, Glurenorm)
- glyburide (DiaBeta, Micronase)
- glyburide and metformin (Glucovance)
- insulin (Humulin, Novolin R)
- metformin (Glucophage, Riomet)
- miglitol (Glyset)
- nateglinide (Starlix)
- pioglitazone (Actos)
- repaglinide (GlucoNorm, Prandin)
- rosiglitazone (Avandia)
- rosiglitazone and metformin (Avandamet)
- tolazamide (Tolinase)
- tolbutamide (Apo-Tolbutamide, Tol-Tab)

Taking devil's claw with these drugs may increase the risk of hypotension (excessively low blood pressure):

- acebutolol (Novo-Acebutolol, Sectral)
- amlodipine (Norvasc)
- atenolol (Apo-Atenol, Tenormin)
- benazepril (Lotensin)
- betaxolol (Betoptic S, Kerlone)
- bisoprolol (Monocor, Zebeta)
- bumetanide (Bumex, Burinex)
- candesartan (Atacand)
- captopril (Capoten, Novo-Captopril)
- carteolol (Cartrol, Ocupress)
- carvedilol (Coreg)
- chlorothiazide (Diuril)
- chlorthalidone (Apo-Chlorthalidone, Thalitone)
- clonidine (Catapres, Duraclon)
- diazoxide (Hyperstat, Proglycem)
- diltiazem (Cardizem, Tiazac)
- doxazosin (Alti-Doxazosin, Cardura)
- enalapril (Vasotec)
- eplerenone (Inspra)
- eprosartan (Teveten)
- esmolol (Brevibloc)
- felodipine (Plendil, Renedil)
- fenoldopam (Corlopam)
- fosinopril (Monopril)
- furosemide (Apo-Furosemide, Lasix)
- guanabenz (Wytensin)
- guanadrel (Hylorel)
- guanfacine (Tenex)
- hydralazine (Apresoline, Novo-Hylazin)
- hydrochlorothiazide (Apo-Hydro, Microzide)
- hydrochlorothiazide and triamterene (Dyazide, Maxzide)
- indapamide (Lozol, Nu-Indapamide)
- irbesartan (Avapro)
- isradipine (DynaCirc)
- labetalol (Normodyne, Trandate)
- lisinopril (Prinivil, Zestril)
- losartan (Cozaar)
- mecamylamine (Inversine)
- mefruside (Baycaron)
- methyclothiazide (Aquatensen, Enduron)
- methyldopa (Apo-Methyldopa, Nu-Medopa)
- metolazone (Mykrox, Zaroxolyn)
- metoprolol (Betaloc, Lopressor)
- minoxidil (Loniten, Rogaine)
- moexipril (Univasc)
- nadolol (Apo-Nadol, Corgard)
- nicardipine (Cardene)
- nifedipine (Adalat CC, Procardia)
- nisoldipine (Sular)
- nitroglycerin (Minitran, Nitro-Dur)
- nitroprusside (Nipride, Nitropress)
- olmesartan (Benicar)
- oxprenolol (Slow-Trasicor, Trasicor)

- perindopril erbumine (Aceon, Coversyl)
- phenoxybenzamine (Dibenzyline)
- phentolamine (Regitine, Rogitine)
- pindolol (Apo-Pindol, Novo-Pindol)
- polythiazide (Renese)
- prazosin (Minipress, Nu-Prazo)
- propranolol (Inderal, InnoPran XL)
- quinapril (Accupril)
- ramipril (Altace)
- reserpine
- spironolactone (Aldactone, Novo-Spiroton)
- telmisartan (Micardis)
- terazosin (Alti-Terazosin, Hytrin)
- timolol (Betimol, Timoptic)
- torsemide (Demadex)
- trandolapril (Mavik)
- triamterene (Dyrenium)
- trichlormethiazide (Metatensin, Naqua)
- valsartan (Diovan)
- verapamil (Calan, Isoptin SR)

Lab Tests That May Be Altered by Devil's Claw
None known

Diseases That May Be Worsened or Triggered by Devil's Claw
- May worsen cardiovascular ailments by affecting the heart rate and blood pressure.
- May worsen ulcers and gastroesophageal reflux disease (GERD) by increasing stomach acid.
- May interfere with attempts to control blood sugar in diabetes.

Foods That May Interact with Devil's Claw
None known

Supplements That May Interact with Devil's Claw
None known

DIGITALIS

The medicinal effects of digitalis, one of our most important heart medicines, were first noted in 1775 by an English doctor, William Withering. He observed that a tea made from the leaves of the foxglove plant, which contains digitalis, had diuretic properties and relieved water retention. Researchers later discovered that digitalis acted primarily on the heart, strengthening and regulating the heartbeat.

Scientific Name
Digitalis lanata

Digitalis Is Also Commonly Known As
Dead men's bells, fairy cap, finger flower, foxglove, lion's mouth

Medicinal Parts
Leaf, seed

Digitalis's Uses
To treat headaches, paralysis, ulcers, heart failure, asthma, and constipation

Typical Dose
There is no typical dose of digitalis, which today is considered obsolete because its effects vary so widely.

Possible Side Effects
❶ Digitalis's side effects include loss of appetite, vomiting, diarrhea, headache, and acute confusion. Digitalis contains cardiac glycosides, which can help control irregular heartbeat, reduce the backup of blood and fluid in the body, and increase blood flow through the kidneys, helping to excrete sodium and relieve swelling in body tis-

sues. However, a buildup of cardiac glycosides can occur, especially when the herb is combined with certain medications or other herbs that contain cardiac glycosides, causing arrhythmias, abnormally slow heartbeat, heart failure, and even death.

Drugs That May Interact with Digitalis

Taking digitalis with these drugs may increase the risk of arrhythmia (irregular heartbeat):

- albuterol (Proventil, Ventolin)
- brimonidine (Alphagan P, PMS-Brimonidine Tartrate)
- cilostazol (Pletal)
- dobutamine (Dobutrex)
- dopamine (Intropin)
- dopexamine (Dopacard)
- enoximone (Perfan)
- ephedrine (Pretz-D)
- inamrinone
- isoetharine (Beta-2, Bronkosol)
- isoproterenol (Isuprel)
- metaproterenol (Alupent)
- metaraminol (Aramine)
- milrinone (Primacor)
- norepinephrine (Levophed)
- pentoxifylline (Pentoxil, Trental)
- phenylephrine (Neo-Synephrine Extra Strength, Vicks Sinex Nasal Spray)
- pseudoephedrine (Dimetapp Decongestant, Sudafed)
- quinidine (Novo-Quinidin, Quinaglute Dura-Tabs)
- sildenafil (Viagra)
- tadalafil (Cialis)
- terbutaline (Brethine)
- theophylline (Elixophyllin, Theochron)
- theophylline and guaifenesin (Elixophyllin-GC, Quibron)
- vardenafil (Levitra)

Taking digitalis with these drugs may increase the risk of cardiac glycoside toxicity:

- acetazolamide (Apo-Acetazolamide, Diamox Sequels)
- azosemide (Diat)
- bumetanide (Bumex, Burinex)
- chlorothiazide (Diuril)
- chlorthalidone (Apo-Chlorthalidone, Thalitone)
- ethacrynic acid (Edecrin)
- etozolin (Elkapin)
- furosemide (Apo-Furosemide, Lasix)
- hydrochlorothiazide (Apo-Hydro, Microzide)
- hydroflumethiazide (Diucardin, Saluron)
- indapamide (Lozol, Nu-Indapamide)
- mannitol (Osmitrol, Resectisol)
- mefruside (Baycaron)
- methazolamide (Apo-Methazolamide, Neptazane)
- methyclothiazide (Aquatensen, Enduron)
- metolazone (Mykrox, Zaroxolyn)
- olmesartan and hydrochlorothiazide (Benicar HCT)
- polythiazide (Renese)
- quinine (Quinine-Odan)
- torsemide (Demadex)
- trichlormethiazide (Metatensin, Naqua)
- urea (Amino-Cerv, UltraMide)
- xipamide (Diurexan, Lumitens)

Lab Tests That May Be Altered by Digitalis

May normalize arrhythmias and electrocardiogram (ECG) readings.

Diseases That May Be Worsened or Triggered by Digitalis

Overdose of digitalis may trigger irregular heartbeat, heart failure.

Foods That May Interact with Digitalis
None known

Supplements That May Interact with Digitalis
- Increased risk of cardiac glycoside toxicity when used with other herbs that contain cardiac glycosides, such as black hellebore, calotropis, motherwort, and others. (For a list of cardiac glycoside–containing herbs and supplements, see Appendix B.)
- Increased risk of potassium depletion when used in conjunction with horsetail plant or licorice.
- Increased risk of cardiotoxicity due to potassium depletion when taken with cardioactive herbs, such as adonis, lily-of-the-valley, and squill. (For a list of cardioactive herbs and supplements, see Appendix B.)
- Increased risk of potassium depletion when used with other stimulant laxative herbs, such as black root, cascara sagrada, castor oil, and senna. (For a list of stimulant laxative herbs and supplements, see Appendix B.)

DONG QUAI

Widely used in China to regulate estrogen levels, dong quai has hormonelike compounds that appear to relieve menstrual disorders and ease the symptoms of menopause. The name "dong quai" (actually "dang gui") means "to return." It is said that a woman who is feeling irritable and doesn't want to be near her husband should take this herb; once she feels better, she will want to return to him. Preliminary scientific research has suggested that dong quai may reduce blood pressure, inhibit certain kinds of irregular heartbeat, protect against clogging of the arteries, combat pain and inflammation, and encourage the death of tumor cells.

Scientific Name
Angelica sinensis

Dong Quai Is Also Commonly Known As
Chinese angelica, dang-gui, tang-kuei, women's ginseng

Medicinal Parts
Root

Dong Quai's Uses
To treat symptoms of menopause, asthma, irregular heartbeat, bronchitis, infections, infertility, and kidney and liver disorders

Typical Dose
A typical dose of dong quai may range from 1 to 2 gm of powdered root taken three times a day; or, in tincture form, 5 to 20 drops of a 1:5 concentration taken up to three times a day.

Possible Side Effects
Dong quai's side effects include gastrointestinal disturbances, fever, and increased bleeding.

Drugs That May Interact with Dong Quai
Taking dong quai with these drugs may increase the risk of bleeding and bruising:
- abciximab (ReoPro)
- alteplase (Activase, Cathflo Activase)
- antithrombin III (Thrombate III)
- argatroban

- aspirin (Bufferin, Ecotrin)
- aspirin and dipyridamole (Aggrenox)
- bivalirudin (Angiomax)
- celecoxib (Celebrex)
- choline magnesium trysalicylate (Trilisate)
- clopidogrel (Plavix)
- dalteparin (Fragmin)
- danaparoid (Orgaran)
- diclofenac (Cataflam, Voltaren)
- diflunisal (Apo-Diflunisal, Dolobid)
- dipyridamole (Novo-Dipiradol, Persantine)
- drotrecogin alfa (Xigris)
- enoxaparin (Lovenox)
- eptifibatide (Integrillin)
- etodolac (Lodine, Utradol)
- fenoprofen (Nalfon)
- flurbiprofen (Ansaid, Ocufen)
- fondaparinux (Arixtra)
- heparin (Hepalean, Hep-Lock)
- hydrocodone and aspirin (Damason-P)
- hydrocodone and ibuprofen (Vicoprofen)
- ibritumomab (Zevalin)
- ibuprofen (Advil, Motrin)
- indobufen (Ibustrin)
- indomethacin (Indocin, Novo-Methacin)
- ketoprofen (Orudis, Rhodis)
- ketorolac (Acular, Toradol)
- lepirudin (Refludan)
- meloxicam (MOBIC, Mobicox)
- nabumetone (Apo-Nabumetone, Relefan)
- nadroparin (Fraxiparine)
- naproxen (Aleve, Naprosyn)
- oxaprozin (Apo-Oxaprozin, Daypro)
- piroxicam (Feldene, Nu-Pirox)
- reteplase (Retavase)
- rofecoxib (Vioxx)
- salsalate (Amgesic, Salflex)

- streptokinase (Streptase)
- sulindac (Clinoril, Nu-Sundac)
- tenecteplase (TNKase)
- tiaprofenic acid (Dom-Tiaprofenic, Surgam)
- ticlopidine (Alti-Ticlopidine, Ticlid)
- tinzaparin (Innohep)
- tirofiban (Aggrastat)
- tolmetin (Tolectin)
- urokinase (Abbokinase)
- valdecoxib (Bextra)
- warfarin (Coumadin, Jantoven)

Taking dong quai with these drugs may enhance the drug's therapeutic and/or adverse effects:
- acebutolol (Novo-Acebutolol, Sectral)
- amiodarone (Cordarone, Pacerone)
- atenolol (Apo-Atenol, Tenormin)
- benazepril (Lotensin)
- bepridil (Vascor)
- betaxolol (Betoptic S, Kerlone)
- bisoprolol (Monocor, Zebeta)
- bumetanide (Bumex, Burinex)
- candesartan (Atacand)
- captopril (Capoten, Novo-Captopril)
- carteolol (Cartrol, Ocupress)
- carvedilol (Coreg)
- cilazapril (Inhibace)
- clonidine (Catapres, Duraclon)
- cyproterone and ethinyl estradiol (Diane-35)
- diltiazem (Cardizem, Tiazac)
- doxazosin (Alti-Doxazosin, Cardura)
- enalapril (Vasotec)
- eprosartan (Teveten)
- estradiol (Climara, Estrace)
- estrogens (conjugated A/synthetic) (Cenestin)
- estrogens (conjugated/equine) (Cenestin, Premarin)

- estrogens (esterified) (Estratab, Menest)
- estropipate (Ogen, Ortho-Est)
- ethinyl estradiol (Estinyl)
- ethinyl estradiol and ethynodiol diacetate (Demulen, Zovia)
- ethinyl estradiol and etonogestrel (NuvaRing)
- ethinyl estradiol and levonorgestrel (Alesse, Triphasil)
- ethinyl estradiol and norenthindrone (Brevicon, Ortho-Novum)
- ethinyl estradiol and norgestimate (Cyclen, Ortho Tri-Cyclen)
- ethinyl estradiol and norgestrel (Cryselle, Ovral)
- felodipine (Plendil, Renedil)
- fosfomycin (Monurol)
- furosemide (Apo-Furosemide, Lasix)
- hydralazine (Apresoline, Novo-Hylazin)
- hydrochlorothiazide (Apo-Hydro, Microzide)
- indapamide (Lozol, Nu-Indapamide)
- irbesartan (Avapro)
- isradipine (DynaCirc)
- labetalol (Normodyne, Trandate)
- lisinopril (Prinivil, Zestril)
- losartan (Cozaar)
- metolazone (Mykrox, Zaroxolyn)
- metoprolol (Betaloc, Lopressor)
- moexipril (Univasc)
- nadolol (Apo-Nadol, Corgard)
- nicardipine (Cardene)
- nifedipine (Adalat CC, Procardia)
- nimodipine (Nimotop)
- nisoldipine (Sular)
- norgestrel (Ovrette)
- oxprenolol (Slow-Trasicor, Trasicor)
- perindopril erbumine (Aceon, Coversyl)
- pindolol (Apo-Pindolol, Novo-Pindol)
- prazosin (Minipress, Nu-Prazo)
- propranolol (Inderal, InnoPran XL)

- quinapril (Accupril)
- ramipril (Altace)
- telmisartan (Micardis)
- terazosin (Hytrin, Novo-Terazosin)
- torsemide (Demadex)
- trandolapril (Mavik)
- valsartan (Diovan)
- verapamil (Calan, Isoptin SR)

Taking dong quai with these drugs may alter/interfere with the action of the drug, and is best avoided by those with estrogen-dependent tumors:
- anastrozole (Arimidex)
- carbocysteine (Mucopront, Rhinatiol)
- cisplatin (Platinol-AQ)
- cyclophosphamide (Cytoxan, Neosar)
- doxorubicin (Adriamycin, Rubex)
- epirubicin (Ellence, Pharmorubicin)
- exemestane (Aromasin)
- fluorouracil (Adrucil, Efudex)
- megestrol (Lin-Megestrol, Megace)
- mitomycin (Mutamycin)
- mitoxantrone (Novantrone)
- paclitaxel (Onxol, Taxol)
- tamoxifen (Nolvadex, Tamofen)
- thiotepa (Thioplex)
- vinblastine (Velban)

Taking dong quai with these drugs may increase skin sensitivity to sunlight:
- bexarotene (Targretin)
- bumetanide (Bumex, Burinex)
- celecoxib (Celebrex)
- chlorpromazine (Thorazine)
- ciprofloxacin (Ciloxan, Cipro)
- dacarbazine (DTIC, DTIC-Dome)
- demeclocycline (Declomycin)
- doxycycline (Apo-Doxy, Vibramycin)

- enalapril (Vasotec)
- etodolac (Lodine, Utradol)
- fluocinonole, hydroquinone, and tretinoin (Tri-Luma)
- fluphenazine (Modecate, Prolixin)
- fosinopril (Monopril)
- furosemide (Apo-Furosemide, Lasix)
- gatifloxacin (Tequin, Zymar)
- gemifloxacin (Factive)
- hydrochlorothiazide (Apo-Hydro, Microzide)
- hydrochlorothiazide and triamterene (Dyazide, Maxzide)
- ibuprofen (Advil, Motrin)
- isotretinoin (Accutane, Caravis)
- ketoprofen (Orudis, Rhodis)
- ketorolac (Acular, Toradol)
- lansoprazole (Prevacid)
- levofloxacin (Levaquin, Quixin)
- lisinopril (Prinivil, Zestril)
- lomefloxacin (Maxaquin)
- loratadine (Alavert, Claritin)
- methotrexate (Rheumatrex, Trexall)
- methotrimeprazine (Novo-Meprazine, Nozain)
- metolazone (Mykrox, Zaroxolyn)
- minocycline (Dynacin, Minocin)
- naproxen (Aleve, Naprosyn)
- nortriptyline (Aventyl HCl, Pamelor)
- ofloxacin (Floxin, Ocuflox)
- olanzapine (Zydis, Zyprexa)
- omeprazole (Losec, Prilosec)
- phenytoin (Dilantin, Phenytek)
- piroxicam (Feldene, Nu-Pirox)
- prochlorperazine (Compazine, Compro)
- quinapril (Accupril)
- risperidone (Risperdal)
- rofecoxib (Vioxx)
- sparfloxacin (Zagam)
- sulfadiazine (Microsulfon)
- sulfamethoxazole and trimethoprim (Bactrim, Septra)
- sulfasalazine (Alti-Sulfasalazine, Azulfidine)
- sulfinpyrazone (Apo-Sulfinpyrazone, Nu-Sulfinpyrazone)
- sulfisoxazole (Gantrisin)
- tetracycline (Novo-Tetra, Sumycin)
- thioridazine (Mellaril)
- tretinoin, oral (Vesanoid)
- trifluoperazine (Novo-Trifluzine, Stelazine)
- trovafloxacin (Trovan)
- zuclopenthixol (Clopixol)

Lab Tests That May Be Altered by Dong Quai
May increase prothrombin time (PT) and plasma international normalized ratio (INR) in those who are also taking warfarin.

Diseases That May Be Worsened or Triggered by Dong Quai
None known

Foods That May Interact with Dong Quai
None known

Supplements That May Interact with Dong Quai
- Increased risk of bleeding when used with herbs and supplements that might affect platelet aggregation, such as angelica, garlic, ginger, ginkgo biloba, turmeric, and others. (For a list of herbs and supplements with anticoagulant/antiplatelet effects, see Appendix B.)
- May increase photosensitivity when combined with St. John's wort.

ECHINACEA

Scientifically proven to have antibiotic effects, echinacea (also known as the purple coneflower) was used by Native Americans to treat snakebites and skin wounds. Today research has shown that echinacea stimulates the production of the infection-fighting white blood cells, has antiviral activity, and is helpful in easing allergies, making it an excellent immune system enhancer.

Scientific Name

Echinacea species (*Echinacea angustifolia, Echinacea pallida, Echinacea purpurea*)

Echinacea Is Also Commonly Known As

Black Sampson, hedgehog, purple coneflower

Medicinal Parts

Leaf, root, whole plant

Echinacea's Uses

To treat colds, infections, wounds, and leg ulcers; to stimulate the immune system. Germany's Commission E has approved the use of *Echinacea purpurea* to treat the common cold, cough, bronchitis, fevers, wounds, burns, infections of the urinary tract, and inflammation of the mouth and throat, and to reduce the risk of infection in susceptible people. It has also approved the use of *Echinacea pallida* to treat colds and fevers.

Typical Dose

A typical daily dose of echinacea (either *purpurea* or *pallida*) is 500 to 1,000 mg in capsule form taken three times a day.

Possible Side Effects

Echinacea's side effects include allergic reactions, nausea, vomiting, fever, heartburn, and constipation.

Drugs That May Interact with Echinacea

Taking echinacea with these drugs may cause or increase liver damage:

- abacavir (Ziagen)
- acarbose (Prandase, Precose)
- acetaminophen (Genapap, Tylenol)
- allopurinol (Aloprim, Zyloprim)
- atorvastatin (Lipitor)
- celecoxib (Celebrex)
- cidofovir (Vistide)
- ciprofloxacin (Cipro, Ciloxan)
- colchicine (ratio-Colchicine)
- cyclosporine (Neoral, Sandimmune)
- diazepam (Apo-Diazepam, Valium)
- docetaxel (Taxotere)
- dofetilide (Tikosyn)
- doxycycline (Apo-Doxy, Vibramycin)
- erythromycin (Erythrocin, Staticin)
- famotidine (Apo-Famotidine, Pepcid)
- fluconazole (Apo-Fluconazole, Diflucan)
- fluphenazine (Modecate, Prolixin)
- fluvastatin (Lescol)
- foscarnet (Foscavir)
- fosphenytoin (Cerebyx)
- ganciclovir (Cytovene, Vitrasert)
- gemfibrozil (Apo-Gemfibrozil, Lopid)
- gentamicin (Alcomicin, Gentacidin)
- glipizide (Glucotrol)
- glyburide (DiaBeta, Micronase)
- ibuprofen (Advil, Motrin)
- indinavir (Crixivan)
- ketoconazole (Apo-Ketoconazole, Nizoral)
- ketoprofen (Orudis, Rhodis)
- ketorolac (Acular, Toradol)
- lamivudine (Epivir, Heptovir)
- levodopa-carbidopa (Nu-Levocarb, Sinemet)
- lovastatin (Altocor, Mevacor)
- meloxicam (MOBIC, Mobicox)

- methotrexate (Rheumatrex, Trexall)
- methyldopa (Apo-Methyldopa, Nu-Medopa)
- methylprednisolone (Depo-Medrol, Medrol)
- moxifloxacin (Avelox, Vigamox)
- naproxen (Aleve, Naprosyn)
- nelfinavir (Viracept)
- nitrofurantoin (Furadantin, Macrobid)
- ofloxacin (Floxin, Ocuflox)
- ondansetron (Zofran)
- paclitaxel (Onxol, Taxol)
- pantoprazole (Pantoloc, Protonix)
- phenytoin (Dilantin, Phenytek)
- piroxicam (Feldene, Nu-Pirox)
- pravastatin (Novo-Pravastatin, Pravachol)
- prochlorperazine (Compazine, Compro)
- rifampin (Rifadin, Rimactane)
- rifapentine (Priftin)
- ritonavir (Norvir)
- saquinavir (Fortovase, Invirase)
- simvastatin (Apo-Simvastatin, Zocor)
- stavudine (Zerit)
- tamoxifen (Nolvadex, Tamofen)
- temazepam (Novo-Temazepam, Restoril)
- tetracycline (Novo-Tetra, Sumycin)
- triazolam (Apo-Triazo, Halcion)
- zidovudine (Novo-AZT, Retrovir)

Taking echinacea with these drugs may worsen HIV or AIDS:
- abacavir (Ziagen)
- acyclovir (Alti-Acyclovir, Zovirax)
- allopurinol (Aloprim, Zyloprim)
- amprenavir (Agenerase)
- cidofovir (Vistide)
- famciclovir (Famvir)
- ganciclovir (Cytovene, Vitrasert)
- indinavir (Crixivan)
- nelfinavir (Viracept)

- rifabutin (Mycobutin)
- ritonavir (Norvir)
- saquinavir (Fortovase, Invirase)
- valganciclovir (Valcyte)
- zidovudine (Novo-AZT, Retrovir)

Taking echinacea with these drugs may interfere with the action of the drug:
- antithymocyte globulin, equine (Atgam)
- antithymocyte globulin, rabbit (Thymoglobulin)
- azathioprine (Imuran)
- basiliximab (Simulect)
- betamethasone (Betatrex, Maxivate)
- cyclosporine (Neoral, Sandimmune)
- daclizumab (Zenapax)
- dexamethasone (Decadron, Dexasone)
- efalizumab (Raptiva)
- hydrocortisone (Cetacort, Locoid)
- methotrexate (Rheumatrex, Trexall)
- methylprednisolone (Depo-Medrol, Medrol)
- muromonab-CD3 (Orthoclone OKT 3)
- mycophenolate (CellCept)
- pimecrolimus (Elidel)
- prednisolone (Inflamase Forte, Pred Forte)
- prednisone (Apo-Prednisone, Deltasone)
- sirolimus (Rapamune)
- tacrolimus (Prograf, Protopic)
- thalidomide (Thalomid)
- triamcinolone (Aristocort, Trinasal)

Taking echinacea with these drugs may worsen tuberculosis:
- doxycycline (Apo-Doxy, Vibramycin)
- isoniazid (Isotamine, Nydrazid)
- tetracycline (Novo-Tetra, Sumycin)

Taking echinacea with these drugs may be harmful:
- etodolac (Lodine, Utradol)—may cause or increase gastrointestinal irritation

Lab Tests That May Be Altered by Echinacea

- May increase alanine aminotransferase (ALT), aspartate aminotransferase (AST), lymphocyte counts, serum immunoglobulin E (IgE), and blood erythrocyte sedimentation rate (ESR).
- May interfere with sperm enzyme activity, when echinacea is taken in high doses.

Diseases That May Be Worsened or Triggered by Echinacea

May trigger allergic reactions in those who typically do not show allergic responses to skin testing.

Foods That May Interact with Echinacea

None known

Supplements That May Interact with Echinacea

None known

ELECAMPANE

Elecampane's scientific name, *Inula helenium*, was taken from Helen of Troy, who was said to be carrying a handful of these sunflowers when the Trojan prince Paris stole her from Sparta, igniting the Trojan War. Favored by the Romans, Greeks, and Celts as a way to treat poor digestion and the effects of overeating, elecampane is used today for these same purposes, as well as for treating respiratory tract infections.

Scientific Name

Inula helenium

Elecampane Is Also Commonly Known As

Elfdock, elfwort, velvet dock, wild sunflower

Medicinal Parts

Rhizome

Elecampane's Uses

To treat colds, menstrual complaints, whooping cough, bronchitis, urinary tract infections, and worm infestation; to stimulate the appetite and digestion

Typical Dose

A typical dose of elecampane is approximately 3g dried root three times a day.

Possible Side Effects

Elecampane's side effects include irritation of mucous membranes and allergic reactions.

Drugs That May Interact with Elecampane

Taking elecampane with these drugs may cause excessive sedation and mental depression and impairment:

- acetaminophen and codeine (Capital and Codeine, Tylenol with Codeine)
- alfentanil (Alfenta)
- alprazolam (Apo-Alpraz, Xanax)
- amobarbital (Amytal)
- amobarbital and secobarbital (Tuinal)
- aspirin and codeine (Coryphen Codeine)
- belladonna and opium (B&O Supprettes)
- bromazepam (Apo-Bromazepam, Gen-Bromazepam)
- brotizolam (Lendorm, Sintonal)
- buprenorphine (Buprenex, Subutex)
- buprenorphine and naloxone (Suboxone)

- butabarbital (Butisol Sodium)
- butalbital, acetaminophen, and caffeine (Esgic, Fioricet)
- butalbital, aspirin, and caffeine (Fiorinal)
- butorphanol (Apo-Butorphanol, Stadol)
- chloral hydrate (Aquachloral Supprettes, Somnote)
- chlordiazepoxide (Apo-Chlordiazepoxide, Librium)
- clobazam (Alti-Clobazam, Frisium)
- clonazepam (Klonopin, Rivotril)
- clorazepate (Tranxene, T-Tab)
- codeine (Codeine Contin)
- dexmedetomidine (Precedex)
- diazepam (Apo-Diazepam, Valium)
- dihydrocodeine, aspirin, and caffeine (Synalgos-DC)
- diphenhydramine (Benadryl Allergy, Nytol)
- estazolam (ProSom)
- fentanyl (Actiq, Duragesic)
- flurazepam (Apo-Flurazepam, Dalmane)
- glutethimide
- haloperidol (Haldol, Novo-Peridol)
- hydrocodone and acetaminophen (Vicodin, Zydone)
- hydrocodone and aspirin (Damason-P)
- hydrocodone and ibuprofen (Vicoprofen)
- hydromorphone (Dilaudid, PMS-Hydro-morphone)
- hydroxyzine (Atarax, Vistaril)
- levomethadyl acetate hydrochloride
- levorphanol (LevoDromoran)
- loprazolam (Dormonoct, Havlane)
- lorazepam (Ativan, Nu-Loraz)
- meperidine (Demerol, Meperitab)
- meperidine and promethazine
- mephobarbital (Mebaral)
- methadone (Dolophine, Methadose)
- methohexital (Brevital, Brevital Sodium)
- midazolam (Apo-Midazolam, Versed)
- morphine sulfate (Kadian, MS Contin)
- nalbuphine (Nubain)
- opium tincture
- oxycodone (OxyContin, Roxicodone)
- oxycodone and acetaminophen (Endocet, Percocet)
- oxycodone and aspirin (Endodan, Percodan)
- oxymorphone (Numorphan)
- paregoric
- pentazocine (Talwin)
- pentobarbital (Nembutal)
- phenobarbital (Luminal Sodium, PMS-Phenobarbital)
- phenoperidine
- prazepam
- primidone (Apo-Primidone, Mysoline)
- promethazine (Phenergan)
- propofol (Diprivan)
- propoxyphene (Darvon, Darvon-N)
- propoxyphene and acetaminophen (Darvocet-N 50, Darvocet-N 100)
- propoxyphene, aspirin, and caffeine (Darvon Compound)
- quazepam (Doral)
- remifentanil (Ultiva)
- secobarbital (Seconal)
- sufentanil (Sufenta)
- s-zopiclone (Lunesta)
- temazepam (Novo-Temazepam, Restoril)
- tetrazepam (Mobiforton, Musapam)
- thiopental (Pentothal)
- triazolam (Apo-Triazo, Halcion)
- zaleplon (Sonata, Stamoc)
- zolpidem (Ambien)
- zopiclone (Alti-Zopiclone, Gen-Zopiclone)

Lab Tests That May Be Altered by Elecampane

None known

Diseases That May Be Worsened or Triggered by Elecampane

- May interfere with blood sugar control in diabetics.
- May interfere with blood pressure control in those with elevated or lowered blood pressure.

Foods That May Interact with Elecampane

None known

Supplements That May Interact with Elecampane

May enhance therapeutic and adverse effects of herbs and supplements that have sedative properties, such as 5-HTP, kava kava, St. John's wort, and valerian. (For a list of herbs and supplements that have sedative properties, see Appendix B.)

ENGLISH HAWTHORN

> English hawthorn, a spring-flowering shrub often grown as an impenetrable hedge, is traditionally used to decorate maypoles for May Day celebrations. Numerous human studies have shown that English hawthorn is helpful in treating the symptoms of mild chronic heart failure and may be helpful in treating hypertension when combined with standard medicines such as ACE inhibitors and calcium channel blockers.

Scientific Name

Crataegus laevigata

English Hawthorn Is Also Commonly Known As

Hawthorn, haw, may bush, mayflower, whitehorn

Medicinal Parts

Flower, leaf, fruit

English Hawthorn's Uses

To treat elevated blood pressure and certain kinds of irregular heartbeat; as a sedative; to prevent the destruction of collagen in the joints. Germany's Commission E has approved the use of English hawthorn to treat a decrease in cardiac output.

Typical Dose

A typical daily dose of English hawthorn is approximately 5 mg of the herb, taken in divided doses three times daily.

Possible Side Effects

English hawthorn's side effects include palpitations, dizziness, headache, and flatulence.

Drugs That May Interact with English Hawthorn

Taking English hawthorn with these drugs may enhance the drug's therapeutic and adverse effects:

- amiodarone (Cordarone, Pacerone)
- amlodipine (Norvasc)
- bepridil (Vascor)
- bretylium
- digitalis (Digitek, Lanoxin)
- diltiazem (Cardizem, Tiazac)
- dofetilide (Tikosyn)
- felodipine (Plendil, Renedil)
- ibutilide (Corvert)
- isosorbide dinitrate (Apo-ISDN, Isordil)
- isosorbide mononitrate (Imdur, Ismo)
- isradipine (DynaCirc)
- lacidipine (Aponil, Caldine)
- lercanidipine (Cardiovasc, Carmen)
- manidipine (Calslot, Iperten)

- nicardipine (Cardene)
- nifedipine (Adalat CC, Procardia)
- nilvadipine
- nimodipine (Nimotop)
- nisoldipine (Sular)
- nitrendipine
- nitroglycerin (Nitro-Bid, Nitro-Dur)
- pinaverium (Dicetel)
- sotalol (Betapace, Sorine)
- verapamil (Calan, Isoptin SR)

Taking English hawthorn with these drugs may increase the risk of bleeding and bruising:
- abciximab (ReoPro)
- aspirin (Bufferin, Ecotrin)
- aspirin and dipyridamole (Aggrenox)
- clopidogrel (Plavix)
- dipyridamole (Novo-Dipiradol, Persantine)
- eptifibatide (Integrillin)
- indobufen (Ibustrin)
- ticlopidine (Alti-Ticlopidine, Ticlid)
- tirofiban (Aggrastat)

Taking English hawthorn with these drugs may decrease drug absorption:
- ferrous sulfate (Feratab, Fer-Iron)
- iron-dextran complex (Dexferrum, INFeD)

Taking English hawthorn with this drug may be harmful:
- digitalis (Digitek, Lanoxin)—may increase the risk of drug toxicity

Lab Tests That May Be Altered by English Hawthorn
None known

Diseases That May Be Worsened or Triggered by English Hawthorn
None known

Foods That May Interact with English Hawthorn
None known

Supplements That May Interact with English Hawthorn
- Increased risk of cardiotoxicity due to potassium depletion when taken with cardioactive herbs, such as digitalis, lily-of-the-valley, and squill. (For a list of cardioactive herbs and supplements, see Appendix B.)
- Increases the action of adonis when taken concurrently.
- Increases the action of lily-of-the-valley when taken concurrently.
- Increases the action of squill when taken concurrently.

ENGLISH LAVENDER

Known for its calming, heavenly scent, English lavender is also an excellent antibacterial that, in oil form, has been used to kill heavyweight bacteria such as streptococcus, pneumococcus, diphtheria, and typhoid. Applied topically, English lavender is also a remedy for cuts, burns, and stings; when inhaled with steam, it eases coughs, colds, and chest infections.

Scientific Name
Lavandula angustifolia, Lavandula officinalis

English Lavender Is Also Commonly Known As
Aspic, French lavender, lavanda, Spanish lavender

Medicinal Parts
Flower, oil of flower

English Lavender's Uses

To treat loss of appetite, insomnia, migraines, asthma, and rheumatic ailments. Germany's Commission E has approved the use of English lavender to treat insomnia, nervousness, loss of appetite, stomach complaints, and circulatory problems.

Typical Dose

A typical dose of English lavender may be up to 2 ml of tincture taken three times a day, or 1 to 2 tsp of dried flowers steeped in 1 cup of boiling water for 10 to 15 minutes and taken as a tea.

Possible Side Effects

Lavender's more common side effects (when taken internally) include constipation, headache, and increased appetite.

Drugs That May Interact with English Lavender

Taking English lavender internally with these drugs may increase sedation:

- acetaminophen and codeine (Capital and Codeine, Tylenol with Codeine)
- acetaminophen, chlorpheniramine, and pseudoephedrine (Children's Tylenol Plus Cold, Sinutab Sinus Allergy Maximum Strength)
- acetaminophen, dextromethorphan, and pseudoephedrine (Alka-Seltzer Plus Flu Liqui-Gels, Sudafed Severe Cold)
- acrivastine and pseudoephedrine (Semprex-D)
- alfentanil (Alfenta)
- amobarbital (Amytal)
- aspirin and codeine (Coryphen Codeine)
- azatadine (Optimine)
- azatadine and pseudoephedrine (Rynatan Tablet, Trinalin)
- azelastine (Astelin, Optivar)

- belladonna and opium (B&O Supprettes)
- brompheniramine and pseudoephedrine (Children's Dimetapp Elixir Cold & Allergy, Lodrane)
- buprenorphine (Buprenex, Subutex)
- buprenorphine and naloxone (Suboxone)
- butabarbital (Butisol Sodium)
- butorphanol (Apo-Butorphanol, Stadol)
- carbinoxamine (Histex CT, Histex PD)
- carbinoxamine and pseudoephedrine (Rondec Drops, Sildec)
- carbinoxamine, pseudoephedrine, and dextromethorphan (Rondec DM Drops, Tussafed)
- cetirizine (Reactine, Zyrtec)
- chloral hydrate (Aquachloral Supprettes, Somnote)
- chlordiazepoxide (Apo-Chlordiazepoxide, Librium)
- chlorpheniramine and acetaminophen (Coricidin HBP Cold and Flu)
- chlorpheniramine and phenylephrine (Histatab Plus, Rynatan)
- chlorpheniramine, ephedrine, phenylephrine, and carbetapentane (Rynatuss, Tynatuss Pediatric)
- chlorpheniramine, phenylephrine, and dextromethorphan (Alka-Seltzer Plus Cold and Cough)
- chlorpheniramine, phenylephrine, and methscopolamine (AH-Chew, Extendryl)
- chlorpheniramine, phenylephrine, and phenyltoloxamine (Comhist, NalexA)
- chlorpheniramine, phenylephrine, codeine, and potassium iodide (Pediacof)
- chlorpheniramine, pseudoephedrine, and codeine (Dihistine DH, RynaC)
- chlorpheniramine, pseudoephedrine, and dextromethorphan (Robitussin Pediatric Night Relief, Vicks Pediatric 44M)

- cimetidine (Nu-Cimet, Tagamet)
- clemastine (Tavist Allergy)
- clorazepate (Tranxene, T-Tab)
- codeine (Codeine Contin)
- cyproheptadine (Periactin)
- deptropine (Deptropine FNA)
- desloratadine (Aerius, Clarinex)
- dexbrompheniramine and pseudoephedrine (Drixomed, Drixoral Cold & Allergy)
- dexchlorpheniramine (Polaramine)
- dexmedetomidine (Precedex)
- diazepam (Apo-Diazepam, Valium)
- dihydrocodeine, aspirin, and caffeine (Synalgos-DC)
- dimethindene (Fenistil)
- diphenhydramine (Benadryl Allergy, Nytol)
- diphenhydramine and pseudoephedrine (Benadryl Allergy/Decongestant, Benadryl Children's Allergy and Sinus)
- doxylamine and pyridoxine (Diclectin)
- epinastine (Elestat)
- estazolam (ProSom)
- famotidine (Apo-Famotidine, Pepcid)
- fentanyl (Actiq, Duragesic)
- fexofenadine (Allegra)
- fexofenadine and pseudoephedrine (Allegra D)
- flurazepam (Apo-Flurazepam, Dalmane)
- haloperidol (Haldol, Novo-Peridol)
- hydrocodone and acetaminophen (Vicodin, Zydone)
- hydrocodone and aspirin (Damason-P)
- hydrocodone and chlorpheniramine (Tussionex)
- hydrocodone and ibuprofen (Vicoprofen)
- hydrocodone, carbinoxamine, and pseudo-ephedrine (Histex HC, TriVent HC)
- hydromorphone (Dilaudid, PMS-Hydromorphone)
- hydroxyzine (Atarax, Vistaril)
- ketotifen (Novo-Ketotifen, Zaditor)
- levocabastine (Livostin)
- levomethadyl acetate hydrochloride
- levorphanol (LevoDromoran)
- loratadine (Alavert, Claritin)
- loratadine and pseudoephedrine (Claritin-D 12 Hour, Claritin-D 24 Hour)
- lorazepam (Ativan, Nu-Loraz)
- mebhydrolin (Bexidal, Incidal)
- meperidine (Demerol, Meperitab)
- meperidine and promethazine
- mephobarbital (Mebaral)
- methadone (Dolophine, Methadose)
- midazolam (Apo-Midazolam, Versed)
- mizolastine (Elina, Mizollen)
- morphine sulfate (Kadian, MS Contin)
- nalbuphine (Nubain)
- nizatidine (Axid, PMS-Nizatidine)
- olopatadine (Patanol)
- opium tincture
- oxatomide (Cenacert, Tinset)
- oxycodone (OxyContin, Roxicodone)
- oxycodone and acetaminophen (Endocet, Percocet)
- oxycodone and aspirin (Endodan, Percodan)
- oxymorphone (Numorphan)
- paregoric
- pentazocine (Talwin)
- pentobarbital (Nembutal)
- phenobarbital (Luminal Sodium, PMS-Pheno-barbital)
- phenoperidine
- promethazine (Phenergan)
- promethazine and codeine (Phenergan with Codeine)
- promethazine and dextromethorphan (Promatussin DM)
- promethazine and phenylephrine
- promethazine, phenylephrine, and codeine

- propofol (Diprivan)
- propoxyphene (Darvon, Darvon-N)
- propoxyphene and acetaminophen (Darvocet-N 50, Darvocet-N 100)
- propoxyphene, aspirin, and caffeine (Darvon Compound)
- quazepam (Doral)
- ranitidine (Alti-Ranitidine, Zantac)
- remifentanil (Ultiva)
- secobarbital (Seconal)
- sufentanil (Sufenta)
- temazepam (Novo-Temazepam, Restoril)
- thiopental (Pentothal)
- triazolam (Apo-Triazo, Halcion)
- tripelennamine (PBZ, PBZ-SR)
- triprolidine and pseudoephedrine (Actifed Cold and Allergy, Silafed)
- triprolidine, pseudoephedrine, and codeine (CoActifed, Covan)
- zolpidem (Ambien)

Taking English lavender (in the form of tea) with these drugs may interfere with drug absorption:
- ferric gluconate (Ferrlecit)
- ferrous fumarate (Femiron, Feostat)
- ferrous gluconate (Fergon, Novo-Ferrogluc)
- ferrous sulfate (Feratab, Fer-Iron)
- ferrous sulfate and ascorbic acid (FeroGrad 500, Vitelle Irospan)
- iron-dextran complex (Dexferrum, INFeD)
- polysaccharide-iron complex (Hytinic, Niferex)

Lab Tests That May Be Altered by English Lavender
May decrease blood cholesterol levels.

Diseases That May Be Worsened or Triggered by English Lavender
None known

Foods That May Interact with English Lavender
None known

Supplements That May Interact with English Lavender
None known

ENGLISH PLANTAIN

The English plantain, a common weed that was brought to North America with the first European settlers and spread throughout almost the entire continent, has lance-shaped leaves and spiky flowers. Farmers planted it in their meadows and pastures as a preferred food for sheep. Medicinally, the juice taken from the leaves was used to calm fevers and promote wound healing, while plantain tea was used to treat congestion.

Scientific Name
Plantago lanceolata

English Plantain Is Also Commonly Known As
Buckhorn, chimney-sweeps, rib grass, ribwort, soldier's herb

Medicinal Parts
Leaf, whole plant

English Plantain's Uses
To treat liver disease, diarrhea, stomach cramps, and various respiratory tract ailments

Typical Dose
A typical daily dose of English plantain ranges from 3 to 6 gm of the herb.

Possible Side Effects

English plantain's side effects include possible allergic reactions.

Drugs That May Interact with English Plantain

Taking English plantain with these drugs may reduce or prevent drug absorption:

- carbamazepine (Carbatrol, Tegretol)
- digitalis (Digitek, Lanoxin)
- ferrous sulfate (Feratab, Fer-Iron)
- iron-dextran complex (Dexferrum, INFeD)
- lithium (Eskalith, Carbolith)

Lab Tests That May Be Altered by English Plantain

None known

Diseases That May Be Worsened or Triggered by English Plantain

None known

Foods That May Interact with English Plantain

None known

Supplements That May Interact with English Plantain

None known

ERGOT

> Ergot is a fungus that infects grains of rye and related grasses. It may be most famous for containing the alkaloid ergine (d-lysergic acid amide), better known as natural LSD. During the Middle Ages, tens of thousands of people in Europe who ate rye bread infested with ergot fungus were afflicted with a disease called St. Anthony's fire, which caused gangrene, convulsions, madness, and death. In modern medicine, two of ergot's alkaloids are commonly used: ergonovine, to induce labor and control hemorrhaging, and ergotamine, to relieve migraine headaches.

Scientific Name

Claviceps purpurea

Ergot Is Also Commonly Known As

Cockspur rye, hornseed, mother of rye, spurred rye

Medicinal Parts

Body of the plant

Ergot's Uses

Ergot was formerly used for migraines and various gynecological and obstetric problems, but is now considered too dangerous to use. In homeopathy, it may be used to treat paralysis, circulatory problems, bleeding, and other ailments.

Typical Dose

A typical homeopathic dose of ergot is approximately 5 drops, 1 tablet, or 10 globules once a day or more, depending on the ailment.

Possible Side Effects

Ergot's side effects include queasiness, vomiting, weakness in the legs, numbness in the fingers, angina, and rapid or slow heartbeat.

Drugs That May Interact with Ergot

Taking ergot with these drugs may cause or increase serotonergic side effects or serotonin syndrome (with symptoms including agitation, rapid heart rate, flushing, heavy sweating, and possibly even death):

- amitriptyline (Elavil, Levate)
- amitriptyline and chlordiazepoxide (Limbitrol)
- amitriptyline and perphenazine (Etrafon, Triavil)

- amoxapine (Asendin)
- bupropion (Wellbutrin, Zyban)
- citalopram (Celexa)
- clomipramine (Anafranil, Novo-Clopramine)
- desipramine (Alti-Desipramine, Norpramin)
- dextromethorphan (found in various formulations of Alka-Seltzer, Contac, PediaCare, Robitussin, Sudafed, Triaminic, and other over-the-counter medications)
- doxepin (Sinequan, Zonalon)
- fluoxetine (Prozac, Sarafem)
- fluvoxamine (Alti-Fluvoxamine, Luvox)
- imipramine (Apo-Imipramine, Tofranil)
- iproniazid (Marsilid)
- lofepramine (Feprapax, Gamanil)
- maprotiline (Novo-Maprotiline)
- melitracen (Dixeran)
- meperidine (Demerol, Meperitab)
- milnacipran (Dalcipran, Lixel)
- mirtazapine (Remeron, Remeron SolTab)
- moclobemide (Alti-Moclobemide, Nu-Moclobemide)
- nefazodone (Serzone)
- nortriptyline (Aventyl HCl, Pamelor)
- paroxetine (Paxil)
- pentazocine (Talwin)
- phenelzine (Nardil)
- protriptyline (Vivactil)
- reboxetine (Davedax, Integrex)
- s-citalopram (Lexapro)
- selegiline (Eldepryl)
- sertraline (Apo-Sertraline, Zoloft)
- tramadol (Ultram)
- tranylcypromine (Parnate)
- trazodone (Desyrel, Novo-Trazodone)
- trimipramine (Apo-Trimip, Surmontil)
- venlafaxine (Effexor)

Taking ergot with these drugs may increase the adverse effects of the drug:

- belladonna, phenobarbital, and ergotamine (Bellamine S, Bel-Tabs)
- bromocriptine (Apo-Bromocriptine, Parlodel)
- cabergoline (Dostinex)
- dihydroergotamine (Migranal)
- ergoloid mesylates (Hydergine)
- ergonovine
- ergotamine (Cafergor, Cafergot)
- methylergonovine (Methergine)
- methysergide (Sansert)
- pergolide (Permax)

Lab Tests That May Be Altered by Ergot
None known

Diseases That May Be Worsened or Triggered by Ergot
May worsen heart problems and peripheral vascular disease by causing the arteries to constrict, hampering blood flow.

Foods That May Interact with Ergot
None known

Supplements That May Interact with Ergot
- May increase positive and negative effects of herbs and supplements that have serotonergic properties, such as 5-hydroxytryptophan (5-HTP), S-adenosylmethionine (SAMe), and St. John's wort. (For a list of herbs and supplements that have serotonergic properties, see Appendix B.)
- May increase positive and negative effects of herbs and supplements that have sympathomimetic activity (stimulate the

central nervous system), such as bitter orange, country mallow, and ma-huang. (For a list of herbs and supplements that have sympathomimetic activity, see Appendix B.)

ETHANOL

> Ethanol (alcohol) is not an herb, of course, but is found in various herbal preparations and other supplements and interacts with a great many medicines. Before using any herb or supplement, read the ingredient list carefully to see if ethanol is included.

Drugs That May Interact with Ethanol

Taking ethanol with these drugs may increase sedation and mental depression and impairment:

- acetaminophen and codeine (Capital and Codeine, Tylenol with Codeine)
- acetophenazine
- aldesleukin (Proleukin)
- alfentanil (Alfenta)
- alprazolam (Apo-Alpraz, Xanax)
- amantadine (Endantadine, Symmetrel)
- amitriptyline (Elavil, Levate)
- amitriptyline and chlordiazepoxide (Limbitrol)
- amitriptyline and perphenazine (Etrafon, Triavil)
- amobarbital (Amytal)
- amobarbital and secobarbital (Tuinal)
- amoxapine (Asendin)
- aspirin and codeine (Coryphen Codeine)
- azelastine (Astelin, Optivar)
- belladonna and opium (B&O Supprettes)
- benztropine (Apo-Benztropine, Cogentin)
- bromazepam (Apo-Bromazepam, Gen-Bromazepam)
- brotizolam (Lendorm, Sintonal)
- buprenorphine (Buprenex, Subutex)
- buprenorphine and naloxone (Suboxone)
- butabarbital (Butisol Sodium)
- butalbital, acetaminophen, and caffeine (Esgic, Fioricet)
- butalbital, aspirin, and caffeine (Fiorinal)
- butorphanol (Apo-Butorphanol, Stadol)
- chloral hydrate (Aquachloral Supprettes, Somnote)
- chlordiazepoxide (Apo-Chlordiazepoxide, Librium)
- chlorzoxazone (Strifion Forte)
- clemastine (Tavist Allergy)
- clobazam (Alti-Clobazam, Frisium)
- clomipramine (Anafranil, Novo-Clopramine)
- clonazepam (Klonopin, Rivotril)
- clorazepate (Tranxene, T-Tab)
- codeine (Codeine Contin)
- cyclobenzaprine (Flexeril, Novo-Cycloprine)
- desipramine (Alti-Desipramine, Norpramin)
- dexmedetomidine (Precedex)
- diazepam (Apo-Diazepam, Valium)
- dihydrocodeine, aspirin, and caffeine (Synalgos-DC)
- diphenhydramine (Benadryl Allergy, Nytol)
- diphenoxylate and atropine (Lomotil, Lonox)
- disopyramide (Norpace, Rhythmodan)
- doxepin (Sinequan, Zonalon)
- doxylamine and pyridoxine (Diclectin)
- dronabinol (Marinol)
- estazolam (ProSom)
- felbamate (Felbatol)
- fentanyl (Actiq, Duragesic)
- fluoxetine (Prozac, Sarafem)

- fluphenazine (Prolixin, Modecate)
- flurazepam (Apo-Flurazepam, Dalmane)
- fluvoxamine (Alti-Fluvoxamine, Luvox)
- galantamine (Razadyne)
- glutethimide
- haloperidol (Haldol, Novo-Peridol)
- hydralazine (Apresoline, Novo-Hylazin)
- hydrocodone and acetaminophen (Vicodin, Zydone)
- hydrocodone and aspirin (Damason-P)
- hydrocodone and ibuprofen (Vicoprofen)
- hydromorphone (Dilaudid, PMS-Hydromorphone)
- hydroxyzine (Atarax, Vistaril)
- imipramine (Apo-Imipramine, Tofranil)
- iproniazid (Marsilid)
- lamotrigine (Lamictal)
- levetiracetam (Keppra)
- levodopa (Dopar, Laradopa)
- levomethadyl acetate hydrochloride
- levorphanol (Levo-Dromoran)
- lofepramine (Feprapax, Gamanil)
- loprazolam (Dormonoct, Havlane)
- lorazepam (Ativan, Nu-Loraz)
- loxapine (Loxitane, Nu-Loxapine)
- meclizine (Antivert, Bonine)
- melitracen (Dixeran)
- meperidine (Demerol, Meperitab)
- meperidine and promethazine
- mephobarbital (Mebaral)
- meprobamate (Miltown, Movo-Mepro)
- mesoridazine (Serentil)
- methadone (Dolophine, Methadose)
- methamphetamine (Desoxyn)
- methocarbamol (Robaxin)
- methohexital (Brevital, Brevital Sodium)
- methotrimeprazine (Novo-Meprazine, Nozain)
- methylphenidate (Concerta, Ritalin)
- metoclopramide (Apo-Metoclop, Reglan)
- midazolam (Apo-Midazolam, Versed)
- mirtazapine (Remeron)
- mitotane (Lysodren)
- moclobemide (Alti-Moclobemide, Nu-Moclobemide)
- molindone (Moban)
- morphine sulfate (Kadian, MS Contin)
- nalbuphine (Nubain)
- nefazodone (Serzone)
- nicardipine (Cardene)
- nifedipine (Adalat CC, Procardia)
- nitrofurantoin (Furadantin, Macrobid)
- nortriptyline (Aventyl HCl, Pamelor)
- olanzapine (Zydis, Zyprexa)
- opium tincture
- oxazepam (Novoxapam, Serax)
- oxcarbazepine (Trileptal)
- oxprenolol (Slow-Trasicor, Trasicor)
- oxybutynin (Ditropan, Oxytrol)
- oxycodone (OxyContin, Roxicodone)
- oxycodone and acetaminophen (Endocet, Percocet)
- oxycodone and aspirin (Endodan, Percodan)
- oxymorphone (Numorphan)
- paregoric
- paroxetine (Paxil)
- pemoline (Cylert, PemADD)
- pentamidine (NebuPent, Pentacarinat)
- pentazocine (Talwin)
- pentobarbital (Nembutal)
- pergolide (Permax)
- perphenazine (Apo-Perphenazine, Trilafon)
- phenelzine (Nardil)
- phenobarbital (Luminal Sodium, PMS-Phenobarbital)
- phenoperidine
- pizotifen (Sandomigran)

- pramipexole (Mirapex)
- prazepam
- primidone (Apo-Primidone, Mysoline)
- procarbazine (Matulane, Natulan)
- prochlorperazine (Compazine, Compro)
- promethazine (Phenergan)
- propofol (Diprivan)
- propoxyphene (Darvon, Darvon-N)
- propoxyphene and acetaminophen (Darvocet-N 50, Darvocet-N 100)
- propoxyphene, aspirin, and caffeine (Darvon Compound)
- protriptyline (Vivactil)
- quazepam (Doral)
- quetiapine (Seroquel)
- remifentanil (Ultiva)
- riluzole (Rilutek)
- risperidone (Risperdal)
- ropinirole (Requip)
- s-citalopram (Lexapro)
- secobarbital (Seconal)
- selegiline (Eldepryl)
- sertraline (Apo-Sertraline, Zoloft)
- sodium oxybate (Xyrem)
- sufentanil (Sufenta)
- s-zopiclone (Lunesta)
- temazepam (Novo-Temazepam, Restoril)
- tetrazepam (Mobiforton, Musapam)
- thalidomide (Thalomid)
- thiethylperazine (Torecan)
- thiopental (Pentothal)
- thioridazine (Mellaril)
- thiothixene (Navane)
- tiagabine (Gabitril)
- tizanidine (Zanaflex)
- tolcapone (Tasmar)
- topiramate (Topamax)
- tramadol (Ultram)

- tranylcypromine (Parnate)
- trazodone (Desyrel, Novo-Trazodone)
- tretinoin (oral) (Vesanoid)
- triazolam (Apo-Triazo, Halcion)
- trifluoperazine (Novo-Trifluzine, Stelazine)
- trihexyphenidyl (Artane)
- trimebutine (Apo-Trimebutine, Modulon)
- trimipramine (Apo-Trimip, Surmontil)
- valproic acid (Depacon, Depakote ER)
- venlafaxine (Effexor)
- vigabatrin (Sabril)
- zaleplon (Sonata, Starnoc)
- zileuton (Zyflo)
- ziprasidone (Geodon)
- zolpidem (Ambien)
- zonisamide (Zonegran)
- zopiclone (Alti-Zopiclone, Gen-Zopiclone)
- zuclopenthixol (Clopixol)

Taking ethanol with these drugs increases the risk of gastric irritation:

- chloroquine (Aralen)
- cladribine (Leustatin)
- dacarbazine (DTIC, DTIC-Dome)
- daunorubicin hydrochloride (Cerubidine)
- dexamethasone (Decadron, Dexasone)
- diclofenac (Cataflam, Voltaren)
- diflunisal (Apo-Diflunisal, Dolobid)
- docetaxel (Taxotere)
- epirubicin (Ellence, Pharmorubicin)
- etodolac (Lodine, Utradol)
- etoposide (Toposar, VePesid)
- etoposide phosphate (Etopophos)
- famotidine (Apo-Famotidine, Pepcid)
- fenoprofen (Nalfon)
- fludarabine (Fludara)
- fluorouracil (Adrucil, Efudex)
- flurbiprofen (Ansaid, Ocufen)

- hydrocodone and acetaminophen (Anexsia, Vicodin)
- hydrocodone and aspirin (Damason-P)
- hydrocodone and ibuprofen (Vicoprofen)
- hydrocortisone (Cetacort, Locoid)
- hydroxychloroquine (Apo-Hydroxyquine, Plaquenil)
- ibuprofen (Advil, Motrin)
- indomethacin (Indocin, Novo-Methacin)
- ketorolac (Acular, Toradol)
- lansoprazole (Prevacid)
- levamisole (Ergamisol)
- mechlorethamine (Mustargen)
- meclofenamate (Meclomen)
- mefenamic acid (Ponstan, Ponstel)
- meloxicam (MOBIC, Mobicox)
- melphalan (Alkeran)
- methylprednisolone (Depo-Medrol, Medrol)
- nabumetone (Apo-Nabumetone, Relefan)
- naproxen (Aleve, Naprosyn)
- nizatidine (Axid, PMS-Nizatidine)
- omeprazole (Losec, Prilosec)
- oxaprozin (Apo-Oxaprozin, Daypro)
- pantoprazole (Pantoloc, Protonix)
- piroxicam (Feldene, Nu-Pirox)
- prednisolone (Inflamase Forte, Pred Forte)
- prednisone (Apo-Prednisone, Deltasone)
- primaquine
- rabeprazole (Aciphex, Pariet)
- ranitidine (Alti-Ranitidine, Zantac)
- rivastigmine (Exelon)
- salsalate (Amgesic, Salflex)
- sulindac (Clinoril, Nu-Sundac)
- thiotepa (Thioplex)
- tiaprofenic acid (Dom-Tiaprofenic, Surgam)
- tolmetin (Tolectin)
- topotecan (Hycamtin)

- triamcinolone (Aristocort, Trinasal)
- valdecoxib (Bextra)

Taking ethanol with these drugs may cause headache, nausea, vomiting, or chest pain:
- cefamandole (Mandol)
- cefotetan (Cefotan)
- disulfiram (Antabuse)
- gliclazide (Diamicron, Novo-Gliclazide)
- glipizide (Glucotrol)
- metronidazole (Flagyl, Noritate)

Taking ethanol with these drugs may cause or increase liver damage:
- acetaminophen (Genapap, Tylenol)
- efavirenz (Sustiva)
- erythromycin (Erythrocin, Staticin)
- fluvastatin (Lescol)
- isoniazid (Isotamine, Nydrazid)
- lovastatin (Altocor, Mevacor)
- methotrexate (Rheumatrex, Trexall)
- peginterferon alfa-2a (Pegasys)
- peginterferon alfa-2b (PEG-Intron)
- pravastatin (Novo-Pravastatin, Pravachol)
- rifampin (Rifadin, Rimactane)
- rosuvastatin (Crestor)
- simvastatin (Apo-Simvastatin, Zocor)

Taking ethanol with these may increase risk of breast cancer and/or osteoporosis:
- estradiol (Climara, Estrace)
- estrogens (conjugated A/synthetic) (Cenestin)
- estrogens (conjugated/equine) (Cenestin, Premarin)
- estrogens (esterified) (Estratab, Menest)
- estropipate (Ogen, Ortho-Est)

- ethinyl estradiol (Estinyl)
- enthinyl estradiol and norenthindrone (Brevicon, Ortho-Novum)
- raloxifene (Evista)
- risedronate (Actonel)
- teriparatide (Forteo)

Taking ethanol with these may increase risk of hypoglycemia (low blood sugar):

- acarbose (Prandase, Precose)
- gliclazide (Diamicron, Novo-Gliclazide)
- glimepiride (Amaryl)
- glipizide (Glucotrol)
- glyburide (DiaBeta, Micronase)
- metformin (Glucophage, Riomet)
- nateglinide (Starlix)
- pentamidine (NebuPent, Pentacarinat)
- pioglitazone (Actos)
- repaglinide (GlucoNorm, Prandin)
- rosiglitazone (Avandia)

Taking ethanol with these may increase risk of hypotension (excessively low blood pressure):

- isosorbide dinitrate (Apo-ISDN, Isordil)
- isosorbide mononitrate (Imdur, Ismo)
- tadalafil (Cialis)

Taking ethanol with these may decrease drug levels:

- procainamide (Procanbid, Pronestyl-SR)
- propranolol (Inderal, InnoPran XL)

Taking ethanol with these may increase the therapeutic and adverse effects of the drug:

- alprostadil (Caverject, Muse)
- diltiazem (Cardizem, Tiazac)
- prazosin (Minipress, Nu-Prazo)

Taking ethanol with these drugs may be harmful:

- acitretin (Soriatane)—causes formation of etretinate, which is harmful to a fetus
- didanosine (Videx, Videx EC)—may increase risk of pancreatitis
- doxycycline (Apo-Doxy, Vibramycin)—may reduce blood levels of the drug
- erythromycin (Erythrocin, Staticin)—may decrease drug absorption
- isotretinoin (Accutane, Caravis)—may increase triglyceride levels
- linezolid (Zyvox)—if ethanol is taken in conjunction with tyramine (found in red wine), hypertensive crisis can result
- nilutamide (Nilandron, Anadron)—may cause flushing, hypotension (low blood pressure), malaise, and other symptoms of a systemic reaction
- phenelzine (Nardil)—may cause severe hypertensive response (increase in blood pressure)
- phenytoin (Dilantin, Phenytek)—may increase or decrease drug metabolism
- tranylcypromine (Parnate)—may cause severe hypertensive response
- verapamil (Calan, Isoptin SR)—may increase ethanol levels
- warfarin (Coumadin, Jantoven)—may interfere with action of the drug
- zolmitriptan (Zomig)—may contribute to central nervous system toxicity

Lab Tests That May Be Altered by Ethanol

May increase values on liver function tests including alanine aminotransferase (ALT), alkaline phosphatase (ALK PHOS), aspartic acid transaminase (AST), bilirubin, and gamma-glutamyltransferase (GGT).

Diseases That May Be Worsened or Triggered by Ethanol

May worsen angina, cardiomyopathy, elevated blood fat levels, gastroesophageal reflux disease (GERD), gout, heart failure, hypertension, insomnia, liver disease, neurological ailments, pancreatitis, peptic ulcer disease, porphyria, and psychiatric ailments.

Foods That May Interact with Ethanol

Chronic alcohol use hampers the absorption of B-vitamins and other nutrients.

Supplements That May Interact with Ethanol

May enhance therapeutic and adverse effects of herbs and supplements that have sedative properties, such as 5-HTP, St. John's wort, and valerian. (For a list of herbs and supplements that have sedative properties, see Appendix B.)

EUCALYPTUS

A favorite meal of koala bears, the leaves of the eucalyptus tree contain a pungent oil that can clear a cold-stuffed head with just a whiff or two. Eucalyptus oil is commonly found in steam-inhalation preparations for colds and flu and in chest rubs, snifters, and cough drops. It can also be rubbed on skin to ease the pain of arthritis and rheumatism.

Scientific Name

Eucalyptus globulus

Eucalyptus Is Also Commonly Known As

Blue gum, fever tree, gum tree, Tasmanian blue gum

Medicinal Parts

Leaf, oil extracted from leaf and branch tips

Eucalyptus's Uses

Eucalyptus leaf is used to treat asthma, fever, whooping cough, loss of appetite, diabetes, and fever. Eucalyptus oil is used to treat asthma, emphysema, cough, ulcers, wounds, burns, and rheumatism. Germany's Commission E has approved the use of eucalyptus leaf to treat coughs and bronchitis and eucalyptus oil to treat rheumatism, bronchitis, and cough.

Typical Dose

The average daily dose of eucalyptus is 1.5 gm of the leaf taken several times a day. A typical internal dose of eucalyptus oil may range from 0.3 to 0.6 gm, while externally several drops of the essential oil may be rubbed onto the skin.

Possible Side Effects

Eucalyptus's side effects include dizziness, seizures, nausea, loss of appetite, and confusion.

Drugs That May Interact with Eucalyptus

Taking eucalyptus with these drugs may increase the risk of hypoglycemia (low blood sugar):

- acarbose (Prandase, Precose)
- acetohexamide
- chlorpropamide (Diabinese, Novo-Propamide)
- gliclazide (Diamicron, Novo-Gliclazide)
- glimepiride (Amaryl)
- glipizide (Glucotrol)
- glipizide and metformin (Metaglip)
- gliquidone (Beglynor, Glurenorm)
- glyburide (DiaBeta, Micronase)
- glyburide and metformin (Glucovance)

- insulin (Humulin, Novolin R)
- metformin (Glucophage, Riomet)
- miglitol (Glyset)
- nateglinide (Starlix)
- pioglitazone (Actos)
- repaglinide (GlucoNorm, Prandin)
- rosiglitazone (Avandia)
- rosiglitazone and metformin (Avandamet)
- tolazamide (Tolinase)
- tolbutamide (Apo-Tolbutamide, Tol-Tab)

Taking eucalyptus with these drugs may reduce the effectiveness of the drug:
- amobarbital (Amytal)
- amobarbital and secobarbital (Tuinal)
- butabarbital (Butisol Sodium)
- butalbital, acetaminophen, and caffeine (Esgic, Fioricet)
- butalbital, aspirin, and caffeine (Fiorinal)
- mephobarbital (Mebaral)
- methohexital (Brevital, Brevital Sodium)
- pentobarbital (Nembutal)
- phenobarbital (Luminal Sodium, PMS-Phenobarbital)
- primidone (Apo-Primidone, Mysoline)
- secobarbital (Seconal)
- thiopental (Pentothal)

Lab Tests That May Be Altered by Eucalyptus
None known

Diseases That May Be Worsened or Triggered by Eucalyptus
- May interfere with attempts to control blood sugar in diabetes.
- May worsen disease of the liver or gastrointestinal tract.

Foods That May Interact with Eucalyptus
None known

Supplements That May Interact with Eucalyptus
Increased risk of additive toxicity when eucalyptus oil is used with herbs and supplements containing unsaturated pyrrolizidine alkaloids (UPAs), such as butterbur, comfrey, and colt's foot. (For a list of herbs containing unsaturated pyrrolizidine alkaloids, see Appendix B.)

EUROPEAN ELDER

The black berries taken from the European elder tree, also known as elderberries, have long been used as a remedy for colds, the flu, and sinus infections. During a flu outbreak in the early 1990s, elderberry extract was compared to a placebo in a group of people living in a farming community. In just two to three days, the elderberry extract produced a significant improvement in fever and other symptoms in nearly 90 percent of those taking it, compared to the six days it took to see similar results among those taking the placebo.

Scientific Name
Sambucus nigra

European Elder Is Also Commonly Known As
Black elder, boor tree, elder, elderberry, ellanwood

Medicinal Parts
Bark, flower, leaf, fruit, and root

European Elder's Uses
To treat colds, laryngitis, shortness of breath, and inflammation

Typical Dose

A typical daily dose of European elder is approximately 10 to 15 gm taken as a tea.

Possible Side Effects

European elder's side effects include dizziness, convulsions, vomiting, and rapid heart rate.

Drugs That May Interact with European Elder

Taking European elder with these drugs may reduce or prevent drug absorption:

- ferric gluconate (Ferrlecit)
- ferrous fumarate (Femiron, Feostat)
- ferrous gluconate (Fergon, Novo-Ferrogluc)
- ferrous sulfate (Feratab, Fer-Iron)
- ferrous sulfate and ascorbic acid (Fero-Grad 500, Vitelle Irospan)
- iron-dextran complex (Dexferrum, INFeD)
- polysaccharide-iron complex (Hytinic, Niferex)

Lab Tests That May Be Altered by European Elder

None known

Diseases That May Be Worsened or Triggered by European Elder

None known

Foods That May Interact with European Elder

None known

Supplements That May Interact with European Elder

None known

EUROPEAN MISTLETOE

European mistletoe is available as a prescription medication in Europe, where it is sometimes used in conjunction with other medications to delay the progression of solid tumors in the breast, colon, and stomach. It has also been used to improve immune function and to lower blood pressure by slowing the heart rate and dilating the arteries.

Scientific Name

Viscum album

European Mistletoe Is Also Commonly Known As

All-Heal, birdlime, devil's fuge, mistletoe, visci

Medicinal Parts

Leaf, stem, fruit, whole plant

European Mistletoe's Uses

European mistletoe fruit is used to treat epilepsy, gout, cramps, tumors, rheumatism, and hardening of the arteries. The stem of European mistletoe is used to treat physical and mental exhaustion and as a tranquilizer. Germany's Commission E has approved the use of the European mistletoe herb as a treatment for rheumatism and a supportive therapy in the treatment of tumors.

Typical Dose

A typical dose of European mistletoe may range from 2 to 6 gm of dried leaves taken three times a day.

Possible Side Effects

European mistletoe's side effects include fever, chills, headache, and chest pain.

Drugs That May Interact with European Mistletoe

Taking European mistletoe with these drugs may reduce or prevent drug absorption:

- ferric gluconate (Ferrlecit)
- ferrous fumarate (Femiron, Feostat)
- ferrous gluconate (Fergon, Novo-Ferrogluc)
- ferrous sulfate (Feratab, Fer-Iron)
- ferrous sulfate and ascorbic acid (Fero-Grad 500, Vitelle Irospan)
- iron-dextran complex (Dexferrum, INFeD)
- polysaccharide-iron complex (Hytinic, Niferex)

Taking European mistletoe with these drugs may interfere with the action of the drug:

- atenolol (Apo-Atenol, Tenormin)
- cyclosporine (Neoral, Sandimmune)
- dexamethasone (Decadron, Dexasone)
- methylprednisolone (Depo-Medrol, Medrol)
- prednisone (Apo-Prednisone, Deltasone)

Taking European mistletoe with these drugs may increase the risk of hypotension (low blood pressure):

- acebutolol (Novo-Acebutolol, Sectral)
- amlodipine (Norvasc)
- atenolol (Apo-Atenol, Tenormin)
- benazepril (Lotensin)
- betaxolol (Betoptic S, Kerlone)
- bisoprolol (Monocor, Zebeta)
- bumetanide (Bumex, Burinex)
- candesartan (Atacand)
- captopril (Capoten, Novo-Captopril)
- carteolol (Cartrol, Ocupress)
- carvedilol (Coreg)
- chlorothiazide (Diuril)
- chlorthalidone (Apo-Chlorthalidone, Thalitone)
- clonidine (Catapres, Duraclon)
- diazoxide (Hyperstat, Proglycem)
- diltiazem (Cardizem, Tiazac)

- doxazosin (Alti-Doxazosin, Cardura)
- enalapril (Vasotec)
- eplerenone (Inspra)
- eprosartan (Teveten)
- esmolol (Brevibloc)
- felodipine (Plendil, Renedil)
- fenoldopam (Corlopam)
- fosinopril (Monopril)
- furosemide (Apo-Furosemide, Lasix)
- guanabenz (Wytensin)
- guanadrel (Hylorel)
- guanfacine (Tenex)
- hydralazine (Apresoline, Novo-Hylazin)
- hydrochlorothiazide (Apo-Hydro, Microzide)
- hydrochlorothiazide and triamterene (Dyazide, Maxzide)
- indapamide (Lozol, Nu-Indapamide)
- irbesartan (Avapro)
- isradipine (DynaCirc)
- labetalol (Normodyne, Trandate)
- lisinopril (Prinivil, Zestril)
- losartan (Cozaar)
- mecamylamine (Inversine)
- mefruside (Baycaron)
- methyclothiazide (Aquatensen, Enduron)
- methyldopa (Apo-Methyldopa, Nu-Medopa)
- metolazone (Mykrox, Zaroxolyn)
- metoprolol (Betaloc, Lopressor)
- minoxidil (Loniten, Rogaine)
- moexipril (Univasc)
- nadolol (Apo-Nadol, Corgard)
- nicardipine (Cardene)
- nifedipine (Adalat CC, Procardia)
- nisoldipine (Sular)
- nitroglycerin (Minitran, Nitro-Dur)
- nitroprusside (Nipride, Nitropress)
- olmesartan (Benicar)

- oxprenolol (Slow-Trasicor, Trasicor)
- perindopril erbumine (Aceon, Coversyl)
- phenoxybenzamine (Dibenzyline)
- phentolamine (Regitine, Rogitine)
- pindolol (Apo-Pindol, Novo-Pindol)
- polythiazide (Renese)
- prazosin (Minipress, Nu-Prazo)
- propranolol (Inderal, InnoPran XL)
- quinapril (Accupril)
- ramipril (Altace)
- reserpine
- spironolactone (Aldactone, Novo-Spiroton)
- telmisartan (Micardis)
- terazosin (Alti-Terazosin, Hytrin)
- timolol (Betimol, Timoptic)
- torsemide (Demadex)
- trandolapril (Mavik)
- triamterene (Dyrenium)
- trichlormethiazide (Matatensin, Naqua)
- valsartan (Diovan)
- verapamil (Calan, Isoptin SR)

Lab Tests That May Be Altered by European Mistletoe

- May increase values on liver function tests including aspartic acid transaminase (AST), alanine aminotransferase (ALT), total bilirubin, and urine bilirubin.
- May increase lymphocyte counts.
- When injected, may contribute to eosinophilia (abnormally high amounts of a certain kind of white blood cell).
- May cause decreased red blood cells.

Diseases That May Be Worsened or Triggered by European Mistletoe

- May worsen cardiovascular ailments.
- May worsen cases of potential transplant rejection by stimulating the immune system.

Foods That May Interact with European Mistletoe

None known

Supplements That May Interact with European Mistletoe

- May be cardiotoxic and have negative effects on the strength of heart contractions.
- May decrease the effectiveness of agents such as English hawthorn that have positive effects on the strength of heart contractions.

EVENING PRIMROSE OIL

Used for medicinal purposes for centuries, the oil taken from the seed of the evening primrose contains gamma-linolenic acid (GLA), an essential fatty acid thought to be in short supply in many people's diets. Evening primrose oil has been used to treat breast tenderness associated with premenstrual syndrome, arthritis, eczema, allergies, hyperactivity in children, dry eyes, and numbness and tingling in the hands and feet.

Scientific Name

Oenothera biennis

Evening Primrose Oil Is Also Commonly Known As

EPO, fever plant, gamma-linolenic acid (GLA), king's cureall, night willow-herb, sun drop

Medicinal Parts

Oil taken from the seed

Evening Primrose Oil's Uses

To treat elevated cholesterol levels, premenstrual syndrome, perimenopausal hot flashes, elevated blood pressure, rheumatoid arthritis, and multiple sclerosis

Typical Dose

A typical daily dose of evening primrose oil may range from 540 mg to 6 gm.

Possible Side Effects

Evening primrose oil's side effects include bloating, nausea, vomiting, diarrhea, and flatulence. It may also increase the risk of pregnancy complications.

Drugs That May Interact with Evening Primrose Oil

Taking evening primrose oil with these drugs may increase the risk of bleeding or bruising:

- abciximab (ReoPro)
- alteplase (Activase, Cathflo Activase)
- antithrombin III (Thrombate III)
- argatroban
- aspirin (Bufferin, Ecotrin)
- aspirin and dipyridamole (Aggrenox)
- bivalirudin (Angiomax)
- clopidogrel (Plavix)
- dalteparin (Fragmin)
- danaparoid (Orgaran)
- dipyridamole (Novo-Dipiradol, Persantine)
- drotrecogin alfa (Xigris)
- enoxaparin (Lovenox)
- eptifibatide (Integrillin)
- fondaparinux (Arixtra)
- heparin (Hepalean, Hep-Lock)
- hydrocodone and aspirin (Damason-P)
- hydrocodone and ibuprofen (Vicoprofen)
- ibritumomab (Zevalin)
- indobufen (Ibustrin)
- lepirudin (Refludan)
- nadroparin (Fraxiparine)
- reteplase (Retavase)
- streptokinase (Streptase)
- tenecteplase (TNKase)
- ticlopidine (Alti-Ticlopidine, Ticlid)
- tinzaparin (Innohep)
- tirofiban (Aggrastat)
- urokinase (Abbokinase)
- warfarin (Coumadin, Jantoven)

Taking evening primrose oil with these drugs may lower the seizure threshold:

- acetazolamide (Apo-Acetazolamide, Diamox Sequels)
- amobarbital (Amytal)
- barbexaclone (Maliasin)
- carbamazepine (Carbatrol, Tegretol)
- chlorpromazine (Largactil, Thorazine)
- clonazepam (Klonopin, Rivotril)
- clorazepate (Tranxene, T-Tab)
- diazepam (Apo-Diazepam, Valium)
- ethosuximide (Zarontin)
- felbamate (Felbatol)
- fluphenazine (Modecate, Prolixin)
- fosphenytoin (Cerebyx)
- gabapentin (Neurontin, Nu-Gabapentin)
- lamotrigine (Lamictal)
- levetiracetam (Keppra)
- lorazepam (Ativan, Nu-Loraz)
- mephobarbital (Mebaral)
- mesoridazine (Serentil)
- methsuximide (Celontin)
- metronidazole (Flagyl, Noritate)
- moxifloxacin (Avelox, Vigamox)
- nortriptyline (Aventyl HCl, Pamelor)
- ofloxacin (Floxin, Ocuflox)
- olanzapine (Zydis, Zyprexa)

- oxazepam (Novoxapam, Serax)
- oxcarbazepine (Trileptal)
- pentobarbital (Nembutal)
- perphenazine (Apo-Perphenazine, Trilafon)
- phenobarbital (Luminal Sodium, PMS-Phenobarbital)
- phenytoin (Dilantin, Phenytek)
- primidone (Apo-Primidone, Mysoline)
- prochlorperazine (Compazine, Compro)
- promethazine (Phenergan)
- quetiapine (Seroquel)
- thiethylperazine (Torecan)
- thiopental (Pentothal)
- thioridazine (Mellaril)
- thiothixene (Navane)
- tiagabine (Gabitril)
- topiramate (Topamax)
- tramadol (Ultram)
- trifluoperazine (Novo-Trifluzine, Stelazine)
- valproic acid (Depacon, Depakote ER)
- venlafaxine (Effexor)
- vigabatrin (Sabril)
- zonisamide (Zonegran)

Lab Tests That May Be Altered by Evening Primrose Oil
- May increase bleeding time, due to gamma-linolenic acid (GLA) content.
- May lower plasma triglycerides and increase HDL "good" cholesterol due to GLA content.

Diseases That May Be Worsened or Triggered by Evening Primrose Oil
None known

Foods That May Interact with Evening Primrose Oil
None known

Supplements That May Interact with Evening Primrose Oil
Increased risk of bleeding when used with herbs and supplements that might affect platelet aggregation, such as angelica, danshen, garlic, ginger, ginkgo biloba, red clover, turmeric, white willow, and others. (For a list of herbs and supplements with anticoagulant/antiplatelet effects, see Appendix B.)

EYEBRIGHT

> Eyebright has been used since the Middle Ages to relieve eye strain, eye inflammation or irritation, and itchy watery eyes due to allergies or colds. It is taken internally in the form of the fresh herb, a tea, or a tincture, or used externally as a compress or an ingredient in eyewash.

Scientific Name
Euphrasia officinalis

Eyebright Is Also Commonly Known As
Meadow eyebright, red eyebright

Medicinal Parts
Above-ground parts

Eyebright's Uses
To treat eye infections, eye fatigue, and hay fever

Typical Dose
A typical dose of eyebright is approximately 2 to 4 gm of the dried herb, taken as an infusion, three times a day.

Possible Side Effects

Eyebright's side effects include weakness, fatigue, sneezing, and headache.

Drugs That May Interact with Eyebright

Taking eyebright with these drugs may interfere with drug absorption:

- ferric gluconate (Ferrlecit)
- ferrous fumarate (Femiron, Feostat)
- ferrous gluconate (Fergon, Novo-Ferrogluc)
- ferrous sulfate (Feratab, Fer-Iron)
- ferrous sulfate and ascorbic acid (FeroGrad 500, Vitelle Irospan)
- iron-dextran complex (Dexferrum, INFeD)
- polysaccharide-iron complex (Hytinic, Niferex)

Lab Tests That May Be Altered by Eyebright

None known

Diseases That May Be Worsened or Triggered by Eyebright

None known

Foods That May Interact with Eyebright

None known

Supplements That May Interact with Eyebright

None known

FENNEL

In the seventeenth century, this aromatic herb gained a reputation for being a slimming aid, and some still believe this holds true. Fennel seeds were once placed in keyholes to keep out ghosts. Today they are valued for their antiseptic and anti-inflammatory properties and are also used to treat arthritis, diabetes, flatulence, and ulcers.

Scientific Name

Foeniculum vulgare

Fennel Is Also Commonly Known As

Bitter fennel, fenkel, fenouil, sweet fennel, wild fennel

Medicinal Parts

Fruit, seed, oil of seed

Fennel's Uses

To treat various skin ailments, fish tapeworms, bronchitis, and menstrual irregularities; to aid digestion; to increase the libido. Germany's Commission E has approved the use of fennel oil and seed to treat cough, bronchitis, and dyspeptic complaints such as heartburn and bloating.

Typical Dose

A typical dose of fennel may range from 0.1 to 0.6 ml of fennel oil, taken three times a day following meals.

Possible Side Effects

Fennel's side effects include lack of appetite, skin sensitivity to light, nausea, and vomiting.

Drugs That May Interact with Fennel

Taking fennel with these drugs may lower the seizure threshold:

- amitriptyline (Elavil, Levate)
- amoxapine (Asendin)

- bupropion (Wellbutrin, Zyban)
- ciprofloxacin (Ciloxan, Cipro)
- desipramine (Alti-Desipramine, Norpramin)
- doxepin (Sinequan, Zonalon)
- fosphenytoin (Cerebyx)
- carbamazepine (Carbatrol, Tegretol)
- ganciclovir (Cytovene, Vitrasert)
- imipramine (Apo-Imipramine, Tofranil)
- levetiracetam (Keppra)
- methylphenidate (Concerta, Ritalin)
- metoclopramide (Apo-Metoclop, Reglan)
- metronidazole (Flagyl, Noritate)
- moxifloxacin (Avelox, Vigamox)
- nortriptyline (Aventyl HCl, Pamelor)
- ofloxacin (Floxin, Ocuflox)
- olanzapine (Zydis, Zyprexa)
- oxcarbazepine (Trileptal)
- phenytoin (Dilantin, Phenytek)
- prochlorperazine (Compazine, Compro)
- quetiapine (Seroquel)
- tramadol (Ultram)
- venlafaxine (Effexor)

Taking fennel with these drugs may increase skin sensitivity to sunlight:
- bumetanide (Bumex, Burinex)
- celecoxib (Celebrex)
- ciprofloxacin (Ciloxan, Cipro)
- doxycycline (Apo-Doxy, Vibramycin)
- enalapril (Vasotec)
- etodolac (Lodine, Utradol)
- fluphenazine (Modecate, Prolixin)
- fosinopril (Monopril)
- furosemide (Apo-Furosemide, Lasix)
- gatifloxacin (Tequin, Zymar)
- hydrochlorothiazide (Apo-Hydro, Microzide)
- hydrochlorothiazide and triamterene (Dyazide, Maxzide)

- ibuprofen (Advil, Motrin)
- indomethacin (Indocin, Novo-Methacin)
- ketoprofen (Orudis, Rhodis)
- ketorolac (Acular, Toradol)
- lansoprazole (Prevacid)
- levofloxacin (Levaquin, Quixin)
- lisinopril (Prinivil, Zestril)
- loratadine (Alavert, Claritin)
- methotrexate (Rheumatrex, Trexall)
- naproxen (Aleve, Naprosyn)
- nortriptyline (Aventyl HCl, Pamelor)
- ofloxacin (Floxin, Ocuflox)
- omeprazole (Losec, Prilosec)
- phenytoin (Dilantin, Phenytek)
- piroxicam (Feldene, Nu-Pirox)
- prochlorperazine (Compazine, Compro)
- quinapril (Accupril)
- risperidone (Risperdal)
- rofecoxib (Vioxx)
- tetracycline (Novo-Tetra, Sumycin)

Taking fennel with these drugs may reduce blood levels of the drug:
- ciprofloxacin (Ciloxan, Cipro)
- levofloxacin (Levaquin, Quixin)
- moxifloxacin (Avelox, Vigamox)

Lab Tests That May Be Altered by Fennel
None known

Diseases That May Be Worsened or Triggered by Fennel
❗ This herb may have estrogen-like effects and should not be used by women with estrogen-sensitive breast cancer or other hormone-sensitive conditions.

Foods That May Interact with Fennel
None known

Supplements That May Interact with Fennel
None known

FENUGREEK

Fenugreek, a popular spice and cousin to the pea that is grown in the Mediterranean area of Europe and western Asia, was used by the ancient Egyptians for incense and embalming. The Romans preferred it as an aid in childbirth, while the Chinese employed it in cases of weakness and swelling of the legs. Today fenugreek is used to treat a number of ailments, including diabetes. In studies, an extract of fenugreek seeds was shown to lower blood sugar in people with type 1 and type 2 diabetes.

Scientific Name
Trigonella foenum-graecum

Fenugreek Is Also Commonly Known As
Bird's foot, Greek hay seed, trigonella

Medicinal Parts
Seed

Fenugreek's Uses
To treat constipation, diabetes, eczema, upper respiratory catarrh, skin ulcers, and inflammation; to stimulate production of milk. Germany's Commission E has approved the use of fenugreek to treat inflammation of the skin and loss of appetite.

Typical Dose
A typical daily dose of fenugreek seed is approximately 6 gm.

Possible Side Effects
Fenugreek's side effects include bruising and bleeding. It may also cause premature labor.

Drugs That May Interact with Fenugreek
Taking fenugreek with these drugs may increase the risk of hypoglycemia (low blood sugar):

- acarbose (Prandase, Precose)
- acetohexamide
- chlorpropamide (Diabinese, Novo-Propamide)
- gliclazide (Diamicron, Novo-Gliclazide)
- glimepiride (Amaryl)
- glipizide (Glucotrol)
- glipizide and metformin (Metaglip)
- gliquidone (Beglynor, Glurenorm)
- glyburide (DiaBeta, Micronase)
- glyburide and metformin (Glucovance)
- insulin (Humulin, Novolin R)
- metformin (Glucophage, Riomet)
- miglitol (Glyset)
- nateglinide (Starlix)
- pioglitazone (Actos)
- repaglinide (GlucoNorm, Prandin)
- rosiglitazone (Avandia)
- rosiglitazone and metformin (Avandamet)
- tolazamide (Tolinase)
- tolbutamide (Apo-Tolbutamide, Tol-Tab)

Taking fenugreek with these drugs may cause or increase liver damage:

- abacavir (Ziagen)
- acarbose (Prandase, Precose)
- acetaminophen (Genapap, Tylenol)
- allopurinol (Aloprim, Zyloprim)
- atorvastatin (Lipitor)
- celecoxib (Celebrex)
- cidofovir (Vistide)
- cyclosporine (Neoral, Sandimmune)

- meloxicam (MOBIC, Mobicox)
- methotrexate (Rheumatrex, Trexall)
- methyldopa (Apo-Methyldopa, Nu-Medopa)
- modafinil (Alertec, Provigil)
- morphine hydrochloride
- morphine sulfate (Kadian, MS Contin)
- naproxen (Aleve, Naprosyn)
- nelfinavir (Viracept)
- nevirapine (Viramune)
- nitrofurantoin (Furadantin, Macrobid)
- ondansetron (Zofran)
- paclitaxel (Onxol, Taxol)
- pantoprazole (Pantoloc, Protonix)
- phenytoin (Dilantin, Phenytek)
- pioglitazone (Actos)
- piroxicam (Feldene, Nu-Pirox)
- pravastatin (Novo-Pravastatin, Pravachol)
- prochlorperazine (Compazine, Compro)
- propoxyphene (Darvon, Darvon-N)
- repaglinide (GlucoNorm, Prandin)
- rifampin (Rifadin, Rimactane)
- rifapentine (Priftin)
- ritonavir (Norvir)
- rofecoxib (Vioxx)
- rosiglitazone (Avandia)
- saquinavir (Fortovase, Invirase)
- simvastatin (Apo-Simvastatin, Zocor)
- stavudine (Zerit)
- tamoxifen (Nolvadex, Tamofen)
- tramadol (Ultram)
- zidovudine (Novo-AZT, Retrovir)

Taking fenugreek with these drugs may increase the risk of bleeding or bruising:
- abciximab (ReoPro)
- aspirin (Bufferin, Ecotrin)
- celecoxib (Celebrex)

- enoxaparin (Lovenox)
- etodolac (Lodine, Utradol)
- fondaparinux (Arixtra)
- heparin (Hepalean, Hep-Lock)
- ibuprofen (Advil, Motrin)
- indomethacin (Indocin, Novo-Methacin)
- ketoprofen (Orudis, Rhodis)
- ketorolac (Acular, Toradol)

Taking fenugreek with these drugs may be harmful:
- digitalis (Digitek, Lanoxin)—may interfere with absorption of the drug and decrease drug effects
- prazosin (Minipress, Nu-Prazo)—may increase the risk of hypotension (excessively low blood pressure)

Lab Tests That May Be Altered by Fenugreek
- May decrease total cholesterol and LDL "bad" cholesterol.
- May decrease blood glucose.
- May cause urine to develop a maple syrup odor (not to be confused with Maple Syrup Urine Disease).

Diseases That May Be Worsened or Triggered by Fenugreek
May interfere with blood sugar control in diabetes.

Foods That May Interact with Fenugreek
Those allergic to fenugreek may be more likely to develop an allergy to foods from the *Fabaceae* family, such as chickpeas, green peas, peanuts, and soybeans.

Supplements That May Interact with Fenugreek
- Increased risk of bleeding when used with herbs and supplements that might affect platelet

aggregation, such as angelica, danshen, garlic, ginger, ginkgo biloba, red clover, turmeric, white willow, and others. (For a list of herbs and supplements with anticoagulant/antiplatelet effects, see Appendix B.)

- May increase blood glucose–lowering effects and risk of hypoglycemia (low blood sugar) when used with herbs and supplements that lower glucose levels, such as alpha-lipoic acid, chromium, devil's claw, Panax ginseng, and psyllium. (For a list of herbs and supplements that lower blood glucose levels, see Appendix B.)

FEVER BARK

The bark of this evergreen tree native to Australia is sometimes used to reduce fever, although there is no scientific evidence that it works. Fever bark has also been used as a uterine stimulant and a treatment for diarrhea and rheumatism. Some herbalists consider it a superior treatment for malaria, but evidence has not borne this out.

Scientific Name
Alstonia constricta

Fever Bark Is Also Commonly Known As
Alstonia bark, Australian quinine, devil tree, fever bush, pale mara

Medicinal Parts
Bark

Fever Bark's Uses
To treat rheumatism, malaria, and diarrhea.

Typical Dose
A typical daily dose of fever bark has not been established.

Possible Side Effects
Fever bark's side effects include depression, irritability, nasal congestion, and lethargy.

Drugs That May Interact with Fever Bark
Taking fever bark with these drugs may increase or decrease the effects of the drug:

- albuterol (Proventil, Ventolin)
- brimonidine (Alphagan P, PMS-Brimonidine Tartrate)
- dobutamine (Dobutrex)
- dopamine (Intropin)
- dopexamine (Dopacard)
- ephedrine (PretzD)
- isoetharine (Beta2, Bronkosol)
- isoproterenol (Isuprel)
- metaproterenol (Alupent)
- metaraminol (Aramine)
- norepinephrine (Levophed)
- phenylephrine (Neo-Synephrine, Vicks Sinex Nasal Spray)
- pseudoephedrine (Dimetapp Decongestant, Sudafed)
- terbutaline (Brethine)

Taking fever bark with this drug may be harmful:
- naloxone (Narcan)—may enhance the drug's therapeutic and/or adverse effects

Lab Tests That May Be Altered by Fever Bark
Due to the reserpine content in fever bark, the herb:
- May increase 5-HIAA (5-hydroxyindolefacetic acid).
- May increase FFA (free fatty acids).

- May increase urine levels of homovanillic acid.
- May increase levels of gastric pepsin.
- May increase plasma prolactin.
- May decrease urine levels of 17-hydroxycorticosteroids.
- May decrease plasma prothrombin time.
- May decrease plasma 5-HT (5-hydroxytryptamine).
- May decrease serum T-4 (thyroxine).
- May decrease urine levels of vanillylmandelic acid.
- May decrease blood platelet levels.
- May alter results of Guaiacols spot test.
- May trigger a false positive reading on tyramine test.

Diseases That May Be Worsened or Triggered by Fever Bark

None known

Foods That May Interact with Fever Bark

None known

Supplements That May Interact with Fever Bark

None known

FEVERFEW

Used by the ancient Greeks to treat "female problems," nausea, allergies, asthma, and a number of other ailments, feverfew is prized by today's herbalists for its ability to relieve headache pain. Some studies have shown that feverfew can effectively reduce the pain and nausea associated with migraines and is a significant migraine preventive when taken for at least four months.

Scientific Name

Tanacetum parthenium

Feverfew Is Also Commonly Known As

Bachelors' button, featherfew, featherfoil, midsummer daisy, wild chamomile

Medicinal Parts

Leaf

Feverfew's Uses

To treat migraine, allergies, arthritis, fever, headaches, insect bites, rheumatic disease, problems with digestion, and gynecological ailments.

Typical Dose

A typical daily dose of feverfew to treat migraine headaches may range from 200 to 250 mg.

Possible Side Effects

Feverfew's side effects include increased risk of allergic reactions in those who are sensitive to plants in the *Asteraceae/Compositae* family, such as chrysanthemums, daisies, marigolds, ragweed, and others. (For a list of herbs from the Asteraceae family, see Appendix B.)

Drugs That May Interact with Feverfew

Taking feverfew with these drugs may increase the risk of bleeding and bruising:

- abciximab (ReoPro)
- alteplase (Activase, Cathflo Activase)
- antithrombin III (Thrombate III)
- argatroban
- aspirin and dipyridamole (Aggrenox)
- bivalirudin (Angiomax)
- clopidogrel (Plavix)

- dalteparin (Fragmin)
- danaparoid (Orgaran)
- dipyridamole (Novo-Dipiradol, Persantine)
- drotrecogin alfa (Xigris)
- enoxaparin (Lovenox)
- eptifibatide (Integrillin)
- fondaparinux (Arixtra)
- heparin (Hepalean, Hep-Lock)
- hydrocodone and aspirin (Damason-P)
- hydrocodone and ibuprofen (Vicoprofen)
- ibritumomab (Zevalin)
- indobufen (Ibustrin)
- lepirudin (Refludan)
- nadroparin (Fraxiparine)
- reteplase (Retavase)
- streptokinase (Streptase)
- tenecteplase (TNKase)
- ticlopidine (Alti-Ticlopidine, Ticlid)
- tinzaparin (Innohep)
- tirofiban (Aggrastat)
- urokinase (Abbokinase)
- warfarin (Coumadin, Jantoven)

- flurbiprofen (Ansaid, Ocufen)
- ibuprofen (Advil, Motrin)
- indomethacin (Indocin, Novo-Methacin)
- ketoprofen (Orudis, Rhodis)
- ketorolac (Acular, Toradol)
- magnesium salicylate (Doan's, Mobidin)
- meclofenamate (Meclomen)
- mefenamic acid (Ponstan, Ponstel)
- meloxicam (MOBIC, Mobicox)
- nabumetone (Apo-Nabumetone, Relafen)
- naproxen (Aleve, Naprosyn)
- niflumic acid (Niflam, Nifluril)
- nimesulide (Areuma, Aulin)
- oxaprozin (Apo-Oxaprozin, Daypro)
- piroxicam (Feldene, Nu-Pirox)
- rofecoxib (Vioxx)
- salsalate (Amgesic, Salflex)
- sulindac (Clinoril, Nu-Sundac)
- tenoxicam (Dolmen, Mobiflex)
- tiaprofenic acid (Dom-Tiaprofenic, Surgam)
- tolmetin (Tolectin)
- valdecoxib (Bextra)

Taking feverfew with these drugs may increase adverse effects:

- acemetacin (Acemetacin Heumann, Acemetacin Sandoz)
- aspirin (Bufferin, Ecotrin)
- celecoxib (Celebrex)
- choline magnesium trisalicylate (Trilisate)
- choline salicylate (Teejel)
- diclofenac (Cataflam, Voltaren)
- diflunisal (Apo-Diflunisal, Dolobid)
- dipyrone (Analgina, Dinador)
- etodolac (Lodine, Utradol)
- etoricoxib (Arcoxia)
- fenoprofen (Nalfon)

Taking feverfew with these drugs may decrease absorption of the drug:

- ferrous sulfate (Feratab, Fer-Iron)
- iron-dextran complex (Dexferrum, INFeD)

Taking feverfew with these drugs may raise heart rate and blood pressure to dangerous levels:

- rizatriptan benzoate (Maxalt)
- zolmitriptan (Zomig)

Lab Tests That May Be Altered by Feverfew
May increase plasma partial thromboplastin time (PTT) and prothrombin time (PT) in those who are also taking warfarin.

Diseases That May Be Worsened or Triggered by Feverfew

None known

Foods That May Interact with Feverfew

None known

Supplements That May Interact with Feverfew

Increased risk of bleeding when used with herbs and supplements that might affect platelet aggregation, such as angelica, danshen, garlic, ginger, ginkgo biloba, red clover, turmeric, white willow, and others. (For a list of herbs and supplements with anticoagulant/antiplatelet effects, see Appendix B.)

FLAX

One of the earliest cultivated plants, flax was valued by ancient Egyptians and Greeks for the fibers taken from its stem, which were woven into cloth (known as linen). Studies have shown that flaxseed oil, a rich source of omega-3 fatty acids, may help lower total cholesterol and blood fat levels, fight inflammation, decrease atherosclerosis, inhibit clot formation, and increase HDL "good" cholesterol levels.

Scientific Name

Linum usitatissimum

Flax Is Also Commonly Known As

Linseed, lint bells, linum, winterlien

Medicinal Parts

Stem, seed, flowering plant, oil extracted from plant or seed

Flax's Uses

To treat constipation, diverticulitis, irritable bowel syndrome, lupus-related kidney inflammation, high cholesterol, and skin inflammation. Germany's Commission E has approved the use of flax to treat constipation and inflammation of the skin. Flaxseed oil is a rich source of omega-3 fatty acids. Some studies have shown that people who supplement with omega-3 fatty acids may be at lower risk of developing Alzheimer's disease. Omega-3's may also decrease the formation of plaque in the coronary arteries.

Typical Dose

A daily internal dose of flax may range from 35 to 50 mg of crushed seeds or 1,000 to 3,000 mg of flaxseed oil. For external use, 30 to 50 gm of flaxseed flour might be combined with a small amount of water, heated, cooled until it is warm to the touch, then applied to a wound to stimulate healing.

Possible Side Effects

Flax's side effects include diarrhea and intestinal obstruction, if taken with insufficient amounts of water.

Drugs That May Interact with Flax

Taking flax with these drugs may increase the risk of hypoglycemia (low blood sugar):

- acarbose (Prandase, Precose)
- acetohexamide
- chlorpropamide (Diabinese, Novo-Propamide)
- gliclazide (Diamicron, Novo-Gliclazide)
- glimepiride (Amaryl)
- glipizide (Glucotrol)
- glipizide and metformin (Metaglip)

- gliquidone (Beglynor, Glurenorm)
- glyburide (DiaBeta, Micronase)
- glyburide and metformin (Glucovance)
- insulin (Humulin, Novolin R)
- metformin (Glucophage, Riomet)
- miglitol (Glyset)
- nateglinide (Starlix)
- pioglitazone (Actos)
- repaglinide (GlucoNorm, Prandin)
- rosiglitazone (Avandia)
- rosiglitazone and metformin (Avandamet)
- tolazamide (Tolinase)
- tolbutamide (Apo-Tolbutamide, Tol-Tab)

Taking flaxseed with these drugs may reduce or prevent drug absorption:

- all drugs taken orally
- digitalis (Digitek, Lanoxin)

Lab Tests That May Be Altered by Flaxseed

- May decrease total cholesterol and LDL "bad" cholesterol.
- May decrease blood glucose.
- May increase triglyceride levels (when partially defatted flaxseed is used).

By Flaxseed Oil

- May increase prothrombin time (PT) test results.
- May decrease triglyceride levels in those with hyperlipoproteinemia.

Diseases That May Be Worsened or Triggered by Flaxseed

- May worsen bleeding disorders by interfering with platelet aggregation.

- May worsen diabetes by pushing blood sugar levels too low.
- This herb may have estrogen-like effects and should not be used by women with estrogen-sensitive breast cancer or other hormone-sensitive conditions.
- May worsen cases of intestinal inflammation.

Foods That May Interact with Flaxseed

None known

Supplements That May Interact with Flaxseed

None known

FOLIC ACID

First extracted from a spinach leaf in 1941, folic acid gets its name from the Latin word for leaf, *folium*, because it is so often found in green leafy vegetables. A member of the B-family of vitamins, folic acid helps the body manufacture red blood cells and DNA. It also helps protect cells against changes to the DNA that could convert them into cancer cells. A lack of folic acid can cause fetal abnormalities, irritability, diarrhea, and headaches.

Typical Dose

The Food and Nutrition Board has set the RDA for folic acid at 400 mcg per day for adult men and women.

Possible Side Effects

Folic acid is considered to be safe and well tolerated in doses less than 1,000 mcg (1 mg) per day. However, doses of 5 mg per day may cause diarrhea, rash, and abdominal cramps, and extremely high doses of 15 mg or more per day may damage the central nervous system.

Drugs That May Interact with Folic Acid

Taking folic acid with these drugs may reduce drug levels and/or effectiveness:

- fosphenytoin (Cerebyx)
- methotrexate (Rheumatrex, Trexall)
- phenobarbital (Luminal Sodium, PMS-Phenobarbital)
- phenytoin (Dilantin, Phenytek)
- primidone (Apo-Primidone, Mysoline)
- pyrimethamine (Daraprim)
- raltitrexed (Tomudex)

Drugs That May Interfere with the Absorption, Utilization, or Excretion of Folic Acid

- aluminum hydroxide (AlternaGel, Alu-Cap)
- aluminum hydroxide and magnesium carbonate (Gaviscon Liquid)
- aluminum hydroxide and magnesium hydroxide (Maalox, Mylanta)
- aluminum hydroxide, magnesium hydroxide, and simethicone (Mylanta Liquid)
- aluminum hydroxide and magnesium trisilicate (Gaviscon Tablet)
- amiloride (Midamor)
- aminosalicylic acid (Nemasol Sodium, Paser)
- aspirin (Bufferin, Ecotrin)
- aspirin and dipyridamole (Aggrenox)
- balsalazide (Colazal)
- betamethasone (Betatrex, Maxivate)
- budesonide (Entocort, Rhinocort)
- butabarbital (Butisol Sodium)
- butalbital, acetaminophen, and caffeine (Esgic, Fioricet)
- butalbital, aspirin, and caffeine (Fiorinal)
- carbamazepine (Carbatrol, Tegretol)
- carisoprodol and aspirin (Soma Compound)
- carisoprodol, aspirin, and codeine (Soma Compound with Codeine)
- celecoxib (Celebrex)
- chloramphenicol (Diochloram, Pentamycetin)
- cholestyramine (Prevalite, Questran)
- choline magnesium trisalicylate (Trilisate)
- choline salicylate (Teejel)
- cimetidine (Nu-Cimet, Tagamet)
- colchicine (ratio-Colchicine)
- colesevelam (WelChol)
- colestipol (Colestid)
- cortisone (Cortone)
- cycloserine (Seromycin Pulvules)
- demeclocycline (Declomycin)
- dexamethasone (Decadron, Dexasone)
- diclofenac (Cataflam, Voltaren)
- diclofenac and misoprostol (Arthrotec)
- diflorasone (Florone, Maxiflor)
- diflunisal (Apo-Diflunisal, Dolobid)
- doxycycline (Apo-Doxy, Vibramycin)
- erythromycin (Erythrocin, Staticin)
- ethosuximide (Zarontin)
- ethotoin (Peganone)
- etodolac (Lodine, Ultradol)
- famotidine (Apo-Famotidine, Pepcid)
- fenoprofen (Nalfon)
- flunisolide (AeroBid-M, Nasarel)
- flurbiprofen (Ansaid, Ocufen)
- fluticasone (Cutivate, Flonase)
- fosphenytoin (Cerebyx)
- glyburide and metformin (Glucovance)
- halobetasol (Ultravate)
- hydrochlorothiazide and tiamterene (Dyazide, Maxzide)

- hydrocodone and aspirin (Azdone, Lortab ASA)
- hydrocortisone (Cetacort, Locoid)
- ibuprofen (Advil, Motrin)
- indomethacin (Indocin, Novo-Methacin)
- isoniazid (Laniazid Oral, PMS-Isoniazid)
- ketoprofen (Orudis, Rhodis)
- ketorolac (Acular, Toradol)
- lansoprazole (Prevacid)
- levonorgestrel (Norplant Implant, Plan B)
- magnesium hydroxide (Dulcolax Milk of Magnesia, Phillips' Milk of Magnesia)
- meclofenamate (Meclomen)
- mefenamic acid (Ponstan, Ponstel)
- meloxicam (MOBIC, Mobicox)
- mephenytoin (Mesantoin)
- mesalamine (Asacol Oral, Rowasa Rectal)
- metformin (Glucophage, Riomet)
- methocarbamol and aspirin (Robaxisal)
- methotrexate (Folex PFS, Rheumatrex)
- methsuximide (Celontin)
- methylprednisolone (Depoject Injection, Medrol Oral)
- minocycline (Dynacin, Minocin)
- mometasone furoate (Elocom, Nasonex)
- nabumetone (Apo-Nabumetone, Relafen)
- naproxen (Aleve, Naprosyn)
- nitrous oxide
- nizatidine (Apo-Nizatidine, Axid)
- norethindrone (Aygestin, Micronor)
- olsalazine (Dipentum)
- omeprazole (Losec, Prilosec)
- oxaprozin (Apo-Oxaprozin, Daypro)
- oxcarbazepine (Trileptal)
- oxycodone and aspirin (Oxycodan, Percodan)
- pentamidine (NebuPent, Pentacarinat)
- phenobarbital (Luminal Sodium, PMS-Phenobarbital)
- phenytoin (Dilantin, Phenytek)
- piroxicam (Feldene, Nu-Pirox)
- prednisolone (Inflamase Forte, Pred Forte)
- prednisone (Apo-Prednisone, Deltasone)
- primidone (Mysoline, Sertan)
- pseudoephedrine and ibuprofen (Advil Cold & Sinus Caplets, Dimetapp Sinus Caplets)
- rabeprazole (Aciphex, Pariet)
- ranitidine (Alti-Ranitidine, Zantac)
- rofecoxib (Vioxx)
- salsalate (Amgesic, Salflex)
- sevelamer (Renagel)
- sulfasalazine (Azulfidine, Salazopyrin)
- sulindac (Clinoril, Nu-Sundac)
- tetracycline (Novo-Tetra, Sumycin)
- tolmetin (Tolectin)
- triamcinolone (Aristocort, Trinasal)
- triamterene (Dyrenium)
- trimethoprim (Primsol, Trimpex)
- valproic acid (Depacon, Depakote ER)
- zonisamide (Zonegran)

Lab Tests That May Be Altered by Folic Acid

- May normalize megaloblastic anemia in those with vitamin B_{12} deficiency or folic acid deficiency.
- Normalizes hematological findings in those with vitamin B_{12} deficiency or pernicious anemia but does not prevent neurological damage.

Diseases That May Be Worsened or Triggered by Folic Acid

Taking supplemental folic acid may worsen seizures in certain people.

Foods That May Interact with Folic Acid

Slightly decreased absorption of supplemental folic acid when taken with food.

Supplements That May Interact with Folic Acid

None known

Fo-ti

The dried or cured root of a vine in the knotweed family, fo-ti is grown throughout China and considered a superior addition to traditional Chinese medicine. The dried (unprocessed) root, which is sometimes called white fo-ti, and the cured (processed) root, which is sometimes called red fo-ti, are considered to be two different herbs. White fo-ti is used to detoxify the blood and relax the bowels; red fo-ti is used to increase energy, invigorate the liver and kidneys, and lower cholesterol.

Scientific Name

Polygonum multiflorum

Fo-ti Is Also Commonly Known As

Chinese cornbind, Chinese knotweed, he-shou-wu

Medicinal Parts

Root

Fo-ti's Uses

To treat insomnia, diabetes mellitus, autoimmune disorders, hemorrhoids, and diverticular disease; as a general tonic

Typical Dose

There is no typical dose of fo-ti.

Possible Side Effects

Fo-ti's side effects include nausea, vomiting, diarrhea, anorexia, and allergic reactions.

Drugs That May Interact with Fo-ti

Taking fo-ti with these drugs may increase the risk of hypokalemia (low levels of potassium in the blood):

- acetazolamide (Apo-Acetazolamide, Diamox Sequels)
- azosemide (Diat)
- bumetanide (Bumex, Burinex)
- chlorothiazide (Diuril)
- chlorthalidone (Apo-Chlorthalidone, Thalitone)
- ethacrynic acid (Edecrin)
- etozolin (Elkapin)
- furosemide (Apo-Furosemide, Lasix)
- hydrochlorothiazide (Apo-Hydro, Microzide)
- hydroflumethiazide (Diucardin, Saluron)
- indapamide (Lozol, Nu-Indapamide)
- mannitol (Osmitrol, Resectisol)
- mefruside (Baycaron)
- methazolamide (Apo-Methazolamide, Neptazane)
- methyclothiazide (Aquatensen, Enduron)
- metolazone (Mykrox, Zaroxolyn)
- olmesartan and hydrochlorothiazide (Benicar HCT)
- polythiazide (Renese)
- torsemide (Demadex)
- trichlormethiazide (Metatensin, Naqua)
- urea (Amino-Cerv, UltraMide)
- xipamide (Diurexan, Lumitens)

Lab Tests That May Be Altered by Fo-ti

None known

Diseases That May Be Worsened or Triggered by Fo-ti

None known

Foods That May Interact with Fo-ti

None known

Supplements That May Interact with Fo-ti

None known

FRANGULA

> Used for centuries in northern and central Europe as a cathartic laxative, the bark of the frangula shrub contains chemicals that attract water to the intestines and stimulate intestinal movement, resulting in the emptying of the bowels. Before it can be used medically, frangula bark must be aged properly, which includes a one-year drying process. The fresh bark is not used because it contains chemicals, including emodin, that cause severe vomiting.

Scientific Name

Rhamnus frangula

Frangula Is Also Commonly Known As

Alder buckthorn, alder dogwood, black alder, black dogwood

Medicinal Parts

Bark

Frangula's Uses

To treat hemorrhoids and poor digestion. Germany's Commission E has approved the use of frangula to treat constipation.

Typical Dose

A typical dose of frangula for constipation may range from 1 to 2 cups of frangula tea per day, using the smallest amount of herb needed to relieve symptoms.

Possible Side Effects

Frangula's side effects include loss of electrolytes, particularly potassium, with long-term use.

Drugs That May Interact with Frangula

Taking frangula with these drugs may increase the risk of hypokalemia (low levels of potassium in the blood):

- acetazolamide (Apo-Acetazolamide, Diamox Sequels)
- azosemide (Diat)
- beclomethasone (Beconase, Vanceril)
- betamethasone (Celestone, Diprolene)
- budesonide (Entocort, Rhinocort)
- budesonide and formoterol (Symbicort)
- bumetanide (Bumex, Burinex)
- chlorothiazide (Diuril)
- chlorthalidone (Apo-Chlorthalidone, Thalitone)
- cortisone (Cortone)
- deflazacort (Calcort, Dezacor)
- dexamethasone (Decadron, Dexasone)
- ethacrynic acid (Edecrin)
- etozolin (Elkapin)
- flunisolide (AeroBid, Nasarel)
- fluorometholone (Eflone, Flarex)
- fluticasone (Cutivate, Flonase)
- furosemide (Apo-Furosemide, Lasix)
- hydrochlorothiazide (Apo-Hydro, Microzide)
- hydrocortisone (Anusol-HC, Locoid)
- hydroflumethiazide (Diucardin, Saluron)
- indapamide (Lozol, Nu-Indapamide)
- mannitol (Osmitrol, Resectisol)
- mefruside (Baycaron)
- methazolamide (Apo-Methazolamide, Neptazane)
- methyclothiazide (Aquatensen, Enduron)
- methylprednisolone (Depo-Medrol, Medrol)
- metolazone (Mykrox, Zaroxolyn)

- olmesartan and hydrochlorothiazide (Benicar HCT)
- polythiazide (Renese)
- prednisolone (Inflamase Forte, Pred Forte)
- prednisone (Apo-Prednisone, Deltasone)
- torsemide (Demadex)
- triamcinolone (Aristocort, Trinasal)
- trichlormethiazide (Metatensin, Naqua)
- urea (Amino-Cerv, UltraMide)
- xipamide (Diurexan, Lumitens)

Taking frangula with these drugs may increase fluid and electrolyte loss:
- cascara
- docusate and senna (Peri-Colace, Senokot-S)

Taking frangula with this drug may be harmful:
- digitalis (Digitek, Lanoxin)—may increase therapeutic and adverse effects of the drug

Lab Tests That May Be Altered by Frangula
May confound results of diagnostic urine tests that rely on a color change by discoloring urine (pink, red, purple, or orange).

Diseases That May Be Worsened or Triggered by Frangula
May worsen irritable bowel syndrome, Crohn's disease, and other intestinal ailments.

Foods That May Interact with Frangula
None known

Supplements That May Interact with Frangula
Increased risk of potassium depletion when used with licorice, horsetail plant, or other stimulant laxative herbs, such as black root, cascara sagrada, castor oil, and senna. (For a list of stimulant laxative herbs and supplements, see Appendix B.)

FUMITORY

Also known as earth smoke, fumitory gets its name because its blue-green color makes the plant look like smoke rising from the ground. Pliny, the famous Roman scholar, wrote that the juice of the fumitory plant made the eyes fill with tears to such an extent that the vision became dim as if peering through smoke. This may explain why it was considered useful in treating afflictions of the eye.

Scientific Name
Fumaria officinalis

Fumitory Is Also Commonly Known As
Beggary, earth smoke, fumus, hedge fumitory, vapor

Medicinal Parts
Leaf, flowering parts

Fumitory's Uses
To treat constipation, scabies, psoriasis, eczema, and liver problems; as a diuretic. Germany's Commission E has approved the use of fumitory to treat liver and gallbladder complaints.

Typical Dose
A typical daily dose of fumitory may range from 2 to 6 gm of the herb.

Possible Side Effects
Fumitory's side effects include lowered blood pressure, nausea, and vomiting.

Drugs That May Interact with Fumitory

Taking fumitory with these drugs may cause or increase kidney damage:

- etodolac (Lodine, Utradol)
- ibuprofen (Advil, Motrin)
- indomethacin (Indocin, Novo-Methacin)
- ketoprofen (Orudis, Rhodis)
- ketorolac (Acular, Toradol)
- meloxicam (MOBIC, Mobicox)
- metformin (Glucophage, Riomet)
- methotrexate (Rheumatrex, Trexall)
- miglitol (Glyset)
- morphine hydrochloride
- morphine sulfate (Kadian, MS Contin)
- naproxen (Aleve, Naprosyn)
- nitrofurantoin (Furadantin, Macrobid)
- ofloxacin (Floxin, Ocuflox)
- penicillin (Pfizerpen, Wycillin)
- piroxicam (Feldene, Nu-Pirox)
- propoxyphene (Darvon, Darvon-N)
- rifampin (Rifadin, Rimactane)
- sucralfate (Carafate, Sulcrate)
- tramadol (Ultram)
- valacyclovir (Valtrex)
- valganciclovir (Valcyte)
- vancomycin (Vancocin)
- zidovudine (Novo-AZT, Retrovir)

Taking fumitory with these drugs may increase the action of the drug:

- acebutolol (Novo-Acebutolol, Sectral)
- adenosine (Adenocard, Adenoscan)
- amiodarone (Cordarone, Pacerone)
- atenolol (Apo-Atenol, Tenormin)
- befunolol (Bentos, Betaclar)
- betaxolol (Betoptic S, Kerlone)
- bisoprolol (Monocor, Zebeta)
- bretylium
- carteolol (Cartrol, Ocupress)
- carvedilol (Coreg)
- celiprolol
- digitalis (Digitek, Lanoxin)
- diltiazem (Cardizem, Tiazac)
- disopyramide (Norpace, Rhythmodan)
- dofetilide (Tikosyn)
- esmolol (Brevibloc)
- flecainide (Tambocor)
- ibutilide (Corvert)
- labetalol (Normodyne, Trandate)
- levobetaxolol (Betaxon)
- levobunolol (Betagan, Novo-Levobunolol)
- lidocaine (Lidoderm, Xylocaine)
- metipranolol (OptiPranolol)
- metoprolol (Betaloc, Lopressor)
- mexiletine (Mexitil, Novo-Mexiletine)
- moricizine (Ethmozine)
- nadolol (Apo-Nadol, Corgard)
- oxprenolol (Slow-Trasicor, Trasicor)
- phenytoin (Dilantin, Phenytek)
- pindolol (Apo-Pindol, Novo-Pindol)
- procainamide (Procanbid, Pronestyl-SR)
- propafenone (GenPropafenone, Rhythmol)
- propranolol (Inderal, InnoPran XL)
- quinidine (Novo-Quinidin, Quinaglute Dura-Tabs)
- sotalol (Betapace, Sorine)
- timolol (Betimol, Timoptic)
- tocainide (Tonocard)
- verapamil (Calan, Isoptin SR)

Taking fumitory with this drug may be harmful:

- digitalis (Digitek, Lanoxin)—may increase risk of drug toxicity due to potassium loss

Lab Tests That May Be Altered by Fumitory

None known

Diseases That May Be Worsened or Triggered by Fumitory

None known

Foods That May Interact with Fumitory

None known

Supplements That May Interact with Fumitory

None known

GAMBOGE

Gamboge is a gum resin obtained from the sap of trees of the genus *Garcinia*, which are cultivated primarily in Cambodia and India. Gamboge is best known as a highly esteemed yellow-orange pigment found in Chinese and Japanese manuscript paintings dating back to the eighth century and still used today. It was also used in European watercolors from the early seventeenth through the twentieth centuries. Medicinally, gamboge is used as a cathartic. In 2005, Japanese researchers isolated substances in gamboge that have antibacterial actions, some of which are specifically effective against *Staphylococcus aureus* bacteria that have grown resistant to modern-day antibiotics.

Scientific Name

Garcinia hanburyi

Gamboge Is Also Commonly Known As

Camboge, Gambodia, gutta Cambodia, gutta gamba, tom rong

Medicinal Parts

Resin

Gamboge's Uses

To treat constipation and intestinal worms.

Typical Dose

There is no typical dose of gamboge.

Possible Side Effects

❶ Gamboge's side effects include abdominal pain, which may occur with as little as 200 mg of the herb. Ingestion of 4 gm may be fatal.

Drugs That May Interact with Gamboge

Taking gamboge with these drugs may increase the risk of hypokalemia (low levels of potassium in the blood):

- acetazolamide (Apo-Acetazolamide, Diamox Sequels)
- azosemide (Diat)
- bumetanide (Bumex, Burinex)
- chlorothiazide (Diuril)
- chlorthalidone (Apo-Chlorthalidone, Thalitone)
- ethacrynic acid (Edecrin)
- etozolin (Elkapin)
- furosemide (Apo-Furosemide, Lasix)
- hydrochlorothiazide (Apo-Hydro, Microzide)
- hydroflumethiazide (Diucardin, Saluron)
- indapamide (Lozol, Nu-Indapamide)
- mannitol (Osmitrol, Resectisol)
- mefruside (Baycaron)
- methazolamide (Apo-Methazolamide, Neptazane)
- methyclothiazide (Aquatensen, Enduron)
- metolazone (Mykrox, Zaroxolyn)
- olmesartan and hydrochlorothiazide (Benicar HCT)
- polythiazide (Renese)
- torsemide (Demadex)
- trichlormethiazide (Metatensin, Naqua)

- urea (Amino-Cerv, UltraMide)
- xipamide (Diurexan, Lumitens)

Taking gamboge with these drugs may increase the risk of electrolyte and fluid loss:
- cascara
- docusate and senna (Peri-Colace, Senokot-S)

Taking gamboge with this drug may be harmful:
- digitalis (Digitek, Lanoxin)—may increase risk of drug toxicity

Lab Tests That May Be Altered by Gamboge
None known

Diseases That May Be Worsened or Triggered by Gamboge
- May worsen cases of potassium loss.
- May worsen cases of Crohn's disease, ulcerative colitis, and other intestinal ailments.

Foods That May Interact with Gamboge
None known

Supplements That May Interact with Gamboge
- Increased risk of potassium depletion when used in conjunction with horsetail plant or licorice.
- Increased risk of potassium depletion when used with other stimulant laxative herbs, such as black root, cascara sagrada, castor oil, and senna. (For a list of stimulant laxative herbs and supplements, see Appendix B.)
- Increased risk of cardiac glycoside toxicity when gamboge is overused and taken with herbs that contain cardiac glycosides, such as black hellebore, calotropis, motherwort, and others.

(For a list of cardiac glycoside–containing herbs and supplements, see Appendix B.)

GARLIC

The juice of this aromatic, healing bulb has such amazing antibiotic properties that it was used on the battlefield during World Wars I and II to disinfect wounds and ward off gangrene. The Soviet army used garlic in this manner so often the herb became known as Russian penicillin. Today garlic is used to lower blood pressure and blood fats, fight infection, destroy certain kinds of cancer cells, and aid in digestion.

Scientific Name
Allium sativum

Garlic Is Also Commonly Known As
Allium, clove garlic, poor man's treacle, stinking rose

Medicinal Parts
Oil, dried or fresh bulb

Garlic's Uses
To treat elevated cholesterol levels, elevated blood pressure, menstrual pains, diabetes, whooping cough, bronchitis, warts, corns, calluses, muscle pain, and arthritis. Germany's Commission E has approved the use of garlic to treat arteriosclerosis, elevated blood pressure, and high cholesterol levels.

Typical Dose
A typical daily dose of garlic is approximately 4 gm of the fresh herb, 8 mg of essential oil, or 1/2 to 3 fresh garlic cloves.

Possible Side Effects

Garlic's side effects include breath and body odor, irritation of the mouth and/or gastrointestinal tract, heartburn, flatulence, and nausea.

Drugs That May Interact with Garlic

Taking garlic with these drugs may increase the risk of bleeding or bruising:

- abciximab (ReoPro)
- acemetacin (Acemetacin Heumann, Acemetacin Sandoz)
- alteplase (Activase, Cathflo Activase)
- antithrombin-III (Thrombate III)
- argatroban
- aspirin (Bufferin, Ecotrin)
- aspirin and dipyridamole (Aggrenox)
- bivalirudin (Angiomax)
- celecoxib (Celebrex)
- choline magnesium trisalicylate (Trilisate)
- choline salicylate (Teejel)
- clopidogrel (Plavix)
- dalteparin (Fragmin)
- danaparoid (Orgaran)
- diclofenac (Cataflam, Voltaren)
- diflunisal (Apo-Diflunisal, Dolobid)
- dipyridamole (Novo-Dipiradol, Persantine)
- dipyrone (Analgina, Dinador)
- drotrecogin alfa (Xigris)
- enoxaparin (Lovenox)
- eptifibatide (Integrillin)
- etodolac (Lodine, Utradol)
- etoricoxib (Arcoxia)
- fenoprofen (Nalfon)
- flurbiprofen (Ansaid, Ocufen)
- fondaparinux (Arixtra)
- heparin (Hepalean, Hep-Lock)
- hydrocodone and aspirin (Damason-P)
- hydrocodone and ibuprofen (Vicoprofen)
- ibritumomab (Zevalin)
- ibuprofen (Advil, Motrin)
- indobufen (Ibustrin)
- indomethacin (Indocin, Novo-Methacin)
- ketoprofen (Orudis, Rhodis)
- ketorolac (Acular, Toradol)
- lepirudin (Refludan)
- magnesium salicylate (Doan's, Mobidin)
- meclofenamate (Meclomen)
- mefenamic acid (Ponstan, Ponstel)
- meloxicam (MOBIC, Mobicox)
- nabumetone (Apo-Nabumetone, Relafen)
- nadroparin (Fraxiparine)
- naproxen (Aleve, Naprosyn)
- niflumic acid (Niflam, Nifluril)
- nimesulide (Areuma, Aulin)
- oxaprozin (Apo-Oxaprozin, Daypro)
- piroxicam (Feldene, Nu-Pirox)
- reteplase (Retavase)
- rofecoxib (Vioxx)
- salsalate (Amgesic, Salflex)
- streptokinase (Streptase)
- sulindac (Clinoril, Nu-Sundac)
- tenecteplase (TNKase)
- tenoxicam (Dolmen, Mobiflex)
- tiaprofenic acid (Dom-Tiaprofenic, Surgam)
- ticlopidine (Alti-Ticlopidine, Ticlid)
- tinzaparin (Innohep)
- tirofiban (Aggrastat)
- tolmetin (Tolectin)
- urokinase (Abbokinase)
- valdecoxib (Bextra)
- warfarin (Coumadin, Jantoven)

Taking garlic with these drugs may increase the risk of hypotension (excessively low blood pressure):

- amlodipine (Norvasc)
- atenolol (Apo-Atenol, Tenormin)
- benazepril (Lotensin)
- bepridil (Vascor)
- betaxolol (Betoptic S, Kerlone)
- bisoprolol (Monocor, Zebeta)
- bumetanide (Bumex, Burinex)
- candesartan (Atacand)
- captopril (Capoten, Novo-Captopril)
- carteolol (Cartrol, Ocupress)
- carvedilol (Coreg)
- cilazapril (Inhibace)
- diltiazem (Cardizem, Tiazac)
- doxazosin (Alti-Doxazosin, Cardura)
- enalapril (Vasotec)
- eprosartan (Teveten)
- felodipine (Plendil, Renedil)
- hydralazine (Apresoline, Novo-Hylazin)
- hydrochlorothiazide (Apo-Hydro, Microzide)
- indapamide (Lozol, Nu-Indapamide)
- irbesartan (Avapro)
- isradipine (DynaCirc)
- labetalol (Normodyne, Trandate)
- lisinopril (Prinivil, Zestril)
- lopinavir and ritonavir (Kaletra)
- losartan (Cozaar)
- metolazone (Mykrox, Zaroxolyn)
- metoprolol (Betaloc, Lopressor)
- moexipril (Univasc)
- nadolol (Apo-Nadol, Corgard)
- nicardipine (Cardene)
- nifedipine (Adalat CC, Procardia)
- nimodipine (Nimotop)
- nisoldipine (Sular)
- olmesartan (Benicar)
- perindopril erbumine (Aceon, Coversyl)
- prazosin (Minipress, Nu-Prazo)

- propranolol (Inderal, InnoPran XL)
- quinapril (Accupril)
- ramipril (Altace)
- telmisartan (Micardis)
- terazosin (Hytrin, Novo-Terazosin)
- torsemide (Demadex)
- trandolapril (Mavik)
- valsartan (Diovan)
- verapamil (Calan, Isoptin SR)

Taking garlic with these drugs may increase the risk of hypoglycemia (low blood sugar):
- acarbose (Prandase, Precose)
- acetohexamide
- chlorpropamide (Diabinese, Novo-Propamide)
- gliclazide (Diamicron, Novo-Gliclazide)
- glimepiride (Amaryl)
- glipizide (Glucotrol)
- glipizide and metformin (Metaglip)
- gliquidone (Beglynor, Glurenorm)
- glyburide (DiaBeta, Micronase)
- glyburide and metformin (Glucovance)
- insulin (Humulin, Novolin R)
- metformin (Glucophage, Riomet)
- miglitol (Glyset)
- nateglinide (Starlix)
- pioglitazone (Actos)
- repaglinide (GlucoNorm, Prandin)
- rosiglitazone (Avandia)
- rosiglitazone and metformin (Avandamet)
- tolazamide (Tolinase)
- tolbutamide (Apo-Tolbutamide, Tol-Tab)

Taking garlic with these drugs may exacerbate hypertension (high blood pressure):
- fosfomycin (Monurol)
- furosemide (Apo-Furosemide, Lasix)

Taking garlic with these drugs may reduce blood levels and/or the effectiveness of the drug:

- amprenavir (Agenerase)
- indinavir (Crixivan)
- lopinavir and ritonavir (Kaletra)
- nelfinavir (Viracept)
- ritonavir (Norvir)
- saquinavir (Fortovase, Invirase)

Taking garlic with these drugs may cause severe gastrointestinal toxicity:

- amprenavir (Agenerase)
- indinavir (Crixivan)
- lopinavir and ritonavir (Kaletra)
- nelfinavir (Viracept)
- ritonavir (Norvir)
- saquinavir (Fortovase, Invirase)

Lab Tests That May Be Altered by Garlic

- May decrease serum cholesterol, LDL "bad" cholesterol, triglycerides, blood lipid profile.
- May decrease platelet aggregation.
- May increase prothrombin time (PT) and serum immunoglobulin E (IgE).
- May increase plasma international normalized ratio (INR) in those who are also taking warfarin.
- May decrease blood pressure.
- May elevate ALMA (S-allyl-mercapturic acid) levels in urine or cause false positive in ALMA determination.

Diseases That May Be Worsened or Triggered by Garlic

- May worsen cases of bleeding disorders by encouraging bleeding.
- May worsen gastrointestinal ailments by irritating the gastrointestinal tract.

Foods That May Interact with Garlic

None known

Supplements That May Interact with Garlic

- Decreased absorption of garlic when taken with acidophilus.
- Increased risk of bleeding when used with herbs and supplements that might affect platelet aggregation. (For a list of herbs and supplements with anticoagulant/antiplatelet effects, see Appendix B.)
- Increased antithrombotic effects when taken with fish oil (eicosapentaenoic acid [EPA]).
- Increased risk of bleeding when garlic is taken with forskolin.

GERMAN CHAMOMILE

Used since ancient times, this beautiful light-blue oil taken from flowers of the German chamomile plant contains constituents with powerful antiseptic, anti-inflammatory, and antimicrobial effects. It's also used for menstrual problems and digestive upsets and as a sleep aid.

Scientific Name

Matricaria recutita

German Chamomile Is Also Commonly Known As

Chamomilla, Hungarian chamomile, pin heads, true chamomile

Medicinal Parts

Flower, whole flowering herb

German Chamomile's Uses

To treat flatulence, diarrhea, inflammation of the gastrointestinal tract and anogenital area, irritation of the upper respiratory tract, gingivitis, hemorrhoids, and acne. Germany's Commission E has approved the use of German chamomile to treat the common cold; fevers; coughs; bronchitis; inflammation of the skin, mouth, and throat; burns and wounds; and to help ward off infections.

Typical Dose

A typical dose of German chamomile is approximately 3 gm of the herb steeped in 150 ml boiling water for five to ten minutes, strained and taken as a tea. This dosage may be repeated three to four times daily.

Possible Side Effects

German chamomile's side effects include allergic reactions.

Drugs That May Interact with German Chamomile

Taking German chamomile with these drugs may increase the risk of bleeding or bruising:
- antithrombin III (Thrombate III)
- argatroban
- aspirin (Bufferin, Ecotrin)
- bivalirudin (Angiomax)
- celecoxib (Celebrex)
- dalteparin (Fragmin)
- danaparoid (Orgaran)
- enoxaparin (Lovenox)
- etodolac (Lodine, Utradol)
- fondaparinux (Arixtra)
- heparin (Hepalean, Hep-Lock)
- ibuprofen (Advil, Motrin)

- indomethacin (Indocin, Novo-Methacin)
- ketoprofen (Orudis, Rhodis)
- ketorolac (Acular, Toradol)
- lepirudin (Refludan)
- tinzaparin (Innohep)
- warfarin (Coumadin, Jantoven)

Taking German chamomile with these drugs may increase the action of the drug:
- alprazolam (Apo-Alpraz, Xanax)
- amobarbital (Amytal)
- bromazepam (Apo-Bromazepam, Gen-Bromazepam)
- brotizolam (Lendorm, Sintonal)
- butabarbital (Butisol Sodium)
- chloral hydrate (Aquachloral Supprettes, Somnote)
- chlordiazepoxide (Apo-Chlordiazepoxide, Librium)
- clobazam (Alti-Clobazam, Frisium)
- clonazepam (Klonopin, Rivotril)
- clorazepate (Tranxene, T-Tab)
- dexmedetomidine (Precedex)
- diazepam (Apo-Diazepam, Valium)
- diphenhydramine (Benadryl Allergy, Nytol)
- estazolam (ProSom)
- flurazepam (Apo-Flurazepam, Dalmane)
- haloperidol (Haldol, Novo-Peridol)
- hydroxyzine (Atarax, Vistaril)
- loprazolam (Dormonoct, Havlane)
- lorazepam (Ativan, Nu-Loraz)
- mephobarbital (Mebaral)
- midazolam (Apo-Midazolam, Versed)
- oxazepam (Novoxapam, Serax)
- pentazocine (Talwin)
- phenobarbital (Luminal Sodium, PMS-Phenobarbital)

- prazepam
- promethazine (Phenergan)
- propofol (Diprivan)
- quazepam (Doral)
- s-zopiclone (Lunesta)
- secobarbital (Seconal)
- temazepam (Novo-Temazepam, Restoril)
- tetrazepam (Mobiforton, Musapam)
- thiopental (Pentothal)
- triazolam (Apo-Triazo, Halcion)
- zolpidem (Ambien)

Taking German chamomile with these drugs may interfere with absorption of the drug:
- ferrous sulfate (Feratab, Fer-Iron)
- iron-dextran complex (Dexferrum, INFeD)

Lab Tests That May Be Altered by German Chamomile
None known

Diseases That May Be Worsened or Triggered by German Chamomile
May worsen cases of asthma

Foods That May Interact with German Chamomile
None known

Supplements That May Interact with German Chamomile
May enhance therapeutic and adverse effects of herbs and supplements that have sedative properties, such as 5-HTP, kava kava, St. John's wort, and valerian. (For a list of herbs and supplements that have sedative properties, see Appendix B.)

GINGER

Native to India and China, ginger is an excellent digestive aid. The root of the ginger plant promotes the secretion of gastric juices, enhancing the absorption of food and easing colic, indigestion, and flatulence. Several studies have shown that ginger also reduces nausea and vomiting during pregnancy.

Scientific Name
Zingiber officinale

Ginger Is Also Commonly Known As
Black ginger, imber, race ginger, zingiber

Medicinal Parts
Root

Ginger's Uses
To treat flatulence, motion sickness, morning sickness, rheumatoid arthritis, loss of appetite, upper respiratory infections, bronchitis, cholera, and burns; to relieve pain. Germany's Commission E has approved the use of ginger to treat loss of appetite, motion sickness, and dyspeptic complaints such as heartburn and bloating.

Typical Dose
A typical dose of ginger may range from 1 to 4 gm per day in capsule or powder form.

Possible Side Effects
Ginger's side effects include bloating, flatulence, and heartburn.

Drugs That May Interact with Ginger

Taking ginger with these drugs may increase the risk of bleeding or bruising:

- abciximab (ReoPro)
- alteplase (Activase, Cathflo Activase)
- antithrombin III (Thrombate III)
- argatroban
- aspirin (Bufferin, Ecotrin)
- aspirin and dipyridamole (Aggrenox)
- bivalirudin (Angiomax)
- celecoxib (Celebrex)
- choline magnesium trysalicylate (Trilisate)
- clopidogrel (Plavix)
- dalteparin (Fragmin)
- danaparoid (Orgaran)
- diclofenac (Cataflam, Voltaren)
- diflunisal (Apo-Diflunisal, Dolobid)
- dipyridamole (Novo-Dipiradol, Persantine)
- drotrecogin alfa (Xigris)
- enoxaparin (Lovenox)
- eptifibatide (Integrillin)
- etodolac (Lodine, Utradol)
- fenoprofen (Nalfon)
- flurbiprofen (Ansaid, Ocufen)
- fondaparinux (Arixtra)
- heparin (Hepalean, Hep-Lock)
- hydrocodone and aspirin (Damason-P)
- hydrocodone and ibuprofen (Vicoprofen)
- ibritumomab (Zevalin)
- ibuprofen (Advil, Motrin)
- indobufen (Ibustrin)
- indomethacin (Indocin, Novo-Methacin)
- ketoprofen (Orudis, Rhodis)
- ketorolac (Acular, Toradol)
- lepirudin (Refludan)
- meloxicam (MOBIC, Mobicox)
- nabumetone (Apo-Nabumetone, Relefan)
- nadroparin (Fraxiparine)
- naproxen (Aleve, Naprosyn)
- oxaprozin (Apo-Oxaprozin, Daypro)
- piroxicam (Feldene, Nu-Pirox)
- reteplase (Retavase)
- rofecoxib (Vioxx)
- salsalate (Amgesic, Salflex)
- streptokinase (Streptase)
- sulindac (Clinoril, Nu-Sundac)
- tenecteplase (TNKase)
- tiaprofenic acid (Dom-Tiaprofenic, Surgam)
- ticlopidine (Alti-Ticlopidine, Ticlid)
- tinzaparin (Innohep)
- tirofiban (Aggrastat)
- tolmetin (Tolectin)
- urokinase (Abbokinase)
- valdecoxib (Bextra)
- warfarin (Coumadin, Jantoven)

Taking ginger with these drugs may reduce the effectiveness of the drug:

- aluminum hydroxide (AlternaGel, Alu-Cap)
- alumnum hydroxide and magnesium carbonate (Gaviscon Extra Strength, Gaviscon Liquid)
- aluminum hydroxide and magnesium hydroxide (Maalox, Rulox)
- aluminum hydroxide and magnesium trisilicate (Gaviscon Tablet)
- aluminum hydroxide, magnesium hydroxide, and simethicone (Maalox, Mylanta Liquid)
- calcium carbonate (Rolaids Extra Strength, Tums)
- calcium carbonate and magnesium hydroxide (Mylanta Gelcaps, Rolaids Extra Strength)
- cimetidine (Nu-Cimet, Tagamet)
- esomeprazole (Nexium)
- famotidine (Apo-Famotidine, Pepcid)

- famotidine, calcium carbonate, and magnesium hydroxide (Pepcid Complete)
- lansoprazole (Prevacid)
- magaldrate and simethicone (Riopan Plus, Riopan Plus Double Strength)
- magnesium hydroxide (Dulcolax Milk of Magnesia, Phillips' Milk of Magnesia)
- magnesium oxide (Mag-Ox 400, Uro-Mag)
- magnesium sulfate (Epsom salts)
- nizatidine (Axid, PMS-Nizatidine)
- omeprazole (Losec, Prilosec)
- pantoprazole (Pantoloc, Protonix)
- rabeprazole (Aciphex, Pariet)
- ranitidine (Alti-Ranitidine, Zantac)
- sodium bicarbonate (Brioschi, Neut)
- sucralfate (Carafate, Sulcrate)

Taking ginger with these drugs may increase the risk of hypoglycemia (low blood sugar):
- acarbose (Prandase, Precose)
- acetohexamide
- chlorpropamide (Diabinese, Novo-Propamide)
- gliclazide (Diamicron, Novo-Gliclazide)
- glimepiride (Amaryl)
- glipizide (Glucotrol)
- glipizide and metformin (Metaglip)
- gliquidone (Beglynor, Glurenorm)
- glyburide (DiaBeta, Micronase)
- glyburide and metformin (Glucovance)
- insulin (Humulin, Novolin R)
- metformin (Glucophage, Riomet)
- miglitol (Glyset)
- nateglinide (Starlix)
- pioglitazone (Actos)
- repaglinide (GlucoNorm, Prandin)
- rosiglitazone (Avandia)
- rosiglitazone and metformin (Avandamet)

- tolazamide (Tolinase)
- tolbutamide (Apo-Tolbutamide, Tol-Tab)

Taking ginger with these drugs may interfere with the action of the drug:
- atenolol (Apo-Atenol, Tenormin)
- benazepril (Lotensin)
- captopril (Capoten, Novo-Captopril)
- carvedilol (Coreg)
- enalapril (Vasotec)
- fosinopril (Monopril)
- labetalol (Normodyne, Trandate)
- lisinopril (Prinivil, Zestril)

Taking ginger with these drugs may alter the effects of the drug:
- bepridil (Vascor)
- diltiazem (Cardizem, Tiazac)
- felodipine (Plendil, Renedil)
- isradipine (DynaCirc)
- nifedipine (Adalat CC, Procardia)

Taking ginger with this drug may be harmful:
- digitalis (Digitek, Lanoxin)—may increase drug effects

Lab Tests That May Be Altered by Ginger
May increase plasma partial thromboplastin time (PTT), prothrombin time (PT), and international normalized ratio (INR) levels in those who are also taking warfarin.

Diseases That May Be Worsened or Triggered by Ginger
- May interfere with attempts to control blood sugar in diabetes.
- May worsen bleeding disorders and increase the risk of bruising and bleeding.

- May worsen cases of high or low blood pressure by interfering with attempts to control blood pressure.

Foods That May Interact with Ginger
None known

Supplements That May Interact with Ginger
Increased risk of bleeding when used with herbs and supplements that might affect platelet aggregation, such as angelica, danshen, garlic, ginkgo biloba, red clover, turmeric, white willow, and others. (For a list of herbs and supplements with anticoagulant/antiplatelet effects, see Appendix B.)

GINKGO BILOBA

Taken from a tree native to China and Japan that dates back 200 million years, ginkgo biloba has been used for thousands of years by practitioners of traditional Chinese medicine for coughs, allergies, and asthma. Today ginkgo biloba has a reputation for being able to improve the memory and ward off signs of senility, possibly through its ability to increase blood flow to the brain.

Scientific Name
Ginkgo biloba

Ginkgo Biloba Is Also Commonly Known As
Maidenhair tree, rokan, tanakan, tebonin

Medicinal Parts
Leaf, seed

Ginkgo Biloba's Uses
To treat asthma, angina, tonsillitis, dizziness, headache; to combat inflammation; to improve concentration and memory deficits due to peripheral arterial disease. Germany's Commission E has approved the use of ginkgo biloba to treat the symptoms of organic brain dysfunction, cramplike calf pain (intermittent claudication), vertigo caused by vascular problems, and ringing in the ears (tinnitus) due to vascular problems.

Typical Dose
A typical dose of ginkgo biloba may range from 40 to 80 mg.

Possible Side Effects
Ginkgo biloba's side effects include headache, anxiety, restlessness, and mild gastrointestinal complaints.

Drugs That May Interact with Ginkgo Biloba
Taking ginkgo biloba with these drugs may increase the risk of bleeding or bruising:

- abciximab (ReoPro)
- acemetacin (Acemetacin Heumann, Acemetacin Sandoz)
- alteplase (Activase, Cathflo Activase)
- antithrombin III (Thrombate III)
- argatroban
- aspirin (Bufferin, Ecotrin)
- aspirin and dipyridamole (Aggrenox)
- bivalirudin (Angiomax)
- celecoxib (Celebrex)
- choline magnesium trisalicylate (Trilisate)
- choline salicylate (Teejel)
- clopidogrel (Plavix)
- dalteparin (Fragmin)

- danaparoid (Orgaran)
- diclofenac (Cataflam, Voltaren)
- diflunisal (Apo-Diflunisal, Dolobid)
- dipyridamole (Novo-Dipiradol, Persantine)
- dipyrone (Analgina, Dinador)
- drotrecogin alfa (Xigris)
- enoxaparin (Lovenox)
- eptifibatide (Integrillin)
- etodolac (Lodine, Utradol)
- etoricoxib (Arcoxia)
- fenoprofen (Nalfon)
- flurbiprofen (Ansaid, Ocufen)
- fondaparinux (Arixtra)
- heparin (Hepalean, Hep-Lock)
- hydrocodone and aspirin (Damason-P)
- hydrocodone and ibuprofen (Vicoprofen)
- ibritumomab (Zevalin)
- ibuprofen (Advil, Motrin)
- indobufen (Ibustrin)
- indomethacin (Indocin, Novo-Methacin)
- ketoprofen (Orudis, Rhodis)
- ketorolac (Acular, Toradol)
- lepirudin (Refludan)
- magnesium salicylate (Doan's, Mobidin)
- meclofenamate (Meclomen)
- mefenamic acid (Ponstan, Ponstel)
- meloxicam (MOBIC, Mobicox)
- nabumetone (Apo-Nabumetone, Relafen)
- nadroparin (Fraxiparine)
- naproxen (Aleve, Naprosyn)
- niflumic acid (Niflam, Nifluril)
- nimesulide (Areuma, Aulin)
- oxaprozin (Apo-Oxaprozin, Daypro)
- piroxicam (Feldene, Nu-Pirox)
- reteplase (Retavase)
- rofecoxib (Vioxx)
- salsalate (Amgesic, Salflex)

- streptokinase (Streptase)
- sulindac (Clinoril, Nu-Sundac)
- tenecteplase (TNKase)
- tenoxicam (Dolmen, Mobiflex)
- tiaprofenic acid (Dom-Tiaprofenic, Surgam)
- ticlopidine (Alti-Ticlopidine, Ticlid)
- tinzaparin (Innohep)
- tirofiban (Aggrastat)
- tolmetin (Tolectin)
- urokinase (Abbokinase)
- valdecoxib (Bextra)
- warfarin (Coumadin, Jantoven)

Taking ginkgo biloba with these drugs may reduce the effectiveness of the drug and worsen hypertension (elevated blood pressure):

- chlorothiazide (Diuril)
- hydrochlorothiazide (Apo-Hydro, Microzide)
- hdrochlorothiazide and triamterene (Dyazide, Maxzide)
- hydroflumethiazide (Diucardin, Saluron)
- methyclothiazide (Aquatensen, Enduron)
- olmesartan and hydrochlorothiazide (Benicar HCT)
- polythiazide (Renese)
- trichlormethiazide (Metatensin, Naqua)
- xipamide (Diurexan, Lumitens)

Taking ginkgo biloba with these drugs may increase the risk of seizures:

- acetazolamide (Apo-Acetazolamide, Diamox Sequels)
- amitriptyline (Elavil, Levate)
- amobarbital (Amytal)
- amoxapine (Asendin)
- barbexaclone (Maliasin)
- bupropion (Wellbutrin, Zyban)

- carbamazepine (Carbatrol, Tegretol)
- ciprofloxacin (Ciloxan, Cipro)
- clonazepam (Klonopin, Rivotril)
- clorazepate (Tranxene, T-Tab)
- desipramine (Alti-Desipramine, Norpramin)
- diazepam (Apo-Diazepam, Valium)
- doxepin (Sinequan, Zonalon)
- ethosuximide (Zarontin)
- felbamate (Felbatol)
- fosphenytoin (Cerebyx)
- gabapentin (Neurontin, Nu-Gabapentin)
- ganciclovir (Cytovene, Vitrasert)
- imipramine (Apo-Imipramine, Tofranil)
- lamotrigine (Lamictal)
- levetiracetam (Keppra)
- lorazepam (Ativan, Nu-Loraz)
- mephobarbital (Mebaral)
- methsuximide (Celontin)
- methylphenidate (Concerta, Ritalin)
- metoclopramide (Apo-Metoclop, Reglan)
- metronidazole (Flagyl, Noritate)
- moxifloxacin (Avelox, Vigamox)
- nortriptyline (Aventyl HCl, Pamelor)
- ofloxacin (Floxin, Ocuflox)
- olanzapine (Zydis, Zyprexa)
- oxazepam (Novoxapam, Serax)
- oxcarbazepine (Trileptal)
- pentobarbital (Nembutal)
- phenobarbital (Luminal Sodium, PMS-Phenobarbital)
- phenytoin (Dilantin, Phenytek)
- primidone (Apo-Primidone, Mysoline)
- prochlorperazine (Compazine, Compro)
- quetiapine (Seroquel)
- thiopental (Pentothal)
- tiagabine (Gabitril)
- topiramate (Topamax)
- tramadol (Ultram)
- valproic acid (Depacon, Depakote ER)
- venlafaxine (Effexor)
- vigabatrin (Sabril)
- zonisamide (Zonegran)

Taking ginkgo biloba with these drugs may disrupt blood sugar control:

- acarbose (Prandase, Precose)
- glipizide (Glucotrol)
- glyburide (DiaBeta, Micronase)
- insulin (Humulin, Novolin R)
- metformin (Glucophage, Riomet)
- miglitol (Glyset)
- pioglitazone (Actos)
- repaglinide (GlucoNorm, Prandin)
- rosiglitazone (Avandia)

Using ginkgo biloba with these drugs may increase the effects of the drug:

- iproniazid (Marsilid)
- moclobemide (Alti-Moclobemide, Nu-Moclobemide)
- phenelzine (Nardil)
- selegiline (Eldepryl)
- tranylcypromine (Parnate)

Using ginkgo biloba with these drugs may be harmful:

- fluoxetine (Prozac, Sarafem)—may cause or increase serotonin syndrome (symptoms of which include agitation, rapid heart rate, flushing, heavy sweating, and possibly even death)
- nifedipine (Adalat CC, Procardia)—may increase blood levels of the drug
- papaverine (Para-Time S.R.)—may increase the risk of adverse effects

Lab Tests That May Be Altered by Ginkgo Biloba

May increase plasma partial thromboplastin time (PTT), prothrombin time (PT), and international normalized ratio (INR) levels and decrease platelet activity.

Diseases That May Be Worsened or Triggered by Ginkgo Biloba

- Small increase in risk of seizures in some patients due to ginkgotoxin content of ginkgo leaf and ginkgo leaf extract.
- Increased risk of mild levels of mania (hyperexcitability) in patients with depression when taken with melatonin or St. John's wort.
- May worsen bleeding disorders by interfering with platelet aggregation.

Foods That May Interact with Ginkgo Biloba

None known

Supplements That May Interact with Ginkgo Biloba

Increased risk of bleeding when used with herbs and supplements that might affect platelet aggregation. (For a list of herbs and supplements with anticoagulant/antiplatelet effects, see Appendix B.)

GINSENG, AMERICAN

In the eighteenth century, a Jesuit missionary living in North America noticed that a plant sometimes used by Native American tribes was almost exactly the same as the Chinese ginseng plant, which was considered a virtual cure-all and aphrodisiac. Thus began a high demand for American ginseng, which continues to this day and has driven it nearly into extinction. Some studies have shown that American ginseng can help lower blood sugar.

Scientific Name

Panax quinquefolius

American Ginseng Is Also Commonly Known As

Canadian ginseng, ginseng root, North American ginseng, red berry, ren shen

Medicinal Parts

Root

American Ginseng's Uses

To treat anemia, diabetes, insomnia, impotence, fever, and attention-deficit hyperactivity disorder (ADHD); to improve stamina; to protect against acute respiratory illness

Typical Dose

A typical dose of American ginseng is approximately 200 mg twice daily to protect against acute respiratory illness, or 3 to 9 gm before a meal to reduce postprandial glucose levels in those with type 2 diabetes.

Possible Side Effects

American ginseng's side effects include nausea, vomiting, anxiety, and insomnia.

Drugs That May Interact with American Ginseng

Taking American ginseng with these drugs may increase the risk of hypoglycemia (low blood sugar):

- acarbose (Prandase, Precose)
- acetohexamide

- chlorpropamide (Diabinese, Novo-Propamide)
- gliclazide (Diamicron, Novo-Gliclazide)
- glimepiride (Amaryl)
- glipizide (Glucotrol)
- glipizide and metformin (Metaglip)
- gliquidone (Beglynor, Glurenorm)
- glyburide (DiaBeta, Micronase)
- glyburide and metformin (Glucovance)
- insulin (Humulin, Novolin R)
- metformin (Glucophage, Riomet)
- miglitol (Glyset)
- nateglinide (Starlix)
- pioglitazone (Actos)
- repaglinide (GlucoNorm, Prandin)
- rosiglitazone (Avandia)
- rosiglitazone and metformin (Avandamet)
- tolazamide (Tolinase)
- tolbutamide (Apo-Tolbutamide, Tol-Tab)

Taking American ginseng with these drugs may increase the risk of bleeding or bruising:

- abciximab (ReoPro)
- alteplase (Activase, Cathflo Activase)
- antithrombin III (Thrombate III)
- argatroban
- aspirin (Bufferin, Ecotrin)
- aspirin and dipyridamole (Aggrenox)
- bivalirudin (Angiomax)
- clopidogrel (Plavix)
- dalteparin (Fragmin)
- danaparoid (Orgaran)
- dipyridamole (Novo-Dipiradol, Persantine)
- drotrecogin alfa (Xigris)
- enoxaparin (Lovenox)
- eptifibatide (Integrillin)
- fondaparinux (Arixtra)
- heparin (Hepalean, Hep-Lock)
- hydrocodone and aspirin (Damason-P)

- hydrocodone and ibuprofen (Vicoprofen)
- ibritumomab (Zevalin)
- indobufen (Ibustrin)
- lepirudin (Refludan)
- ticlopidine (Alti-Ticlopidine, Ticlid)
- tinzaparin (Innohep)
- tirofiban (Aggrastat)
- warfarin (Coumadin, Jantoven)

Lab Tests That May Be Altered by American Ginseng
- May decrease postprandial blood glucose.
- May increase thrombin time (TT) and activated partial thromboplastin time (aPTT).

Diseases That May Be Worsened or Triggered by American Ginseng
- May worsen bleeding diseases by interfering with coagulation.
- This herb may have estrogen-like effects and should not be used by women with estrogen-sensitive breast cancer or other hormone-sensitive conditions.
- May worsen schizophrenia if taken in large doses.

Foods That May Interact with American Ginseng
Increased stimulant effects when taken with caffeine-containing foods and drinks such as coffee, tea, and caffeinated soft drinks. (For a list of caffeine-containing herbs, foods, and supplements, see Appendix B.)

Supplements That May Interact with American Ginseng
Increased stimulant effects when taken with herbs and supplements containing caffeine, such as cola nut, guarana, and maté. (For a list of caffeine-containing herbs, foods, and supplements, see Appendix B.)

GINSENG, PANAX

Panax means "cure for all ills" and ginseng means "man root," referring to the human shape of the root. In traditional Chinese medicine, Panax ginseng is used to strengthen the immune system, increase vitality, boost resistance to stress-related maladies, and treat chronic illnesses. Its active ingredients are the ginsenosides, which have been shown to have anti-inflammatory, antioxidant, and anticancer effects.

Scientific Name
Panax ginseng

Panax Ginseng Is Also Commonly Known As
Chinese ginseng, five-fingers, Korean ginseng, red berry

Medicinal Parts
Root

Panax Ginseng's Uses
To treat anxiety, nerve pain, insomnia, stomach upset, and loss of appetite

Typical Dose
A typical dose of Panax ginseng may range from 100 to 400 mg.

Possible Side Effects
Panax ginseng's side effects include insomnia, nervousness, and vomiting.

Drugs That May Interact with Panax Ginseng
Taking Panax ginseng with these drugs may increase the risk of bleeding or bruising:

- abciximab (ReoPro)
- alteplase (Activase, Cathflo Activase)
- antithrombin III (Thrombate III)
- argatroban
- aspirin (Bufferin, Ecotrin)
- aspirin and dipyridamole (Aggrenox)
- bivalirudin (Angiomax)
- clopidogrel (Plavix)
- dalteparin (Fragmin)
- danaparoid (Orgaran)
- dipyridamole (Novo-Dipiradol, Persantine)
- drotrecogin alfa (Xigris)
- enoxaparin (Lovenox)
- eptifibatide (Integrillin)
- fondaparinux (Arixtra)
- heparin (Hepalean, Hep-Lock)
- hydrocodone and aspirin (Damason-P)
- hydrocodone and ibuprofen (Vicoprofen)
- ibritumomab (Zevalin)
- indobufen (Ibustrin)
- lepirudin (Refludan)
- nadroparin (Fraxiparine)
- streptokinase (Streptase)
- ticlopidine (Alti-Ticlopidine, Ticlid)
- tinzaparin (Innohep)
- tirofiban (Aggrastat)
- warfarin (Coumadin, Jantoven)

Taking Panax ginseng with these drugs may increase the risk of hypoglycemia (low blood sugar):
- acarbose (Prandase, Precose)
- acetohexamide
- chlorpropamide (Diabinese, Novo-Propamide)
- gliclazide (Diamicron, Novo-Gliclazide)
- glimepiride (Amaryl)
- glipizide (Glucotrol)
- glipizide and metformin (Metaglip)
- gliquidone (Beglynor, Glurenorm)

- glyburide (DiaBeta, Micronase)
- glyburide and metformin (Glucovance)
- insulin (Humulin, Novolin R)
- metformin (Glucophage, Riomet)
- miglitol (Glyset)
- nateglinide (Starlix)
- pioglitazone (Actos)
- repaglinide (GlucoNorm, Prandin)
- rosiglitazone (Avandia)
- rosiglitazone and metformin (Avandamet)
- tolazamide (Tolinase)
- tolbutamide (Apo-Tolbutamide, Tol-Tab)

Taking Panax ginseng with these drugs may trigger agitation, headache, insomnia, and tremor and may worsen depression:

- iproniazid (Marsilid)
- moclobemide (Alti-Moclobemide, Nu-Moclobemide)
- phenelzine (Nardil)
- selegiline (Eldepryl)
- tranylcypromine (Parnate)

Taking Panax ginseng with these drugs may increase the risk of bleeding or bruising:

- antithrombin III (Thrombate III)
- argatroban
- bivalirudin (Angiomax)
- dalteparin (Fragmin)
- danaparoid (Orgaran)
- drotrecogin alfa (Xigris)
- enoxaparin (Lovenox)
- fondaparinux (Arixtra)
- heparin (Hepalean, Hep-Lock)
- hydrocodone and aspirin (Damason-P)
- hydrocodone and ibuprofen (Vicoprofen)
- ibritumomab (Zevalin)
- lepirudin (Refludan)

- tinzaparin (Innohep)
- warfarin (Coumadin, Jantoven)

Taking Panax ginseng with these drugs may lead to symptoms of estrogen excess (such as breakthrough bleeding or breast pain):

- estrogens (conjugated A/synthetic) (Cenestin)
- estrogens (conjugated/equine) (Cenestin, Premarin)

Taking Panax ginseng with these drugs may be harmful:

- albendazole (Albenza)—may reduce the effectiveness of the drug
- nifedipine (Adalat CC, Procardia)—may increase drug levels in the body

Lab Tests That May Be Altered by Panax Ginseng

- May decrease fasting blood glucose concentrations.
- May decrease glycosylated hemoglobin (HbA1c) levels and improve glucose control in those with type 2 diabetes.
- May increase thrombin time (TT), international normalized ratio (INR) levels, plasma partial thromboplastin time (PTT), and activated partial thromboplastin time (aPTT).
- May increase serum and twenty-four-hour urine estrogens.
- May cause falsely increased or decreased serum digoxin levels, depending on the type of test used.

Diseases That May Be Worsened or Triggered by Panax Ginseng

- May worsen bleeding conditions by interfering with coagulation.
- May interfere with attempts to control blood sugar in diabetes by lowering blood sugar too far.

- This herb may have estrogen-like effects and should not be used by women with estrogen-sensitive breast cancer or other hormone-sensitive conditions.
- May worsen schizophrenia if taken in large doses.

Foods That May Interact with Panax Ginseng

Increased stimulant effects when taken together with caffeine-containing foods and drinks such as coffee, tea, and caffeinated soft drinks. (For a list of caffeine-containing herbs, foods, and supplements, see Appendix B.)

Supplements That May Interact with Panax Ginseng

- Increased hypertension, central nervous system stimulation, and risk of life-threatening ventricular arrhythmias when taken with ma-huang.
- Increased stimulant effects when taken with herbs and supplements containing caffeine, such as cola nut, guarana, and maté. (For a list of caffeine-containing herbs, foods, and supplements, see Appendix B.)
- Increased blood glucose–lowering effects and risk of hypoglycemia (low blood sugar) when used with herbs and supplements that lower glucose levels, such as alpha-lipoic acid, chromium, devil's claw, and psyllium. (For a list of herbs and supplements that lower blood glucose levels, see Appendix B.)

GINSENG, SIBERIAN

Siberian ginseng, which originated in the Russian province of Siberia, has long been valued in China as an "adaptogen," an herb that helps people handle physical and emotional stress. Although it is a member of the ginseng family, this herb is not considered a true ginseng because it is of a different genus from the Panax and American varieties. The Siberian ginseng root, which is not harvested until it is at least two years old, is thought to become more effective the older it gets.

Scientific Name

Eleutherococcus senticosus

Siberian Ginseng Is Also Commonly Known As

Ciwujia, devil's bush, Eleuthero ginseng, Russian root, untouchable, ussuri, wild pepper, wu-jia

Medicinal Parts

Root, root rind, fluid extract of root and rhizome

Siberian Ginseng's Uses

To treat atherosclerosis (hardening of the arteries), rheumatic heart disease, high blood pressure, and herpes simplex virus type 2; to improve athletic performance and protect against environmental stress. Germany's Commission E has approved the use of Siberian ginseng to treat a tendency toward infection and lack of stamina.

Typical Dose

A typical daily dose of Siberian ginseng to treat herpes simplex type 2 infections is approximately 400 mg of extract (standardized to contain eleutheroside E 0.3 percent).

Possible Side Effects

Siberian ginseng's side effects include drowsiness, irritability, anxiety, breast pain, and depression.

Drugs That May Interact with Siberian Ginseng

Taking Siberian ginseng with these drugs may increase the risk of hypoglycemia (low blood sugar):

- acarbose (Prandase, Precose)
- acetohexamide
- chlorpropamide (Diabinese, Novo-Propamide)
- gliclazide (Diamicron, Novo-Gliclazide)
- glimepiride (Amaryl)
- glipizide (Glucotrol)
- glipizide and metformin (Metaglip)
- gliquidone (Beglynor, Glurenorm)
- glyburide (DiaBeta, Micronase)
- glyburide and metformin (Glucovance)
- insulin (Humulin, Novolin R)
- metformin (Glucophage, Riomet)
- miglitol (Glyset)
- nateglinide (Starlix)
- pioglitazone (Actos)
- repaglinide (GlucoNorm, Prandin)
- rosiglitazone (Avandia)
- rosiglitazone and metformin (Avandamet)
- tolazamide (Tolinase)
- tolbutamide (Apo-Tolbutamide, Tol-Tab)

Taking Siberian ginseng with these drugs may increase the risk of bleeding or bruising:

- abciximab (ReoPro)
- alteplase (Activase, Cathflo Activase)
- antithrombin III (Thrombate III)
- argatroban
- aspirin (Bufferin, Ecotrin)
- aspirin and dipyridamole (Aggrenox)
- bivalirudin (Angiomax)
- clopidogrel (Plavix)
- dalteparin (Fragmin)
- danaparoid (Orgaran)
- dipyridamole (Novo-Dipiradol, Persantine)
- drotrecogin alfa (Xigris)
- enoxaparin (Lovenox)
- eptifibatide (Integrillin)
- fondaparinux (Arixtra)
- heparin (Hepalean, Hep-Lock)
- hydrocodone and aspirin (Damason-P)
- hydrocodone and ibuprofen (Vicoprofen)
- ibritumomab (Zevalin)
- indobufen (Ibustrin)
- lepirudin (Refludan)
- reteplase (Retavase)
- streptokinase (Streptase)
- tenecteplase (TNKase)
- ticlopidine (Alti-Ticlopidine, Ticlid)
- tinzaparin (Innohep)
- tirofiban (Aggrastat)
- urokinase (Abbokinase)
- warfarin (Coumadin, Jantoven)

Taking Siberian ginseng with this drug may be harmful:

- digitalis (Digitek, Lanoxin)—may increase blood levels of the drug

Lab Tests That May Be Altered by Siberian Ginseng
- May decrease blood glucose concentrations.
- May increase serum androstenedione.

Diseases That May Be Worsened or Triggered by Siberian Ginseng
- May worsen cardiovascular ailments by triggering elevated blood pressure, rapid heart rate, or irregular heartbeat.
- May worsen hypertension.
- This herb may have estrogen-like effects and should not be used by women with estrogen-sensitive breast cancer or other hormone-sensitive conditions.

Foods That May Interact with Siberian Ginseng
None known

Supplements That May Interact with Siberian Ginseng
- ❶ Increased hypertension, central nervous system stimulation, and risk of life-threatening ventricular arrhythmias when taken with ma-huang.
- May increase blood glucose–lowering effects and risk of hypoglycemia (low blood sugar) when used with herbs and supplements that lower glucose levels, such as alpha-lipoic acid, chromium, devil's claw, Panax ginseng, and psyllium. (For a list of herbs and supplements that lower blood glucose levels, see Appendix B.)
- Increased risk of bleeding when used with herbs and supplements that might affect platelet aggregation, such as angelica, danshen, garlic, ginger, ginkgo biloba, red clover, turmeric, white willow, and others. (For a list of herbs and supplements with anticoagulant/antiplatelet effects, see Appendix B.)
- May enhance therapeutic and adverse effects of herbs and supplements that have sedative properties, such as 5-HTP, kava kava, St. John's wort, and valerian. (For a list of herbs and supplements that have sedative properties, see Appendix B.)

GLUCOMANNAN

> A soluble dietary fiber, glucomannan is used in China and Japan as a general health remedy and thickening agent for foods. Because glucomannan bulks the intestinal contents and slows gastric emptying and the absorption of glucose, it is sometimes used as an antidiabetic agent, a laxative, or a method of weight reduction.

Scientific Name
Amorphophallus konjac

Glucomannan Is Also Commonly Known As
Konjac, konjac mannan

Medicinal Parts
Fiber extracted from the konjac root

Glucomannan's Uses
To treat constipation, type 2 diabetes, and high cholesterol; to assist in weight loss and blood glucose control

Typical Dose
A typical dose of glucomannan for adult weight loss is approximately 1 gm three times a day.

Possible Side Effects
Glucomannan's side effects include hypoglycemia (low blood sugar), cramping, and esophageal and gastrointestinal obstructions.

Drugs That May Interact with Glucomannan
Taking glucomannan with these drugs may increase the risk of hypoglycemia (low blood sugar):
- acarbose (Prandase, Precose)
- acetohexamide
- chlorpropamide (Diabinese, Novo-Propamide)
- gliclazide (Diamicron, Novo-Gliclazide)
- glimepiride (Amaryl)
- glipizide (Glucotrol)
- glipizide and metformin (Metaglip)
- gliquidone (Beglynor, Glurenorm)
- glyburide (DiaBeta, Micronase)
- glyburide and metformin (Glucovance)
- insulin (Humulin, Novolin R)

- metformin (Glucophage, Riomet)
- miglitol (Glyset)
- nateglinide (Starlix)
- pioglitazone (Actos)
- repaglinide (Prandin, GlucoNorm)
- rosiglitazone (Avandia)
- rosiglitazone and metformin (Avandamet)
- tolazamide (Tolinase)
- tolbutamide (Apo-Tolbutamide, Tol-Tab)

Lab Tests That May Be Altered by Glucomannan
- May lower total cholesterol and LDL "bad" cholesterol in adults with type 2 diabetes and adults who are obese.
- May lower serum triglycerides in adults who are obese.
- May lower blood glucose in those with type 2 diabetes.

Diseases That May Be Worsened or Triggered by Glucomannan
None known

Foods That May Interact with Glucomannan
None known

Supplements That May Interact with Glucomannan
May increase blood glucose–lowering effects and risk of hypoglycemia (low blood sugar) when used with herbs and supplements that lower glucose levels, such as alpha-lipoic acid, chromium, devil's claw, Panax ginseng, and psyllium. (For a list of herbs and supplements that lower blood glucose levels, see Appendix B.)

GOAT'S RUE

Goat's rue, which probably takes its name from the unpleasant odor released by its leaves when crushed, was used in the Middle Ages to "sweat out" the plague and in nineteenth-century France to promote milk production in cows. Known to reduce blood sugar and stimulate the production of milk in lactating women (increasing milk output by up to 50 percent in some cases), extracts of goat's rue have also been shown to inhibit the growth of certain bacteria and slow the clumping of platelets that could lead to dangerous blood clots.

Scientific Name
Galega officinalis

Goat's Rue Is Also Commonly Known As
French honeysuckle, French lilac, Italian fitch

Medicinal Parts
Leaf, tip of branch

Goat's Rue's Uses
As a supportive therapy for diabetes, to increase production of milk, and as a diuretic

Typical Dose
A typical dose of goat's rue is approximately 1 tsp of dried leaves mixed with 8 oz boiling water, steeped for 15 minutes, then strained, and taken as a tea.

Possible Side Effects
There are no known side effects when goat's rue is taken in recommended therapeutic dosages.

Drugs That May Interact with Goat's Rue

Taking goat's rue with these drugs may increase the risk of hypoglycemia (low blood sugar):

- acarbose (Prandase, Precose)
- acetohexamide
- chlorpropamide (Diabinese, Novo-Propamide)
- gliclazide (Diamicron, Novo-Gliclazide)
- glimepiride (Amaryl)
- glipizide (Glucotrol)
- glipizide and metformin (Metaglip)
- gliquidone (Beglynor, Glurenorm)
- glyburide (DiaBeta, Micronase)
- glyburide and metformin (Glucovance)
- insulin (Humulin, Novolin R)
- metformin (Glucophage, Riomet)
- miglitol (Glyset)
- nateglinide (Starlix)
- pioglitazone (Actos)
- repaglinide (GlucoNorm, Prandin)
- rosiglitazone (Avandia)
- rosiglitazone and metformin (Avandamet)
- tolazamide (Tolinase)
- tolbutamide (Apo-Tolbutamide, Tol-Tab)

Lab Tests That May Be Altered by Goat's Rue

May decrease blood glucose concentrations.

Diseases That May Be Worsened or Triggered by Goat's Rue

May complicate diabetes therapy by pushing blood sugar down too far.

Foods That May Interact with Goat's Rue

None known

Supplements That May Interact with Goat's Rue

May increase blood glucose–lowering effects and risk of hypoglycemia (low blood sugar) when used with herbs and supplements that lower glucose levels, such as alpha-lipoic acid, chromium, devil's claw, Panax ginseng, and psyllium. (For a list of herbs and supplements that lower blood glucose levels, see Appendix B.)

GOLDENSEAL

Named for its bright-yellow roots, goldenseal was used by the Cherokee Indians as a wash for wounds and skin diseases and as a treatment for sore, inflamed eyes. Because it effectively calms inflammation of the mucous membranes, it is used today as a soothing ingredient in many lotions. The berberine in goldenseal also fights various species of chlamydia, staphylococcus and streptococcus, and the herb has been shown to increase the activity of immune system cells called macrophages, which literally engulf and devour invading cells and cellular debris.

Scientific Name

Hydrastis canadensis

Goldenseal Is Also Commonly Known As

Eye balm, eye root, Indian dye, turmeric root, wild curcuma, yellow root

Medicinal Parts

Rhizome

Goldenseal's Uses

To treat gastrointestinal ulcers, gastritis, bladder infections, sore throat, postpartum hemorrhage, tuberculosis, and skin disorders such as eczema, boils, and pruritis

Typical Dose

A typical dose of goldenseal to treat bladder infections may range from 500 to 1,000 mg of freeze-dried root taken three times daily.

Possible Side Effects

Goldenseal's side effects include mucous membrane irritation, constipation, and digestive disorders.

Drugs That May Interact with Goldenseal

Taking goldenseal with these drugs may cause excessive sedation and mental depression and impairment:

- alprazolam (Apo-Alpraz, Xanax)
- amitriptyline (Elavil, Levate)
- amoxapine (Asendin)
- bupropion (Wellbutrin, Zyban)
- buspirone (BuSpar, Nu-Buspirone)
- clonazepam (Klonopin, Rivotril)
- cyclobenzaprine (Flexeril, Novo-Cycloprine)
- desipramine (Alti-Desipramine, Norpramin)
- diazepam (Apo-Diazepam, Valium)
- diphenhydramine (Benadryl Allergy, Nytol)
- doxepin (Sinequan, Zonalon)
- fluoxetine (Prozac, Sarafem)
- fluphenazine (Prolixin, Modecate)
- flurazepam (Apo-Flurazepam, Dalmane)
- imipramine (Apo-Imipramine, Tofranil)
- lorazepam (Ativan, Nu-Loraz)
- metoclopramide (Apo-Metoclop, Reglan)
- midazolam (Apo-Midazolam, Versed)
- morphine hydrochloride
- morphine sulfate (Kadian, MS Contin)

- nefazodone (Serzone)
- nortriptyline (Aventyl HCl, Pamelor)
- olanzapine (Zydis, Zyprexa)
- oxazepam (Novoxapam, Serax)
- oxcarbazepine (Trileptal)
- prochlorperazine (Compazine, Compro)
- propoxyphene (Darvon, Darvon-N)
- quetiapine (Seroquel)
- risperidone (Risperdal)
- temazepam (Novo-Temazepam, Restoril)
- tramadol (Ultram)
- triazolam (Apo-Triazo, Halcion)
- zolpidem (Ambien)

Taking goldenseal with these drugs may interfere with the action of the drug:

- atenolol (Apo-Atenol, Tenormin)
- benazepril (Lotensin)
- captopril (Capoten, Novo-Captopril)
- carvedilol (Coreg)
- cimetidine (Nu-Cimet, Tagamet)
- diltiazem (Cardizem, Tiazac)
- enalapril (Vasotec)
- enoxaparin (Lovenox)
- famotidine (Apo-Famotidine, Pepcid)
- felodipine (Plendil, Renedil)
- fosinopril (Monopril)
- heparin (Hepalean, Hep-Lock)
- isradipine (DynaCirc)
- labetalol (Normodyne, Trandate)
- lansoprazole (Prevacid)
- lisinopril (Prinivil, Zestril)
- metoprolol (Betaloc, Lopressor)
- nadolol (Apo-Nadol, Corgard)
- nifedipine (Adalat CC, Procardia)
- omeprazole (Losec, Prilosec)
- pantoprazole (Pantoloc, Protonix)

- prazosin (Minipress, Nu-Prazo)
- propranolol (Inderal, InnoPran XL)
- quinapril (Accupril)
- ranitidine (Alti-Ranitidine, Zantac)
- sucralfate (Carafate, Sulcrate)
- timolol (Betimol, Timoptic)
- valsartan (Diovan)
- verapamil (Calan, Isoptin SR)

Taking goldenseal with these drugs may increase the risk of hypokalemia (low levels of potassium in the blood):
- bumetanide (Bumex, Burinex)
- hydrochlorothiazide (Apo-Hydro, Microzide)

Taking goldenseal with these drugs may increase vasoconstriction (narrowing of the blood vessels):
- ephedrine (Pretz-D)
- ergotamine (Cafergor, Cafergot)
- rizatriptan benzoate (Maxalt)
- zolmitriptan (Zomig)

Taking goldenseal with these drugs may increase drug effects:
- digitalis (Digitek, Lanoxin)
- furosemide (Apo-Furosemide, Lasix)

Lab Tests That May Be Altered by Goldenseal
- May increase blood osmolality.
- May increase serum or urine plasma sodium.

Diseases That May Be Worsened or Triggered by Goldenseal
May worsen inflammatory or infectious gastrointestinal diseases by irritating the gastrointestinal tract.

Foods That May Interact with Goldenseal
None known

Supplements That May Interact with Goldenseal
May reduce absorption of B vitamins when the herb is taken in large doses.

GOSSYPOL

Gossypol is a compound found in unrefined cottonseed oil that inhibits male fertility. In 1929, investigators found a correlation between low fertility rates for couples in China's Jiangxi Province and the use of crude cottonseed oil for cooking. In extensive tests conducted in China, gossypol has been shown to lower the production of sperm and/or cause sperm to become immobile, without affecting hormone levels or libido. In one study, this male contraceptive action lasted many weeks after the last dose of gossypol was taken.

Scientific Name
Gossypium hirsutum

Gossypol Is Also Commonly Known As
Cotton, cottonseed oil, upland cotton, wild cotton

Medicinal Parts
Extract derived from the plant

Gossypol's Uses
To treat uterine bleeding, HIV, and endometriosis; as a male contraceptive and a vaginal spermicide; to induce labor and delivery

Typical Dose

A typical dose of gossypol as a male contraceptive may range from 15 to 20 mg per day for up to sixteen weeks, then reduced to half that amount for maintenance.

Possible Side Effects

Gossypol's side effects include fatigue, appetite changes, diarrhea, and sloughing of gastrointestinal mucosal cells.

Drugs That May Interact with Gossypol

Taking gossypol with these drugs may increase the risk of hypokalemia (low levels of potassium in the blood):

- acetazolamide (Apo-Acetazolamide, Diamox Sequels)
- azosemide (Diat)
- bumetanide (Bumex, Burinex)
- chlorothiazide (Diuril)
- chlorthalidone (Apo-Chlorthalidone, Thalitone)
- ethacrynic acid (Edecrin)
- etozolin (Elkapin)
- furosemide (Apo-Furosemide, Lasix)
- hydrochlorothiazide (Apo-Hydro, Microzide)
- hydroflumethiazide (Diucardin, Saluron)
- indapamide (Lozol, Nu-Indapamide)
- mannitol (Osmitrol, Resectisol)
- mefruside (Baycaron)
- methazolamide (Apo-Methazolamide, Neptazane)
- methyclothiazide (Aquatensen, Enduron)
- metolazone (Mykrox, Zaroxolyn)
- olmesartan and hydrochlorothiazide (Benicar HCT)
- polythiazide (Renese)
- torsemide (Demadex)
- trichlormethiazide (Metatensin, Naqua)
- urea (Amino-Cerv, UltraMide)
- xipamide (Diurexan, Lumitens)

Taking gossypol with these drugs may cause or increase kidney damage:

- amorolfine (Loceryl, Locetar)
- amphotericin B cholesteryl sulfate complex (Amphotec)
- amphotericin B conventional (Amphocin, Fungizone)
- amphotericin B lipid complex (Abelcet)
- amphotericin B liposomal (AmBisome)
- bifonazole (Amycor, Canesten)
- butenafine (Lotrimin Ultra, Mentax)
- butoconazole (Gynazole-1, Mycelex-3)
- caspofungin (Cancidas)
- ciclopirox (Loprox, Penlac)
- clotrimazole (Gyne-Lotrimin 3, Mycelex)
- econazole (Spectazole)
- etodolac (Lodine, Utradol)
- fluconazole (Apo-Fluconazole, Diflucan)
- flucytosine (Ancobon)
- gentian violet
- griseofulvin (Fulvicin-U/F, Grifulvin V)
- iodoquinol and hydrocortisone (Dermazene, Vytone)
- isoconazole (Fazol, Gyno-Travogen)
- itraconazole (Sporanox)
- ketoconazole (Apo-Ketoconazole, Nizoral)
- meloxicam (MOBIC, Mobicox)
- metformin (Glucophage, Riomet)
- methotrexate (Rheumatrex, Trexall)
- metronidazole (Flagyl, Noritate)
- miconazole (Femizol-M, Monistat 3)
- miglitol (Glyset)
- morphine hydrochloride
- morphine sulfate (Kadian, MS Contin)

- naftifine (Naftin)
- natamycin (Natacyn)
- nitrofurantoin (Furadantin, Macrobid)
- nystatin (Mycostatin, Nystat-RX)
- ofloxacin (Floxin, Ocuflox)
- omoconazole (Afongan, Fongamil)
- oxiconazole (Oxistat)
- penicillin (Pfizerpen, Wycillin)
- povidone-iodine (Betadine, Vagi-Gard)
- propoxyphene (Darvon, Darvon-N)
- rifampin (Rifadin, Rimactane)
- stavudine (Zerit)
- sucralfate (Carafate, Sulcrate)
- sulconazole (Exelderm)
- terbinafine (Lamisil, Lamisil AT)
- terconazole (Terazol 3, Terazol 7)
- tioconazole (1-Day, Vagistat)
- tolciclate (Fungifos, Tolmicol)
- tolnaftate (Gold Bond Antifungal, Tinactin Antifungal Jock Itch)
- tramadol (Ultram)
- valacyclovir (Valtrex)
- vancomycin (Vancocin)
- voriconazole (VFEND)
- zidovudine (Novo-AZT, Retrovir)

- etodolac (Lodine, Utradol)
- etoricoxib (Arcoxia)
- fenoprofen (Nalfon)
- flurbiprofen (Ansaid, Ocufen)
- ibuprofen (Advil, Motrin)
- indomethacin (Indocin, Novo-Methacin)
- ketoprofen (Orudis, Rhodis)
- ketorolac (Acular, Toradol)
- magnesium salicylate (Doan's, Mobidin)
- meclofenamate (Meclomen)
- mefenamic acid (Ponstar, Ponstel)
- meloxicam (MOBIC, Mobicox)
- nabumetone (Apo-Nabumetone, Relafen)
- naproxen (Aleve, Naprosyn)
- niflumic acid (Niflam, Nifluril)
- nimesulide (Areuma, Aulin)
- oxaprozin (Apo-Oxaprozin, Daypro)
- piroxicam (Feldene, Nu-Pirox)
- rofecoxib (Vioxx)
- salsalate (Amgesic, Salflex)
- sulindac (Clinoril, Nu-Sundac)
- tenoxicam (Dolmen, Mobiflex)
- tiaprofenic acid (Dom Tiaprofenic, Surgam)
- tolmetin (Tolectin)
- valdecoxib (Bextra)

Taking gossypol with these drugs may increase gastrointestinal adverse effects:

- acemetacin (Acemetacin Heumann, Acemetacin Sandoz)
- aspirin (Bufferin, Ecotrin)
- celecoxib (Celebrex)
- choline magnesium trisalicylate (Trilisate)
- choline salicylate (Teejel)
- diclofenac (Cataflam, Voltaren)
- diflunisal (Apo-Diflunisal, Dolobid)
- dipyrone (Analgina, Dinador)

Taking gossypol with these drugs may reduce or prevent absorption of the drug:

- ferrous sulfate (Feratab, Fer-Iron)
- iron-dextran complex (Dexferrum, INFeD)

Lab Tests That May Be Altered by Gossypol
None known

Diseases That May Be Worsened or Triggered by Gossypol
May cause or worsen potassium depletion.

Foods and Drinks That May Interact with Gossypol

When taken with alcohol, may inhibit certain enzymes that break down alcohol in the body, allowing levels of a by-product of alcohol metabolism called acetaldehyde to accumulate. High levels of acetaldehyde can damage tissues.

Supplements That May Interact with Gossypol

- Increased risk of cardiac glycoside toxicity when used with other herbs that contain cardiac glycosides, such as black hellebore, calotropis, motherwort, and others. (For a list of cardiac glycoside–containing herbs and supplements, see Appendix B.)
- Increased risk of potassium depletion when used in conjunction with horsetail plant or licorice.
- Increased risk of potassium depletion when used with stimulant laxative herbs, such as black root, cascara sagrada, castor oil, and senna. (For a list of stimulant laxative herbs and supplements, see Appendix B.)

GOTU KOLA

Gotu kola is a creeping plant that grows in hot, swampy areas of the world, such as India, Sri Lanka, and South Africa. It produces fan-shaped leaves that look something like an old British penny, thus its common name, pennywort. Used for centuries by Ayurvedic healers, gotu kola contains triterpenes, which are believed to encourage the production of collagen in blood vessel walls, strengthen the veins, improve blood circulation in the legs, and accelerate the healing of burns and wounds.

Scientific Name

Centella asiatica

Gotu Kola Is Also Commonly Known As

Hydrocotyle, Indian pennywort, marsh penny, white rot

Medicinal Parts

Leaf, stem

Gotu Kola's Uses

To treat depression, rheumatism, skin diseases, poor circulation, scabies, and poorly healing wounds.

Typical Dose

A typical dose of gotu kola is approximately 0.3 to 0.6 gm of dried leaves.

Possible Side Effects

When used internally, gotu kola's side effects include sensitivity of the skin to sunlight, and infertility. When used externally, gotu kola may cause skin irritation.

Drugs That May Interact with Gotu Kola

Taking gotu kola with these drugs may cause excessive sedation and mental depression and impairment:

- alprazolam (Apo-Alpraz, Xanax)
- aripiprazole (Abilify)
- baclofen (Lioresal, Nu-Baclo)
- bromazepam (Apo-Bromazepam, Novo-Bromazepam)
- buprenorphine (Buprenex, Subutex)
- bupropion (Wellbutrin, Zyban)
- buspirone (BuSpar, Nu-Buspirone)

- butabarbital (Butisol Sodium)
- butorphanol (Apo-Butorphanol, Stadol)
- carbamazepine (Carbatrol, Tegretol)
- chloral hydrate (Aquachloral Supprettes, Somnote)
- chlordiazepoxide (Apo-Chlordiazepoxide, Librium)
- chlorpromazine (Thorazine)
- citalopram (Celexa)
- clobazam (Alti-Clobazam, Frisium)
- clonazepam (Klonopin, Rivotril)
- clonidine (Catapres, Duraclon)
- clorazepate (Tranxene, T-Tab)
- clozapine (Clozaril, Gen-Clozapine)
- codeine (Codeine Contin)
- cyclobenzaprine (Flexeril, Novo-Cycloprine)
- dantrolene (Dantrium)
- diazepam (Apo-Diazepam, Valium)
- diphenhydramine (Benadryl Allergy, Nytol)
- doxylamine and pyridoxine (Diclectin)
- fentanyl (Actiq, Duragesic)
- fluoxetine (Prozac, Sarafem)
- fluphenazine (Modecate, Prolixin)
- flurazepam (Apo-Flurazepam, Dalmane)
- gabapentin (Neurontin, Nu-Gabapentin)
- haloperidol (Haldol, Novo-Peridol)
- hydromorphone (Dilaudid, PMS-Hydromorphone)
- hydroxyzine (Atarax, Vistaril)
- levorphanol (Levo-Dromoran)
- lorazepam (Ativan, Nu-Loraz)
- loxapine (Loxitane, Nu-Loxapine)
- meperidine (Demerol, Meperitab)
- meprobamate (Miltown, Movo-Mepro)
- mesoridazine (Serentil)
- methadone (Dolophine, Methadose)
- methocarbamol (Robaxin)
- methotrimeprazine (Novo-Meprazine, Nozain)
- midazolam (Apo-Midazolam, Versed)
- mirtazapine (Remeron)
- molindone (Moban)
- morphine sulfate (Kadian, MS Contin)
- nalbuphine (Nubain)
- olanzapine (Zydis, Zyprexa)
- oxazepam (Novoxapam, Serax)
- oxcarbazepine (Trileptal)
- oxycodone (OxyContin, Roxicodone)
- oxymorphone (Numorphan)
- paclitaxel (Onxol, Taxol)
- perphenazine (Apo-Perphenazine, Trilafon)
- phenobarbital (Luminal Sodium, PMS-Phenobarbital)
- phenytoin (Dilantin, Phenytek)
- pizotifen (Sandomigran)
- prazepam
- primidone (Apo-Primidone, Mysoline)
- prochlorperazine (Compazine, Compro)
- promethazine (Phenergan)
- quetiapine (Seroquel)
- risperidone (Risperdal)
- ropinirole (Requip)
- s-citalopram (Lexapro)
- sertraline (Apo-Sertraline, Zoloft)
- sodium oxybate (Xyrem)
- temazepam (Novo-Temazepam, Restoril)
- thiethylperazine (Torecan)
- thioridazine (Mellaril)
- thiothixene (Navane)
- tiagabine (Gabitril)
- tizanidine (Zanaflex)
- tolcapone (Tasmar)
- tramadol (Ultram)
- triazolam (Apo-Triazo, Halcion)
- trifluoperazine (Novo-Trifluzine, Stelazine)

- vigabatrin (Sabril)
- zaleplon (Sonata, Starnoc)
- zolpidem (Ambien)
- zopiclone (Alti-Zopiclone, Gen-Zopiclone)
- zuclopenthixol (Clopixol)

Taking gotu kola with these drugs may interfere with the action of the drug:

- acarbose (Prandase, Precose)
- acetohexamide
- acipimox (Acipimox, Olbetam)
- aspirin and pravastatin (Pravigard PAC)
- atorvastatin (Lipitor)
- bezafibrate (Bezalip, PMS-Bezafibrate)
- chlorpropamide (Diabinese, Novo-Propamide)
- cholestyramine (Prevalite, Questran)
- ciprofibrate (Estaprol, Modalim)
- clofibrate (Claripex, Novo-Fibrate)
- colesevelam (WelChol)
- colestipol (Colestid)
- fenofibrate (Lofibra, TriCor)
- fluvastatin (Lescol)
- gemfibrozil (Apo-Gemfibrozil, Lopid)
- gliclazide (Diamicron, Novo-Gliclazide)
- glimepiride (Amaryl)
- glipizide (Glucotrol)
- glipizide and metformin (Metaglip)
- gliquidone (Beglynor, Glurenorm)
- glyburide (DiaBeta, Micronase)
- glyburide and metformin (Glucovance)
- insulin (Humulin, Novolin R)
- lovastatin (Altocor, Mevacor)
- metformin (Glucophage, Riomet)
- miglitol (Glyset)
- nateglinide (Starlix)
- niacin (Niacor, Nicotinex)
- niacin and lovastatin (Advicor)

- pioglitazone (Actos)
- pravastatin (Novo-Pravastatin, Pravachol)
- probucol
- repaglinide (GlucoNorm, Prandin)
- rosiglitazone (Avandia)
- rosiglitazone and metformin (Avandamet)
- rosuvastatin (Crestor)
- simvastatin (Apo-Simvastatin, Zocor)
- tolazamide (Tolinase)
- tolbutamide (Apo-Tolbutamide, Tol-Tab)

Lab Tests That May Be Altered by Gotu Kola

None known

Diseases That May Be Worsened or Triggered by Gotu Kola

May increase blood sugar, cholesterol, or blood fat levels.

Foods That May Interact with Gotu Kola

None known

Supplements That May Interact with Gotu Kola

May enhance therapeutic and adverse effects of herbs and supplements that have sedative properties, such as 5-HTP, kava kava, St. John's wort, and valerian. (For a list of herbs and supplements that have sedative properties, see Appendix B.)

GRAPEFRUIT

Grapefruit is included in this book not because it is a particularly important "herb," but because it can interact with certain drugs in a unique and dangerous way. A metabolic system

continued

called cytochrome p450 helps break down many drugs in the intestines before they are absorbed. Grapefruit contains substances called furano-coumarins that interfere with this process. As a result, when such drugs are taken together with grapefruit or grapefruit juice, greater amounts of the drug will reach the circulation. This leads to higher blood levels of the drug and may increase the drug's therapeutic and/or toxic effects.

Scientific Name
Citrus paradisi

Grapefruit Is Also Commonly Known As
Paradisapfel, pomelo, toronja

Medicinal Parts
Fruit, juice of fruit, seed

Grapefruit's Uses
To treat psoriasis; to lower cholesterol and "unclog" the arteries; to aid in weight reduction.

Typical Dose
There is no typical dose of grapefruit.

Possible Side Effects
Grapefruit may cause occasional heartburn, nausea, and other symptoms of dyspepsia.

Drugs That May Interact with Grapefruit
Taking grapefruit or grapefruit juice with these drugs may increase absorption and/or blood levels of the drug:

- alprazolam (Apo-Alpraz, Xanax)
- amlodipine (Norvasc)
- atorvastatin (Lipitor)
- bepridil (Vascor)
- bromazepam (Apo-Bromazepam, Gen-Bromazepam)
- brotizolam (Lendorm, Sintonal)
- buspirone (BuSpar, Nu-Buspirone)
- carbamazepine (Carbatrol, Tegretol)
- carvedilol (Coreg)
- chlordiazepoxide (Apo-Chlordiazepoxide, Librium)
- cisapride (Propulsid)
- clobazam (Alti-Clobazam, Frisium)
- clomipramine (Anafranil, Novo-Clopramine)
- clonazepam (Klonopin, Rivotril)
- clorazepate (Tranxene, T-Tab)
- cyclosporine (Neoral, Sandimmune)
- dextromethorphan (found in various formulations of Alka-Seltzer, Contac, PediaCare, Robitussin, Sudafed, Triaminic, and other over-the-counter medications)
- diazepam (Apo-Diazepam, Valium)
- diltiazem (Cardizem, Tiazac)
- erythromycin (Erythrocin, Staticin)
- estazolam (ProSom)
- estrogens (conjugated A/synthetic) (Cenestin)
- estrogens (conjugated/equine) (Congest, Premarin)
- estrogens (conjugated/equine) and medroxy-progesterone (Premprase, Prempro)
- estrogens (esterified) and methyltestosterone (Estratest, Estratest H.S.)
- estrogens (esterified) (Menest, Estratab)
- ethinyl estradiol and desogestrel (Cyclessa, Ortho-Cept)
- ethinyl estradiol and ethynodiol diacetate (Demulen, Zovia)
- ethinyl estradiol and etonogestrel (NuvaRing)

- ethinyl estradiol and levonorgestrel (Alesse, Triphasil)
- ethinyl estradiol and norelgestromin (Evra, Ortho Evra)
- ethinyl estradiol and norethindrone (Brevicon, Ortho-Novum)
- ethinyl estradiol and norgestimate (Cyclen, Ortho Tri-Cyclen)
- ethinyl estradiol and norgestrel (Cryselle, Ovral)
- felodipine (Plendil, Renedil)
- flurazepam (Apo-Flurazepam, Dalmane)
- fluvastatin (Lescol)
- isradipine (DynaCirc)
- lacidipine (Aponil, Caldine)
- lercanidipine (Cardiovasc, Carmen)
- loprazolam (Dormonoct, Havlane)
- lorazepam (Ativan, Nu-Loraz)
- lovastatin (Altocor, Mevacor)
- manidipine (Calslot, Iperten)
- mestranol and norethindrone (Necon 1/50, Ortho-Novum 1/50)
- methylprednisolone (Depo-Medrol, Medrol)
- midazolam (Apo-Midazolam, Versed)
- nicardipine (Cardene)
- nifedipine (Adalat CC, Procardia)
- nilvadipine
- nimodipine (Nimotop)
- nisoldipine (Sular)
- nitrendipine
- pinaverium (Dicetel)
- prazepam
- praziquantel (Biltricide)
- quazepam (Doral)
- quinidine (Novo-Quinidin, Quinaglute Dura-Tabs)
- rosuvastatin (Crestor)
- saquinavir (Fortovase, Invirase)

- scopolamine (Scopace, Transderm Scop)
- sildenafil (Viagra)
- simvastatin (Apo-Simvastatin, Zocor)
- temazepam (Novo-Temazepam, Restoril)
- tetrazepam (Mobiforton, Musapam)
- triazolam (Apo-Triazo, Halcion)
- verapamil (Calan, Isoptin SR)

Taking grapefruit or grapefruit juice with these drugs may decrease absorption and blood levels of the drug:

- etoposide (Toposar, VePesid)
- fexofenadine (Allegra)
- itraconazole (Sporanox)
- theophylline (Elixophyllin, Theochron)

Taking grapefruit or grapefruit juice with this drug may increase therapeutic and/or adverse effects of the drug:

- warfarin (Coumadin, Jantoven)

Lab Tests That May Be Altered by Grapefruit

- Decreased metabolism and increased plasma concentrations of amlodipine, atorvastatin, buspirone, carbamazepine, cyclosporine, diazepam, diltiazem, ethinyl-estradiol, felodipine, losartan, lovastatin, midazolam, nicardipine, nifedipine, nimodipine, nisoldipine, saquinavir, simvastatin, 17-beta-estradiol, terfenadine, triazolam, and verapamil.
- May lower hematocrit in those with elevated levels and increase hematocrit in those with low levels.

Diseases That May Be Worsened or Triggered by Grapefruit

None known

Foods That May Interact with Grapefruit

- May interfere with the metabolism of quinine in tonic water, worsening rhythm disorders such as long QT syndrome.
- When taken with red wine, may exert an additive inhibitory effect on cytochrome P450, increasing risk for interactions with other drugs.

Supplements That May Interact with Grapefruit

Increased serum levels of lovastatin when taken together with red yeast rice (Cholestin).

GRAPE SEED

Grape seed extract is high in compounds called procyanidolic oligomers (PCOs), which are powerful antioxidants, perhaps even stronger than vitamins C and E. It is thought to be able to reduce free radical damage, strengthen and repair connective tissue, and help moderate allergic and inflammatory responses by reducing histamine production. Grape seed extract is currently marketed as a preventive for heart disease, a treatment for allergic conditions, and a revitalizing agent for aging skin.

Scientific Name

Vitis vinifera

Grape Seed Is Also Commonly Known As

Activin, grape seed extract, grape seed oil, proanthodyn

Medicinal Parts

Seed

Grape Seed's Uses

To treat atherosclerosis, varicose veins, fragile capillaries, elevated blood pressure, hemorrhoids, macular degeneration, and premenstrual syndrome; as an antioxidant

Typical Dose

A typical daily dose of grape seed extract may range from 75 to 300 mg.

Possible Side Effects

Grape seed's side effects include headache and sore throat.

Drugs That May Interact with Grape Seed

Taking grape seed with these drugs may increase the risk of bleeding and bruising:

- abciximab (ReoPro)
- aspirin (Bufferin, Ecotrin)
- enoxaparin (Lovenox)
- fondaparinux (Arixtra)
- heparin (Hepalean, Hep-Lock)
- ticlopidine (Alti-Ticlopidine, Ticlid)
- urokinase (Abbokinase)
- warfarin (Coumadin, Jantoven)

Lab Tests That May Be Altered by Grape Seed

None known

Diseases That May Be Worsened or Triggered by Grape Seed

None known

Foods That May Interact with Grape Seed

None known

Supplements That May Interact with Grape Seed

None known

GREEN TEA

> Green tea, which is made from the fresh, unfermented leaves of the *Camellia sinensis* bush, contains powerful antioxidants called catechins and other health-enhancing substances. Mounting scientific evidence indicates that green tea may help reduce total cholesterol and LDL "bad" cholesterol while raising HDL "good" cholesterol, ward off certain kinds of cancer, assist in weight loss, fight bacteria, and slow the aging process.

Scientific Name
Camellia sinensis

Green Tea Is Also Commonly Known As
Chinese green tea, gunpowder tea, Japanese green tea

Medicinal Parts
Leaf

Green Tea's Uses
To treat elevated cholesterol, diabetes, migraine headaches, fatigue, and stomach disorders; to reduce the risk of heart disease; to prevent dental caries.

Typical Dose
A typical daily dose of green tea may range from 300 to 400 mg of polyphenols (green tea's active ingredient) in the form of tea or extract. One cup of tea contains 50 to 100 mg of polyphenols.

Possible Side Effects
Green tea's side effects include heartburn, gastric irritation, and reduction of appetite.

Drugs That May Interact with Green Tea
Taking green tea with these drugs may increase the risk of bleeding or bruising:

- abciximab (ReoPro)
- alteplase (Activase, Cathflo Activase)
- antithrombin III (Thrombate III)
- argatroban
- aspirin (Bufferin, Ecotrin)
- bivalirudin (Angiomax)
- choline magnesium trisalicylate (Trilisate)
- clopidogrel (Plavix)
- danaparoid (Orgaran)
- dipyridamole (Novo-Dipiradol, Persantine)
- drotrecogin alfa (Xigris)
- enoxaparin (Lovenox)
- etodolac (Lodine, Utradol)
- fenoprofen (Nalfon)
- flurbiprofen (Ansaid, Ocufen)
- fondaparinux (Arixtra)
- heparin (Hepalean, Hep-Lock)
- hydrocodone and aspirin (Damason-P)
- hydrocodone and ibuprofen (Vicoprofen)
- ibritumomab (Zevalin)
- ibuprofen (Advil, Motrin)
- indobufen (Ibustrin)
- indomethacin (Indocin, Novo-Methacin)
- ketorolac (Acular, Toradol)
- lepirudin (Refludan)
- nabumetone (Apo-Nabumetone, Relefan)
- nadroparin (Fraxiparine)
- naproxen (Aleve, Naprosyn)
- oxaprozin (Apo-Oxaprozin, Daypro)
- piroxicam (Feldene, Nu-Pirox)
- salsalate (Amgesic, Salflex)
- streptokinase (Streptase)
- sulindac (Clinoril, Nu-Sundac)
- tiaprofenic acid (Dom-Tiaprofenic, Surgam)

- ticlopidine (Alti-Ticlopidine, Ticlid)
- tolmetin (Tolectin)
- valdecoxib (Bextra)
- warfarin (Coumadin, Jantoven)

Green tea contains caffeine, so see Caffeine and Caffeine-Containing Herbs on p. 111 for an additional list of drugs that may interact with this herb.

Lab Tests That May Be Altered by Green Tea
See Caffeine and Caffeine-Containing Herbs on p. 112 for a list of lab tests that may interact with the caffeine in this herb.

Diseases That May Be Worsened or Triggered by Green Tea
See Caffeine and Caffeine-Containing Herbs on p. 113 for a list of diseases that may be worsened or triggered by the caffeine in this herb.

Foods That May Interact with Green Tea
- May increase therapeutic and adverse effects of caffeine when taken together with caffeine-containing foods and drinks. (For a list of caffeine-containing foods and drinks, see Appendix B.)
- May interfere with the absorption of nonheme iron (iron from sources other than meat) and/or iron supplements in the diet.
- Increased risk of microcytic anemia in infants who are given tea.
- Milk can bind the antioxidants in green tea and decrease their beneficial effects.

Supplements That May Interact with Green Tea
See Caffeine and Caffeine-Containing Herbs on p. 113 for a list of supplements that may interact with the caffeine in this herb.

GUARANA

A tropical plant native to Venezuela and northern Brazil, guarana produces a small red fruit with a high caffeine content. Many Brazilians enjoy chewing guarana seeds for the energy boost, or drinking fizzy, fruity guarana soft drinks, which are second in popularity only to cola drinks. Some people also claim that guarana is an aphrodisiac.

Scientific Name
Paullinia cupana

Guarana Is Also Commonly Known As
Brazilian cocoa, guarana bread, paullinia, zoom

Medicinal Parts
Seed

Guarana's Uses
To treat digestion problems, headache, fever, and dysmenorrhea; to ease fatigue, hunger, and thirst; as a diuretic

Typical Dose
A typical dose of guarana is approximately 1 gm of the powdered form.

Possible Side Effects
Guarana's side effects include restlessness, nervousness, insomnia, gastric irritation, and diuresis.

Drugs That May Interact with Guarana
Taking guarana with this drug may interfere with the action of the drug:
- alprazolam (Apo-Alpraz, Xanax)

Taking guarana with these drugs may increase the risk of hypokalemia (low levels of potassium in the blood):

- bepridil (Vascor)
- digitalis (Digitek, Lanoxin)
- diltiazem (Cardizem, Tiazac)
- dofetilide (Tikosyn)
- flecainide (Tambocor)
- insulin (Humulin, Novolin R)
- quinidine (Novo-Quinidin, Quinaglute Dura-Tabs)
- sildenafil (Viagra)
- sotalol (Betapace, Sorine)
- verapamil (Calan, Isoptin SR)

Guarana contains caffeine, so see Caffeine and Caffeine-Containing Herbs on p. 111 for an additional list of drugs that may interact with this herb.

Lab Tests That May Be Altered by Guarana

May cause a reduction in serum ferritin, hemoglobin, and/or serum iron concentration in those who are iron-deficient.

See also Caffeine and Caffeine-Containing Herbs on p. 112 for a list of lab tests that may interact with the caffeine in this herb.

Diseases That May Be Worsened or Triggered by Guarana

See Caffeine and Caffeine-Containing Herbs on p. 113 for a list of diseases that may be worsened or triggered by the caffeine in this herb.

Foods That May Interact with Guarana

May increase therapeutic and adverse effects of caffeine when taken together with caffeine-containing foods and drinks. (For a list of caffeine-containing foods and supplements, see Appendix B.)

Supplements That May Interact with Guarana

See Caffeine and Caffeine-Containing Herbs on p. 113 for a list of supplements that may interact with the caffeine in this herb.

GUAR GUM

A soluble dietary fiber taken from the seed of the guar plant native to India, guar gum expands when combined with liquid in the intestines, providing more bulk to the feces and promoting bowel action. But because it absorbs fluid, guar gum may also be helpful in treating diarrhea. In manufacturing, guar gum is used as a thickener, binding agent, or stabilizer in foods, beverages, creams, and lotions.

Scientific Name

Cyamopsis tetragonoloba

Guar Gum Is Also Commonly Known As

Aconite bean, Calcutta lucerne, clusterbean, guar

Medicinal Parts

Whole plant

Guar Gum's Uses

To treat night blindness, loss of appetite, constipation, and diabetes; to aid digestion.

Typical Dose

A typical dose of guar gum is approximately 5 gm in tablet or granule form, taken three times daily.

Possible Side Effects

Guar gum's side effects include nausea, flatulence, diarrhea, and gastrointestinal discomfort.

Drugs That May Interact with Guar Gum

Taking guar gum with these drugs may increase the risk of hypoglycemia (low blood sugar):

- acarbose (Prandase, Precose)
- acetohexamide
- chlorpropamide (Diabinese, Novo-Propamide)
- gliclazide (Diamicron, Novo-Gliclazide)
- glimepiride (Amaryl)
- glipizide (Glucotrol)
- glipizide and metformin (Metaglip)
- gliquidone (Beglynor, Glurenorm)
- glyburide (DiaBeta, Micronase)
- glyburide and metformin (Glucovance)
- insulin (Humulin, Novolin R)
- metformin (Glucophage, Riomet)
- miglitol (Glyset)
- nateglinide (Starlix)
- pioglitazone (Actos)
- repaglinide (GlucoNorm, Prandin)
- rosiglitazone (Avandia)
- rosiglitazone and metformin (Avandamet)
- tolazamide (Tolinase)
- tolbutamide (Apo-Tolbutamide, Tol-Tab)

Taking guar gum with these drugs may be harmful:

- all drugs taken orally—may reduce or prevent drug absorption

Lab Tests That May Be Altered by Guar Gum

- Decreased total cholesterol and LDL "bad" cholesterol.
- Decreased "after-eating" (postprandial) blood glucose.

Diseases That May Be Worsened or Triggered by Guar Gum

May worsen narrowings of or obstructions in the gastrointestinal tract.

Foods That May Interact with Guar Gum

Decreased nutrient absorption when taken with meals over the long term.

Supplements That May Interact with Guar Gum

Decreased nutrient absorption when taken concurrently with vitamin/mineral supplements.

GUGGUL

> Guggul, a resin produced by the mukul mirth tree, is a traditional Indian remedy that has been used to treat skin diseases, urinary problems, joint pain, and other ailments. When further refined, it becomes guggulipid, which contains various substances that may lower cholesterol and help combat obesity.

Scientific Name

Commiphora mukluk

Guggul Is Also Commonly Known As

Guggal, guggulipid, gum guggal, mukul, myrrh tree

Medicinal Parts

Extract of gum resin

Guggul's Uses

To treat arthritis, skin diseases, and atherosclerosis; to lower cholesterol; to aid in weight loss.

Typical Dose

A typical dose of guggul may range from 1,000 to 2,000 mg of guggul extract (guggulipid) providing 75 to 150 mg of guggulsterones.

Possible Side Effects

Guggul's side effects include nausea, vomiting, diarrhea, bloating, belching, and hiccups.

Drugs That May Interact with Guggul

Taking guggul with these drugs may reduce or prevent drug absorption and effects:

- diltiazem (Cardizem, Tiazac)
- propranolol (Inderal, InnoPran XL)

Taking guggul with these drugs may be harmful:

- fondaparinux (Arixtra)—may increase the risk of bleeding or bruising
- levothyroxine (Levothroid, Synthroid)—may alter drug effects

Lab Tests That May Be Altered by Guggul

- Decreased total cholesterol and LDL "bad" cholesterol levels.
- Decreased triglyceride levels.
- Decreased thyroid-stimulating hormone (TSH) levels.
- Increased triiodothyronine (T3) levels.

Diseases That May Be Worsened or Triggered by Guggul

None known

Foods That May Interact with Guggul

None known

Supplements That May Interact with Guggul

Increased risk of bleeding when used with herbs and supplements that might affect platelet aggregation.

(For a list of herbs and supplements with anticoagulant/antiplatelet effects, see Appendix B.)

GYMNEMA

> *Gymnema sylvestre*, a woody, climbing plant grown in India, was given the Hindu name of *gurmar*, which means "sugar destroyer," because chewing the leaves takes away the ability to taste sweetness. A small number of studies suggest that the herb lowers blood sugar in diabetics.

Scientific Name

Gymnema sylvestre

Gymnema Is Also Commonly Known As

Gurmar, merasingi, meshashringi, miracle plant

Medicinal Parts

Leaf

Gymnema's Uses

To treat coughs, malaria, constipation, and diabetes; as a diuretic and digestive stimulant

Typical Dose

A typical dose of gymnema is approximately 200 mg of extract taken twice a day.

Possible Side Effects

Gymnema's side effects include nausea, vomiting, anorexia, and allergic reactions.

Drugs That May Interact with Gymnema

Taking gymnema with these drugs may increase the risk of hypoglycemia (low blood sugar):

- acarbose (Prandase, Precose)
- acetohexamide
- chlorpropamide (Diabinese, Novo-Propamide)
- gliclazide (Diamicron, Novo-Gliclazide)
- glimepiride (Amaryl)
- glipizide (Glucotrol)
- glipizide and metformin (Metaglip)
- gliquidone (Beglynor, Glurenorm)
- glyburide (DiaBeta, Micronase)
- glyburide and metformin (Glucovance)
- insulin (Humulin, Novolin R)
- metformin (Glucophage, Riomet)
- miglitol (Glyset)
- nateglinide (Starlix)
- pioglitazone (Actos)
- repaglinide (GlucoNorm, Prandin)
- rosiglitazone (Avandia)
- rosiglitazone and metformin (Avandamet)
- tolazamide (Tolinase)
- tolbutamide (Apo-Tolbutamide, Tol-Tab)

Lab Tests That May Be Altered by Gymnema

- Decreased blood glucose levels.
- Decreased total cholesterol LDL "bad" cholesterol levels.

Diseases That May Be Worsened or Triggered by Gymnema

May interfere with blood sugar control in diabetes.

Foods That May Interact with Gymnema

None known

Supplements That May Interact with Gymnema

None known

HAWAIIAN BABY WOODROSE

Hawaiian baby woodrose is a perennial climbing vine native to India, with large furry seeds that grow in seed pods resembling blooming roses carved out of wood. The leaves and roots of this plant have been used traditionally in India for their ability to combat inflammation and germs. In some areas of the world, Hawaiian baby woodrose seeds are used as a hallucinogen, as they contain substances similar to those found in LSD.

Scientific Name

Argyreia nervosa

Hawaiian Baby Woodrose Is Also Commonly Known As

Baby Hawaiian woodrose, elephant-climber, elephant creeper, silver-morning-glory, wood-rose

Medicinal Parts

Leaf, root

Hawaiian Baby Woodrose's Uses

To relieve pain; to increase sweating; as a hallucinogen and for sacred rituals.

Typical Dose

There is no typical dose of Hawaiian baby woodrose.

Possible Side Effects

Hawaiian baby woodrose's side effects include nausea, vomiting, dizziness, blurred vision, visual and auditory hallucinations, sweating, and increased heart rate.

Drugs That May Interact with Hawaiian Baby Woodrose

Taking Hawaiian baby woodrose with these drugs may increase the risk of serotonergic side effects (such as insomnia, anxiety, agitation, and nausea):
- iproniazid (Marsilid)
- meperidine (Demerol, Meperitab)
- moclobemide (Alti-Moclobemide, Nu-Moclobemide)
- pentazocine (Talwin)
- phenelzine (Nardil)
- selegiline (Eldepryl)
- tramadol (Ultram)
- tranylcypromine (Parnate)

Lab Tests That May Be Altered by Hawaiian Baby Woodrose

None known

Diseases That May Be Worsened or Triggered by Hawaiian Baby Woodrose

None known

Foods That May Interact with Hawaiian Baby Woodrose

None known

Supplements That May Interact with Hawaiian Baby Woodrose

May increase positive and negative effects of herbs and supplements that have serotonergic properties, such as 5-HTP, S-adenosylmethionine (SAMe), and St. John's wort. (For a list of herbs and supplements that have serotonergic properties, see Appendix B.)

HEARTSEASE

Heartsease, a beautiful little wild pansy that was a staple in medieval gardens, was once believed to be a potent love charm. Its flowers are an old remedy for heart disease, and an infusion of the herb was reputedly the cure for a broken heart. Heartsease contains salicylates and rutin, both of which are anti-inflammatories, and may explain the herb's ability to calm skin inflammation.

Scientific Name

Viola tricolor

Heartsease Is Also Commonly Known As

Heart's ease, johnny-jump-up, look-up-and-kiss-me, pansy, pansy viscum, wild pansy

Medicinal Parts

Flower

Heartsease's Uses

To treat eczema, seborrhea, cradle cap, and constipation. Germany's Commission E has approved the use of heartsease to treat skin inflammation.

Typical Dose

A typical daily dose of heartsease has not been established.

Possible Side Effects

Heartsease's side effects include anorexia and diarrhea.

Drugs That May Interact with Heartsease

Taking heartsease with these drugs may increase the action of the drug:

- aminosalicylic acid (Nemasol Sodium, Paser)
- aspirin (Bufferin, Ecotrin)
- choline magnesium trisalicylate (Trilisate)
- choline salicylate (Teejel)
- salsalate (Amgesic, Salflex)

Lab Tests That May Be Altered by Heartsease
None known

Diseases That May Be Worsened or Triggered by Heartsease
None known

Foods That May Interact with Heartsease
None known

Supplements That May Interact with Heartsease
None known

HEDGE MUSTARD

Hedge mustard is a very common weed with a small yellow flower that grows on vacant lots and hillsides throughout the United States and Europe. It becomes a dry, wiry tumbleweed in the winter. The French named hedge mustard the "singer's plant," considering it an infallible remedy for the loss of voice. A strong infusion of the entire plant, which has expectorant properties, has been used traditionally for all diseases of the throat.

Scientific Name
Sisymbrium officinale

Hedge Mustard Is Also Commonly Known As
Bank cress, bank mustard, English watercress, singer's plant

Medicinal Parts
Above-ground parts, flower

Hedge Mustard's Uses
To treat laryngitis, pharyngitis, loss of voice, severe hoarseness, chronic bronchitis, and gallbladder inflammation

Typical Dose
A typical daily dose of hedge mustard in herb form may range from 0.5 to 1.0 gm, or the same amount can be made into an infusion (producing three to four cups of tea).

Possible Side Effects
❶ Hedge mustard's side effects include vomiting, diarrhea, headache, and irregular heartbeat. Hedge mustard contains cardiac glycosides, which can help control irregular heartbeat, reduce the backup of blood and fluid in the body, and increase blood flow through the kidneys, helping to excrete sodium and relieve swelling in body tissues. However, a buildup of cardiac glycosides can occur, especially when the herb is combined with certain medications or other herbs that contain cardiac glycosides, causing arrhythmias, abnormally slow heartbeat, heart failure, and even death.

Drugs That May Interact with Hedge Mustard
Taking hedge mustard with this drug may be harmful:
- digitalis (Digitek, Lanoxin)—may increase therapeutic and/or adverse effects of the drug

Lab Tests That May Be Altered by Hedge Mustard
None known

Diseases That May Be Worsened or Triggered by Hedge Mustard
None known

Foods That May Interact with Hedge Mustard
None known

Supplements That May Interact with Hedge Mustard
- Increased risk of cardiac glycoside toxicity when used with other herbs that contain cardiac glycosides, such as black hellebore, calotropis, motherwort, and others. (For a list of cardiac glycoside–containing herbs and supplements, see Appendix B.)
- Increased risk of cardiotoxicity due to potassium depletion when taken with cardioactive herbs, such as adonis, digitalis, lily-of-the-valley, and squill. (For a list of cardioactive herbs and supplements, see Appendix B.)
- Increased risk of potassium depletion when used in conjunction with horsetail plant or licorice.
- Increased risk of potassium depletion when used with stimulant laxative herbs, such as black root, cascara sagrada, castor oil, and senna. (For a list of stimulant laxative herbs and supplements, see Appendix B.)

HENBANE

Henbane, which literally means "killer of poultry," is a weed native to the Mediterranean area that has antispasmodic, hypnotic, and mild diuretic effects. Its leaves and seeds contain the alkaloids hyoscyamine, hyoscine, and scopolamine, which relax spasms of the involuntary muscles, lessen pain, and induce drowsiness. The pharmaceutical industry uses the henbane alkaloids as a basis for certain painkillers and antispasmodics.

Scientific Name
Hyoscyamus niger

Henbane Is Also Commonly Known As
Black henbane, devil's eye, hogbean, poison tobacco, stinking nightshade

Medicinal Parts
Leaf

Henbane's Uses
To treat toothache, facial pain, lower abdominal pain, and other kinds of pain; to help reduce existing scar tissue. Germany's Commission E has approved the use of henbane to treat dyspeptic complaints such as heartburn and bloating.

Typical Dose
A typical dose of henbane is approximately 0.5 gm of the standardized powder (0.25 to 0.35 mg total alkaloids).

Possible Side Effects
Henbane's side effects include constipation, dry mouth, reduced sweating, overheating, and difficulty in urinating.

Drugs That May Interact with Henbane
Taking henbane with these drugs may increase some of the effects of the drug:

- acetaminophen, chlorpheniramine, and pseudoephedrine (Children's Tylenol Plus Cold, Sinutab Sinus Allergy Maximum Strength)
- acetaminophen, dextromethorphan, and pseudoephedrine (Alka-Seltzer Plus Flu Liqui-Gels, Sudafed Severe Cold)
- acrivastine and pseudoephedrine (Semprex-D)
- amantadine (Endantadine, Symmetrel)
- amitriptyline (Elavil, Levate)
- amitriptyline and chlordiazepoxide (Limbitrol)
- amitriptyline and perphenazine (Etrafon, Triavil)
- azatadine (Optimine)
- azatadine and pseudoephedrine (Rynatan Tablet, Trinalin)
- azelastine (Astelin, Optivar)
- brompheniramine and pseudoephedrine (Children's Dimetapp Elixir Cold & Allergy, Lodrane)
- carbinoxamine (Histex CT, Histex PD)
- carbinoxamine and pseudoephedrine (Rondec Drops, Sildec)
- carbinoxamine, pseudoephedrine, and dextromethorphan (Rondec-DM Drops, Tussafed)
- cetirizine (Reactine, Zyrtec)
- chlorpheniramine and acetaminophen (Coricidin HBP Cold and Flu)
- chlorpheniramine and phenylephrine (Histatab Plus, Rynatan)
- chlorpheniramine, ephedrine, phenylephrine, and carbetapentane (Rynatuss, Tynatuss Pediatric)
- chlorpheniramine, phenylephrine, and dextromethorphan (Alka-Seltzer Plus Cold and Cough)
- chlorpheniramine, phenylephrine, and methscopolamine (AH-Chew, Extendryl)
- chlorpheniramine, phenylephrine, and phenyltoloxamine (Comhist, Nalex-A)
- chlorpheniramine, phenylephrine, codeine, and potassium iodide (Pediacof)
- chlorpheniramine, pseudoephedrine, and codeine (Dihistine DH, Ryna-C)
- chlorpheniramine, pseudoephedrine, and dextromethorphan (Robitussin Pediatric Night Relief, Vicks Pediatric 44M)
- chlorpromazine (Largactil, Thorazine)
- cimetidine (Nu-Cimet, Tagamet)
- clemastine (Tavist Allergy)
- clomipramine (Anafranil, Novo-Clopramine)
- clozapine (Clozeril, Gen-Clozapine)
- cyproheptadine (Periactin)
- deptropine (Deptropine FNA)
- desipramine (Alti-Desipramine, Norpramin)
- desloratadine (Aerius, Clarinex)
- dexbrompheniramine and pseudoephedrine (Drixomed, Drixoral Cold & Allergy)
- dexchlorpheniramine (Polaramine)
- dimethindene (Fenistil)
- diphenhydramine (Benadryl Allergy, Nytol)
- diphenhydramine and pseudoephedrine (Benadryl Allergy/Decongestant, Benadryl Children's Allergy and Sinus)
- doxepin (Sinequan, Zonalon)
- doxylamine and pyridoxine (Diclecti)
- epinastine (Elestat)
- famotidine (Apo-Famotidine, Pepcid)
- fexofenadine (Allegra)
- fexofenadine and pseudoephedrine (Allegra-D)
- fluphenazine (Modecate, Prolixin)
- hydrocodone and chlorpheniramine (Tussionex)
- hydrocodone, carbinoxamine, and pseudoephedrine (Histex HC, Tri-Vent HC)
- hydroxyzine (Atarax, Vistaril)
- imipramine (Apo-Imipramine, Tofranil)
- ketotifen (Novo-Ketotifen, Zaditor)
- levocabastine (Livostin)

- lofepramine (Feprapax, Gamanil)
- loratadine (Alaver, Claritin)
- loratadine and pseudoephedrine (Claritin-D 12 Hour, Claritin-D 24 Hour)
- mebhydrolin (Bexidal, Incida)
- melitracen (Dixeran)
- mesoridazine (Serentil)
- mizolastine (Elina, Mizolle)
- nizatidine (Axid, PMS-Nizatidine)
- nortriptyline (Aventyl HCl, Pamelor)
- olopatadine (Patanol)
- oxatomide (Cenacert, Tinset)
- oxybutinin (Ditropan, Oxytrol)
- perphenazine (Apo-Perphenazine, Trilafon)
- procainamide (Procanbid, Pronestyl-SR)
- prochlorperazine (Compazine, Compro)
- promethazine (Phenergan)
- promethazine and codeine (Phenergan with Codeine)
- promethazine and dextromethorphan (Promatussin DM)
- promethazine and phenylephrine
- promethazine, phenylephrine, and codeine
- protriptyline (Vivactil)
- quinidine (Novo-Quinidin, Quinaglute Dura-Tabs)
- ranitidine (Alti-Ranitidine, Zantac)
- thiethylperazine (Torecan)
- thioridazine (Mellaril)
- thiothixene (Navane)
- trifluoperazine (Novo-Trifluzine, Stelazine)
- trimipramine (Apo-Trimip, Surmontil)
- tripelennamine (PBZ, PBZ-SR)
- triprolidine and pseudoephedrine (Actifed Cold and Allergy, Silafed)
- triprolidine, pseudoephedrine, and codeine (CoActifed, Covan)

Lab Tests That May Be Altered by Henbane
None known

Diseases That May Be Worsened or Triggered by Henbane
The hyoscyamine and scopolamine found in the herb may trigger rapid heart rate, and worsen fever, gastroesophageal reflux disease (GERD), congestive heart failure, urinary retention, constipation, narrow-angle glaucoma, stomach ulcers, and diseases involving obstruction of the gastrointestinal tract.

Foods That May Interact with Henbane
None known

Supplements That May Interact with Henbane
May increase positive and negative effects of herbs and supplements that have anticholinergic effects, such as belladonna and scopolia. (For a list of herbs and supplements that have anticholinergic effects, see Appendix B.)

HOPS

Hops exert a calming effect on the nervous system—so calming, in fact, that they may cause temporary impairment of male sexual desire. For this reason, the herb was commonly cultivated in medieval monasteries. Hops are used today as a pain reliever, antidepressant, sleep aid, and a treatment for menopausal symptoms.

Scientific Name
Humulus lupulus

Hops Is Also Commonly Known As

Common hops, European hops, houblon

Medicinal Parts

Flower (female part)

Hops' Uses

To treat nerve pain, tension headaches, insomnia, and nervousness. Germany's Commission E has approved the use of hops to treat anxiety, agitation, nervousness, restlessness, and insomnia.

Typical Dose

A typical dose of hops is 0.5 gm of cut herb.

Possible Side Effects

Hops' side effects include excessive sedation, dizziness, and allergic reactions.

Drugs That May Interact with Hops

Taking hops with these drugs may increase the risk of sedation and mental depression and impairment:

- amobarbital (Amytal)
- amobarbital and secobarbital (Tuinal)
- butabarbital (Butisol Sodium)
- butalbital, acetaminophen, and caffeine (Esgic, Fioricet)
- butalbital, aspirin, and caffeine (Fiorinal)
- mephobarbital (Mebaral)
- methohexital (Brevital, Brevital Sodium)
- pentobarbital (Nembutal)
- phenobarbital (Luminal Sodium, PMS-Phenobarbital)
- primidone (Apo-Primidone, Mysoline)
- secobarbital (Seconal)
- thiopental (Pentothal)

Lab Tests That May Be Altered by Hops

None known

Diseases That May Be Worsened or Triggered by Hops

May worsen depression.

Foods That May Interact with Hops

May increase sedative effects when consumed with alcohol.

Supplements That May Interact with Hops

May enhance therapeutic and adverse effects of herbs and supplements that have sedative properties, such as 5-HTP, kava kava, St. John's wort, and valerian. (For a list of herbs and supplements that have sedative properties, see Appendix B.)

HOREHOUND

Horehound, a plant with small white flowers that grows throughout Europe and Asia, has been used since Roman times as a remedy for coughs and other upper respiratory ailments. Its major active constituent, marrubiin, is an expectorant that also gives horehound its bitter taste, stimulating the flow of saliva and gastric juices and improving digestion.

Scientific Name

Marrubium vulgare

Horehound Is Also Commonly Known As

Houndsbane, marrubium, marvel

Medicinal Parts
Leaf, stem, flower, branch, whole plant

Horehound's Uses
To treat bloating, flatulence, bronchitis, whooping cough, asthma, respiratory infections, diarrhea, painful menstruation, ulcers, and wounds. Also used as a digestive tonic. Germany's Commission E has approved the use of horehound to treat loss of appetite and dyspeptic complaints such as heartburn and bloating.

Typical Dose
A typical daily dose of horehound is approximately 4.5 gm of the herb or 30 to 60 ml of the pressed juice.

Possible Side Effects
Horehound's side effects include nausea, vomiting, diarrhea, decreased blood glucose levels, and arrhythmias.

Drugs That May Interact with Horehound
Taking horehound with these drugs may disrupt blood sugar control:
- acarbose (Prandase, Precose)
- acetohexamide
- chlorpropamide (Diabinese, Novo-Propamide)
- gliclazide (Diamicron, Novo-Gliclazide)
- glimepiride (Amaryl)
- glipizide (Glucotrol)
- glipizide and metformin (Metaglip)
- gliquidone (Beglynor, Glurenorm)
- glyburide (DiaBeta, Micronase)
- glyburide and metformin (Glucovance)
- insulin (Humulin, Novolin R)
- metformin (Glucophage, Riomet)
- miglitol (Glyset)
- nateglinide (Starlix)
- pioglitazone (Actos)
- repaglinide (GlucoNorm, Prandin)
- rosiglitazone (Avandia)
- rosiglitazone and metformin (Avandamet)
- tolazamide (Tolinase)
- tolbutamide (Apo-Tolbutamide, Tol-Tab)

Taking horehound with these drugs may increase the risk of serotonergic effects (such as insomnia, anxiety, agitation, and nausea):
- granisetron (Kytril)
- ondansetron (Zofran)
- rizatriptan benzoate (Maxalt)
- sumatriptan (Imitrex)

Taking horehound with these drugs may interfere with absorption of the drug:
- ferric gluconate (Ferrlecit)
- ferrous fumarate (Femiron, Feostat)
- ferrous gluconate (Fergon, Novo-Ferrogluc)
- ferrous sulfate (Feratab, Fer-Iron)
- ferrous sulfate and ascorbic acid (FeroGrad 500, Vitelle Irospan)
- iron-dextran complex (Dexferrum, INFeD)
- polysaccharide-iron complex (Hytinic, Niferex)

Lab Tests That May Be Altered by Horehound
None known

Diseases That May Be Worsened or Triggered by Horehound
None known

Foods That May Interact with Horehound
None known

Supplements That May Interact with Horehound
None known

HORSE CHESTNUT

Widely cultivated as large shade and street trees, horse chestnut trees line the famous Avenue des Champs-Élysées in Paris. Their fruit, the bitter, highly astringent horse chestnut, contains tannins, saponins, and flavonoids, which are strong anti-inflammatory substances that some believe will strengthen and tone blood vessel walls. This makes horse chestnut a favorite for treating hemorrhoids, phlebitis, and varicose veins.

Scientific Name
Aesculus hippocastanum

Horse Chestnut Is Also Commonly Known As
Buckeye, conqueror tree, Spanish chestnut

Medicinal Parts
Leaf, seed, bark, flower

Horse Chestnut's Uses
Horse chestnut leaf is used to treat leg pain, varicose veins, eczema, hemorrhoids, coughs, arthritis, and rheumatism. Horse chestnut seeds are used to treat sprains, bruises, rheumatism, and varicose veins. Germany's Commission E has approved the use of horse chestnut seeds to treat chronic venous insufficiency.

Typical Dose
A typical daily dose of horse chestnut leaf is approximately 1 tsp of finely cut leaves steeped in 150 ml boiling water for 5 to 10 minutes, then strained and taken as a tea. A typical daily dose of horse chestnut seed in extract form may range from 40 to 120 mg of aescin (its active ingredient).

Possible Side Effects
Horse chestnut's side effects include headache, dizziness, nausea, and gastrointestinal irritation.

Drugs That May Interact with Horse Chestnut
Taking horse chestnut with these drugs may increase the risk of bleeding or bruising:

- abciximab (ReoPro)
- alteplase (Activase, Cathflo Activase)
- aminosalicylic acid (Nemasol Sodium, Paser)
- antithrombin III (Thrombate III)
- argatroban
- aspirin (Bufferin, Ecotrin)
- aspirin and dipyridamole (Aggrenox)
- bivalirudin (Angiomax)
- celecoxib (Celebrex)
- choline magnesium trysalicylate (Trilisate)
- choline salicylate (Teejel)
- clopidogrel (Plavix)
- dalteparin (Fragmin)
- danaparoid (Orgaran)
- diclofenac (Cataflam, Voltaren)
- diflunisal (Apo-Diflunisal, Dolobid)
- dipyridamole (Novo-Dipiradol, Persantine)
- drotrecogin alfa (Xigris)
- enoxaparin (Lovenox)
- eptifibatide (Integrillin)
- etodolac (Lodine, Utradol)
- fenoprofen (Nalfon)
- flurbiprofen (Ansaid, Ocufen)

- fondaparinux (Arixtra)
- heparin (Hepalean, Hep-Lock)
- hydrocodone and aspirin (Damason-P)
- hydrocodone and ibuprofen (Vicoprofen)
- ibritumomab (Zevalin)
- ibuprofen (Advil, Motrin)
- indobufen (Ibustrin)
- indomethacin (Indocin, Novo-Methacin)
- ketoprofen (Orudis, Rhodis)
- ketorolac (Acular, Toradol)
- lepirudin (Refludan)
- meloxicam (MOBIC, Mobicox)
- nabumetone (Apo-Nabumetone, Relefan)
- nadroparin (Fraxiparine)
- naproxen (Aleve, Naprosyn)
- oxaprozin (Apo-Oxaprozin, Daypro)
- piroxicam (Feldene, Nu-Pirox)
- reteplase (Retavase)
- rofecoxib (Vioxx)
- salsalate (Amgesic, Salflex)
- streptokinase (Streptase)
- sulindac (Clinoril, Nu-Sundac)
- tenecteplase (TNKase)
- tiaprofenic acid (Dom-Tiaprofenic, Surgam)
- ticlopidine (Alti-Ticlopidine, Ticlid)
- tinzaparin (Innohep)
- tirofiban (Aggrastat)
- tolmetin (Tolectin)
- urokinase (Abbokinase)
- valdecoxib (Bextra)
- warfarin (Coumadin, Jantoven)

Taking horse chestnut with these drugs may increase the risk of hypoglycemia (low blood sugar):
- acarbose (Prandase, Precose)
- acetohexamide
- chlorpropamide (Diabinese, Novo-Propamide)

- gliclazide (Diamicron, Novo-Gliclazide)
- glimepiride (Amaryl)
- glipizide (Glucotrol)
- glipizide and metformin (Metaglip)
- gliquidone (Beglynor, Glurenorm)
- glyburide (DiaBeta, Micronase)
- glyburide and metformin (Glucovance)
- insulin (Humulin, Novolin R)
- metformin (Glucophage, Riomet)
- miglitol (Glyset)
- nateglinide (Starlix)
- pioglitazone (Actos)
- repaglinide (GlucoNorm, Prandin)
- rosiglitazone (Avandia)
- rosiglitazone and metformin (Avandamet)
- tolazamide (Tolinase)
- tolbutamide (Apo-Tolbutamide, Tol-Tab)

Taking horse chestnut (in the form of tea) with these drugs may interfere with absorption of the drug:
- ferric gluconate (Ferrlecit)
- ferrous fumarate (Femiron, Feostat)
- ferrous gluconate (Fergon, Novo-Ferrogluc)
- ferrous sulfate (Feratab, Fer-Iron)
- ferrous sulfate and ascorbic acid (FeroGrad 500, Vitelle Irospan)
- iron-dextran complex (Dexferrum, INFeD)
- polysaccharide-iron complex (Hytinic, Niferex)

Lab Tests That May Be Altered by Horse Chestnut
None known

Diseases That May Be Worsened or Triggered by Horse Chestnut
- May interfere with blood sugar control in diabetes.
- May worsen cases of inflammatory or infectious

gastrointestinal diseases by irritating the gastrointestinal tract.

- May damage the kidneys.

Foods That May Interact with Horse Chestnut
None known

Supplements That May Interact with Horse Chestnut

- Increased risk of bleeding when used with herbs and supplements that might affect platelet aggregation, such as angelica, danshen, garlic, ginger, ginkgo biloba, red clover, turmeric, white willow, and others. (For a list of herbs and supplements with anticoagulant/antiplatelet effects, see Appendix B.)
- May increase blood glucose–lowering effects and risk of hypoglycemia (low blood sugar) when used with herbs and supplements that lower glucose levels, such as alpha-lipoic acid, chromium, devil's claw, Panax ginseng, and psyllium. (For a list of herbs and supplements that lower blood glucose levels, see Appendix B.)
- The tannins in horse chestnut may cause the alkaloids in certain other herbs to separate and settle, increasing the risk of toxic reactions. (For a list of herbs and other substances high in alkaloids, see Appendix B.)

HORSERADISH

Known primarily as a food condiment, horseradish is used as an herb to lessen joint inflammation and treat whooping cough and infected sinuses. It is also used as a diuretic, a circulatory stimulant, and an antibacterial agent.

Scientific Name
Armoracia rusticana

Horseradish Is Also Commonly Known As
Great Raifort, mountain radish, red cole

Medicinal Parts
Root

Horseradish's Uses
To treat infections of the respiratory and urinary tracts, the flu, gout, rheumatism, digestive problems, and minor muscle aches. Germany's Commission E has approved the use of horseradish to treat cough, bronchitis, and urinary tract infections.

Typical Dose
A typical dose of horseradish taken internally is up to 20 gm of the fresh root (cut or ground); externally, ointment or gel should contain no more than 2 percent mustard oil (an active ingredient in horseradish).

Possible Side Effects
Horseradish's side effects include diarrhea and irritation of gastrointestinal and urinary tracts. Avoid taking horseradish if you have stomach ulcers or kidney disease. The root of the horseradish plant should be freshly grated just before use, but do so outside or risk irritating your eyes when the mustard oil within it is released into the air.

Drugs That May Interact with Horseradish

Taking horseradish with these drugs may be harmful:

- fondaparinux (Arixtra)—may increase the risk of bleeding or bruising
- levothyroxine (Levothroid, Synthroid)—may interfere with drug's actions

Lab Tests That May Be Altered by Horseradish

None known

Diseases That May Be Worsened or Triggered by Horseradish

May worsen cases of inflammatory or infectious gastrointestinal ailments by irritating the gastrointestinal tract.

Foods That May Interact with Horseradish

None known

Supplements That May Interact with Horseradish

Increased risk of bleeding when used with herbs and supplements that might affect platelet aggregation. (For a list of herbs and supplements with anticoagulant/antiplatelet effects, see Appendix B.)

HORSETAIL

Horsetail is so named because its jointed stems produce bristly leaves that resemble a horse's tail. The stems of the horsetail plant contain such high concentrations of silica that they have been used for polishing metal, especially pewter. Horsetail tea, high in organic silicon concentrations, has been used to strengthen connective tissue, fight arthritis, treat urinary tract infections, promote bone and cartilage formation, and revive brittle nails and lifeless hair.

Scientific Name

Equisetum arvense

Horsetail Is Also Commonly Known As

Bottle-brush, field horsetail, horse willow, pewterwort, shave grass

Medicinal Parts

Above-ground parts

Horsetail's Uses

To treat kidney stones, rheumatic disease, gout, brittle fingernails, loss of hair, frostbite, ulcers, and wounds. Germany's Commission E has approved the use of horsetail to treat urinary tract infections, kidney and bladder stones, wounds, and burns.

Typical Dose

A typical daily dose of horsetail is approximately 6 gm of the herb, taken with plenty of fluids.

Possible Side Effects

Horsetail's more common side effects when taken internally include thiamin deficiency. Used externally, it may cause seborrheic dermatitis.

Drugs That May Interact with Horsetail

Taking horsetail with these drugs may increase the risk of hypokalemia (low levels of potassium in the blood):

- acetazolamide (Apo-Acetazolamide, Diamox Sequels)
- azosemide (Diat)
- bumetanide (Bumex, Burinex)
- chlorothiazide (Diuril)
- chlorthalidone (Apo-Chlorthalidone, Thalitone)
- ethacrynic acid (Edecrin)
- etozolin (Elkapin)
- furosemide (Apo-Furosemide, Lasix)
- hydrochlorothiazide (Apo-Hydro, Microzide)
- hydroflumethiazide (Diucardin, Saluron)
- indapamide (Lozol, Nu-Indapamide)
- mannitol (Osmitrol, Resectisol)
- mefruside (Baycaron)
- methazolamide (Apo-Methazolamide, Neptazane)
- methyclothiazide (Aquatensen, Enduron)
- metolazone (Mykrox, Zaroxolyn)
- olmesartan and hydrochlorothiazide (Benicar HCT)
- polythiazide (Renese)
- torsemide (Demadex)
- trichlormethiazide (Metatensin, Naqua)
- urea (Amino-Cerv, UltraMide)
- xipamide (Diurexan, Lumitens)

Taking horsetail with these drugs may increase the risk of drug toxicity:
- digitalis (Digitek, Lanoxin)
- lithium (Carbolith, Eskalith)

Taking horsetail with these drugs may increase stimulation of the central nervous system:
- caffeine-containing drugs (such as Alka-Seltzer Morning Relief Tablets, Cafergot, Excedrin Extra-Strength)
- theophylline (Elixophyllin, Uniphyl)

Lab Tests That May Be Altered by Horsetail

None known

Diseases That May Be Worsened or Triggered by Horsetail

May harm heart and kidney function by encouraging the excretion of too much potassium.

Foods That May Interact with Horsetail

- May cause increased central nervous system stimulation when used with caffeinated beverages such as coffee or tea.
- May break down thiamin (vitamin B_1), increasing risk of thiamin deficiency.
- Increased risk of potassium depletion when used in conjunction with licorice.
- Increased risk of potassium depletion when used with stimulant laxative herbs, such as black root, cascara sagrada, castor oil, and senna. (For a list of stimulant laxative herbs and supplements, see Appendix B.)
- Increased risk of chromium toxicity when taken with chromium supplements due to chromium content of horsetail.
- Increased central nervous system stimulation when used with tobacco or nicotine.

Supplements That May Interact with Horsetail

- Increased risk of cardiac glycoside toxicity when used with other herbs that contain cardiac glycosides, such as black hellebore, calotropis, motherwort, and others. (For a list of cardiac glycoside–containing herbs and supplements, see Appendix B.)
- Increased risk of cardiotoxicity due to potassium depletion when taken with cardioactive herbs, such as adonis, digitalis,

lily-of-the-valley, and squill. (For a list of cardioactive herbs and supplements, see Appendix B.)

- Increased risk of potassium depletion when used in conjunction with licorice.
- Increased risk of potassium depletion when used with stimulant laxative herbs, such as black root, cascara sagrada, castor oil, and senna. (For a list of stimulant laxative herbs and supplements, see Appendix B.)
- Increased risk of chromium toxicity when taken with chromium supplements or herbs containing chromium, such as brewer's yeast and cascara sagrada.

HYSSOP

Hyssop was recommended by the ancient Greek physician Hippocrates as a treatment for chest complaints, and it is still used today to treat colds, flu, bronchitis, and other respiratory disorders. This makes sense, as the herb contains marrubiin, a substance that has antiviral and antibiotic activities and also functions as a strong expectorant.

Scientific Name
Hyssopus officinalis

Hyssop Is Also Commonly Known As
Hissopo, jufa, ysop

Medicinal Parts
Above-ground parts

Hyssop's Uses
To treat colds, diseases of the respiratory tract, liver problems, asthma, colic, and urinary tract inflammation

Typical Dose
A typical dose of hyssop is two 445 mg capsules taken three times daily.

Possible Side Effects
Hyssop's side effects include nausea, vomiting, anorexia, diarrhea, and allergic reactions.

Drugs That May Interact with Hyssop
Taking hyssop with these drugs may interfere with the action of the drug:

- carbamazepine (Carbatrol, Tegretol)
- fluphenazine (Modecate, Prolixin)
- fosphenytoin (Cerebyx)
- levetiracetam (Keppra)
- oxcarbazepine (Trileptal)
- phenytoin (Dilantin, Phenytek)

Lab Tests That May Be Altered by Hyssop
None known

Diseases That May Be Worsened or Triggered by Hyssop
May worsen seizure disorders.

Foods That May Interact with Hyssop
None known

Supplements That May Interact with Hyssop
None known

IBOGA

Iboga, a rain forest shrub native to western Africa, is valued primarily for its root bark, which contains several hallucinogenic alkaloids, most notably ibogaine. When taken in small amounts, iboga stimulates the central nervous system; when taken in larger doses, it induces hallucinations. Used by adherents of the Bwiti religion in west-central Africa for spiritual and ceremonial purposes, iboga (in the form of ibogaine) has been used medically to treat opiate addiction.

Scientific Name
Tabernanthe iboga

Medicinal Parts
Root

Iboga's Uses
To treat opiate addiction, fever, flu, and elevated blood pressure; to prevent drowsiness and fatigue; as an aphrodisiac

Typical Dose
There is no typical dose of iboga.

Possible Side Effects
Iboga's side effects include decreased heart rate, lowered blood pressure, hallucinations, anxiety, and respiratory arrest.

Drugs That May Interact with Iboga
Taking iboga with these drugs may interfere with the action of the drug:
- atropine (Isopto Atropine, Sal-Tropine)
- benztropine (Apo-Benztropine, Cogentin)
- clidinium and chlordiazepoxide (Apo-Chlorax, Librax)
- cyclopentolate (Cyclogyl, Cylate)
- dicyclomine (Bentyl, Lomine)
- glycopyrrolate (Robinul, Robinul Forte)
- homatropine (Isopto Homatropine)
- hyoscyamine (Hyosine, Levsin)
- hyoscyamine, atropine, scopolamine, and phenobarbital (Donnatal, Donnatal Exten-tabs)
- ipratropium (Atrovent, Nu-Ipratropium)
- oxitropium (Oxivent, Tersigat)
- prifinium (Padrin, Riabel)
- procyclidine (Kemadrin, Procyclid)
- propantheline (Propanthel)
- scopolamine (Scopace, Transderm Scop)
- tiotropium (Spiriva)
- tolterodine (Detrol, Detrol LA)
- trihexyphenidyl (Apo-Trihex)
- trimethobenzamide (Tigan)

Taking iboga with these drugs may increase the therapeutic and/or adverse effects of the drug:
- acetylcholine (Miochol-E)
- bethanechol (Duvoid, Urecholine)
- carbachol (Carbastat, Isopto Carbachol)
- cevimeline (Evoxac)
- donepezil (Aricept)
- edrophonium (Enlon, Reversol)
- methacholine (Provocholine)
- neostigmine (Prostigmin)
- physostigmine (Eserine)
- pilocarpine (Isopto Carpine, Salagen)
- pyridostigmine (Mestinon)
- rivastigmine (Exelon)
- tacrine (Cognex)

Lab Tests That May Be Altered by Iboga
None known

Diseases That May Be Worsened or Triggered by Iboga
None known

Foods That May Interact with Iboga
None known

Supplements That May Interact with Iboga
None known

INDIAN HEMP

A poisonous herb native to the United States and best known for the excellent ropes made from its fibers, Indian hemp secretes a milky sap when its leaves or stems are broken. This sap is extremely bitter and repels animals, earning the herb the common name "dogbane." The sap and roots of Indian hemp contain substances that stimulate the heart. A toxic chemical found in the plant's roots, cymarin, was once used as a cardiac stimulant.

Scientific Name
Apocynum cannabinum

Indian Hemp Is Also Commonly Known As
Bitter root, Canadian hemp, dogbane, Indian physic, milkweed, wallflower

Medicinal Parts
Root, juice

Indian Hemp's Uses
To treat rheumatism, asthma, coughs, syphilis, and heart problems; as a diuretic

Typical Dose
A typical daily dose of Indian hemp may range from 10 to 30 drops of liquid extract, or 0.3 to 0.6 ml of tincture (1:10).

Possible Side Effects
❶ Indian hemp's side effects include nausea, vomiting, decreased heart rate, and lowered blood pressure. Indian hemp contains cardiac glycosides, which can help control irregular heartbeat, reduce the backup of blood and fluid in the body, and increase blood flow through the kidneys, helping to excrete sodium and relieve swelling in body tissues. However, a buildup of cardiac glycosides can occur, especially when the herb is combined with certain medications or other herbs that contain cardiac glycosides, causing arrhythmias, abnormally slow heartbeat, heart failure, and even death.

Drugs That May Interact with Indian Hemp
Taking Indian hemp with these drugs may increase the risk of drug toxicity:

- acetazolamide (Apo-Acetazolamide, Diamox Sequels)
- azosemide (Diat)
- bumetanide (Bumex, Burinex)
- chlorothiazide (Diuril)
- chlorthalidone (Apo-Chlorthalidone, Thalitone)
- ethacrynic acid (Edecrin)
- etozolin (Elkapin)
- furosemide (Apo-Furosemide, Lasix)

- hydrochlorothiazide (Apo-Hydro, Microzide)
- hydroflumethiazide (Diucardin, Saluron)
- indapamide (Lozol, Nu-Indapamide)
- mannitol (Osmitrol, Resectisol)
- mefruside (Baycaron)
- methazolamide (Apo-Methazolamide, Neptazane)
- methyclothiazide (Aquatensen, Enduron)
- metolazone (Mykrox, Zaroxolyn)
- olmesartan and hydrochlorothiazide (Benicar HCT)
- polythiazide (Renese)
- torsemide (Demadex)
- trichlormethiazide (Metatensin, Naqua)
- urea (Amino-Cerv, UltraMide)
- xipamide (Diurexan, Lumitens)

Taking Indian hemp with this drug may be harmful:
- digitalis (Digitek, Lanoxin)—may increase drug's therapeutic and adverse effects

Lab Tests That May Be Altered by Indian Hemp
None known

Diseases That May Be Worsened or Triggered by Indian Hemp
None known

Foods That May Interact with Indian Hemp
None known

Supplements That May Interact with Indian Hemp
Increased risk of cardiac glycoside toxicity when used with other herbs that contain cardiac glycosides, such as black hellebore, calotropis, motherwort, and others. (For a list of cardiac glycoside–containing herbs and supplements, see Appendix B.)

INDIAN LONG PEPPER

> Indian long pepper is part of an Ayurvedic medicine called Pippali Rasayana used for the treatment of chronic dysentery and worm infestations. In one study with fifty volunteers, fifteen days' treatment with this medicine reduced the symptoms of giardiasis, a diarrheal illness caused by a microscopic parasite, *Giardia lamblia*.

Scientific Name
Piper longum

Indian Long Pepper Is Also Commonly Known As
Bi bo, jaborandi pepper, kana, long pepper, magadhi

Medicinal Parts
Fruit

Indian Long Pepper's Uses
To treat toothache, headache, cough, diarrhea, heartburn, psoriasis, and tuberculosis; to stimulate menstrual flow; to improve digestion

Typical Dose
There is no typical dose of Indian long pepper.

Possible Side Effects
There are no known side effects attributed to Indian long pepper.

Drugs That May Interact with Indian Long Pepper

Taking Indian long pepper with these drugs may increase absorption and blood levels of the drug:

- phenytoin (Dilantin, Phenytek)
- propranolol (Inderal, InnoPran XL)
- theophylline (Elixophyllin, Theochron)

Lab Tests That May Be Altered by Indian Long Pepper

May increase serum concentrations of phenytoin, propranolol, and theophylline.

Diseases That May Be Worsened or Triggered by Indian Long Pepper

None known

Foods That May Interact with Indian Long Pepper

None known

Supplements That May Interact with Indian Long Pepper

Increased bioavailability of sparteine, a constituent of Scotch broom that causes depression of the nervous system and can be toxic in large amounts.

INDIAN SQUILL

> Indian squill, a highly toxic Mediterranean plant from the lily family, gets its name from the Greek word *scilla*, which means "excite" or "disturb." This is a good description of what squill does to the stomach, as it is known to cause vomiting and diarrhea. The bulb of the Indian squill plant was once used to treat asthma and other breathing problems, increase the flow of urine, and improve heart functioning, although today it is considered too dangerous to use. In India, squill is sometimes used for wart removal.

Scientific Name

Urginea indica

Indian Squill Is Also Commonly Known As

South Indian squill

Medicinal Parts

Bulb

Indian Squill's Uses

To treat asthma, digestive problems, rheumatism, various skin conditions, and menstrual ailments.

Typical Dose

A typical dose ranges from 60 to 200 mg per day.

Possible Side Effects

Indian squill's side effects include loss of appetite, vomiting, headache, and diarrhea.

Drugs That May Interact with Indian Squill

Taking Indian squill with these drugs may increase the risk of arrhythmia (irregular heartbeat):

- albuterol (Proventil, Ventolin)
- brimonidine (Alphagan, P, PMS-Brimonidine Tartrate)
- cilostazol (Pletal)
- dobutamine (Dobutrex)
- dopamine (Intropin)
- dopexamine (Dopacard)

- enoximone (Perfan)
- ephedrine (Pretz-D)
- inamrinone
- isoetharine (Beta-2, Bronkosol)
- isoproterenol (Isuprel)
- metaproterenol (Alupent)
- metaraminol (Aramine)
- milrinone (Primacor)
- norepinephrine (Levophed)
- pentoxifylline (Pentoxil, Trental)
- phenylephrine (Neo-Synephrine Extra Strength, Vicks Sinex Nasal Spray)
- pseudoephedrine (Dimetapp Decongestant, Sudafed)
- quinidine (Novo-Quinidin, Quinaglute Dura-Tabs)
- sildenafil (Viagra)
- tadalafil (Cialis)
- terbutaline (Brethine)
- theophylline and guaifenesin (Elixophyllin-GC, Quibron)
- theophylline (Elixophyllin, Theochron)
- vardenafil (Levitra)

Taking Indian squill with these drugs may increase the therapeutic and/or adverse effects of the drug:

- beclomethasone (Beconase, Vanceril)
- betamethasone (Celestone, Diprolene)
- budesonide (Entocort, Rhinocort)
- budesonide and formoterol (Symbicort)
- cortisone (Cortone)
- deflazacort (Calcort, Dezacor)
- dexamethasone (Decadron, Dexasone)
- flunisolide (AeroBid, Nasarel)
- fluorometholone (Eflone, Flarex)
- fluticasone (Cutivate, Flonase)

- hydrocortisone (Anusol-HC, Locoid)
- loteprednol (Alrex, Lotemax)
- medrysone (HMS Liquifilm)
- methylprednisolone (DepoMedrol, Medrol)
- prednisolone (Inflamase Forte, Pred Forte)
- prednisone (Apo-Prednisone, Deltasone)
- rimexolone (Vexol)
- triamcinolone (Aristocort, Trinasal)

Taking Indian squill with these drugs may increase the risk of drug toxicity:

- cascara
- digitalis (Digitek, Lanoxin)
- docusate and senna (Peri-Colace, Senokot-S)
- quinidine (Novo-Quinidin, Quinaglute Dura-Tabs)

Lab Tests That May Be Altered by Indian Squill
None known

Diseases That May Be Worsened or Triggered by Indian Squill

- May worsen inflammatory or infectious gastrointestinal ailments by irritating the gastrointestinal tract.
- May worsen existing cases of low potassium or calcium levels.
- May worsen various heart ailments.

Foods That May Interact with Indian Squill
None known

Supplements That May Interact with Indian Squill

- Increased risk of cardiac glycoside toxicity when used with other herbs that contain cardiac glycosides, such as black hellebore, calotropis, motherwort and others. (For a list of cardiac glycoside–containing herbs and supplements, see Appendix B.)

- Increased risk of cardiotoxicity due to potassium depletion when taken with cardioactive herbs, such as adonis, digitalis, lily-of-the-valley, and maté. (For a list of cardioactive herbs and supplements, see Appendix B.)
- Increased risk of potassium depletion when used in conjunction with horsetail plant or licorice.
- Increased risk of potassium depletion when used with stimulant laxative herbs, such as black root, cascara sagrada, castor oil, and senna. (For a list of stimulant laxative herbs and supplements, see Appendix B.)

IRON

Iron serves as part of the protein called hemoglobin in red blood cells, which transports oxygen from the lungs to the rest of the body. If you run short of iron, you may feel weak and tired, and your immune system will falter.

Typical Dose

The Food and Nutrition Board has set the RDA at 8 mg per day for adult men, 18 mg per day for women ages nineteen to fifty, and 8 mg per day for women fifty-one years old and up.

Possible Side Effects

Excessive amounts of iron can cause diabetes mellitus and heart damage.

Drugs That May Interact with Iron

Taking iron with these drugs may interfere with the absorption and the action of the drug:

- alendronate (Fosamax, Novo-Alendronate)
- cinoxacin (Cinobac)
- ciprofloxacin (Ciloxan, Cipro)
- clodronate (Bonefos, Ostac)
- demeclocycline (Declomycin)
- doxycycline (Apo-Doxy, Vibramycin)
- etidronate (Didronel)
- gatifloxacin (Tequin, Zymar)
- gemifloxacin (Factive)
- ibandronic acid (Bondronat)
- levodopa (Dopar, Larodopa)
- levofloxacin (Levaquin, Quixin)
- levothyroxine (Levothroid, Synthroid)
- lomefloxacin (Maxaquin)
- methyldopa (Apo-Methyldopa, Nu-Medopa)
- minocycline (Dynacin, Minocin)
- moxifloxacin (Avelox, Vigamox)
- mycophenolate (CellCept)
- nalidixic acid (NegGram)
- norfloxacin (Apo-Norflox, Noroxin)
- ofloxacin (Floxin, Ocuflox)
- oxytetracycline (Terramycin, Terramycin IM)
- pamidronate (Aredia)
- pefloxacin (Peflacine, Perflox)
- penicillamine (Cuprimine, Depen)
- risedronate (Actonel)
- sparfloxacin (Zagam)
- sulfasalazine (Alti-Sulfasalazine, Azulfidine)
- tetracycline (Novo-Tetra, Sumycin)
- tiludronate (Skelid)
- trovafloxacin
- zoledronic acid (Zometa)

Drugs That May Interfere with the Absorption, Utilization, or Excretion of Iron

- aluminum hydroxide (AlternaGel, Alu-Cap)
- aluminum hydroxide and magnesium carbonate (Gaviscon Liquid)

- aluminum hydroxide and magnesium hydroxide (Maalox, Mylanta)
- aluminum hydroxide, magnesium hydroxide, and simethicone (Mylanta Liquid)
- aluminum hydroxide and magnesium trisilicate (Gaviscon Tablet)
- aspirin (Bufferin, Ecotrin)
- aspirin and dipyridamole (Aggrenox)
- butalbital, aspirin, and caffeine (Fiorinal)
- calcium carbonate (Rolaids Extra Strength, Tums)
- carisoprodol and aspirin (Soma Compound)
- carisoprodol, aspirin, and codeine (Soma Compound with Codeine)
- cholestyramine (Prevalite, Questran)
- choline magnesium trisalicylate (Trilisate)
- choline salicylate (Teejel)
- cimetidine (Nu-Cimet, Tagamet)
- clofibrate (Atromid-S, Novo-Fibrate)
- colesevelam (WelChol)
- colestipol (Colestid)
- demeclocycline (Declomycin)
- doxycycline (Apo-Doxy, Vibramycin)
- esomeprazole (Nexium)
- famotidine (Apo-Famotidine, Pepcid)
- hydrocodone and aspirin (Azdone, Lortab ASA)
- indomethacin (Indocin, Novo-Methacin)
- lansoprazole (Prevacid)
- magnesium hydroxide (Dulcolax Milk of Magnesia, Phillips' Milk of Magnesia)
- meclocycline (Meclan Topical)
- methocarbamol and aspirin (Robaxisal)
- minocycline (Dynacin, Minocin)
- neomycin (Myciguent, Neo-Fradin)
- nizatidine (Apo-Nizatidine, Axid)
- omeprazole (Losec, Prilosec)
- oxycodone and aspirin (Oxycodan, Percodan)
- pantoprazole (Pantoloc, Protonix)
- penicillamine (Cuprimine, Depen)
- rabeprazole (Aciphex, Pariet)
- ranitidine (Alti-Ranitidine, Zantac)
- stanzolol (Winstrol)
- tetracycline (Novo-Tetra, Sumycin)

Lab Tests That May Be Altered by Iron

May cause false positive in tests for occult fecal blood (stool guaiac test).

Diseases That May Be Worsened or Triggered by Iron

May worsen ulcerative colitis and other intestinal conditions, such as constipation.

Foods That May Interact with Iron

- Decreased absorption of dietary and supplemental iron when taken concurrently with the calcium in dairy products.
- Decreased absorption of dietary and supplemental iron when taken concurrently with coffee or tea.

Supplements That May Interact with Iron

- Improved hematological response to iron supplements in those with anemia when taken with riboflavin (vitamin B_2).
- Improved absorption of supplementary or dietary nonheme (nonmeat) iron when taken with supplemental or dietary vitamin C.
- Possible decrease in absorption of dietary nonheme (nonmeat) iron when taken with soy protein (especially nonfermented kind).
- Improved nonheme iron absorption from iron-fortified grains when taken with vitamin A and/or beta-carotene, when vitamin A deficiency is present.

- Decreased absorption of dietary iron when high amounts of supplemental zinc are taken on an empty stomach, and vice versa.

JALAP

This twelve-foot, climbing evergreen vine, native to Mexico is dubbed *Ipomoea purgea*. *Ipomoea* means "wormlike," referring to its twisted, wormlike roots, and *purga* means "cleanse," the major reason jalap was used. A powerful intestinal irritant and cathartic, jalap was used for centuries by the Mexicans and introduced into Europe in 1565. The roots, bark, and seeds contain cardiac glycosides that have anti-inflammatory and stimulant properties and may help relieve pain.

Scientific Name
Ipomoea purga

Jalap Is Also Commonly Known As
Ipomoea, jalap bindweed, Mexican jalap, Vera Cruz jalap

Medicinal Parts
Root

Jalap's Uses
Jalap resin (taken from the root) is used for constipation. Jalap root was formerly used as a laxative and a purgative but is now considered obsolete.

Typical Dose
A typical dose of jalap resin is 60 to 300 mg.

Possible Side Effects
Jalap's side effects include nausea, gastroenteritis, and cramplike pains. Jalap contains cardiac glycosides, which can help control irregular heartbeat, reduce the backup of blood and fluid in the body, and increase blood flow through the kidneys, helping to excrete sodium and relieve swelling in body tissues. However, a buildup of cardiac glycosides can occur, especially when the herb is combined with certain medications or other herbs that contain cardiac glycosides, causing arrhythmias, abnormally slow heartbeat, heart failure, and even death.

Drugs That May Interact with Jalap
Taking jalap with these drugs may increase the risk of hypokalemia (low levels of potassium in the blood):

- acetazolamide (Apo-Acetazolamide, Diamox Sequels)
- azosemide (Diat)
- bumetanide (Bumex, Burinex)
- chlorothiazide (Diuril)
- chlorthalidone (Apo-Chlorthalidone, Thalitone)
- ethacrynic acid (Edecrin)
- etozolin (Elkapin)
- furosemide (Apo-Furosemide, Lasix)
- hydrochlorothiazide (Apo-Hydro, Microzide)
- hydroflumethiazide (Diucardin, Saluron)
- indapamide (Lozol, Nu-Indapamide)
- mannitol (Osmitrol, Resectisol)
- mefruside (Baycaron)
- methazolamide (Apo-Methazolamide, Neptazane)
- methyclothiazide (Aquatensen, Enduron)
- metolazone (Mykrox, Zaroxolyn)
- olmesartan and hydrochlorothiazide (Benicar HCT)

- polythiazide (Renese)
- torsemide (Demadex)
- trichlormethiazide (Metatensin, Naqua)
- urea (Amino-Cerv, UltraMide)
- xipamide (Diurexan, Lumitens)

Taking jalap with this drug may be harmful:
- digitalis (Digitek, Lanoxin)—may increase the risk of drug toxicity

Lab Tests That May Be Altered by Jalap
None known

Diseases That May Be Worsened or Triggered by Jalap
May worsen inflammatory or infectious gastrointestinal ailments by irritating the gastrointestinal tract.

Foods That May Interact with Jalap
None known

Supplements That May Interact with Jalap
- Increased risk of cardiac glycoside toxicity when used with other herbs that contain cardiac glycosides, such as black hellebore, calotropis, motherwort, and others. (For a list of cardiac glycoside–containing herbs and supplements, see Appendix B.)
- Increased risk of potassium depletion when used in conjunction with horsetail plant or licorice.
- Increased risk of potassium depletion when used with other stimulant laxative herbs, such as black root, cascara sagrada, castor oil, and senna. (For a list of stimulant laxative herbs and supplements, see Appendix B.)

JIMSON WEED

A native of India and a member of the potato or nightshade family, jimson weed is believed to be named after Jamestown, Virginia, where it was first brought from England. Jimson weed is toxic and contains the alkaloids atropine and scopolamine, psychoactive substances that some people consume to get a high. These alkaloids are also used in pharmaceutical preparations to treat Parkinson's disease, peptic ulcers, diarrhea, bronchial asthma, and motion sickness.

Scientific Name
Datura stramonium

Jimson Weed Is Also Commonly Known As
Datura, Devil's apple, Jamestown weed, nightshade, stinkweed

Medicinal Parts
Leaf, seed, above-ground parts

Jimson Weed's Uses
To treat asthma, convulsive cough, high temperatures, pain, and rheumatism

Typical Dose
A typical dose of jimson weed may range from 0.05 to 0.1 gm of the stabilized leaf powder, taken up to three times a day.

Possible Side Effects
❶ Jimson weed's side effects include drying of the mucous membranes, extreme thirst, rapid heart rate, nausea, vomiting, and auditory and visual hallucinations. Jimson weed is highly

toxic, and it is considered very dangerous to inhale the smoke or put the leaf or seed in the mouth.

Drugs That May Interact with Jimson Weed

Taking jimson weed with these drugs may increase the risk of anticholinergic effects (such as blurred vision, constipation, dry mouth, light-headedness, and urinary problems):

- amantadine (Symmetral)
- amitriptyline (Elavil, Levate)
- amitriptyline and chlordiazepoxide (Limbitrol)
- amitriptyline and perphenazine (Etrafon, Triavil)
- amoxapine (Asendin)
- atropine (Isopto Atropine, SalTropine)
- benztropine (Apo-Benztropine, Cogentin)
- clidinium and chlordiazepoxide (Apo-Chlorax, Librax)
- clomipramine (Anafranil, Novo-Clopramine)
- cyclobenzaprine (Flexeril, Novo-Cycloprine)
- cyclopentolate (Cyclogyl, Cylate)
- desipramine (Alti-Desipramine, Norpramin)
- dicyclomine (Bentyl, Lomine)
- diphenhydramine (Benadryl Allergy, Nytol)
- doxepin (Sinequan, Zonalon)
- fluphenazine (Modecate, Prolixin)
- glycopyrrolate (Robinul, Robinul Forte)
- haloperidol (Haldol, Novo-Peridol)
- homatropine (Isopto Homatropine)
- hyoscyamine (Hyosine, Levsin)
- hyoscyamine, atropine, scopolamine, and phenobarbital (Donnatal, Donnatal Extentabs)
- imipramine (Apo-Imipramine, Tofranil)
- ipratropium (Atrovent, Nu-Ipratropium)
- iproniazid (Marsilid)
- lofepramine (Feprapax, Gamanil)
- loratadine (Alavert, Claritin)
- melitracen (Dixeran)
- moclobemide (Alti-Moclobemide, Nu-Moclobemide)
- nortriptyline (Aventyl HCl, Pamelor)
- oxitropium (Oxivent, Tersigat)
- phenelzine (Nardil)
- prifinium (Padrin, Riabel)
- prochlorperazine (Compazine, Compro)
- procyclidine (Kemadrin, Procyclid)
- propantheline (Propanthel)
- protriptyline (Vivactil)
- scopolamine (Scopace, Transderm Scop)
- selegiline (Eldepryl)
- tiotropium (Spiriva)
- tolterodine (Detrol, Detrol LA)
- tranylcypromine (Parnate)
- trihexyphenidyl (Artane)
- trimethobenzamide (Tigan)
- trimipramine (Apo-Trimip, Surmontil)

Taking jimson weed with these drugs may decrease the action of the drug:

- chlorpromazine (Largactil, Thorazine)
- fluphenazine (Modecate, Prolixin)
- mesoridazine (Serentil)
- perphenazine (Apo-Perphenazine, Trilafon)
- prochlorperazine (Compazine, Compro)
- promethazine (Phenergan)
- thiethylperazine (Torecan)
- thioridazine (Mellaril)
- thiothixene (Navane)
- trifluoperazine (Novo-Trifluzine, Stelazine)

Lab Tests That May Be Altered by Jimson Weed

None known

Diseases That May Be Worsened or Triggered by Jimson Weed

The hyoscyamine and scopolamine found in the herb may trigger rapid heart rate and worsen fever, gastroesophageal reflux disease (GERD), congestive heart failure, urinary retention, constipation, narrow-angle glaucoma, stomach ulcers, and diseases involving obstruction of the gastrointestinal tract.

Foods That May Interact with Jimson Weed

None known

Supplements That May Interact with Jimson Weed

None known

JUNIPER

> Juniper berries are the key flavor ingredient in gin, and indeed the name "juniper" comes from the French word *genievre*, which means "gin." The ancients recommended that those who indulged in too much gin drink a tea made from the juniper berry as a hangover remedy. Juniper is used today as an antiflatulent, diuretic, and treatment for urinary tract infections, gastrointestinal disorders, and inflammation.

Scientific Name

Juniperus communis

Juniper Is Also Commonly Known As

Enebro, ginepro, juniper berry

Medicinal Parts

Berry, oil of berry

Juniper's Uses

To treat digestive problems, gout, arteriosclerosis, halitosis, and menstrual pain; to regulate menstruation. Germany's Commission E has approved the use of juniper to treat dyspeptic complaints, such as heartburn and bloating.

Typical Dose

A typical daily dose of juniper may range from 2 to 10 gm of the dried berry or 20 to 100 mg of the essential oil.

Possible Side Effects

Juniper's side effects include kidney irritation. Topically, juniper can cause eye and skin irritation.

Drugs That May Interact with Juniper

Taking juniper with these drugs may cause or worsen kidney damage:

- etodolac (Lodine, Utradol)
- ibuprofen (Advil, Motrin)
- indomethacin (Indocin, Novo-Methacin)
- ketoprofen (Orudis, Rhodis)
- ketorolac (Acular, Toradol)
- meloxicam (MOBIC, Mobicox)
- methotrexate (Rheumatrex, Trexall)
- miglitol (Glyset)
- morphine hydrochloride
- morphine sulfate (Kadian, MS Contin)
- naproxen (Aleve, Naprosyn)
- nitrofurantoin (Furadantin, Macrobid)
- ofloxacin (Floxin, Ocuflox)
- penicillin (Pfizerpen, Wycillin)
- piroxicam (Feldene, Nu-Pirox)
- propoxyphene (Darvon, Darvon-N)
- rifampin (Rifadin, Rimactane)

- stavudine (Zerit)
- sucralfate (Carafate, Sulcrate)
- valacyclovir (Valtrex)
- vancomycin (Vancocin)
- zidovudine (Novo-AZT, Retrovir)

Taking juniper with these drugs may interfere with the effects of the drug and increase the risk of hyperglycemia (excessively high blood sugar):

- insulin (Humulin, Novolin R)
- metformin (Glucophage, Riomet)
- miglitol (Glyset)
- pioglitazone (Actos)
- repaglinide (GlucoNorm, Prandin)
- rosiglitazone (Avandia)

Taking juniper with this drug may be harmful:
- lithium (Eskalith, Carbolith)—may increase the risk of drug toxicity

Lab Tests That May Be Altered by Juniper
May confound results of diagnostic urine tests that rely on a color change, as large amounts of juniper berry can turn the urine purple.

Diseases That May Be Worsened or Triggered by Juniper
- May worsen inflammatory or infectious gastrointestinal ailments by irritating the gastrointestinal tract.
- May worsen seizure disorders.

Foods That May Interact with Juniper
None known

Supplements That May Interact with Juniper
None known

KAVA KAVA

Kava kava is an herb that comes from the South Pacific, where it has long been used as a tranquilizer. Certain native tribes used an alcoholic drink made from the kava kava root to induce hallucinogenic states during their religious ceremonies. Kava kava contains kavalactones, substances that stimulate and then depress the nervous system, producing a sedative effect that relaxes the skeletal muscles.

Scientific Name
Piper methysticum

Kava Kava Is Also Commonly Known As
Ava, ava pepper, intoxicating pepper, kawa, kew, tonga

Medicinal Parts
Rhizome, root

Kava Kava's Uses
To treat nervousness, insomnia, syphilis, gonorrhea, asthma, rheumatism, heartburn, and bloating; to aid in weight loss. Germany's Commission E has approved the use of kava kava to treat nervous anxiety, stress, restlessness, tension, and agitation.

Typical Dose
A typical dose of kava kava root extract may range from 150 to 300 mg, taken twice daily, with a daily dose of kavalactones ranging from 50 to 240 mg.

Possible Side Effects
Kava kava's side effects include mild gastrointestinal complaints, minor impairment of motor

reflexes, dizziness, headache, and allergic reactions.

Drugs That May Interact with Kava Kava

Taking kava kava with these drugs may increase the risk of bleeding or bruising:

- abciximab (ReoPro)
- alteplase (Activase, Cathflo Activase)
- antithrombin III (Thrombate III)
- argatroban
- aspirin (Bufferin, Ecotrin)
- aspirin and dipyridamole (Aggrenox)
- bivalirudin (Angiomax)
- clopidogrel (Plavix)
- dalteparin (Fragmin)
- danaparoid (Orgaran)
- dipyridamole (Novo-Dipiradol, Persantine)
- enoxaparin (Lovenox)
- eptifibatide (Integrillin)
- fondaparinux (Arixtra)
- heparin (Hepalean, Hep-Lock)
- indobufen (Ibustrin)
- lepirudin (Refludan)
- nadroparin (Fraxiparine)
- reteplase (Retavase)
- streptokinase (Streptase)
- tenecteplase (TNKase)
- ticlopidine (Alti-Ticlopidine, Ticlid)
- tinzaparin (Innohep)
- tirofiban (Aggrastat)
- urokinase (Abbokinase)
- warfarin (Coumadin, Jantoven)

Taking kava kava with these drugs may increase sedation and mental depression and/or impairment:

- acetaminophen and codeine (Capital and Codeine, Tylenol with Codeine)
- alfentanil (Alfenta)
- alprazolam (Apo-Alpraz, Xanax)
- amitriptyline (Elavil, Levate)
- amobarbital (Amytal)
- amobarbital and secobarbital (Tuinal)
- amoxapine (Asendin)
- aripiprazole (Abilify)
- aspirin and codeine (Coryphen Codeine)
- belladonna and opium (B&O Supprettes)
- bromazepam (Apo-Bromazepam, Gen-Bromazepam)
- brotizolam (Lendorm, Sintonal)
- buprenorphine (Buprenex, Subutex)
- buprenorphine and naloxone (Suboxone)
- bupropion (Wellbutrin, Zyban)
- buspirone (BuSpar, Nu-Buspirone)
- butabarbital (Butisol Sodium)
- butalbital, acetaminophen, and caffeine (Esgic, Fioricet)
- butalbital, aspirin, and caffeine (Fiorinal)
- butorphanol (Apo-Butorphanol, Stadol)
- carbamazepine (Carbatrol, Tegretol)
- chloral hydrate (Aquachloral Supprettes, Somnote)
- chlordiazepoxide (Apo-Chlordiazepoxide, Librium)
- chlorpromazine (Thorazine)
- citalopram (Celexa)
- clobazam (Alti-Clobazam, Frisium)
- clomipramine (Anafranil, Novo-Clopramine)
- clonazepam (Klonopin, Rivotril)
- clonidine (Catapres, Duraclon)
- clorazepate (Tranxene, T-Tab)
- clozapine (Clozaril, Gen-Clozapine)
- codeine (Codeine Contin)
- cyclobenzaprine (Flexeril, Novo-Cycloprine)
- dantrolene (Dantrium)
- desipramine (Alti-Desipramine, Norpramin)
- diazepam (Apo-Diazepam, Valium)

- dihydrocodeine, aspirin, and caffeine (Synalgos-DC)
- diphenhydramine (Benadryl Allergy, Nytol)
- doxepin (Sinequan, Zonalon)
- doxylamine and pyridoxine (Diclectin)
- estazolam (ProSom)
- evorphanol (Levo-Dromoran)
- fentanyl (Actiq, Duragesic)
- fexofenadine (Allegra)
- fluoxetine (Prozac, Sarafem)
- fluphenazine (Modecate, Prolixin)
- flurazepam (Apo-Flurazepam, Dalmane)
- gabapentin (Neurontin, Nu-Gabapentin)
- hydrocodone and acetaminophen (Anexsia, Vicodin)
- hydrocodone and aspirin (Damason-P)
- hydrocodone and ibuprofen (Vicoprofen)
- hydromorphone (Dilaudid, PMS-Hydromorphone)
- hydroxyzine (Atarax, Vistaril)
- imipramine (Apo-Imipramine, Tofranil)
- levorphanol (Levo-Dromoran)
- loprazolam (Dormonoct, Havlane)
- lorazepam (Ativan, Nu-Loraz)
- loxapine (Loxitane, Nu-Loxapine)
- meperidine (Demerol, Meperitab)
- meperidine and promethazine
- mephobarbital (Mebaral)
- meprobamate (Miltown, Movo-Mepro)
- mesoridazine (Serentil)
- methadone (Dolophine, Methadose)
- methocarbamol (Robaxin)
- methohexital (Brevital, Brevital Sodium)
- methotrimeprazine (Novo-Meprazine, Nozain)
- metoclopramide (Apo-Metoclop, Reglan)
- midazolam (Apo-Midazolam, Versed)
- mirtazapine (Remeron)
- moclobemide (Alti-Moclobemide, Nu-Moclobemide)
- molindone (Moban)
- morphine hydrochloride
- morphine sulfate (Kadian, MS Contin)
- nalbuphine (Nubain)
- nefazodone (Serzone)
- nortriptyline (Aventyl HCl, Pamelor)
- olanzapine (Zydis, Zyprexa)
- opium tincture
- oxazepam (Novoxapam, Serax)
- oxcarbazepine (Trileptal)
- oxycodone (OxyContin, Roxicodone)
- oxycodone and acetaminophen (Endocet, Percocet)
- oxycodone and aspirin (Endodan, Percodan)
- oxymorphone (Numorphan)
- paclitaxel (Onxol, Taxol)
- paroxetine (Paxil)
- pentazocine (Talwin)
- pentobarbital (Nembutal)
- perphenazine (Apo-Perphenazine, Trilafon)
- phenobarbital (Luminal Sodium, PMS-Phenobarbital)
- phenoperidine
- phenytoin (Dilantin, Phenytek)
- pizotifen (Sandomigran)
- pramipexole (Mirapex)
- prazepam
- primidone (Apo-Primidone, Mysoline)
- prochlorperazine (Compazine, Compro)
- promethazine (Phenergan)
- propoxyphene (Darvon, Darvon-N)
- propoxyphene and acetaminophen (Darvocet-N 50, Darvocet-N 100)
- propoxyphene, aspirin, and caffeine (Darvon Compound)
- protriptyline (Vivactil)
- quazepam (Doral)
- quetiapine (Seroquel)

- remifentanil (Ultiva)
- risperidone (Risperdal)
- ropinirole (Requip)
- s-citalopram (Lexapro)
- secobarbital (Seconal)
- selegiline (Eldepryl)
- sertraline (Apo-Sertraline, Zoloft)
- sodium oxybate (Xyrem)
- sufentanil (Sufenta)
- temazepam (Novo-Temazepam, Restoril)
- tetrazepam (Mobiforton, Musapam)
- thiethylperazine (Torecan)
- thiopental (Pentothal)
- thioridazine (Mellaril)
- thiothixene (Navane)
- tiagabine (Gabitril)
- tizanidine (Zanaflex)
- tolcapone (Tasmar)
- tramadol (Ultram)
- trazodone (Desyrel, Novo-Trazodone)
- triazolam (Apo-Triazo, Halcion)
- trifluoperazine (Novo-Trifluzine, Stelazine)
- trimipramine (Apo-Trimip, Surmontil)
- venlafaxine (Effexor)
- vigabatrin (Sabril)
- zaleplon (Sonata, Starnoc)
- zolpidem (Ambien)
- zopiclone (Alti-Zopiclone, Gen-Zopiclone)

Taking kava kava with these drugs may decrease the effectiveness of the drug:
- amantadine (Endantadine, Symmetrel)
- bromocriptine (Apo-Bromocriptine, Parlodel)
- carbidopa (Lodsoyn)
- chlorpromazine (Largactil, Thorazine)
- fluphenazine (Modecate, Prolixin)
- levodopa (Dopar, Larodopa)

- levodopa-carbidopa (Nu-Levocarb, Sinemet)
- mesoridazine (Serentil)
- methylphenidate (Concerta, Ritalin)
- modafinil (Alertec, Provigil)
- pergolide (Permax)
- perphenazine (Apo-Perphenazine, Trilafon)
- pramipexole (Mirapex)
- prochlorperazine (Compazine, Compro)
- promethazine (Phenergan)
- ropinirole (Requip)
- thiethylperazine (Torecan)
- thioridazine (Mellaril)
- thiothixene (Navane)
- trifluoperazine (Novo-Trifluzine, Stelazine)

Taking kava kava with these drugs may cause or increase liver damage:
- atorvastatin (Lipitor)
- meloxicam (MOBIC, Mobicox)
- methotrexate (Rheumatrex, Trexall)
- methyldopa (Apo-Methyldopa, Nu-Medopa)
- naproxen (Aleve, Naprosyn)
- nevirapine (Viramune)
- nitrofurantoin (Furadantin, Macrobid)
- ofloxacin (Floxin, Ocuflox)
- ondansetron (Zofran)
- paclitaxel (Onxol, Taxol)

❶ Taking kava kava with these drugs may cause or increase serotonin syndrome, symptoms of which include agitation, rapid heart rate, flushing, heavy sweating, and possibly even death:
- desipramine (Alti-Desipramine, Norpramin)
- doxepin (Sinequan, Zonalon)
- fluvoxamine (Alti-Fluvoxamine, Luvox)
- imipramine (Apo-Imipramine, Tofranil)
- nortriptyline (Aventyl HCl, Pamelor)

- pramipexole (Mirapex)
- protriptyline (Vivactil)
- trazodone (Desyrel, Novo-Trazodone)
- trimipramine (Apo-Trimip, Surmontil)
- venlafaxine (Effexor)

Taking kava kava with these drugs may increase the risk of monoamine oxidase inhibitor (MAOI) toxicity (symptoms of which include anxiety, insomnia, restlessness, dizziness, and sweating):

- iproniazid (Marsilid)
- moclobemide (Alti-Moclobemide, Nu-Moclobemide)
- phenelzine (Nardil)
- selegiline (Eldepryl)
- tranylcypromine (Parnate)

Taking kava kava with these drugs may increase the adverse effects of the drug:

- allopurinol (Aloprim, Zyloprim)
- fluphenazine (Modecate, Prolixin)
- risperidone (Risperdal)

Lab Tests That May Be Altered by Kava Kava

- May cause liver damage.
- May increase values on liver function tests including aspartic acid transaminase (AST), alanine aminotransferase (ALT), total bilirubin, and conjugated bilirubin.

Diseases That May Be Worsened or Triggered by Kava Kava

May worsen hepatitis in certain people.

Foods That May Interact with Kava Kava

- Absorption of kava kava increases when taken with food.

- Increased risk of drowsiness, impaired motor skills, and liver damage when combined with alcohol.

Supplements That May Interact with Kava Kava

- May enhance therapeutic and adverse effects of herbs and supplements that have sedative properties, such as 5-HTP, St. John's wort, and valerian. (For a list of herbs and supplements that have sedative properties, see Appendix B.)
- May increase the risk of liver damage when combined with herbs and supplements that can cause hepatotoxicity (destructive effects on the liver), such as bishop's weed, borage, chaparral, uva ursi, and others. (For a list of herbs and supplements that can cause hepatotoxicity, see Appendix B.)

KELP

Kelp, often referred to as seaweed, is a highly nutritious undersea plant that contains nearly thirty minerals. It nourishes the glands (especially the thyroid and pituitary), sensory nerves, spinal cord, and brain tissue. During the nineteenth century, kelp was used as an aid in cervical dilatation, although physicians later adopted steel dilating instruments to avoid infections.

Scientific Name

Laminaria digitata

Kelp Is Also Commonly Known As

Brown algae, horsetail, laminaria, seaweed, tangleweed

Medicinal Parts

Leaflike part of plant body

Kelp's Uses

To treat obesity and hypertension; to help regulate thyroid function; as an anticoagulant.

Typical Dose

A typical daily dose of kelp may range from 500 to 650 mg in capsule/tablet form.

Possible Side Effects

Kelp's side effects include decreased blood pressure, nausea, vomiting, and allergic reactions.

Drugs That May Interact with Kelp

Taking kelp with these drugs may increase the risk of hypotension (excessively low blood pressure):

- acebutolol (Novo-Acebutolol, Sectral)
- amlodipine (Norvasc)
- atenolol (Apo-Atenol, Tenormin)
- benazepril (Lotensin)
- betaxolol (Betoptic S, Kerlone)
- bisoprolol (Monocor, Zebeta)
- bumetanide (Bumex, Burinex)
- candesartan (Atacand)
- captopril (Capoten, Novo-Captopril)
- carteolol (Cartrol, Ocupress)
- carvedilol (Coreg)
- chlorothiazide (Diuril)
- chlorthalidone (Apo-Chlorthalidone, Thalitone)
- clonidine (Catapres, Duraclon)
- diazoxide (Hyperstat, Proglycem)
- diltiazem (Cardizem, Tiazac)
- doxazosin (Alti-Doxazosin, Cardura)
- enalapril (Vasotec)
- eplerenone (Inspra)
- eprosartan (Teveten)
- esmolol (Brevibloc)
- felodipine (Plendil, Renedil)
- fenoldopam (Corlopam)
- fosinopril (Monopril)
- furosemide (Apo-Furosemide, Lasix)
- guanabenz (Wytensin)
- guanadrel (Hylorel)
- guanfacine (Tenex)
- hydralazine (Apresoline, Novo-Hylazin)
- hydrochlorothiazide (Apo-Hydro, Microzide)
- hydrochlorothiazide and triamterene (Dyazide, Maxzide)
- indapamide (Lozol, Nu-Indapamide)
- irbesartan (Avapro)
- isradipine (DynaCirc)
- labetalol (Normodyne, Trandate)
- lisinopril (Prinivil, Zestril)
- losartan (Cozaar)
- mecamylamine (Inversine)
- mefruside (Baycaron)
- methyclothiazide (Aquatensen, Enduron)
- methyldopa (Apo-Methyldopa, Nu-Medopa)
- metolazone (Mykrox, Zaroxolyn)
- metoprolol (Betaloc, Lopressor)
- minoxidil (Loniten, Rogaine)
- moexipril (Univasc)
- nadolol (Apo-Nadol, Corgard)
- nicardipine (Cardene)
- nifedipine (Adalat CC, Procardia)
- nisoldipine (Sular)
- nitroglycerin (Minitran, Nitro-Dur)
- nitroprusside (Nipride, Nitropress)
- olmesartan (Benicar)
- oxprenolol (Slow-Trasicor, Trasicor)
- perindopril erbumine (Aceon, Coversyl)
- phenoxybenzamine (Dibenzyline)
- phentolamine (Regitine, Rogitine)
- pindolol (Apo-Pindol, Novo-Pindol)
- polythiazide (Renese)

- prazosin (Minipress, Nu-Prazo)
- propranolol (Inderal, InnoPran XL)
- quinapril (Accupril)
- ramipril (Altace)
- reserpine
- spironolactone (Aldactone, Novo-Spiroton)
- telmisartan (Micardis)
- terazosin (Alti-Terazosin, Hytrin)
- timolol (Betimol, Timoptic)
- torsemide (Demadex)
- trandolapril (Mavik)
- triamterene (Dyrenium)
- trichlormethiazide (Metatensin, Naqua)
- valsartan (Diovan)
- verapamil (Calan, Isoptin SR)

Taking kelp with these drugs may increase the risk of bleeding or bruising:

- antithrombin III (Thrombate III)
- argatroban
- bivalirudin (Angiomax)
- dalteparin (Fragmin)
- danaparoid (Orgaran)
- fondaparinux (Arixtra)
- heparin (Hepalean, Hep-Lock)
- lepirudin (Refludan)
- tinzaparin (Innohep)
- warfarin (Coumadin, Jantoven)

Lab Tests That May Be Altered by Kelp
- May increase serum potassium levels.
- May increase thyroid-stimulating hormone (TSH) levels due to the iodine content of kelp.

Diseases That May Be Worsened or Triggered by Kelp
May worsen both hyperthyroidism and hypothyroidism, due to iodine in the herb.

Foods That May Interact with Kelp
None known

Supplements That May Interact with Kelp
May increase risk of hyperkalemia (excessively high levels of potassium in the blood) when taken with potassium supplements due to the potassium content of kelp.

KHAT

> The fresh leaves of khat, an evergreen shrub native to east Africa and Saudi Arabia, have been chewed for centuries for their stimulating effects, which are similar to those of amphetamines. Khat, which contains the psychostimulant cathine, is used to increase alertness, reduce fatigue, and suppress the appetite, although regular use can cause insomnia, anxiety, anorexia, and psychological dependence.

Scientific Name
Catha edulis

Khat Is Also Commonly Known As
Abyssinian tea, Arabian-tea, cat, chat, miraa, tschut

Medicinal Parts
Leaf

Khat's Uses
To treat headache, depression, asthma, fever, and coughs; to improve performance and communicative abilities; to suppress hunger and increase sexual desire.

Typical Dose

A typical dose of khat may range from 100 to 200 gm of the fresh raw leaves, which are chewed, then followed with fluids.

Possible Side Effects

Khat's side effects include hyperactivity, euphoria, nervousness, insomnia, constipation, and depression (once effects wear off).

Drugs That May Interact with Khat

Taking khat with these drugs may increase the action of the drug:

- acebutolol (Novo-Acebutolol, Sectral)
- acetaminophen, chlorpheniramine, and pseudoephedrine (Children's Tylenol Plus Cold, Sinutab Sinus Allergy Maximum Strength)
- acetaminophen, dextromethorphan, and pseudoephedrine (Alka-Seltzer Plus Flu Liqui-Gels, Sudafed Severe Cold)
- acrivastine and pseudoephedrine (Semprex-D)
- adenosine (Adenocard, Adenoscan)
- amiodarone (Cordarone, Pacerone)
- amlodipine (Norvasc)
- atenolol (Apo-Atenol, Tenormin)
- azatadine (Optimine)
- azatadine and pseudoephedrine (Rynatan Tablet, Trinalin)
- azelastine (Astelin, Optivar)
- befunolol (Bentos, Betaclar)
- benazepril (Lotensin)
- bepridil (Vascor)
- betaxolol (Betoptic S, Kerlone)
- bisoprolol (Monocor, Zebeta)
- bretylium
- brompheniramine and pseudoephedrine (Children's Dimetapp Elixir Cold & Allergy, Lodrane)

- bumetanide (Bumex, Burinex)
- candesartan (Atacand)
- captopril (Capoten, Novo-Captopril)
- carbinoxamine (Histex CT, Histex PD)
- carbinoxamine and pseudoephedrine (Rondec Drops, Sildec)
- carbinoxamine, pseudoephedrine, and dextromethorphan (Rondec DM Drops, Tussafed)
- carteolol (Cartrol, Ocupress)
- carvedilol (Coreg)
- celiprolol
- cetirizine (Reactine, Zyrtec)
- chlorothiazide (Diuril)
- chlorpheniramine and acetaminophen (Coricidin HBP Cold and Flu)
- chlorpheniramine and phenylephrine (Histatab Plus, Rynatan)
- chlorpheniramine, ephedrine, phenylephrine, and carbetapentane (Rynatuss, Tynatuss Pediatric)
- chlorpheniramine, phenylephrine, and dextromethorphan (Alka-Seltzer Plus Cold and Cough)
- chlorpheniramine, phenylephrine, and methscopolamine (AH-Chew, Extendryl)
- chlorpheniramine, phenylephrine, and phenyltoloxamine (Comhist, NalexA)
- chlorpheniramine, phenylephrine, codeine, and potassium iodide (Pediacof)
- chlorpheniramine, pseudoephedrine, and codeine (Dihistine DH, RynaC)
- chlorpheniramine, pseudoephedrine, and dextromethorphan (Robitussin Pediatric Night Relief, Vicks Pediatric 44M)
- chlorthalidone (Apo-Chlorthalidone, Thalitone)
- cimetidine (Nu-Cimet, Tagamet)
- clemastine (Tavist Allergy)
- clonidine (Catapres, Duraclon)

- cyproheptadine (Periactin)
- deptropine (Deptropine FNA)
- desloratadine (Aerius, Clarinex)
- dexbrompheniramine and pseudoephedrine (Drixomed, Drixoral Cold & Allergy)
- dexchlorpheniramine (Polaramine)
- dextroamphetamine (Dexedrine, Dextrostat)
- dextroamphetamine and amphetamine (Adderall, Adderall XR)
- diazoxide (Hyperstat, Proglycem)
- digitalis (Digitek, Lanoxin)
- diltiazem (Cardizem, Tiazac)
- dimethindene (Fenistil)
- diphenhydramine (Benadryl Allergy, Nytol)
- diphenhydramine and pseudoephedrine (Benadryl Allergy/Decongestant, Benadryl Children's Allergy and Sinus)
- disopyramide (Norpace, Rhythmodan)
- dofetilide (Tikosyn)
- doxazosin (Alti-Doxazosin, Cardura)
- doxylamine and pyridoxine (Diclectin)
- enalapril (Vasotec)
- epinastine (Elestat)
- eplerenone (Inspra)
- eprosartan (Teveten)
- esmolol (Brevibloc)
- famotidine (Apo-Famotidine, Pepcid)
- felodipine (Plendil, Renedil)
- fenoldopam (Corlopam)
- fexofenadine (Allegra)
- fexofenadine and pseudoephedrine (Allegra D)
- flecainide (Tambocor)
- fosinopril (Monopril)
- furosemide (Apo-Furosemide, Lasix)
- guaifenesin and phenylephrine (Endal, Prolex-D)
- guaifenesin and pseudoephedrine (Aquatab, Maxifed)
- guanabenz (Wytensin)
- guanadrel (Hylorel)
- guanfacine (Tenex)
- hydralazine (Apresoline, Novo-Hylazin)
- hydrochlorothiazide (Apo-Hydro, Microzide)
- hydrochlorothiazide and triamterene (Dyazide, Maxzide)
- hydrocodone and chlorpheniramine (Tussionex)
- hydrocodone, carbinoxamine, and pseudoephedrine (Histex HC, TriVent HC)
- hydroxyzine (Atarax, Vistaril)
- ibutilide (Corvert)
- indapamide (Lozol, Nu-Indapamide)
- iproniazid (Marsilid)
- irbesartan (Avapro)
- isradipine (DynaCirc)
- ketotifen (Novo-Ketotifen, Zaditor)
- labetalol (Normodyne, Trandate)
- lacidipine (Aponil, Caldine)
- lercanidipine (Cardiovasc, Carmen)
- levobetaxolol (Betaxon)
- levobunolol (Betagan, Novo-Levobunolol)
- levocabastine (Livostin)
- lidocaine (Lidoderm, Xylocaine)
- lisinopril (Prinivil, Zestril)
- loratadine (Alavert, Claritin)
- loratadine and pseudoephedrine (Claritin-D 12 Hour, Claritin-D 24 Hour)
- losartan (Cozaar)
- manidipine (Calslot, Iperten)
- mebhydrolin (Bexidal, Incidal)
- mecamylamine (Inversine)
  mefruside (Baycaron)
- methamphetamine (Desoxyn)
- methyclothiazide (Aquatensen, Enduron)
- methyldopa (Apo-Methyldopa, Nu-Medopa)
- metipranolol (OptiPranolol)

- metolazone (Mykrox, Zaroxolyn)
- metoprolol (Betaloc, Lopressor)
- mexiletine (Mexitil, Novo-Mexiletine)
- minoxidil (Loniten, Rogaine)
- mizolastine (Elina, Mizollen)
- moclobemide (Alti-Moclobemide, Nu-Moclobemide)
- moexipril (Univasc)
- moricizine (Ethmozine)
- nadolol (Apo-Nadol, Corgard)
- naphazoline (Allersol, Naphcon)
- nicardipine (Cardene)
- nifedipine (Adalat CC, Procardia)
- nilvadipine
- nimodipine (Nimotop)
- nisoldipine (Sular)
- nitrendipine
- nitroglycerin (Minitran, Nitro-Dur)
- nitroprusside (Nipride, Nitropress)
- nizatidine (Axid, PMS-Nizatidine)
- olmesartan (Benicar)
- olopatadine (Patanol)
- oxatomide (Cenacert, Tinset)
- oxprenolol (Slow-Trasicor, Trasicor)
- perindopril erbumine (Aceon, Coversyl)
- phenelzine (Nardil)
- phenoxybenzamine (Dibenzyline)
- phentolamine (Regitine, Rogitine)
- phenytoin (Dilantin, Phenytek)
- pinaverium (Dicetel)
- pindolol (Apo-Pindol, Novo-Pindol)
- polythiazide (Renese)
- prazosin (Minipress, Nu-Prazo)
- procainamide (Procanbid, Pronestyl-SR)
- promethazine (Phenergan)
- promethazine and codeine (Phenergan with Codeine)
- promethazine and dextromethorphan (Promatussin DM)
- promethazine and phenylephrine
- promethazine, phenylephrine, and codeine
- propafenone (GenPropafenone, Rhythmol)
- propranolol (Inderal, InnoPran XL)
- pseudoephedrine (Dimetapp Decongestant, Sudafed 12 Hour)
- quinapril (Accupril)
- quinidine (Novo-Quinidin, Quinaglute DuraTabs)
- ramipril (Altace)
- ranitidine (Alti-Ranitidine, Zantac)
- reserpine
- selegiline (Eldepryl)
- sotalol (Betapace, Sorine)
- spironolactone (Aldactone, Novo-Spiroton)
- telmisartan (Micardis)
- terazosin (Alti-Terazosin, Hytrin)
- timolol (Betimol, Timoptic)
- tocainide (Tonocard)
- torsemide (Demadex)
- trandolapril (Mavik)
- tranylcypromine (Parnate)
- triamterene (Dyrenium)
- trichlormethiazide (Metatensin, Naqua)
- tripelennamine (PBZ, PBZ-SR)
- triprolidine and pseudoephedrine (Actifed Cold and Allergy, Silafed)
- triprolidine, pseudoephedrine, and codeine (CoActifed, Covan)
- valsartan (Diovan)
- verapamil (Calan, Isoptin SR)

Taking khat with these drugs may interfere with the action of the drug:

- nafcillin (Nallpen, Unipen)
- penicillin (Pfizerpen, Wycillin)

Lab Tests That May Be Altered by Khat
None known

Diseases That May Be Worsened or Triggered by Khat
None known

Foods That May Interact with Khat
None known

Supplements That May Interact with Khat
None known

Kudzu

In China and Japan, the root of this fast-growing, flowering vine has been a common ingredient in foods and medications for centuries. More recently, researchers have found that substances in kudzu root interfere with the body's ability to metabolize alcohol, and a drug derived from kudzu root may help in the treatment of alcoholism.

Scientific Name
Pueraria Montana

Kudzu Is Also Commonly Known As
Japanese arrowroot, ge gen, kudzu vine, pueraria root

Medicinal Parts
Flower, root

Kudzu's Uses
To treat the measles, irregular heartbeat, breast pain, fever, diarrhea, diabetes, traumatic injuries, and psoriasis; to relieve the symptoms of alcoholic hangover

Typical Dose
A typical dose of kudzu for treatment of chronic alcoholism is approximately 1.2 gm of kudzu root extract two times daily for four months.

Possible Side Effects
There are no reported side effects with the use of kudzu.

Drugs That May Interact with Kudzu
Taking kudzu with these drugs may enhance the effects of the drug:

- acebutolol (Novo-Acebutolol, Sectral)
- adenosine (Adenocard, Adenoscan)
- amiodarone (Cordarone, Pacerone)
- bretylium
- digitalis (Digitek, Lanoxin)
- diltiazem (Cardizem, Tiazac)
- disopyramide (Norpace, Rhythmodan)
- dofetilide (Tikosyn)
- esmolol (Brevibloc)
- flecainide (Tambocor)
- ibutilide (Corvert)
- lidocaine (Lidoderm, Xylocaine)
- mexiletine (Mexitil, Novo-Mexiletine)
- moricizine (Ethmozine)
- phenytoin (Dilantin, Phenytek)
- procainamide (Procanbid, Pronestyl-SR)
- propafenone (GenPropafenone, Rhythmol)
- propranolol (Inderal, InnoPran XL)
- quinidine (Novo-Quinidin, Quinaglute DuraTabs)
- sotalol (Betapace, Sorine)
- tocainide (Tonocard)
- verapamil (Calan, Isoptin SR)

Taking kudzu with these drugs may increase the risk of hypoglycemia (low blood sugar):

- acarbose (Prandase, Precose)
- acetohexamide
- chlorpropamide (Diabinese, Novo-Propamide)
- gliclazide (Diamicron, Novo-Gliclazide)
- glimepiride (Amaryl)
- glipizide (Glucotrol)
- glipizide and metformin (Metaglip)
- gliquidone (Beglynor, Glurenorm)
- glyburide (DiaBeta, Micronase)
- glyburide and metformin (Glucovance)
- insulin (Humulin, Novolin R)
- metformin (Glucophage, Riomet)
- miglitol (Glyset)
- nateglinide (Starlix)
- pioglitazone (Actos)
- repaglinide (GlucoNorm, Prandin)
- rosiglitazone (Avandia)
- rosiglitazone and metformin (Avandamet)
- tolazamide (Tolinase)
- tolbutamide (Apo-Tolbutamide, Tol-Tab)

Lab Tests That May Be Altered by Kudzu

- May decrease blood glucose levels.
- May decrease blood cholesterol levels.

Diseases That May Be Worsened or Triggered by Kudzu

This herb may have estrogen-like effects and should not be used by women with estrogen-sensitive breast cancer or other hormone-sensitive conditions.

Foods That May Interact with Kudzu

None known

Supplements That May Interact with Kudzu

May increase action of herbs and supplements that have estrogenic activity, such as black cohosh, chaste tree berry, and soy. (For a list of herbs and supplements that have estrogenic activity, see Appendix B.)

LARCH

This tall conifer, native to the northwestern United States, produces a gum underneath its bark that Native Americans chewed for its sweet taste and medicinal qualities. Both the gum and an infusion of the bark have been used as a dressing for wounds and a treatment for sore throats, coughs, colds, and tuberculosis.

Scientific Name

Larix occidentalis

Larch Is Also Commonly Known As

Arabinogalactan, larch arabinogalactan, larch gum, Mongolia larch, western larch, wood gum

Medicinal Parts

Bark

Larch's Uses

To treat colds, flu, ear inflammation in children, HIV, and AIDS; as a dietary fiber supplement; to stimulate the immune system

Typical Dose

A typical dose of larch is approximately 1 tsp larch arabinogalactan powder mixed with water or juice, taken two or three times daily.

Possible Side Effects
Larch's side effects include flatulence and bloating.

Drugs That May Interact with Larch
Taking larch with these drugs may interfere with the action of the drug:
- antithymocyte globulin (equine) (Atgam)
- antithymocyte globulin (rabbit) (Thymoglobulin)
- azathioprine (Imuran)
- basiliximab (Simulect)
- beclomethasone (Beconase, Vanceril)
- betamethasone (Celestone, Diprolene)
- budesonide (Entocort, Rhinocort)
- budesonide and formoterol (Symbicort)
- cortisone (Cortone)
- cyclosporine (Neoral, Sandimmune)
- daclizumab (Zenapax)
- deflazacort (Calcort, Dezacor)
- dexamethasone (Decadron, Dexasone)
- efalizumab (Raptiva)
- flunisolide (AeroBid, Nasarel)
- fluorometholone (Eflone, Flarex)
- fluticasone (Cutivate, Flonase)
- hydrocortisone (Anusol-HC, Locoid)
- loteprednol (Alrex, Lotemax)
- medrysone (HMS Liquifilm)
- methotrexate (Rheumatrex, Trexall)
- methylprednisolone (Medrol, Depo-Medrol)
- muromonab-CD3 (Orthoclone OKT 3)
- mycophenolate (CellCept)
- pimecrolimus (Elidel)
- prednisolone (Inflamase Forte, Pred Forte)
- prednisone (Apo-Prednisone, Deltasone)
- rimexolone (Vexol)
- sirolimus (Rapamune)
- tacrolimus (Prograf, Protopic)
- thalidomide (Thalomid)
- triamcinolone (Aristocort, Trinasal)

Lab Tests That May Be Altered by Larch
None known

Diseases That May Be Worsened or Triggered by Larch
May interfere with therapies that depend on suppressing the immune system.

Foods That May Interact with Larch
None known

Supplements That May Interact with Larch
None known

LAUREL

> A symbol of peace and victory in ancient Greece, laurel leaves (also known as bay leaves) were used to make wreaths of honor for great scholars, artists, soldiers, and athletes. Although therapeutic use is uncommon, the extract or essential oil of laurel leaves is sometimes used to treat rheumatic disorders, amenorrhea, gastric ulcers, and colic.

Scientific Name
Laurus nobilis

Laurel Is Also Commonly Known As
Bay, bay laurel, daphne, noble laurel, sweet bay

Medicinal Parts
Leaf, fruit, oil

Laurel's Uses

To treat rheumatism, dandruff, and flatulence; as a general tonic

Typical Dose

There is no typical dose of laurel.

Possible Side Effects

Laurel's side effects include allergic reactions.

Drugs That May Interact with Laurel

Taking laurel with these drugs may increase the risk of hypoglycemia (low blood sugar):

- acarbose (Prandase, Precose)
- acetohexamide
- chlorpropamide (Diabinese, Novo-Propamide)
- gliclazide (Diamicron, Novo-Gliclazide)
- glimepiride (Amaryl)
- glipizide (Glucotrol)
- glipizide and metformin (Metaglip)
- gliquidone (Beglynor, Glurenorm)
- glyburide (DiaBeta, Micronase)
- glyburide and metformin (Glucovance)
- insulin (Humulin, Novolin R)
- metformin (Glucophage, Riomet)
- miglitol (Glyset)
- nateglinide (Starlix)
- pioglitazone (Actos)
- repaglinide (GlucoNorm, Prandin)
- rosiglitazone (Avandia)
- rosiglitazone and metformin (Avandamet)
- tolazamide (Tolinase)
- tolbutamide (Apo-Tolbutamide, Tol-Tab)

Lab Tests That May Be Altered by Laurel

None known

Diseases That May Be Worsened or Triggered by Laurel

None known

Foods That May Interact with Laurel

None known

Supplements That May Interact with Laurel

None known

LEMON BALM

A member of the mint family, lemon balm has been used since the Middle Ages to lift the spirits, reduce stress and anxiety, promote sleep, ease flatulence, and improve appetite. Lemon balm also has antiviral properties and has been found to be very effective in treating herpes simplex cold sores.

Scientific Name

Melissa officinalis

Lemon Balm Is Also Commonly Known As

Balm, cure-all, dropsy plant, honey plant, melissa, sweet balm

Medicinal Parts

Leaf, whole plant, oil

Lemon Balm's Uses

To treat depression, vomiting, headaches, Alzheimer's disease, elevated blood pressure, menstrual irregularities, muscle stiffness, nerve pain, and rheumatism

Typical Dose
A typical daily dose of lemon balm has not been established.

Possible Side Effects
Lemon balm's side effects include nausea, vomiting, dizziness, and wheezing.

Drugs That May Interact with Lemon Balm
Taking lemon balm with these drugs may increase the risk of excessive sedation and mental depression and impairment:
- alprazolam (Apo-Alpraz, Xanax)
- amitriptyline (Elavil, Levate)
- amobarbital (Amytal)
- amobarbital and secobarbital (Tuinal)
- amoxapine (Asendin)
- bupropion (Wellbutrin, Zyban)
- buspirone (BuSpar, Nu-Buspirone)
- butabarbital (Butisol Sodium)
- butalbital, acetaminophen, and caffeine (Esgic, Fioricet)
- butalbital, aspirin, and caffeine (Fiorinal)
- clonazepam (Klonopin, Rivotril)
- cyclobenzaprine (Flexeril, Novo-Cycloprine)
- desipramine (Alti-Desipramine, Norpramin)
- diazepam (Apo-Diazepam, Valium)
- diphenhydramine (Benadryl Allergy, Nytol)
- doxepin (Sinequan, Zonalon)
- fluoxetine (Prozac, Sarafem)
- fluphenazine (Modecate, Prolixin)
- flurazepam (Apo-Flurazepam, Dalmane)
- imipramine (Apo-Imipramine, Tofranil)
- lorazepam (Ativan, Nu-Loraz)
- mephobarbital (Mebaral)
- methohexital (Brevital, Brevital Sodium)
- metoclopramide (Apo-Metoclop, Reglan)
- midazolam (Apo-Midazolam, Versed)
- morphine hydrochloride
- morphine sulfate (Kadian, MS Contin)
- nefazodone (Serzone)
- nortriptyline (Aventyl HCl, Pamelor)
- olanzapine (Zydis, Zyprexa)
- oxazepam (Novoxapam, Serax)
- oxcarbazepine (Trileptal)
- pentobarbital (Nembutal)
- phenobarbital (Luminal Sodium, PMS-Phenobarbital)
- primidone (Apo-Primidone, Mysoline)
- prochlorperazine (Compazine, Compro)
- propoxyphene (Darvon, Darvon-N)
- quetiapine (Seroquel)
- risperidone (Risperdal)
- secobarbital (Seconal)
- temazepam (Novo-Temazepam, Restoril)
- thiopental (Pentothal)
- tramadol (Ultram)
- triazolam (Apo-Triazo, Halcion)
- zolpidem (Ambien)

Taking lemon balm (in tea form) with these drugs may decrease absorption of the drug:
- ferric gluconate (Ferrlecit)
- ferrous fumarate (Femiron, Feostat)
- ferrous gluconate (Fergon, Novo-Ferrogluc)
- ferrous sulfate (Feratab, Fer-Iron)
- ferrous sulfate and ascorbic acid (FeroGrad 500, Vitelle Irospan)
- iron-dextran complex (Dexferrum, INFeD)
- polysaccharide-iron complex (Hytinic, Niferex)

Lab Tests That May Be Altered by Lemon Balm
None known

Diseases That May Be Worsened or Triggered by Lemon Balm
None known

Foods That May Interact with Lemon Balm
None known

Supplements That May Interact with Lemon Balm
May enhance therapeutic and adverse effects of herbs and supplements that have sedative properties, such as 5-HTP, kava kava, St. John's wort, and valerian. (For a list of herbs and supplements that have sedative properties, see Appendix B.)

LESSER GALANGAL

Lesser galangal, the spicy, aromatic root of a plant native to China, most likely gets its name from the Arabic word *khanlanjan*, a corruption of a Chinese word meaning "mild ginger." Like ginger, lesser galangal is useful in promoting digestion and preventing vomiting, morning sickness, and motion sickness. Some studies have also found that a constituent of lesser galangal inhibits inflammation.

Scientific Name
Alpinia officinarum

Lesser Galangal Is Also Commonly Known As
Alpinia, catarrh root, Chinese ginger, East India root, galanga, India root

Medicinal Parts
Rhizome

Lesser Galangal's Uses
To treat pain, particularly stomach pain. Germany's Commission E has approved the use of lesser galangal to treat loss of appetite and dyspeptic complaints, such as heartburn and bloating.

Typical Dose
A typical dose of lesser galangal may range from 0.5 to 1.0 gm mixed with 150 ml boiling water, allowed to steep ten minutes, drained and taken as a tea.

Possible Side Effects
No side effects are known when lesser galangal is taken in designated therapeutic doses.

Drugs That May Interact with Lesser Galangal
Taking lesser galangal with these drugs may interfere with the action of the drug:
- aluminum hydroxide (AlternaGel, Alu-Cap)
- aluminum hydroxide and magnesium carbonate (Gaviscon Extra Strength, Gaviscon Liquid)
- aluminum hydroxide and magnesium hydroxide (Maalox, Rulox)
- aluminum hydroxide and magnesium trisilicate (Gaviscon Tablet)
- aluminum hydroxide, magnesium hydroxide, and simethicone (Maalox, Mylanta Liquid)
- calcium carbonate (Rolaids Extra Strength, Tums)
- calcium carbonate and magnesium hydroxide (Mylanta Gelcaps, Rolaids Extra Strength)
- cimetidine (Nu-Cimet, Tagamet)
- esomeprazole (Nexium)
- famotidine (Apo-Famotidine, Pepcid)
- famotidine, calcium carbonate, and magnesium hydroxide (Pepcid Complete)

- lansoprazole (Prevacid)
- magaldrate and simethicone (Riopan Plus, Riopan Plus Double Strength)
- magnesium hydroxide (Dulcolax Milk of Magnesia, Phillips' Milk of Magnesia)
- magnesium oxide (Mag-Ox 400, Uro-Mag)
- magnesium sulfate (Epsom salts)
- nizatidine (Axid, PMS-Nizatidine)
- omeprazole (Losec, Prilosec)
- pantoprazole (Pantoloc, Protonix)
- rabeprazole (Aciphex, Pariet)
- ranitidine (Alti-Ranitidine, Zantac)
- sodium bicarbonate (Brioschi, Neut)

Lab Tests That May Be Altered by Lesser Galangal
None known

Diseases That May Be Worsened or Triggered by Lesser Galangal
None known

Foods That May Interact with Lesser Galangal
None known

Supplements That May Interact with Lesser Galangal
None known

LICORICE

Licorice root has a number of medicinal properties, most of which stem from its active ingredient glycyrrhizin, which appears to have anti-inflammatory, antiviral, antiallergic, and estrogenic activities. Licorice is used to soothe sore throats, reduce arthritis pain and stiffness, lessen the pain of ulcers, ease menopausal symptoms, and treat hepatitis B. It may even slow the growth of certain kinds of cancer.

Scientific Name
Glycyrrhiza glabra

Licorice Is Also Commonly Known As
Chinese licorice, licorice root, liquorice, Spanish licorice, sweet root, sweet wort

Medicinal Parts
Root

Licorice's Uses
To treat stomach ulcers, bronchitis, sore throat, dry cough, arthritis, bacterial and viral infections, chronic fatigue syndrome, and constipation

Typical Dose
A typical dose of licorice may range from 1 to 4 gm of powdered root, taken three times daily.

Possible Side Effects
Licorice's side effects include elevated blood pressure, retention of sodium and water, low levels of potassium in the blood, lethargy, and headache. Those with hypertension should avoid it. Licorice is also unsafe for those who have cirrhosis, kidney disease, or heart disease as well as women who are pregnant. For all others, licorice should be used for no longer than six weeks, to minimize the risk of adverse effects.

Drugs That May Interact with Licorice

Taking licorice with these drugs may interfere with the effectiveness of the drug:

- acebutolol (Novo-Acebutolol, Sectral)
- adenosine (Adenocard, Adenoscan)
- amiodarone (Cordarone, Pacerone)
- bretylium
- cyclosporine (Neoral, Sandimmune)
- dexamethasone (Decadron, Dexasone)
- digitalis (Digitek, Lanoxin)
- diltiazem (Cardizem, Tiazac)
- disopyramide (Norpace, Rhythmodan)
- dofetilide (Tikosyn)
- esmolol (Brevibloc)
- flecainide (Tambocor)
- ibutilide (Corvert)
- lidocaine (Lidoderm, Xylocaine)
- mexiletine (Mexitil, Novo-Mexiletine)
- moricizine (Ethmozine)
- phenytoin (Dilantin, Phenytek)
- procainamide (Procanbid, Pronestyl-SR)
- propafenone (GenPropafenone, Rhythmol)
- propranolol (Inderal, InnoPran XL)
- quinidine (Novo-Quinidin, Quinaglute Dura-Tabs)
- sotalol (Betapace, Sorine)
- testosterone (Androderm, Testoderm)
- tocainide (Tonocard)
- verapamil (Calan, Isoptin SR)

Taking licorice with these drugs may increase the risk of hypokalemia (low levels of potassium in the blood):

- acetazolamide (Apo-Acetazolamide, Diamox Sequels)
- azosemide (Diat)
- bumetanide (Bumex, Burinex)
- cascara
- chlorothiazide (Diuril)
- chlorthalidone (Apo-Chlorthalidone, Thalitone)
- digitalis (Digitek, Lanoxin)
- diltiazem (Cardizem, Tiazac)
- docusate (Colace, Ex-Lax Stool Softener)
- docusate and senna (Peri-Colace, Senokot-S)
- dofetilide (Tikosyn)
- enalapril (Vasotec)
- ethacrynic acid (Edecrin)
- etozolin (Elkapin)
- furosemide (Apo-Furosemide, Lasix)
- hydrochlorothiazide (Apo-Hydro, Microzide)
- hydroflumethiazide (Diucardin, Saluron)
- indapamide (Lozol, Nu-Indapamide)
- lactulose (Constulose, Enulose)
- magnesium citrate (CitroMag)
- magnesium hydroxide (Dulcolax Milk of Magnesia, Phillips' Milk of Magnesia)
- magnesium hydroxide and mineral oil (Phillips' M-O)
- magnesium oxide (MagOx 400, Uro-Mag)
- magnesium sulfate (Epsom salts)
- mannitol (Osmitrol, Resectisol)
- mefruside (Baycaron)
- methazolamide (Apo-Methazolamide, Neptazane)
- methyclothiazide (Aquatensen, Enduron)
- metolazone (Mykrox, Zaroxolyn)
- olmesartan and hydrochlorothiazide (Benicar HCT)
- polyethylene glycol-electrolyte solution (Colyte, MiraLax)
- polythiazide (Renese)
- psyllium (Metamucil, Reguloid)
- sildenafil (Viagra)
- sorbitol (Sorbilax)

- torsemide (Demadex)
- trichlormethiazide (Metatensin, Naqua)
- urea (Amino-Cerv, UltraMide)
- verapamil (Calan, Isoptin SR)
- xipamide (Diurexan, Lumitens)

Taking licorice with these drugs may increase the risk of bleeding and bruising:

- abciximab (ReoPro)
- alteplase (Activase, Cathflo Activase)
- antithrombin III (Thrombate III)
- argatroban
- aspirin (Bufferin, Ecotrin)
- aspirin and dipyridamole (Aggrenox)
- bivalirudin (Angiomax)
- celecoxib (Celebrex)
- clopidogrel (Plavix)
- dalteparin (Fragmin)
- danaparoid (Orgaran)
- dipyridamole (Novo-Dipiradol, Persantine)
- enoxaparin (Lovenox)
- eptifibatide (Integrillin)
- fondaparinux (Arixtra)
- heparin (Hepalean, Hep-Lock)
- indobufen (Ibustrin)
- indomethacin (Indocin, Novo-Methacin)
- ketoprofen (Orudis, Rhodis)
- ketorolac (Acular, Toradol)
- lepirudin (Refludan)
- meloxicam (MOBIC, Mobicox)
- nadroparin (Fraxiparine)
- naproxen (Aleve, Naprosyn)
- piroxicam (Feldene, Nu-Pirox)
- reteplase (Retavase)
- rofecoxib (Vioxx)
- streptokinase (Streptase)
- tenecteplase (TNKase)

- ticlopidine (Alti-Ticlopidine, Ticlid)
- tinzaparin (Innohep)
- tirofiban (Aggrastat)
- urokinase (Abbokinase)
- warfarin (Coumadin, Jantoven)

Taking licorice with these drugs may increase the risk of hypertension (high blood pressure):

- acebutolol (Novo-Acebutolol, Sectral)
- amlodipine (Norvasc)
- atenolol (Apo-Atenol, Tenormin)
- benazepril (Lotensin)
- betaxolol (Betoptic S, Kerlone)
- bisoprolol (Monocor, Zebeta)
- bumetanide (Bumex, Burinex)
- candesartan (Atacand)
- captopril (Capoten, Novo-Captopril)
- carteolol (Cartrol, Ocupress)
- carvedilol (Coreg)
- chlorothiazide (Diuril)
- chlorothalidone (Apo-Chlorthalidone, Thalitone)
- clonidine (Catapres, Duraclon)
- diazoxide (Hyperstat, Proglycem)
- diltiazem (Cardizem, Tiazac)
- doxazosin (Alti-Doxazosin, Cardura)
- enalapril (Vasotec)
- ephedrine (Pretz-D)
- eplerenone (Inspra)
- eprosartan (Teveten)
- esmolol (Brevibloc)
- ethinyl estradiol and desogestrel (Cyclessa, Ortho-Cept)
- ethinyl estradiol and drospirenone (Yasmin)
- ethinyl estradiol and ethynodiol diacetate (Demulen, Zovia)
- ethinyl estradiol and levonorgestrel (Alesse, Triphasil)

- ethinyl estradiol and norethindrone (Brevicon, Ortho-Novum)
- ethinyl estradiol and norgestimate (Cyclen, Ortho Tri-Cyclen)
- ethinyl estradiol and norgestrel (Cryselle, Ovral)
- felodipine (Plendil, Renedil)
- fenoldopam (Corlopam)
- fosinopril (Monopril)
- furosemide (Apo-Furosemide, Lasix)
- guanabenz (Wytensin)
- guanadrel (Hylorel)
- guanfacine (Tenex)
- hydralazine (Apresoline, Novo-Hylazin)
- hydrochlorothiazide (Apo-Hydro, Microzide)
- indapamide (Lozol, Nu-Indapamide)
- irbesartan (Avapro)
- isradipine (DynaCirc)
- labetalol (Normodyne, Trandate)
- levalbuterol (Xopenex)
- lisinopril (Prinivil, Zestril)
- losartan (Cozaar)
- mecamylamine (Inversine)
- mefruside (Baycaron)
- mestranol and norethindrone (Necon 1/50, Ortho-Novum 1/50)
- methyclothiazide (Aquatensen, Enduron)
- methyldopa (Apo-Methyldopa, Nu-Medopa)
- metolazone (Mykrox, Zaroxolyn)
- metoprolol (Betaloc, Lopressor)
- minoxidil (Loniten, Rogaine)
- moexipril (Univasc)
- nadolol (Apo-Nadol, Corgard)
- nicardipine (Cardene)
- nifedipine (Adalat CC, Procardia)
- nisoldipine (Sular)
- nitroglycerin (Minitran, Nitro-Dur)
- nitroprusside (Nipride, Nitropress)

- olmesartan (Benicar)
- oxprenolol (Slow-Trasicor, Trasicor)
- perindopril erbumine (Aceon, Coversyl)
- phenoxybenzamine (Dibenzyline)
- phentolamine (Regitine, Rogitine)
- pindolol (Apo-Pindol, Novo-Pindol)
- polythiazide (Renese)
- prazosin (Minipress, Nu-Prazo)
- propranolol (Inderal, InnoPran XL)
- quinapril (Accupril)
- ramipril (Altace)
- reserpine
- telmisartan (Micardis)
- terazosin (Alti-Terazosin, Hytrin)
- timolol (Betimol, Timoptic)
- torsemide (Demadex)
- trandolapril (Mavik)
- trichlormethiazide (Metatensin, Naqua)
- valsartan (Diovan)
- verapamil (Calan, Isoptin SR)

Taking licorice with these drugs may increase the risk of hyperglycemia (high blood sugar):

- acarbose (Prandase, Precose)
- acetohexamide
- chlorpropamide (Diabinese, Novo-Propamide)
- gliclazide (Diamicron, Novo-Gliclazide)
- glimepiride (Amaryl)
- glipizide (Glucotrol)
- glipizide and metformin (Metaglip)
- gliquidone (Beglynor, Glurenorm)
- glyburide (DiaBeta, Micronase)
- glyburide and metformin (Glucovance)
- insulin (Humulin, Novolin R)
- metformin (Glucophage, Riomet)
- miglitol (Glyset)
- nateglinide (Starlix)

- pioglitazone (Actos)
- repaglinide (GlucoNorm, Prandin)
- rosiglitazone (Avandia)
- rosiglitazone and metformin (Avandamet)
- tolazamide (Tolinase)
- tolbutamide (Apo-Tolbutamide, Tol-Tab)

Taking licorice with these drugs may increase the therapeutic and/or adverse effects of the drug:
- beclomethasone (Beconase, Vanceril)
- betamethasone (Celestone, Diprolene)
- budesonide (Entocort, Rhinocort)
- budesonide and formoterol (Symbicort)
- cortisone (Cortone)
- deflazacort (Calcort, Dezacor)
- dexamethasone (Decadron, Dexasone)
- flunisolide (AeroBid, Nasarel)
- fluorometholone (Eflone, Flarex)
- fluticasone (Cutivate, Flonase)
- hydrocortisone (Anusol-HC, Locoid)
- methylprednisolone (DepoMedrol, Medrol)
- prednisolone (Inflamase Forte, Pred Forte)
- prednisone (Deltasone, Apo-Prednisone)
- triamcinolone (Aristocort, Trinasal)

Taking licorice with these drugs may increase the risk of drug toxicity:
- iproniazid (Marsilid)
- moclobemide (Alti-Moclobemide, Nu-Moclobemide)
- phenelzine (Nardil)
- selegiline (Eldepryl)
- tranylcypromine (Parnate)

Taking licorice with these drugs may be harmful:
- choline magnesium trysalicylate (Trilisate)—may increase drug levels

- loratadine (Alavert, Claritin)—may increase risk of arrhythmias and other heart problems

Lab Tests That May Be Altered by Licorice
- May decrease anion gap.
- May decrease potassium levels.
- May decrease serum prolactin levels.
- May decrease serum or urine sodium levels.
- Possible positive test for serum urine myoglobin levels.
- May increase serum 17-hydroxyprogesterone levels.
- May increase blood pressure levels.
- May decrease serum testosterone levels.

Diseases That May Be Worsened or Triggered by Licorice
- May hamper attempts to control blood sugar in diabetes.
- May worsen congestive heart failure by encouraging the body to retain fluid.
- This herb may have estrogen-like effects and should not be used by women with estrogen-sensitive breast cancer or other hormone-sensitive conditions.
- May worsen hypertension by elevating blood pressure.
- May trigger low levels of potassium.
- May worsen existing cases of kidney or liver disease.

Foods That May Interact with Licorice
Grapefruit juice may increase the mineralocorticoid activities of licorice. (See section on grapefruit.)

Supplements That May Interact with Licorice
- Increased risk of cardiotoxicity due to potassium depletion when taken with cardioactive herbs,

such as adonis, digitalis, lily-of-the-valley, and squill. (For a list of cardioactive herbs and supplements, see Appendix B.)

- Increased risk of potassium depletion when used with stimulant laxative herbs, such as black root, cascara sagrada, castor oil, and senna. (For a list of stimulant laxative herbs and supplements, see Appendix B.)
- Decreased response to potassium supplementation.

LILY-OF-THE-VALLEY

> These little white bell-shaped blossoms perched atop delicate stems, sometimes called our lady's tears, were first cultivated in 1420 and are often used in weddings, signifying "a return to happiness." Because lily-of-the-valley contains cardiac glycosides, it has been used as a cardiac tonic to slow the action of a weak, irritable heart, while simultaneously increasing its power.

Scientific Name
Convallaria majalis

Lily-of-the-Valley Is Also Commonly Known As
Constancy, Jacob's ladder, ladder-to-heaven, may lily, our lady's tears

Medicinal Parts
Whole plant

Lily-of-the-Valley's Uses
To treat stroke, leprosy, heart problems, and epilepsy. Germany's Commission E has approved the use of lily-of-the-valley to treat irregular heartbeat and other heart ailments.

Typical Dose
A typical daily dose of lily-of-the-valley is approximately 600 mg of tincture or liquid extract.

Possible Side Effects
Lily-of-the-valley's side effects include nausea, vomiting, irregular heartbeat, and headache. Lily-of-the-valley contains cardiac glycosides, which can help control irregular heartbeat, reduce the backup of blood and fluid in the body, and increase blood flow through the kidneys, helping to excrete sodium and relieve swelling in body tissues. However, a buildup of cardiac glycosides can occur, especially when the herb is combined with certain medications or other herbs that contain cardiac glycosides, causing arrhythmias, abnormally slow heartbeat, heart failure, and even death.

Drugs That May Interact with Lily-of-the-Valley
Taking lily-of-the-valley with these drugs may enhance the therapeutic and/or adverse effects of the drug:

- betamethasone (Betatrex, Maxivate)
- calcium acetate (PhosLo)
- calcium carbonate (Rolaids Extra Strength, Tums)
- calcium chloride
- calcium citrate (Osteocit)
- calcium glubionate
- calcium gluceptate
- calcium gluconate
- cascara
- cortisone (Cortone)
- deflazacort (Calcort, Dezacor)

- dexamethasone (Decadron, Dexasone)
- digitalis (Digitek, Lanoxin)
- docusate (Colace, Ex-Lax Stool Softener)
- docusate and senna (Peri-Colace, Senokot-S)
- hydrocortisone (Cetacort, Locoid)
- lactulose (Constulose, Enulose)
- magnesium citrate (Citro-Mag)
- magnesium hydroxide (Dulcolax Milk of Magnesia, Phillips' Milk of Magnesia)
- magnesium hydroxide and mineral oil (Phillips' M-O)
- magnesium oxide (Mag-Ox 400, Uro-Mag)
- magnesium sulfate (Epsom salts)
- methylprednisolone (Depo-Medrol, Medrol)
- polyethylene glycol-electrolyte solution (Colyte, MiraLax)
- prednisolone (Inflamase Forte, Pred Forte)
- prednisone (Apo-Prednisone, Deltasone)
- psyllium (Metamucil, Reguloid)
- quinidine (Novo-Quinidin, Quinaglute Dura-Tabs)
- sorbitol (Sorbilax)
- triamcinolone (Aristocort, Trinasal)

Taking lily-of-the-valley with these drugs may increase the risk of bradycardia (slow heart rate):
- acebutolol (Novo-Acebutolol, Sectral)
- amlodipine (Norvasc)
- atenolol (Apo-Atenol, Tenormin)
- befunolol (Bentos, Betaclar)
- bepridil (Vascor)
- betaxolol (Betoptic S, Kerlone)
- bisoprolol (Monocor, Zebeta)
- carteolol (Cartrol, Ocupress)
- carvedilol (Coreg)
- celiprolol
- digitalis (Digitek, Lanoxin)

- diltiazem (Cardizem, Tiazac)
- esmolol (Brevibloc)
- felodipine (Plendil, Renedil)
- isradipine (DynaCirc)
- labetalol (Normodyne, Trandate)
- lacidipine (Aponil, Caldine)
- lercanidipine (Cardiovasc, Carmen)
- levobetaxolol (Betaxon)
- levobunolol (Betagan, Novo-Levobunolol)
- manidipine (Calslot, Iperten)
- metipranolol (OptiPranolol)
- metoprolol (Betaloc, Lopressor)
- nadolol (Apo-Nadol, Corgard)
- nicardipine (Cardene)
- nifedipine (Adalat CC, Procardia)
- nilvadipine
- nimodipine (Nimotop)
- nisoldipine (Sular)
- nitrendipine
- oxprenolol (Slow-Trasicor, Trasicor)
- pinaverium (Dicetel)
- pindolol (Apo-Pindol, Novo-Pindol)
- propranolol (Inderal, InnoPran XL)
- sotalol (Betapace, Sorine)
- timolol (Betimol, Timoptic)
- verapamil (Calan, Isoptin SR)

Taking lily-of-the-valley with these drugs may increase the risk of cardiac glycoside toxicity:
- acetazolamide (Apo-Acetazolamide, Diamox Sequels)
- azosemide (Diat)
- bumetanide (Bumex, Burinex)
- chlorothiazide (Diuril)
- chlorthalidone (Apo-Chlorthalidone, Thalitone)
- ethacrynic acid (Edecrin)
- etozolin (Elkapin)

- furosemide (Apo-Furosemide, Lasix)
- hydrochlorothiazide (Apo-Hydro, Microzide)
- hydroflumethiazide (Diucardin, Saluron)
- indapamide (Lozol, Nu-Indapamide)
- mannitol (Osmitrol, Resectisol)
- mefruside (Baycaron)
- methazolamide (Apo-Methazolamide, Neptazane)
- methyclothiazide (Aquatensen, Enduron)
- metolazone (Mykrox, Zaroxolyn)
- olmesartan and hydrochlorothiazide (Benicar HCT)
- polythiazide (Renese)
- torsemide (Demadex)
- trichlormethiazide (Metatensin, Naqua)
- urea (Amino-Cerv, UltraMide)
- xipamide (Diurexan, Lumitens)

Lab Tests That May Be Altered by Lily-of-the-Valley
None known

Diseases That May Be Worsened or Triggered by Lily-of-the-Valley
None known

Foods That May Interact with Lily-of-the-Valley
None known

Supplements That May Interact with Lily-of-the-Valley
- Increased risk of cardiac glycoside toxicity when used with other herbs that contain cardiac glycosides, such as black hellebore, calotropis, motherwort, and others. (For a list of cardiac glycoside–containing herbs and supplements, see Appendix B.)
- Increased risk of potassium depletion when used in conjunction with horsetail plant or licorice.

- Increased risk of cardiotoxicity due to potassium depletion when taken with cardioactive herbs, such as adonis, digitalis, and squill. (For a list of cardioactive herbs and supplements, see Appendix B.)
- Increased risk of potassium depletion when used with stimulant laxative herbs, such as black root, cascara sagrada, castor oil, and senna. (For a list of stimulant laxative herbs and supplements, see Appendix B.)
- Increased action of lily-of-the-valley when taken concurrently with English hawthorn.

LINDEN

The flowers of this large shade and avenue tree, found in the milder areas of Europe, Asia, and North America, have long been used to treat upset stomach, flatulence, and mild gallbladder ailments. At least one human study has confirmed the antispasmodic action of linden, particularly in the intestines. In tea form, linden flowers are used to promote sweating and ease fevers.

Scientific Name
Tilia species

Linden Is Also Commonly Known As
European lime, European linden, linn flowers

Medicinal Parts
Flower

Linden's Uses
To treat cough, bronchitis, fever, infectious diseases, and gallbladder and liver ailments. Ger-

many's Commission E has approved the use of linden flower to treat cough and bronchitis.

Typical Dose
A typical daily dose of linden may range from 2 to 4 gm of the herb.

Possible Side Effects
Linden's side effects include heart damage when the dried flower is taken orally, or the skin eruptions called urticaria (hives) when the dried flower is used topically.

Drugs That May Interact with Linden
Taking linden with these drugs may increase the risk of excessive sedation and mental depression and impairment:
- alprazolam (Apo-Alpraz, Xanax)
- clonazepam (Klonopin, Rivotril)
- diazepam (Apo-Diazepam, Valium)
- flurazepam (Apo-Flurazepam, Dalmane)
- lorazepam (Ativan, Nu-Loraz)
- midazolam (Apo-Midazolam, Versed)
- oxazepam (Novoxapam, Serax)
- temazepam (Novo-Temazepam, Restoril)
- triazolam (Apo-Triazo, Halcion)

Lab Tests That May Be Altered by Linden
None known

Diseases That May Be Worsened or Triggered by Linden
None known

Foods That May Interact with Linden
None known

Supplements That May Interact with Linden
None known

LOVAGE

In ancient times, lovage was planted in front of the house to keep away the plague, snakes, insects, and other evil forces. It was also often used in love potions. Today lovage is used to treat kidney disorders, gastric conditions, and respiratory congestion and as a sedative.

Scientific Name
Levisticum officinale

Lovage Is Also Commonly Known As
Bladder seed, lavose, love parsley, sea parsley, smallage, smellage

Medicinal Parts
Root, rhizome, fruit

Lovage's Uses
To treat indigestion, flatulence, menstrual problems, gastric conditions; to prevent kidney gravel

Typical Dose
A typical dose of lovage may range from 1.5 to 3.0 gm of finely chopped root mixed with 150 ml boiling water, steeped for ten to fifteen minutes, strained, and taken as a tea, two to three times a day.

Possible Side Effects

Lovage's side effects include allergic reactions and skin sensitivity to sun.

Drugs That May Interact with Lovage

Taking lovage with these drugs may increase skin sensitivity to sunlight:

- bumetanide (Bumex, Burinex)
- celecoxib (Celebrex)
- ciprofloxacin (Ciloxan, Cipro)
- doxycycline (Apo-Doxy, Vibramycin)
- enalapril (Vasotec)
- etodolac (Lodine, Utradol)
- fluphenazine (Modecate, Prolixin)
- fosinopril (Monopril)
- furosemide (Apo-Furosemide, Lasix)
- gatifloxacin (Tequin, Zymar)
- hydrochlorothiazide (Apo-Hydro, Microzide)
- ibuprofen (Advil, Motrin)
- indomethacin (Indocin, Novo-Methacin)
- ketoprofen (Orudis, Rhodis)
- ketorolac (Acular, Toradol)
- lansoprazole (Prevacid)
- levofloxacin (Levaquin, Quixin)
- lisinopril (Prinivil, Zestril)
- loratadine (Alavert, Claritin)
- methotrexate (Rheumatrex, Trexall)
- naproxen (Aleve, Naprosyn)
- nortriptyline (Aventyl HCl, Pamelor)
- ofloxacin (Floxin, Ocuflox)
- omeprazole (Losec, Prilosec)
- phenytoin (Dilantin, Phenytek)
- piroxicam (Feldene, Nu-Pirox)
- prochlorperazine (Compazine, Compro)
- quinapril (Accupril)
- risperidone (Risperdal)
- rofecoxib (Vioxx)
- tetracycline (Novo-Tetra, Sumycin)

Taking lovage with these drugs may increase the risk of bleeding or bruising:

- abciximab (ReoPro)
- aminosalicylic acid (Nemasol Sodium, Paser)
- antithrombin III (Thrombate III)
- argatroban
- aspirin (Bufferin, Ecotrin)
- aspirin and dipyridamole (Aggrenox)
- bivalirudin (Angiomax)
- choline magnesium trisalicylate (Trilisate)
- choline salicylate (Teejel)
- clopidogrel (Plavix)
- dalteparin (Fragmin)
- danaparoid (Orgaran)
- dipyridamole (Novo-Dipiradol, Persantine)
- enoxaparin (Lovenox)
- eptifibatide (Integrillin)
- fondaparinux (Arixtra)
- heparin (Hepalean, Hep-Lock)
- indobufen (Ibustrin)
- lepirudin (Refludan)
- salsalate (Amgesic, Salflex)
- ticlopidine (Alti-Ticlopidine, Ticlid)
- tinzaparin (Innohep)
- tirofiban (Aggrastat)
- warfarin (Coumadin, Jantoven)

Lab Tests That May Be Altered by Lovage

None known

Diseases That May Be Worsened or Triggered by Lovage

- May worsen hypertension by increasing sodium retention.
- May worsen kidney inflammation or impaired kidney function.

Foods That May Interact with Lovage
None known

Supplements That May Interact with Lovage
None known

LUNGWORT

Lungwort is so named because of its prowess as an expectorant and its ability to reduce bronchial mucus and restore lung elasticity, and because its speckled leaf somewhat resembles a lung. It is used to treat cough, congestion, and bronchitis as well as menstrual irregularity and diarrhea.

Scientific Name
Pulmonaria officinalis

Lungwort Is Also Commonly Known As
Common lungwort, Jerusalem sage, lungs of oak

Medicinal Parts
Leaf

Lungwort's Uses
To treat respiratory congestion, cough, diarrhea, various urinary and gastrointestinal tract ailments, and wounds

Typical Dose
A typical daily dose of lungwort has not been established.

Possible Side Effects
Lungwort's side effects include nausea, lack of appetite, and an increased tendency toward bleeding.

Drugs That May Interact with Lungwort
Taking lungwort with these drugs may increase the risk of bleeding and bruising:

- aminosalicylic acid (Nemasol Sodium, Paser)
- antithrombin III (Thrombate III)
- argatroban
- aspirin (Bufferin, Ecotrin)
- bivalirudin (Angiomax)
- choline magnesium trisalicylate (Trilisate)
- choline salicylate (Teejel)
- dalteparin (Fragmin)
- danaparoid (Orgaran)
- enoxaparin (Lovenox)
- fondaparinux (Arixtra)
- heparin (Hepalean, Hep-Lock)
- lepirudin (Refludan)
- salsalate (Amgesic, Salflex)
- tinzaparin (Innohep)
- warfarin (Coumadin, Jantoven)

Lab Tests That May Be Altered by Lungwort
None known

Diseases That May Be Worsened or Triggered by Lungwort
None known

Foods That May Interact with Lungwort
None known

Supplements That May Interact with Lungwort
None known

MADAGASCAR PERIWINKLE

This popular garden flower with its star-shaped pink, purple, or white flowers has long been used as a folk remedy for diabetes, wasp stings, coughs, and colds. In recent years, scientists discovered that the Madagascar periwinkle contains as many as seventy alkaloids, some of which lower blood sugar levels, ease hypertension, stop bleeding, fight cancer, and have a powerful tranquilizing effect.

Scientific Name

Catharanthus roseus

Madagascar Periwinkle Is Also Commonly Known As

Cape periwinkle, catharanthus, church-flower, magdalena, myrtle, periwinkle

Medicinal Parts

Above-ground parts

Madagascar Periwinkle's Uses

Internally, it is used as a diuretic and to treat diabetes, cough, inflammation of the throat, and lung congestion. Externally, it is used for insect stings and bites, skin infection, skin inflammation, and eye irritation.

Typical Dose

There is no typical dose of Madagascar periwinkle.

Possible Side Effects

Madagascar periwinkle's side effects include nausea, vomiting, hair loss, vertigo, hallucinations, and seizures.

Drugs That May Interact with Madagascar Periwinkle

Taking Madagascar periwinkle with these drugs may increase the risk of hypoglycemia (low blood sugar):

- acarbose (Prandase, Precose)
- acetohexamide
- chlorpropamide (Diabinese, Novo-Propamide)
- gliclazide (Diamicron, Novo-Gliclazide)
- glimepiride (Amaryl)
- glipizide (Glucotrol)
- glipizide and metformin (Metaglip)
- gliquidone (Beglynor, Glurenorm)
- glyburide (DiaBeta, Micronase)
- glyburide and metformin (Glucovance)
- insulin (Humulin, Novolin R)
- metformin (Glucophage, Riomet)
- miglitol (Glyset)
- nateglinide (Starlix)
- pioglitazone (Actos)
- repaglinide (GlucoNorm, Prandin)
- rosiglitazone (Avandia)
- rosiglitazone and metformin (Avandamet)
- tolazamide (Tolinase)
- tolbutamide (Apo-Tolbutamide, Tol-Tab)

Lab Tests That May Be Altered by Madagascar Periwinkle

May lower blood glucose.

Diseases That May Be Worsened or Triggered by Madagascar Periwinkle

May cause hypoglycemia (low blood sugar).

Foods That May Interact with Madagascar Periwinkle

None known

Supplements That May Interact with Madagascar Periwinkle

None known

MAGNESIUM

> Used by every cell in the body, the mineral magnesium participates in over three hundred biochemical reactions that help produce energy, bind calcium to tooth enamel, manufacture fats and proteins, and flush excess ammonia from the body. It also helps the muscles relax and is vital for proper heart function. Yet only a small amount of the mineral is found in the bloodstream. Should you run short of magnesium, you may develop muscle tremors, elevated blood pressure, gastrointestinal problems, personality and mood changes, generalized weakness, and other problems.

Typical Dose

The Food and Nutrition Board has set the RDA for magnesium at 400 mg per day for men ages nineteen to thirty and at 420 mg per day for men ages thirty-one and up. The RDA is 310 mg per day for women ages nineteen to thirty and 320 mg per day for women ages thirty-one and up.

Possible Side Effects

Taking too much supplemental magnesium can lead to weakness, lethargy, and diarrhea.

Drugs That May Interact with Magnesium

Taking magnesium with these drugs may increase the risk of muscular weakness and/or paralysis:

- amikacin (Amikin)
- dibekacin (Debekacyl, Dikacine)
- gentamicin (Alcomicin, Gentacidin)
- isepamicin (Exacin, Isepacine)
- kanamycin (Kantrex)
- neomycin (Myciguent, Neo-Fradin)
- streptomycin
- tobramycin (Nebcin, Tobrex)

Taking magnesium with these drugs may enhance the effects of the drug:

- atracurium (Tracrium)
- botulinum toxin type A (Botox, Botox Cosmetic)
- botulinum toxin type B (Myobloc)
- cisatracurium (Nimbex)
- doxacurium (Nuromax)
- mivacurium (Mivacron)
- pancuronium
- rocuronium (Zemuron)
- succinylcholine (Quelicin)
- vecuronium (Norcuron)

Taking magnesium with these drugs may increase the risk of hypotension (excessively low blood pressure):

- amlodipine (Norvasc)
- bepridil (Vascor)
- diltiazem (Cardizem, Tiazac)
- felodipine (Plendil, Renedil)
- isradipine (DynaCirc)
- lacidipine (Aponil, Caldine)
- lercanidipine (Cardiovasc, Carmen)
- manidipine (Calslot, Iperten)
- nicardipine (Cardene)
- nifedipine (Adalat CC, Procardia)
- nilvadipine

- nimodipine (Nimotop)
- nisoldipine (Sular)
- nitrendipine
- pinaverium (Dicetel)
- verapamil (Calan, Isoptin SR)

Taking magnesium with these drugs may decrease the absorption and/or effectiveness of the drug:

- alendronate (Fosamax, Novo-Alendronate)
- cinoxacin (Cinobac)
- ciprofloxacin (Ciloxan, Cipro)
- clodronate (Bonefos, Ostac)
- demeclocycline (Declomycin)
- doxycycline (Apo-Doxy, Vibramycin)
- etidronate (Didronel)
- gatifloxacin (Tequin, Zymar)
- gemifloxacin (Factive)
- ibandronic acid (Bondronat)
- levofloxacin (Levaquin, Quixin)
- lomefloxacin (Maxaquin)
- minocycline (Dynacin, Minocin)
- moxifloxacin (Avelox, Vigamox)
- nalidixic acid (NegGram)
- norfloxacin (Apo-Norflox, Noroxin)
- ofloxacin (Floxin, Ocuflox)
- oxytetracycline (Terramycin, Terramycin IM)
- pamidronate (Aredia)
- pefloxacin (Peflacine, Perflox)
- risedronate (Actonel)
- sparfloxacin (Zagam)
- tetracycline (Novo-Tetra, Sumycin)
- tiludronate (Skelid)
- trovafloxacin
- zoledronic acid (Zometa)

Taking magnesium with these drugs may be harmful to the heart:

- labetalol (Normodyne, Trandate)
- levomethadyl acetate hydrochloride

Drugs That May Interfere with the Absorption, Utilization, or Excretion of Magnesium

- acetazolamide (Apo-Acetazolamide, Diamox)
- alendronate (Fosamax, Novo-Alendronate)
- aluminum hydroxide (AlternaGel, Alu-Cap)
- aluminum hydroxide and magnesium carbonate (Gaviscon Liquid)
- aluminum hydroxide and magnesium hydroxide (Maalox, Mylanta)
- aluminum hydroxide, magnesium hydroxide, and simethicone (Mylanta Liquid)
- aluminum hydroxide and magnesium trisilicate (Gaviscon Tablet)
- amikacin (Amikin)
- amiloride and hydrochlorothiazide (Moduret, Nu-Amilzide)
- amphotericin B (Amphocin, Fungizone)
- arsenic trioxide (Trisenox)
- atenolol and chlorthalidone (Tenoretic)
- beclomethasone (Beconase, Vanceril)
- betamethasone (Betatrex, Maxivate)
- budesonide (Entocort, Rhinocort)
- bumetanide (Bumex, Burinex)
- busulfan (Busulfex, Myleran)
- calcium chloride
- candesartan and hydrochlorothiazide (Atacand HCT)
- carboplatin (Paraplatin, Paraplatin-AQ)
- chlorothiazide (Diuril)
- chlorthalidone (Apo-Chlorthalidone, Thalitone)
- cholestyramine (Prevalite, Questran)
- cisplatin (Platinol, Platinol-AQ)
- colchicine (ratio-Colchicine)
- cortisone (Cortone)

- cyclosporine (Neoral, Sandimmune)
- demeclocycline (Declomycin)
- dexamethasone (Decadron, Dexasone)
- diflorasone (Florone, Maxiflor)
- digoxin (Digoxin, Lanoxin)
- doxycycline (Apo-Doxy, Vibramycin)
- enalapril and hydrochlorothiazide (Vaseretic)
- enoxacin (Penetrex)
- ethacrynic acid (Edecrin)
- etidronate (Didronel)
- flucytosine (Ancobon)
- flunisolide (AeroBid-M, Nasarel)
- fluticasone (Cutivate, Flonase)
- foscarnet (Foscavir)
- furosemide (Apo-Furosemide, Lasix)
- gemtuzumab ozogamicin (Mylotarg)
- gentamicin (Alcomicin, Gentacidin)
- halobetasol (Ultravate)
- hydralazine (Apresoline, Novo-Hylazin)
- hydralazine and hydrochlorothiazide (Apresazide)
- hydrochlorothiazide (Apo-Hydro, Microzide)
- hydrochlorothiazide and spironolactone (Aldactazide, Novo-Spirozine)
- hydrochlorothiazide and triamterene (Dyazide, Maxzide)
- hydrocortisone (Cetacort, Locoid)
- indapamide (Lozol, Nu-Indapamide)
- irbesartan and hydrochlorothiazide (Avalide)
- kanamycin (Kantrex)
- levonorgestrel (Norplant Implant, Plan B)
- losartan and hydrochlorothiazide (Hyzaar)
- meclocycline (Meclan Topical)
- methyclothiazide (Aquatensen, Enduron)
- methyldopa and hydrochlorothiazide (Aldoril, PMS-Dopazide)
- methylprednisolone (Depoject Injection, Medrol Oral)
- metolazone (Mykrox, Zaroxolyn)
- minocycline (Dynacin, Minocin)
- moexipril and hydrochlorothiazide (Uniretic)
- mometasone furoate (Elocom, Nasonex)
- mycophenolate (CellCept)
- neomycin (Myciguent, Neo-Fradin)
- norethindrone (Aygestin, Micronor)
- pamidronate (Aredia)
- penicillamine (Cuprimine, Depen)
- pentamidine (NebuPent, Pentacarinat)
- polythiazide (Renese)
- potassium and sodium phosphate (K-Phos Neutral, Uro-KP-Neutral)
- potassium chloride (Apo-K, Micro-K)
- prazosin and polythiazide (Minizide)
- prednisolone (Inflamase Forte, Pred Forte)
- prednisone (Apo-Prednisone, Deltasone)
- propranolol and hydrochlorothiazide (Inderide)
- raloxifene (Evista)
- sodium phosphate (Fleet Enema, Fleet Phospho-Soda)
- spironolactone (Aldactone, Novo-Spiroton)
- streptomycin
- tacrolimus (Prograf, Protopic)
- telmisartan and hydrochlorothiazide (Micardis HCT, Micardis Plus)
- tetracycline (Novo-Tetra, Sumycin)
- tobramycin (Nebcin, Tobrex)
- torsemide (Demadex)
- triamcinolone (Aristocort, Trinasal)
- triamterene (Dyrenium)
- trichlormethiazide (Metahydrin, Naqua)
- valsartan and hydrochlorothiazide (Diovan HCT)
- voriconazole (VFEND)
- zalcitabine (Hivid)
- zoledronic acid (Zometa)

Lab Tests That May Be Altered by Magnesium

- May cause false increase in serum alkaline phosphatase test (when magnesium salts are used).
- May decrease serum angiotensin-converting enzyme levels (when magnesium sulfate is used).
- May lower blood pressure in those with mild to moderate hypertension.

Diseases That May Be Worsened or Triggered by Magnesium

None known

Foods That May Interact with Magnesium

None known

Supplements That May Interact with Magnesium

- In women, urinary excretion of magnesium may be decreased and blood levels of magnesium increased when boron supplements are taken.
- Absorption of dietary magnesium may be decreased when calcium supplements are taken.
- Absorption of magnesium is enhanced by supplemental vitamin D, especially when the vitamin is taken in large doses.
- Magnesium hydroxide taken with malic acid may decrease fibromyalgia-related pain and tenderness.
- Absorption of magnesium and magnesium balance may be decreased by supplemental zinc.

MA-HUANG

This Chinese medicine, used for thousands of years, contains the alkaloid ephedrine, which has been extensively promoted as a way to aid weight loss, enhance sports performance, and increase energy. As of 2004, however, all dietary supplements containing ephedrine were banned in the United States, when it was determined that using this substance could cause serious side effects, including heart attack, seizure, stroke, and death.

Scientific Name

Ephedra sinica

Ma-Huang Is Also Commonly Known As

Desert herb, ephedra, ephedrine, herbal ecstasy, sea grape, yellow horse

Medicinal Parts

Branch, root, rhizomes, whole plant

Ma-Huang's Uses

To treat asthma, cough, bronchitis, nasal congestion, joint ailments, pains in the bones; as a heart and central nervous system stimulant. Germany's Commission E has approved the use of ma-huang to treat cough and bronchitis.

Typical Dose

A typical dose of ma-huang may range from 12 to 30 mg total ephedra alkaloids, calculated as ephedrine, up to a maximum of 120 mg per day.

Possible Side Effects

❶ Ma-huang's side effects include dizziness, anxiety, irritability, insomnia, headache, anorexia, and nausea. It may also be associated with irregular heartbeat, heart attack, and sudden death.

Drugs That May Interact with Ma-Huang

Taking ma-huang with these drugs may increase the risk of hypertension (high blood pressure):

- acebutolol (Novo-Acebutolol, Sectral)
- albuterol (Proventil, Ventolin)
- amlodipine (Norvasc)
- atenolol (Apo-Atenol, Tenormin)
- benazepril (Lotensin)
- betaxolol (Betoptic S, Kerlone)
- bisoprolol (Monocor, Zebeta)
- brimonidine (Alphagan P, PMS-Brimonidine Tartrate)
- bumetanide (Bumex, Burinex)
- candesartan (Atacand)
- captopril (Capoten, Novo-Captopril)
- carteolol (Cartrol, Ocupress)
- carvedilol (Coreg)
- chlorothiazide (Diuril)
- chlorthalidone (Apo-Chlorthalidone, Thalitone)
- clonidine (Catapres, Duraclon)
- diazoxide (Hyperstat, Proglycem)
- diltiazem (Cardizem, Tiazac)
- dobutamine (Dobutrex)
- dopamine (Intropin)
- dopexamine (Dopacard)
- doxazosin (Alti-Doxazosin, Cardura)
- enalapril (Vasotec)
- ephedrine (PretzD)
- eplerenone (Inspra)
- eprosartan (Teveten)
- esmolol (Brevibloc)
- felodipine (Plendil, Renedil)
- fenoldopam (Corlopam)
- fosinopril (Monopril)
- furosemide (Apo-Furosemide, Lasix)
- guanabenz (Wytensin)
- guanadrel (Hylorel)
- guanfacine (Tenex)
- hydralazine (Apresoline, Novo-Hylazin)
- hydrochlorothiazide (Apo-Hydro, Microzide)
- hydrochlorothiazide and triamterene (Dyazide, Maxzide)
- indapamide (Lozol, Nu-Indapamide)
- irbesartan (Avapro)
- isoetharine (Beta2, Bronkosol)
- isoproterenol (Isuprel)
- isradipine (DynaCirc)
- labetalol (Normodyne, Trandate)
- lisinopril (Prinivil, Zestril)
- losartan (Cozaar)
- mecamylamine (Inversine)
- mefruside (Baycaron)
- metaproterenol (Alupent)
- metaraminol (Aramine)
- methyclothiazide (Aquatensen, Enduron)
- methyldopa (Apo-Methyldopa, Nu-Medopa)
- metolazone (Mykrox, Zaroxolyn)
- metoprolol (Betaloc, Lopressor)
- midodrine (Amatine, ProAmatine)
- minoxidil (Loniten, Rogaine)
- moexipril (Univasc)
- nadolol (Apo-Nadol, Corgard)
- nicardipine (Cardene)
- nifedipine (Adalat CC, Procardia)
- nisoldipine (Sular)
- nitroglycerin (Minitran, Nitro-Dur)
- nitroprusside (Nipride, Nitropress)
- norepinephrine (Levophed)
- olmesartan (Benicar)
- oxprenolol (Slow-Trasicor, Trasicor)
- oxytocin (Pitocin, Syntocinon)
- perindopril erbumine (Aceon, Coversyl)
- phenoxybenzamine (Dibenzyline)

- phentolamine (Regitine, Rogitine)
- phenylephrine (Neo-Synephrine, Vicks Sinex Nasal Spray)
- pindolol (Apo-Pindol, Novo-Pindol)
- polythiazide (Renese)
- prazosin (Minipress, Nu-Prazo)
- propranolol (Inderal, InnoPran XL)
- pseudoephedrine (Dimetapp Decongestant, Sudafed 12 Hour)
- pseudoephedrine (Dimetapp Decongestant, Sudafed)
- quinapril (Accupril)
- ramipril (Altace)
- reserpine
- spironolactone (Aldactone, Novo-Spiroton)
- telmisartan (Micardis)
- terazosin (Alti-Terazosin, Hytrin)
- terbutaline (Brethine)
- timolol (Betimol, Timoptic)
- torsemide (Demadex)
- trandolapril (Mavik)
- triamterene (Dyrenium)
- trichlormethiazide (Metatensin, Naqua)
- valsartan (Diovan)
- verapamil (Calan, Isoptin SR)

Taking ma-huang with these drugs may increase the risk of agitation, excessive sweating, hypertensive crisis, and hyperthermia:
- albuterol (Proventil, Ventolin)
- amitriptyline (Elavil, Levate)
- amitriptyline and chlordiazepoxide (Limbitrol)
- amitriptyline and perphenazine (Etrafon, Triavil)
- amoxapine (Asendin)
- brimonidine (Alphagan P, PMS-Brimonidine Tartrate)

- clomipramine (Anafranil, Novo-Clopramine)
- desipramine (Alti-Desipramine, Norpramin)
- dobutamine (Dobutrex)
- dopamine (Intropin)
- dopexamine (Dopacard)
- doxepin (Sinequan, Zonalon)
- ephedrine (PretzD)
- imipramine (Apo-Imipramine, Tofranil)
- iproniazid (Marsilid)
- isoetharine (Beta2, Bronkosol)
- isoproterenol (Isuprel)
- lofepramine (Feprapax, Gamanil)
- melitracen (Dixeran)
- metaproterenol (Alupent)
- metaraminol (Aramine)
- moclobemide (Alti-Moclobemide, Nu-Moclobemide)
- norepinephrine (Levophed)
- nortriptyline (Aventyl HCl, Pamelor)
- phenelzine (Nardil)
- phenylephrine (Neo-Synephrine, Vicks Sinex Nasal Spray)
- protriptyline (Vivactil)
- pseudoephedrine (Dimetapp Decongestant, Sudafed)
- selegiline (Eldepryl)
- terbutaline (Brethine)
- tranylcypromine (Parnate)
- trimipramine (Apo-Trimp, Surmontil)

Taking ma-huang with these drugs may reduce blood levels of the drug:
- beclomethasone (Beconase, Vanceril)
- betamethasone (Celestone, Diprolene)
- budesonide (Entocort, Rhinocort)
- budesonide and formoterol (Symbicort)

- cortisone (Cortone)
- deflazacort (Calcort, Dezacor)
- dexamethasone (Decadron, Dexasone)
- flunisolide (AeroBid, Nasarel)
- fluorometholone (Eflone, Flarex)
- fluticasone (Cutivate, Flonase)
- hydrocortisone (Anusol-HC, Locoid)
- methylprednisolone (DepoMedrol, Medrol)
- prednisolone (Inflamase Forte, Pred Forte)
- prednisone (Apo-Prednisone, Deltasone)
- triamcinolone (Aristocort, Trinasal)

Taking ma-huang with these drugs may increase the effects of the drug:
- albuterol (Proventil, Ventolin)
- brimonidine (Alphagan P, PMS-Brimonidine Tartrate)
- dobutamine (Dobutrex)
- dopamine (Intropin)
- dopexamine (Dopacard)
- ephedrine (PretzD)
- isoetharine (Beta2, Bronkosol)
- isoproterenol (Isuprel)
- metaproterenol (Alupent)
- metaraminol (Aramine)
- norepinephrine (Levophed)
- phenylephrine (Neo-Synephrine, Vicks Sinex Nasal Spray)
- pseudoephedrine (Dimetapp Decongestant, Sudafed, Sudafed 12-Hour)
- terbutaline (Brethine)

Taking ma-huang with these drugs may increase the risk of herb toxicity:
- acetazolamide (Apo-Acetazolamide, Diamox Sequels)
- aluminum hydroxide (AlternaGel, AluCap)
- aluminum hydroxide and magnesium carbonate (Gaviscon Extra Strength, Gaviscon Liquid)
- aluminum hydroxide and magnesium hydroxide (Maalox, Rulox)
- aluminum hydroxide and magnesium trisilicate (Gaviscon Tablet)
- aluminum hydroxide, magnesium hydroxide, and simethicone (Maalox, Mylanta Liquid)
- calcium carbonate (Rolaids Extra Strength, Tums)
- calcium carbonate and magnesium hydroxide (Mylanta Gelcaps, Rolaids Extra Strength)
- dichlorphenamide (Daranide)
- famotidine, calcium carbonate, and magnesium hydroxide (Pepcid Complete)
- magaldrate and simethicone (Riopan Plus, Riopan Plus Double Strength)
- magnesium hydroxide (Dulcolax Milk of Magnesia, Phillips' Milk of Magnesia)
- magnesium oxide (Mag-Ox 400, Uro-Mag)
- magnesium sulfate (Epsom salts)
- sodium bicarbonate (Brioschi, Neut)

Taking ma-huang with these drugs may increase the risk of tachycardia (rapid heart rate):
- chlorpromazine (Thorazine, Largactil)
- fluphenazine (Modecate, Prolixin)
- mesoridazine (Serentil)
- perphenazine (Apo-Perphenazine, Trilafon)
- prochlorperazine (Compazine, Compro)
- promethazine (Phenergan)
- thiethylperazine (Torecan)
- thioridazine (Mellaril)
- thiothixene (Navane)
- trifluoperazine (Novo-Trifluzine, Stelazine)

Taking ma-huang with these drugs may increase the risk of hyperglycemia (low blood sugar):
- acarbose (Prandase, Precose)
- acetohexamide
- chlorpropamide (Diabinese, Novo-Propamide)
- gliclazide (Diamicron, Novo-Gliclazide)
- glimepiride (Amaryl)
- glipizide (Glucotrol)
- glipizide and metformin (Metaglip)
- gliquidone (Beglynor, Glurenorm)
- glyburide (DiaBeta, Micronase)
- glyburide and metformin (Glucovance)
- insulin (Humulin, Novolin R)
- metformin (Glucophage, Riomet)
- miglitol (Glyset)
- nateglinide (Starlix)
- pioglitazone (Actos)
- repaglinide (GlucoNorm, Prandin)
- rosiglitazone (Avandia)
- rosiglitazone and metformin (Avandamet)
- tolazamide (Tolinase)
- tolbutamide (Apo-Tolbutamide, Tol-Tab)

Taking ma-huang with these drugs may be harmful:
- digitalis (Digitek, Lanoxin)—may increase the risk of arrhythmia (irregular heartbeat)
- reserpine—may increase the effects of the herb

Lab Tests That May Be Altered by Ma-Huang
- May cause false positive results in urine amphetamine/methamphetamine tests.
- May increase plasma catecholamine levels.
- May increase blood glucose levels.
- May increase blood lactate levels.
- May cause false positive results in urine ephedrine tests.
- May increase values on liver function tests, including aspartic acid transaminase (AST), alanine aminotransferase (ALT), total bilirubin, and urine bilirubin.

Diseases That May Be Worsened or Triggered by Ma-Huang
- May worsen anxiety.
- May worsen anorexia because it contains ephedra, which can reduce the appetite.
- May worsen diabetes by interfering with blood sugar control.
- May worsen heart disease by triggering rapid or irregular heartbeat.
- May encourage the formation of kidney stones.

Foods That May Interact with Ma-Huang
Increased stimulatory and adverse effects of both ma-huang and caffeine when the two are taken together.

Supplements That May Interact with Ma-Huang
- Increased risk of insomnia, nervousness, dizziness, elevated blood pressure (hypertension), and adverse cardiovascular effects when used with herbs and supplements that have stimulant properties, such as caffeine, coffee, cola nut, and others. (For a list of herbs and supplements that have stimulant properties, see Appendix B.)
- May cause increased vasoconstriction (constriction of blood vessels) and hypertension (elevated blood pressure) when combined with ergot alkaloid derivatives.

- When used with Panax ginseng, may increase the risk of arrhythmia (irregular heartbeat).

Maitake Mushroom

Known by its Japanese name of maitake, this fungus is a time-honored medicine and a delectable culinary item. Its name means "dancing mushroom" because, according to legend, people would dance for joy when they came upon it in the woods. Research has indicated that substances in the maitake mushroom can strengthen the body's defenses by activating immune-system "soldiers" called T-cells, and may shrink certain tumors and protect immune system cells from destruction by HIV.

Scientific Name
Grifola frondosa

Maitake Mushroom Is Also Commonly Known As
Dancing mushroom, king of mushrooms, monkey's bench

Medicinal Parts
Body and mycelium

Maitake Mushroom's Uses
To treat diabetes mellitus, high cholesterol, hypertension (high blood pressure), and obesity

Typical Dose
A typical daily dose of maitake mushroom may range from 200 to 500 mg.

Possible Side Effects
There are no known side effects when maitake mushroom is taken in recommended dosages.

Drugs That May Interact with Maitake Mushroom
Taking maitake mushroom with these drugs may decrease the effectiveness of the drug:
- antithymocyte globulin (equine) (Atgam)
- antithymocyte globulin (rabbit) (Thymoglobulin)
- azathioprine (Imuran)
- basiliximab (Simulect)
- cyclosporine (Neoral, Sandimmune)
- daclizumab (Zenapax)
- efalizumab (Raptiva)
- methotrexate (Rheumatrex, Trexall)
- muromonab-CD3 (Orthoclone OKT 3)
- mycophenolate (CellCept)
- pimecrolimus (Elidel)
- sirolimus (Rapamune)
- tacrolimus (Prograf, Protopic)
- thalidomide (Thalomid)

Taking maitake mushroom with these drugs may increase the risk of hypoglycemia (low blood sugar):
- acarbose (Prandase, Precose)
- acetohexamide
- chlorpropamide (Diabinese, Novo-Propamide)
- gliclazide (Diamicron, Novo-Gliclazide)
- glimepiride (Amaryl)
- glipizide (Glucotrol)
- glipizide and metformin (Metaglip)
- gliquidone (Beglynor, Glurenorm)
- glyburide (DiaBeta, Micronase)
- glyburide and metformin (Glucovance)
- insulin (Humulin, Novolin R)

- metformin (Glucophage, Riomet)
- miglitol (Glyset)
- nateglinide (Starlix)
- pioglitazone (Actos)
- repaglinide (GlucoNorm, Prandin)
- rosiglitazone (Avandia)
- rosiglitazone and metformin (Avandamet)
- tolazamide (Tolinase)
- tolbutamide (Apo-Tolbutamide, Tol-Tab)

Lab Tests That May Be Altered by Maitake Mushroom
May lower blood glucose levels in those with type 2 diabetes.

Diseases That May Be Worsened or Triggered by Maitake Mushroom
May lower blood sugar levels in those with diabetes.

Foods That May Interact with Maitake Mushroom
None known

Supplements That May Interact with Maitake Mushroom
May increase blood glucose–lowering effects and risk of hypoglycemia (low blood sugar) when used with herbs and supplements that lower glucose levels, such as alpha-lipoic acid, chromium, devil's claw, Panax ginseng, and psyllium. (For a list of herbs and supplements that lower blood glucose levels, see Appendix B.)

MANDRAKE

Ancient Israeli tribes, always outnumbered by hostile neighbors, used mandrake to help ensure their marriages would be fruitful and their ranks would increase. During the Middle Ages and Renaissance, mandrake was associated with sex and fertility, which may explain why it's also known as Satan's apple. Used by Native Americans as a laxative and to remove intestinal parasites, in modern times mandrake root has been investigated as a possible treatment for leukemia.

Scientific Name:
Mandragora officinarum

Mandrake Is Also Commonly Known As
Alraunwurzel, mandragora, Satan's apple

Medicinal Parts
Root, whole plant

Mandrake's Uses
To treat stomach ulcers, hay fever, whooping cough, and asthma

Typical Dose
There is no typical dose of mandrake.

Possible Side Effects
Mandrake's side effects include drowsiness, confusion, dry mouth, blurred vision, decreased sweating, overheating, and flushing.

Drugs That May Interact with Mandrake
Taking mandrake with these drugs may increase the therapeutic and/or adverse effects of the drug:

- atropine (Isopto Atropine, Sal-Tropine)
- benztropine (Apo-Benztropine, Cogentin)
- clidinium and chlordiazepoxide (Apo-Chlorax, Librax)
- cyclopentolate (Cyclogyl, Cylate)
- dicyclomine (Bentyl, Lomine)
- glycopyrrolate (Robinul, Robinul Forte)
- homatropine (Isopto Homatropine)
- hyoscyamine (Hyosine, Levsin)
- hyoscyamine, atropine, scopolamine, and phenobarbital (Donnatal, Donnatal Extentabs)
- ipratropium (Atrovent, Nu-Ipratropium)
- oxitropium (Oxivent, Tersigat)
- prifinium (Padrin, Riabel)
- procyclidine (Kemadrin, Procyclid)
- propantheline (Propanthel)
- scopolamine (Scopace, Transderm Scop)
- tiotropium (Spiriva)
- tolterodine (Detrol, Detrol LA)
- trihexyphenidyl (Apo-Trihex)
- trimethobenzamide (Tigan)

Lab Tests That May Be Altered by Mandrake
None known

Diseases That May Be Worsened or Triggered by Mandrake
May worsen coronary artery disease, rapid heart rate, congestive heart failure, elevated blood pressure, stomach ulcers, gastrointestinal ailments, gastroesophageal reflux disease (GERD), narrow-angle glaucoma, benign prostatic hypertrophy (BPH), liver disease, or kidney disease.

Foods That May Interact with Mandrake
None known

Supplements That May Interact with Mandrake
May increase positive and negative effects of herbs and supplements that have anticholinergic effects, such as belladonna, henbane, and scopolia. (For a list of herbs and supplements that have anticholinergic effects, see Appendix B.)

MANNA

Manna is the sugary sap taken from the south European flowering ash, a small tree native to the coasts of the Mediterranean. It is used medicinally as a gentle laxative. Studies have shown that manna has a number of health-enhancing properties, including the ability to fight off viruses, control oxidation, prevent sun-induced damage, quell inflammation, and strengthen the immune system.

Scientific Name
Fraxinus ornus

Manna Is Also Commonly Known As
Flake manna, flowering ash, manna ash

Medicinal Parts
Juice extracted from the bark

Manna's Uses
To soften stool in cases of hemorrhoids and other situations in which easy elimination is desired. Germany's Commission E has approved the use of manna to treat constipation.

Typical Dose

A typical dose of manna may range from 20 to 30 gm.

Possible Side Effects

Manna's side effects include flatulence and nausea.

Drugs That May Interact with Manna

Taking manna with these drugs may increase the risk of hypokalemia (low levels of potassium in the blood):

- acetazolamide (Apo-Acetazolamide, Diamox Sequels)
- azosemide (Diat)
- bumetanide (Bumex, Burinex)
- chlorothiazide (Diuril)
- chlorthalidone (Apo-Chlorthalidone, Thalitone)
- ethacrynic acid (Edecrin)
- etozolin (Elkapin)
- furosemide (Apo-Furosemide, Lasix)
- hydrochlorothiazide (Apo-Hydro, Microzide)
- hydrochlorothiazide and triamterene (Dyazide, Maxzide)
- hydroflumethiazide (Diucardin, Saluron)
- indapamide (Lozol, Nu-Indapamide)
- mannitol (Osmitrol, Resectisol)
- mefruside (Baycaron)
- methazolamide (Apo-Methazolamide, Neptazane)
- methyclothiazide (Aquatensen, Enduron)
- metolazone (Mykrox, Zaroxolyn)
- olmesartan and hydrochlorothiazide (Benicar HCT)
- polythiazide (Renese)
- torsemide (Demadex)
- trichlormethiazide (Metatensin, Naqua)
- urea (Amino-Cerv, UltraMide)
- xipamide (Diurexan, Lumitens)

Lab Tests That May Be Altered by Manna

None known

Diseases That May Be Worsened or Triggered by Manna

May worsen cases of intestinal or bowel obstruction.

Foods That May Interact with Manna

None known

Supplements That May Interact with Manna

- Increased risk of potassium depletion when used in conjunction with horsetail plant or licorice.
- Increased risk of potassium depletion when used with other stimulant laxative herbs, such as black root, cascara sagrada, castor oil, and senna. (For a list of stimulant laxative herbs and supplements, see Appendix B.)

MARIJUANA

Marijuana, a relative of the hops plant, has been used since ancient times as a medicinal and psychoactive agent. The leaves, which are typically smoked but may be ingested, contain hundreds of chemicals, but the main active ingredient is tetrahydrocannabinol (THC). Marijuana has been used to ease the pain, nausea, and vomiting associated with chemotherapy; relieve headaches; ease symptoms of glaucoma; and induce relaxation, among other things.

Scientific Name
Cannabis sativa

Marijuana Is Also Commonly Known As
Cannabis, grass, Indian hemp, pot, weed

Medicinal Parts
Leaf, flower, twig tips

Marijuana's Uses
To treat glaucoma, constipation, beriberi, gout, rheumatism, insomnia, cough, nerve pain, and asthma; to stimulate the appetite; to produce mind-altering effects

Typical Dose
There is no standard dose of marijuana.

Possible Side Effects
Marijuana's side effects include impaired reaction time and motor coordination, nausea, vomiting, dry mouth, panic, rapid heart rate, irregular heartbeat, and depression and other emotional disturbances.

Drugs That May Interact with Marijuana
Taking marijuana with these drugs may increase the heart rate and the risk of delirium:
- amitriptyline (Elavil, Levate)
- amitriptyline and chlordiazepoxide (Limbitrol)
- amitriptyline and perphenazine (Etrafon, Triavil)
- amoxapine (Asendin)
- clomipramine (Anafranil, Novo-Clopramine)
- desipramine (Alti-Desipramine, Norpramin)
- doxepin (Sinequan, Zonalon)
- imipramine (Apo-Imipramine, Tofranil)
- lofepramine (Feprapax, Gamanil)
- melitracen (Dixeran)
- nortriptyline (Aventyl HCl, Pamelor)
- protriptyline (Vivactil)
- trimipramine (Apo-Trimip, Surmontil)

Taking marijuana with these drugs may increase the risk of excessive sedation and mental depression and impairment:
- amobarbital (Amytal)
- amobarbital and secobarbital (Tuinal)
- butabarbital (Butisol Sodium)
- butalbital, acetaminophen, and caffeine (Esgic, Fioricet)
- butalbital, aspirin, and caffeine (Fiorinal)
- mephobarbital (Mebaral)
- methohexital (Brevital, Brevital Sodium)
- pentobarbital (Nembutal)
- phenobarbital (Luminal Sodium, PMS-Phenobarbital)
- primidone (Apo-Primidone, Mysoline)
- secobarbital (Seconal)
- thiopental (Pentothal)

Taking marijuana with these drugs may interfere with absorption of the drug:
- amprenavir (Agenerase)
- indinavir (Crixivan)
- lopinavir and ritonavir (Kaletra)
- nelfinavir (Viracept)
- ritonavir (Norvir)
- saquinavir (Fortovase, Invirase)

Taking marijuana with these drugs may cause symptoms of mania:
- citalopram (Celexa)
- fluoxetine (Prozac, Sarafem)

- fluvoxamine (Alti-Fluvoxamine, Luvox)
- paroxetine (Paxil)
- s-citalopram (Lexapro)
- sertraline (Apo-Sertraline, Zoloft)

Taking marijuana with these drugs may be harmful:

- disulfiram (Antabuse)—may increase the risk of low-level mania (excitability, hyperactivity, talkativeness, quick anger, and other symptoms)
- theophylline (Elixophyllin, Theochron)—may speed clearance of theophylline from the bloodstream, necessitating an increased dose of the drug

Lab Tests That May Be Altered by Marijuana

May decrease intraocular pressure and glaucoma test results.

Diseases That May Be Worsened or Triggered by Marijuana

- May cause rapid heartbeat and temporarily elevated blood pressure.
- May increase susceptibility to infections by suppressing the immune system.
- May worsen respiratory ailments.
- May encourage development of psychosis in both psychosis-free and psychosis-prone individuals.

Foods That May Interact with Marijuana

Increased or synergistic central nervous system effects (for example, impaired reaction time, motor coordination, and visual perception) with concurrent ingestion of alcohol.

Supplements That May Interact with Marijuana

May enhance therapeutic and adverse effects of herbs and supplements that have sedative properties, such as 5-HTP, kava kava, St. John's wort, and valerian. (For a list of herbs and supplements that have sedative properties, see Appendix B.)

MARSHMALLOW

The names are the same, but this herb is *not* related to the soft sugary thing roasted over campfires. The herb marshmallow, which is grown near salt marshes, contains a gummy substance called mucilage that can relieve inflamed tissues and soothe coughs. Studies suggest that the pectin in marshmallow can help control blood sugar and combat constipation, while other ingredients may stimulate immune cells to fight off invaders.

Scientific Name

Althaea officinalis

Marshmallow Is Also Commonly Known As

Althea, Moorish mallow, mortification root, sweet weed, wymote

Medicinal Parts

Flower, leaf, root

Marshmallow's Uses

Marshmallow leaf and marshmallow root are used to treat cough, bronchitis, diarrhea, ulcers, and insect bites. Germany's Commission E has approved the use of marshmallow leaf to treat cough and bronchitis and marshmallow root to treat irritation of the mouth and throat and inflammation of the gastric mucosa.

Typical Dose

A typical dose of marshmallow is approximately 5 gm of the root or 6 gm of the leaf.

Possible Side Effects

Marshmallow's side effects include hypoglycemia (low blood sugar), nausea, vomiting, anorexia, and allergic reactions.

Drugs That May Interact with Marshmallow

Taking marshmallow with these drugs may increase the risk of hypoglycemia (low blood sugar):

- acarbose (Prandase, Precose)
- acetohexamide
- chlorpropamide (Diabinese, Novo-Propamide)
- gliclazide (Diamicron, Novo-Gliclazide)
- glimepiride (Amaryl)
- glipizide (Glucotrol)
- glipizide and metformin (Metaglip)
- gliquidone (Beglynor, Glurenorm)
- glyburide (DiaBeta, Micronase)
- glyburide and metformin (Glucovance)
- insulin (Humulin, Novolin R)
- metformin (Glucophage, Riomet)
- miglitol (Glyset)
- nateglinide (Starlix)
- pioglitazone (Actos)
- repaglinide (GlucoNorm, Prandin)
- rosiglitazone (Avandia)
- rosiglitazone and metformin (Avandamet)
- tolazamide (Tolinase)
- tolbutamide (Apo-Tolbutamide, Tol-Tab)

Taking marshmallow with these drugs may interfere with drug absorption:

- all drugs taken orally

Lab Tests That May Be Altered by Marshmallow

May lower blood glucose results.

Diseases That May Be Worsened or Triggered by Marshmallow

None known

Foods That May Interact with Marshmallow

None known

Supplements That May Interact with Marshmallow

May decrease absorption of other herbs or supplements when taken concurrently.

MATÉ

Maté (also called yerba maté, which means "herb cup") is a species of holly originating in parts of South America. Its leaves, which contain caffeine, theophylline, and theobromine, are brewed into tea, and the drink is taken as a stimulant. A 2005 study found that maté can slow glycation, the improper linking of sugars and proteins that lays the foundation for many of the health complications seen in elevated blood sugar and diabetes. An earlier study showed that maté extract triggers the destruction of certain cancer cells.

Scientific Name

Ilex paraguariensis

Maté Is Also Commonly Known As

Chimarro, Jesuit's tea, maté folium, St. Bartholomew's tea, yerba maté

Medicinal Parts

Leaf

Maté's Uses

To treat depression, fatigue, ulcers, inflammation, rheumatism, diabetes, and anemia. Germany's Commission E has approved the use of maté to treat lack of stamina.

Typical Dose

A typical daily dose of maté may range from 2 to 3 gm of the herb.

Possible Side Effects

Maté's side effects may include insomnia, nausea, and rapid heart rate. Prolonged use of maté may increase the risk of mouth, esophageal, kidney, bladder, and lung cancer.

Drugs That May Interact with Maté

Taking maté with these drugs may cause or increase liver damage:

- abacavir (Ziagen)
- acarbose (Prandase, Precose)
- acetaminophen (Genapap, Tylenol)
- allopurinol (Aloprim, Zyloprim)
- atorvastatin (Lipitor)
- celecoxib (Celebrex)
- cidofovir (Vistide)
- cimetidine (Nu-Cimet, Tagamet)
- ciprofloxacin (Ciloxan, Cipro)
- cyclosporine (Neoral, Sandimmune)
- meloxicam (MOBIC, Mobicox)

- methotrexate (Rheumatrex, Trexall)
- methyldopa (Apo-Methyldopa, Nu-Medopa)
- modafinil (Alertec, Provigil)
- morphine hydrochloride
- morphine sulfate (Kadian, MS Contin)
- naproxen (Aleve, Naprosyn)
- nelfinavir (Viracept)
- nevirapine (Viramune)
- nitrofurantoin (Macrobid, Furadantin)
- ondansetron (Zofran)
- paclitaxel (Onxol, Taxol)
- pantoprazole (Pantoloc, Protonix)
- phenytoin (Dilantin, Phenytek)
- pioglitazone (Actos)
- piroxicam (Feldene, Nu-Pirox)
- pravastatin (Novo-Pravastatin, Pravachol)
- prochlorperazine (Compazine, Compro)
- propoxyphene (Darvon, Darvon-N)
- repaglinide (GlucoNorm, Prandin)
- rifampin (Rifadin, Rimactane)
- rifapentine (Priftin)
- ritonavir (Norvir)
- rofecoxib (Vioxx)
- rosiglitazone (Avandia)
- saquinavir (Fortovase, Invirase)
- simvastatin (Apo-Simvastatin, Zocor)
- stavudine (Zerit)
- tamoxifen (Nolvadex, Tamofen)
- tramadol (Ultram)
- zidovudine (Novo-AZT, Retrovir)

Taking maté with these drugs may interfere with the actions of the drug:

- acetaminophen and codeine (Capital and Codeine, Tylenol with Codeine)
- alfentanil (Alfenta)

- alprazolam (Apo-Alpraz, Xanax)
- amobarbital (Amytal)
- amobarbital and secobarbital (Tuinal)
- aspirin and codeine (Coryphen Codeine)
- belladonna and opium (B&O Supprettes)
- bromazepam (Apo-Bromazepam, Gen-Bromazepam)
- brotizolam (Lendorm, Sintonal)
- buprenorphine (Buprenex, Subutex)
- buprenorphine and naloxone (Suboxone)
- butabarbital (Butisol Sodium)
- butalbital, acetaminophen, and caffeine (Esgic, Fioricet)
- butalbital, aspirin, and caffeine (Fiorinal)
- butorphanol (Apo-Butorphanol, Stadol)
- chloral hydrate (Aquachloral Supprettes, Somnote)
- chlordiazepoxide Apo-Chlordiazepoxide, Librium)
- clobazam (Alti-Clobazam, Frisium)
- clonazepam (Klonopin, Rivotril)
- clorazepate (Tranxene, T-Tab)
- codeine (Codeine Contin)
- dexmedetomidine (Precedex)
- diazepam (Apo-Diazepam, Valium)
- dihydrocodeine, aspirin, and caffeine (Synalgos-DC)
- diphenhydramine (Benadryl Allergy, Nytol)
- estazolam (ProSom)
- fentanyl (Actiq, Duragesic)
- flurazepam (Apo-Flurazepam, Dalmane)
- glutethimide
- haloperidol (Haldol, Novo-Peridol)
- hydrocodone and acetaminophen (Vicodin, Zydone)
- hydrocodone and aspirin (Damason-P)
- hydrocodone and ibuprofen (Vicoprofen)
- hydromorphone (Dilaudid, PMS-Hydromorphone)
- hydroxyzine (Atarax, Vistaril)
- levomethadyl acetate hydrochloride
- levorphanol (LevoDromoran)
- loprazolam (Dormonoct, Havlane)
- lorazepam (Ativan, Nu-Loraz)
- meperidine (Demerol, Meperitab)
- meperidine and promethazine
- mephobarbital (Mebaral)
- methadone (Dolophine, Methadose)
- methohexital (Brevital, Brevital Sodium)
- midazolam (Apo-Midazolam, Versed)
- morphine sulfate (Kadian, MS Contin)
- nalbuphine (Nubain)
- opium tincture
- oxazepam (Novoxapam, Serax)
- oxycodone (OxyContin, Roxicodone)
- oxycodone and acetaminophen (Endocet, Percocet)
- oxycodone and aspirin (Endodan, Percodan)
- oxymorphone (Numorphan)
- paregoric
- pentazocine (Talwin)
- pentobarbital (Nembutal)
- phenobarbital (Luminal Sodium, PMS-Phenobarbital)
- phenoperidine
- prazepam
- primidone (Apo-Primidone, Mysoline)
- promethazine (Phenergan)
- propofol (Diprivan)
- propoxyphene (Darvon, Darvon-N)
- propoxyphene and acetaminophen (Darvocet-N 50, Darvocet-N 100)
- propoxyphene, aspirin, and caffeine (Darvon Compound)

- quazepam (Doral)
- remifentanil (Ultiva)
- secobarbital (Seconal)
- sufentanil (Sufenta)
- s-zopiclone (Lunesta)
- temazepam (Novo-Temazepam, Restoril)
- tetrazepam (Mobiforton, Musapam)
- thiopental (Pentothal)
- triazolam (Apo-Triazo, Halcion)
- zaleplon (Sonata, Stamoc)
- zolpidem (Ambien)
- zopiclone (Alti-Zopiclone, Gen-Zopiclone)

Taking maté with these drugs may increase the diuretic effects of the drug:
- acetazolamide (Apo-Acetazolamide, Diamox Sequels)
- amiloride (Midamor)
- azosemide (Diat)
- bumetanide (Bumex, Burinex)
- chlorothiazide (Diuril)
- chlorthalidone (Apo-Chlorthalidone, Thalitone)
- ethacrynic acid (Edecrin)
- etozolin (Elkapin)
- furosemide (Apo-Furosemide, Lasix)
- hydrochlorothiazide (Apo-Hydro, Microzide)
- hydrochlorothiazide and triamterene (Dyazide, Maxzide)
- hydroflumethiazide (Diucardin, Saluron)
- indapamide (Lozol, Nu-Indapamide)
- mannitol (Osmitrol, Resectisol)
- mefruside (Baycaron)
- methazolamide (Apo-Methazolamide, Neptazane)
- methyclothiazide (Aquatensen, Enduron)
- metolazone (Mykrox, Zaroxolyn)

- olmesartan and hydrochlorothiazide (Benicar HCT)
- polythiazide (Renese)
- spironolactone (Aldactone, Novo-Spiroton)
- torsemide (Demadex)
- triamterene (Dyrenium)
- trichlormethiazide (Metatensin, Naqua)
- urea (Amino-Cerv, UltraMide)
- xipamide (Diurexan, Lumitens)

Taking maté with these drugs may increase the therapeutic and/or adverse effects of the drug:
- dexmethylphenidate (Focalin)
- dextroamphetamine (Dexedrine, Dextrostat)
- dextroamphetamine and amphetamine (Adderall, Adderall XR)
- doxapram (Dopram)
- methamphetamine (Desoxyn)
- methylphenidate (Concerta, Ritalin)
- modafinil (Alertec, Provigil)
- pemoline (Cylert, PemADD)

Maté contains caffeine, so see Caffeine and Caffeine-Containing Herbs on p. 111 for an additional list of drugs that may interact with this herb.

Lab Tests That May Be Altered by Maté
See Caffeine and Caffeine-Containing Herbs on p. 112 for a list of lab tests that may interact with the caffeine in this herb.

Diseases That May Be Worsened or Triggered by Maté
May increase the risk of cancer among smokers. See Caffeine and Caffeine-Containing Herbs on p. 113 for a list of diseases that may be worsened or triggered by the caffeine in this herb.

Foods That May Interact with Maté

May increase therapeutic and adverse effects of caffeine when taken together with caffeine-containing foods and drinks. (For a list of caffeine-containing herbs, foods, and supplements, see Appendix B.)

Supplements That May Interact with Maté

See Caffeine and Caffeine-Containing Herbs on p. 113 for a list of supplements that may interact with the caffeine in this herb.

MAYAPPLE

The mayapple, native to the woodlands of Canada and the eastern United States, is a small plant that produces a single white flower in May, which later turns into a yellow berry that resembles a tiny apple. The mayapple rhizome contains high amounts of the compounds podophyllotoxin and alpha and beta peltatin, which have cancer-fighting properties. Extracts of mayapple are currently used in certain topical medications for genital warts and some forms of skin cancer.

Scientific Name

Podophyllum peltatum

Mayapple Is Also Commonly Known As

Duck's foot, hog apple, mandrake, raccoon berry, wild lemon

Medicinal Parts

Rhizome, resin extracted from rhizome

Mayapple's Uses

To treat warts, fever, snakebite, and syphilis; and as a laxative. Germany's Commission E has approved the use of mayapple to treat warts.

Typical Dose

A typical daily dose of mayapple root may range from 1.5 to 3.0 gm per day, applied to the skin.

Possible Side Effects

Mayapple's side effects may include severe skin irritation.

Drugs That May Interact with Mayapple

Taking mayapple with these drugs may increase the risk of hypokalemia (low levels of potassium in the blood):

- acetazolamide (Apo-Acetazolamide, Diamox Sequels)
- azosemide (Diat)
- bumetanide (Bumex, Burinex)
- chlorothiazide (Diuril)
- chlorthalidone (Apo-Chlorthalidone, Thalitone)
- ethacrynic acid (Edecrin)
- etozolin (Elkapin)
- furosemide (Apo-Furosemide, Lasix)
- hydrochlorothiazide (Apo-Hydro, Microzide)
- hydroflumethiazide (Diucardin, Saluron)
- indapamide (Lozol, Nu-Indapamide)
- mannitol (Osmitrol, Resectisol)
- mefruside (Baycaron)
- methazolamide (Apo-Methazolamide, Neptazane)
- methyclothiazide (Aquatensen, Enduron)
- metolazone (Mykrox, Zaroxolyn)
- olmesartan and hydrochlorothiazide (Benicar HCT)

- polythiazide (Renese)
- torsemide (Demadex)
- trichlormethiazide (Metatensin, Naqua)
- urea (Amino-Cerv, UltraMide)
- xipamide (Diurexan, Lumitens)

Taking mayapple with these drugs may decrease the laxative effect of the herb:
- belladonna and opium (B&O Supprettes)
- belladonna, phenobarbital, and ergotamine (Bellamine S, Bel-Tabs)
- ipecac

Lab Tests That May Be Altered by Mayapple

May decrease red blood cell concentration.

Diseases That May Be Worsened or Triggered by Mayapple

May worsen gastrointestinal ailments by irritating the gastrointestinal tract.

Foods That May Interact with Mayapple

Increased laxative effect of mayapple when used concurrently with salt.

Supplements That May Interact with Mayapple
- Increased risk of cardiac glycoside toxicity when used with other herbs that contain cardiac glycosides, such as black hellebore, calotropis, motherwort, and others. (For a list of cardiac glycoside–containing herbs and supplements, see Appendix B.)
- Increased risk of potassium depletion when used in conjunction with horsetail plant or licorice.
- Increased risk of potassium depletion when used with other stimulant laxative herbs, such as black root, cascara sagrada, castor oil, and senna. (For a list of stimulant laxative herbs and supplements, see Appendix B.)
- Decreased laxative effect of mayapple when used concurrently with hyoscyamus, leptandra, or lobelia.

MEADOWSWEET

A member of the rose family, this sweet-smelling, fuzzy white flower was one of the three most sacred herbs of the Druids. It contains aspirin-like chemicals that help reduce fever and relieve pain and is also used to soothe the digestive tract, reduce excessive acidity, and ease nausea. In various studies, the herb has demonstrated the ability to destroy bacteria, control oxidation, and help keep the blood thin and less likely to clot unnecessarily.

Scientific Name

Filipendula ulmaria

Meadowsweet Is Also Commonly Known As

Bridewort, dolloff, dropwort, meadsweet, queen of the meadow

Medicinal Parts

Flower, whole plant

Meadowsweet's Uses

To treat cough, bronchitis, gout, headaches, stomach ulcers, diarrhea, and rheumatism of the joints. Germany's Commission E has approved the use of meadowsweet flower to treat cough, bronchitis, colds, and fever and the use of meadowsweet herb to treat cough and bronchitis.

Typical Dose

A typical daily dose of meadowsweet may range from 2.5 to 3.5 gm of meadowsweet flower or 4 to 5 gm of meadowsweet herb.

Possible Side Effects

Meadowsweet's more common side effects (flower or herb) include nausea, vomiting, anorexia, and allergic reactions.

Drugs That May Interact with Meadowsweet

Taking meadowsweet with these drugs may increase the risk of bleeding or bruising:
- abciximab (ReoPro)
- antithrombin III (Thrombate III)
- argatroban
- aspirin (Bufferin, Ecotrin)
- bivalirudin (Angiomax)
- celecoxib (Celebrex)
- dalteparin (Fragmin)
- danaparoid (Orgaran)
- enoxaparin (Lovenox)
- etodolac (Lodine, Utradol)
- fondaparinux (Arixtra)
- heparin (Hepalean, Hep-Lock)
- ibuprofen (Advil, Motrin)
- indomethacin (Indocin, Novo-Methacin)
- ketoprofen (Orudis, Rhodis)
- ketorolac (Acular, Toradol)
- lepirudin (Refludan)
- meloxicam (MOBIC, Mobicox)
- naproxen (Aleve, Naprosyn)
- piroxicam (Feldene, Nu-Pirox)
- rofecoxib (Vioxx)
- ticlopidine (Alti-Ticlopidine, Ticlid)
- tinzaparin (Innohep)
- urokinase (Abbokinase)
- warfarin (Coumadin, Jantoven)

Taking meadowsweet with these drugs may interfere with absorption of the drug:
- ferric gluconate (Ferrlecit)
- ferrous fumarate (Femiron, Feostat)
- ferrous gluconate (Fergon, Novo-Ferrogluc)
- ferrous sulfate (Feratab, Fer-Iron)
- ferrous sulfate and ascorbic acid (FeroGrad 500, Vitelle Irospan)
- iron-dextran complex (Dexferrum, INFeD)
- polysaccharide-iron complex (Hytinic, Niferex)

Lab Tests That May Be Altered by Meadowsweet

None known

Diseases That May Be Worsened or Triggered by Meadowsweet

None known

Foods That May Interact with Meadowsweet

None known

Supplements That May Interact with Meadowsweet

None known

MILK THISTLE

An ancient medicinal herb used to protect and purify the liver as early as A.D. 23, milk thistle's active ingredient is silymarin. Scientific research has shown that silymarin helps guard against the

continued

liver damage caused by ethanol and other substances, prevent blockages that can interfere with the flow of bile from the liver to the small intestines, and spur the production of new liver cells. It also has been found to quell inflammation and control the oxidation that can damage body cells and tissues.

Scientific Name
Silybum marianum

Milk Thistle Is Also Commonly Known As
Holy thistle, lady's thistle, Marian thistle, Mediterranean milk thistle, St. Mary thistle

Medicinal Parts
Seed, above-ground parts

Milk Thistle's Uses
Milk thistle herb is used to treat liver ailments, diseases of the spleen, dyspepsia, and gallbladder complaints. It is also used to protect the liver from toxins and to stimulate menstrual flow and the production of breast milk. Germany's Commission E has approved the use of milk thistle seed to treat liver and gallbladder complaints as well as dyspeptic symptoms, such as heartburn and bloating.

Typical Dose
A typical dose of milk thistle herb is approximately 1/2 tsp of the herb mixed with 150 ml boiling water, steeped for five to ten minutes, then strained and taken as a tea. A typical daily dose of milk thistle seed in capsule form may range from 140 to 420 mg, divided into two to three doses.

Possible Side Effects
Milk thistle's side effects include nausea, vomiting, anorexia, menstrual changes, and allergic reactions.

Drugs That May Interact with Milk Thistle
Taking milk thistle with these drugs may be harmful:
- acarbose (Prandase, Precose)—may increase the risk of loose stools and adverse effects of the drug
- phentolamine (Regitine, Rogitine)—may interfere with the action of the drug

Lab Tests That May Be Altered by Milk Thistle
None known

Diseases That May Be Worsened or Triggered by Milk Thistle
This herb may have estrogen-like effects and should not be used by women with estrogen-sensitive breast cancer or other hormone-sensitive conditions.

Foods That May Interact with Milk Thistle
None known

Supplements That May Interact with Milk Thistle
None known

MOTHERWORT

Motherwort, a plant that belongs to the mint family, has a shaggy leaf resembling a lion's tail, from which it gets its scientific name: *Leonurus*, a combination of the Latin word *leo*, meaning "lion," and the Greek word *oura*, meaning "tail." The second part of its name, *cardiaca*, comes from the Greek word for heart. Together they describe motherwort's major functions. It helps relieve the pain of childbirth, stimulate uterine contractions after delivery, and ease postpartum anxiety. It also calms heart palpitations, irregular heartbeat, and rapid heartbeat.

Scientific Name
Leonurus cardiaca

Motherwort Is Also Commonly Known As
Lion's ear, lion's tail, Roman motherwort, throwwort

Medicinal Parts
Above-ground parts

Motherwort's Uses
To treat asthma, lack of menstruation, menopausal symptoms, flatulence, and hyperthyroidism. Germany's Commission E has approved the use of motherwort to treat a poorly functioning thyroid gland and nervous heart complaints.

Typical Dose
A typical daily dose of motherwort is approximately 4.5 gm of the herb or 2 to 4 ml of liquid extract (1:1) taken three times daily.

Possible Side Effects
Motherwort's side effects include allergic reactions, uterine bleeding, diarrhea, and stomach irritation. Motherwort contains cardiac glycosides, which can help control irregular heartbeat, reduce the backup of blood and fluid in the body, and increase blood flow through the kidneys, helping to excrete sodium and relieve swelling in body tissues. However, a buildup of cardiac glycosides can occur, especially when the herb is combined with certain medications or other herbs that contain cardiac glycosides, causing arrhythmia, abnormally slow heartbeat, heart failure, and even death.

Drugs That May Interact with Motherwort
Taking motherwort with these drugs may increase skin sensitivity to sunlight:
- bumetanide (Bumex, Burinex)
- celecoxib (Celebrex)
- ciprofloxacin (Ciloxan, Cipro)
- doxycycline (Apo-Doxy, Vibramycin)
- enalapril (Vasotec)
- etodolac (Lodine, Utradol)
- fluphenazine (Modecate, Prolixin)
- fosinopril (Monopril)
- furosemide (Apo-Furosemide, Lasix)
- gatifloxacin (Tequin, Zymar)
- hydrochlorothiazide (Apo-Hydro, Microzide)
- ibuprofen (Advil, Motrin)
- indomethacin (Indocin, Novo-Methacin)
- ketoprofen (Orudis, Rhodis)
- ketorolac (Acular, Toradol)
- lansoprazole (Prevacid)
- levofloxacin (Levaquin, Quixin)
- lisinopril (Prinivil, Zestril)
- loratadine (Alavert, Claritin)
- methotrexate (Rheumatrex, Trexall)
- naproxen (Aleve, Naprosyn)
- nortriptyline (Aventyl HCl, Pamelor)
- ofloxacin (Floxin, Ocuflox)
- omeprazole (Losec, Prilosec)

- phenytoin (Dilantin, Phenytek)
- piroxicam (Feldene, Nu-Pirox)
- prochlorperazine (Compazine, Compro)
- quinapril (Accupril)
- risperidone (Risperdal)
- rofecoxib (Vioxx)
- tetracycline (Novo-Tetra, Sumycin)

Taking motherwort with these drugs may increase the risk of bleeding and bruising:
- antithrombin III (Thrombate III)
- argatroban
- bivalirudin (Angiomax)
- dalteparin (Fragmin)
- danaparoid (Orgaran)
- enoxaparin (Lovenox)
- fondaparinux (Arixtra)
- heparin (Hepalean, Hep-Lock)
- lepirudin (Refludan)
- tinzaparin (Innohep)
- warfarin (Coumadin, Jantoven)

Taking motherwort with these drugs may increase the risk of bradycardia (slow heart rate):
- acebutolol (Novo-Acebutolol, Sectral)
- atenolol (Apo-Atenol, Tenormin)
- befunolol (Bentos, Betaclar)
- betaxolol (Betoptic S, Kerlone)
- bisoprolol (Monocor, Zebeta)
- carteolol (Cartrol, Ocupress)
- carvedilol (Coreg)
- celiprolol
- digitalis (Digitek, Lanoxin)
- esmolol (Brevibloc)
- labetalol (Normodyne, Trandate)
- levobetaxolol (Betaxon)
- levobunolol (Betagan, Novo-Levobunolol)

- metipranolol (OptiPranolol)
- metoprolol (Betaloc, Lopressor)
- nadolol (Apo-Nadol, Corgard)
- oxprenolol (Slow-Trasicor, Trasicor)
- pindolol (Apo-Pindol, Novo-Pindol)
- propranolol (Inderal, InnoPran XL)
- sotalol (Betapace, Sorine)
- timolol (Betimol, Timoptic)

Taking motherwort with these drugs may interfere with absorption of the drug:
- ferric gluconate (Ferrlecit)
- ferrous fumarate (Femiron, Feostat)
- ferrous gluconate (Fergon, Novo-Ferrogluc)
- ferrous sulfate (Feratab, Fer-Iron)
- ferrous sulfate and ascorbic acid (FeroGrad 500, Vitelle Irospan)
- iron-dextran complex (Dexferrum, INFeD)
- polysaccharide-iron complex (Hytinic, Niferex)

Taking motherwort with these drugs may be harmful:
- digitalis (Digitek, Lanoxin)—may increase the risk of excessively low blood pressure and irregular heartbeat

Lab Tests That May Be Altered by Motherwort
May increase thyroid function and test results in those with hyperthyroidism.

Diseases That May Be Worsened or Triggered by Motherwort
May interfere with treatment for heart ailments.

Foods That May Interact with Motherwort
None known

Supplements That May Interact with Motherwort

Increased risk of cardiac glycoside toxicity when used with other herbs that contain cardiac glycosides, such as black hellebore, calotropis, and others. (For a list of cardiac glycoside–containing herbs and supplements, see Appendix B.)

MYRRH

So prized that the three wise men presented it to the infant Jesus as a gift, myrrh has been known since ancient times as the herbalist's cleanser. Traditionally it has been used to treat upper respiratory conditions, leg ulcers, and stomatitis and as a prime ingredient in gargles and mouthwashes for the treatment of mouth sores, infected gums, sore throats, coughs, and thrush.

Scientific Name
Commiphora molmol

Myrrh Is Also Commonly Known As
African myrrh, Arabian myrrh, bal, bol, didin, guggal gum, guggal resin

Medicinal Parts
Resin

Myrrh's Uses
To treat cough, intestinal infections, lack of menstruation, stomach ailments, and inflammation of the mucosa of the mouth and throat. Germany's Commission E has approved the use of myrrh to treat inflammation of the mouth and throat.

Typical Dose
A typical dose of myrrh may range from 1 to 4 ml of tincture applied to the affected area two to three times daily, or in mouthwash form, 5 to 10 drops in a glass of water.

Possible Side Effects
Myrrh's side effects include diarrhea and changes in heart rate.

Drugs That May Interact with Myrrh
Taking myrrh with these drugs may increase the risk of hypoglycemia (low blood sugar):

- acarbose (Prandase, Precose)
- acetohexamide
- chlorpropamide (Diabinese, Novo-Propamide)
- gliclazide (Diamicron, Novo-Gliclazide)
- glimepiride (Amaryl)
- glipizide (Glucotrol)
- glipizide and metformin (Metaglip)
- gliquidone (Beglynor, Glurenorm)
- glyburide (DiaBeta, Micronase)
- glyburide and metformin (Glucovance)
- insulin (Humulin, Novolin R)
- metformin (Glucophage, Riomet)
- miglitol (Glyset)
- nateglinide (Starlix)
- pioglitazone (Actos)
- repaglinide (GlucoNorm, Prandin)
- rosiglitazone (Avandia)
- rosiglitazone and metformin (Avandamet)
- tolazamide (Tolinase)
- tolbutamide (Apo-Tolbutamide, Tol-Tab)

Lab Tests That May Be Altered by Myrrh
May decrease blood glucose levels.

Diseases That May Be Worsened or Triggered by Myrrh

- May interfere with diabetes therapy by lowering blood sugar.
- May worsen fever, inflammation, and uterine bleeding.

Foods That May Interact with Myrrh

None known

Supplements That May Interact with Myrrh

None known

NERVE ROOT

Also known as lady's slipper because its delicate bloom looks like a ballet slipper, this mildly stimulating and antispasmodic herb was used by Native Americans to calm nervous tension, ease cramps, and banish headaches. It has also been used to treat depression related to female problems. Unfortunately, nerve root has been overcollected to the point of near extinction and is now a protected species, making it difficult to find.

Scientific Name

Cypripedium calceolus

Nerve Root Is Also Commonly Known As

American valerian, bleeding heart, lady's slipper, slipper root, Venus shoe, yellow lady's slipper

Medicinal Parts

Root, rhizome

Nerve Root's Uses

To treat nervousness, emotional tension, insomnia, diarrhea, and menstrual difficulties

Typical Dose

A typical dose of nerve root may range from 2 to 4 gm of the dried root/rhizome mixed with 150 ml of boiling water, steeped for five to ten minutes and taken as a tea three times a day.

Possible Side Effects

Nerve root's side effects include hallucinations, restlessness, headache, and giddiness.

Drugs That May Interact with Nerve Root

Taking nerve root with these drugs may increase the risk of excessive sedation and mental depression and impairment:

- alprazolam (Apo-Alpraz, Xanax)
- amitriptyline (Elavil, Levate)
- amoxapine (Asendin)
- bupropion (Wellbutrin, Zyban)
- buspirone (BuSpar, Nu-Buspirone)
- clonazepam (Klonopin, Rivotril)
- cyclobenzaprine (Flexeril, Novo-Cycloprine)
- desipramine (Alti-Desipramine, Norpramin)
- diazepam (Apo-Diazepam, Valium)
- diphenhydramine (Benadryl Allergy, Nytol)
- doxepin (Sinequan, Zonalon)
- fluoxetine (Prozac, Sarafem)
- fluphenazine (Modecate, Prolixin)
- flurazepam (Apo-Flurazepam, Dalmane)
- imipramine (Apo-Imipramine, Tofranil)
- lorazepam (Ativan, Nu-Loraz)
- metoclopramide (Apo-Metoclop, Reglan)
- midazolam (Apo-Midazolam, Versed)
- morphine hydrochloride

- morphine sulfate (Kadian, MS Contin)
- nefazodone (Serzone)
- nortriptyline (Aventyl HCl, Pamelor)
- olanzapine (Zydis, Zyprexa)
- oxazepam (Novoxapam, Serax)
- oxcarbazepine (Trileptal)
- prochlorperazine (Compazine, Compro)
- propoxyphene (Darvon, Darvon-N)
- quetiapine (Seroquel)
- risperidone (Risperdal)
- temazepam (Novo-Temazepam, Restoril)
- tramadol (Ultram)
- triazolam (Apo-Triazo, Halcion)
- zolpidem (Ambien)

Lab Tests That May Be Altered by Nerve Root
None known

Diseases That May Be Worsened or Triggered by Nerve Root
None known

Foods That May Interact with Nerve Root
None known

Supplements That May Interact with nerve Root
None known

NIACIN

A member of the B-family of vitamins formerly known as vitamin B_3, niacin participates in nearly every cellular metabolic pathway in the body. It helps keep the skin, mouth, nerves, and intestines healthy and aids in the extraction of energy from food. Since the mid-1950s, doctors have been using a form of niacin called nicotinic acid to reduce elevated cholesterol. A lack of niacin can trigger diarrhea, dermatitis, dementia, insomnia, nausea, and fatigue.

Typical Dose
The Food and Nutrition Board has set the RDA for niacin at 16 mg per day for adult men and 14 mg per day for adult women.

Possible Side Effects
Excessive amounts of niacin can cause flushing of the skin, abnormal glucose metabolism, nausea, and liver damage.

Drugs That May Interact with Niacin (taken in the form of high-dose nicotinic acid)
Taking niacin with these drugs may interfere with the action of the drug:
- acarbose (Prandase, Precose)
- acetohexamide
- chlorpropamide (Diabinese, Novo-Propamide)
- glimepride (Amaryl)
- glipizide (Glucotrol)
- glyburide (DiaBeta, Micronase)
- metformin (Glucophage, Riomet)
- miglitol (Glyset)
- nateglinide (Starlix)
- pioglitazone (Actos)
- repaglinide (GlucoNorm, Prandin)
- rosiglitazone (Avandia)
- rosiglitazone and metformin (Avandamet)
- tolazamide (Tolinase)
- tolbutamide (Apo-Tolbutamide, Tol-Tab)

Taking niacin with these drugs may increase the risk of rhabdomyolysis (a potentially fatal muscle disease):

- atorvastatin (Lipitor)
- fluvastatin (Lescol)
- lovastatin (Altocor, Mevacor)
- pravastatin (Novo-Pravastatin, Pravachol)
- rosuvastatin (Crestor)
- simvastatin (Apo-Simvastatin, Zocor)

Taking niacin with these drugs may increase the risk of hypotension (excessively low blood pressure):

- amlodipine (Norvasc)
- bepridil (Vascor)
- diltiazem (Cardizem, Tiazac)
- felodipine (Plendil, Renedil)
- isosorbide dinitrate (Dilatrate-SR, Isordil)
- isosorbide mononitrate (Imdur, Ismo)
- isradipine (DynaCirc)
- lacidipine (Aponil, Caldine)
- lercanidipine (Cardiovasc, Carmen)
- manidipine (Calslot, Iperten)
- nicardipine (Cardene)
- nifedipine (Adalat CC, Procardia)
- nilvadipine
- nimodipine (Nimotop)
- nisoldipine (Sular)
- nitrendipine
- nitroglycerin (Nitro-Dur, Nitro-Bid)
- pinaverium (Dicetel)
- verapamil (Calan, Isoptin SR)

Taking niacin with these drugs may interfere with the absorption of the vitamin:

- cholestyramine (Prevalite, Questran)
- colestipol (Colestid)

Taking niacin with these drugs may reduce the niacin flush seen with high doses of nicotinic acid:

- acemetacin (Acemetacin Heumann, Acemetacin Sandoz)
- aspirin (Bufferin, Ecotrin)
- celecoxib (Celebrex)
- choline magnesium trisalicylate (Trilisate)
- choline salicylate (Teejel)
- diclofenac (Cataflam, Voltaren)
- diflunisal (Apo-Diflunisal, Dolobid)
- dipyrone (Analgina, Dinador)
- etodolac (Lodine, Utradol)
- etoricoxib (Arcoxia)
- fenoprofen (Nalfon)
- flurbiprofen (Ansaid, Ocufen)
- ibuprofen (Advil, Motrin)
- indomethacin (Indocin, Novo-Methacin)
- ketoprofen (Orudis, Rhodis)
- ketorolac (Acular, Toradol)
- magnesium salicylate (Doan's, Mobidin)
- meclofenamate (Meclomen)
- mefenamic acid (Ponstan, Ponstel)
- meloxican (MOBIC, Mobicox)
- nabumetone (Apo-Nabumetone, Relafen)
- naproxen (Aleve, Naprosyn)
- niflumic acid (Niflam, Nifluril)
- nimesulide (Areuma, Aulin)
- oxaprozin (Apo-Oxaprozin, Daypro)
- piroxicam (Feldene, Nu-Pirox)
- rofecoxib (Vioxx)
- salsalate (Amgesic, Salflex)
- sulindac (Clinoril, Nu-Sundac)
- tenoxicam (Dolmen, Mobiflex)
- tiaprofenic acid (DomTiaprofenic, Surgam)
- tolmetin (Tolectin)
- valdecoxib (Bextra)

Taking niacin with these drugs may cause the following effects:

- gemfibrozil (Lopid, Apo-Gemfibrozil)—both the drug and the vitamin may increase each other's ability to reduce blood cholesterol when taken together
- mecamylamine (Inversine)—may cause low blood pressure when standing up (postural hypotension)
- nicotine (NicoDerm CQ, Nicotrol)—may increase the risk of dizziness and flushing
- warfarin (Coumadin, Jantoven)—may increase the risk of bleeding and bruising

Drugs That May Interfere with the Absorption, Utilization, or Excretion of Niacin

- amikacin (Amikin)
- amoxicillin (Amoxil, Novamoxin)
- ampicillin (Omnipen, Totacillin)
- azithromycin (Zithromax)
- carbenicillin (Geocillin)
- cefaclor (Ceclor)
- cefadroxil (Duricef)
- cefamandole (Mandol)
- cefazolin (Ancef, Kefzol)
- cefdinir (Omnicef)
- cefditoren (Spectracef)
- cefepime (Maxipime)
- cefonicid (Monocid)
- cefoperazone (Cefobid)
- cefotaxime (Claforan)
- cefotetan (Cefotan)
- cefoxitin (Mefoxin)
- cefpodoxime (Vantin)
- cefprozil (Cefzil)
- ceftazidime (Ceptaz, Fortaz)
- ceftibuten (Cedax)
- ceftizoxime (Cefizox)
- ceftriaxone (Rocephin)
- cefuroxime (Ceftin, Kefurox)
- cephalexin (Biocef, Keftab)
- cephalothin (Ceporacin)
- cephapirin (Cefadyl)
- cepharadine (Velosef)
- cinoxacin (Cinobac)
- ciprofloxacin (Ciloxan, Cipro)
- clarithromycin (Biaxin, Biaxin XL)
- cloxacillin (Cloxapen, Nu-Cloxi)
- demeclocycline (Declomycin)
- dicloxacillin (Dycill, Pathocil)
- dirithromycin (Dynabac)
- doxycycline (Apo-Doxy, Vibramycin)
- erythromycin (Erythrocin, Staticin)
- gatofloxacin (Tequin, Zymar)
- gentamicin (Alcomicin, Gentacidin)
- isoniazid (Laniazid Oral, PMS-Isoniazid)
- kanamycin (Kantrex)
- levofloxacin (Levaquin, Quixin)
- linezolid (Zyvox)
- lomefloxacin (Maxaquin)
- loracarbef (Lorabid)
- meclocycline (Meclan Topical)
- minocycline (Dynacin, Minocin)
- moxifloxacin (Avelox)
- nafcillin (Nafcil Injection, Unipen Oral)
- nalidixic acid (NegGram)
- norfloxacin (Chibroxin Ophthalmic, Noroxin Oral)
- ofloxacin (Floxin, Ocuflox)
- penicillin G benzathine (Bicillin L-A, Permapen)
- penicillin G benzathine and penicillin G procaine (Bicicillin C-R)
- penicillin G procaine (Pfizerpen-AS, Wycillin)
- penicillin V potassium (Suspen, Truxcillin)

- piperacillin (Pipracil)
- piperacillin and tazobactam sodium (Zosyn)
- rifampin and isoniazid (Rifamate)
- sparfloxacin (Zagam)
- sulfadiazine (Microsulfon)
- sulfisoxazole (Gantrisin)
- tetracycline (Novo-Tetra, Sumycin)
- ticarcillin (Ticar)
- ticarcillin and clavulanate potassium (Timentin)
- tobramycin (Nebcin, Tobrex)
- trimethoprim (Primsol, Trimpex)
- trovafloxacin (Trovan)

Lab Tests That May Be Altered by Niacin
- May increase homocysteine levels when taken in doses of 1,000 to 3,000 mg.
- May increase liver function tests, including alanine aminotransferase (ALT), aspartic acid transaminase (AST), serum bilirubin, and lactate dehydrogenase (LDH).
- May cause false increase in urinary catecholamine fluorometric assays, due to niacin's production of fluorescent substances.
- May cause false positive results in urinary glucose tests using cupric sulfate (Benedict's solution, Clinitest, Fehling's solution).

Diseases That May Be Worsened or Triggered by Niacin
- May increase the risk of irregular heartbeat if taken in large amounts.
- May worsen allergies by triggering the release of histamine.
- May worsen diabetes by raising blood sugar levels.
- May worsen gallbladder disease, gout, kidney

disease, liver disease, peptic ulcer disease, and low blood pressure.

Foods That May Interact with Niacin
Taking niacin with a hot drink can increase niacin flushing.

Supplements That May Interact with Niacin
- Niacin's positive effect on HDL "good" cholesterol can be decreased by concurrent use of the antioxidants beta-carotene, vitamin C, vitamin E, and/or selenium.
- The beneficial effect of sustained-release niacin and simvastatin (Zocor) on the risk of heart disease may be decreased by use of the antioxidants beta-carotene, vitamin C, vitamin E, and/or selenium.
- Increased risk of liver damage when combined with herbs and supplements that can cause hepatotoxicity (destructive effects on the liver), such as bishop's weed, borage, chaparral, uva ursi, and others. (For a list of herbs and supplements that can cause hepatotoxicity, see Appendix B.)

NONI

The noni plant is a tropical evergreen tree growing in the Pacific Islands that produces a fruit about the size of a potato. The noni fruit, juice, bark, and leaves are all used in herbal remedies and Polynesian folk medicine. Test-tube studies indicate that noni may be able to kill the bacteria that cause tuberculosis, inhibit the activity of *E. coli*, and reduce blood pressure. However, there are few well-designed human studies on noni.

Scientific Name
Morinda citrifolia

Noni Is Also Commonly Known As
Hog apple, mengkudu, morinda, wild pine

Medicinal Parts
Leaf, fruit, juice

Noni's Uses
To treat diabetes, fever, and stomachache; to purify the blood

Typical Dose
There is no typical dose of noni.

Possible Side Effects
Noni's side effects include nausea, vomiting, anorexia, sedation, allergic reactions, and hyperkalemia (high levels of potassium in the blood).

Drugs That May Interact with Noni
Taking noni with these drugs may increase the risk of hyperkalemia (high blood levels of potassium):
- amiloride (Midamor)
- hydrochlorothiazide and triamterene (Dyazide, Maxzide)
- spironolactone (Aldactone, Novo-Spiroton)
- triamterene (Dyrenium)

Taking noni with these drugs may interfere with the action of the drug:
- cyclosporine (Neoral, Sandimmune)
- dexamethasone (Decadron, Dexasone)
- prednisone (Apo-Prednisone, Deltasone)

Lab Tests That May Be Altered by Noni
May confound results of diagnostic urine tests that rely on a color change by discoloring urine (pink, red, purple, or orange).

Diseases That May Be Worsened or Triggered by Noni
May worsen cases of elevated potassium levels (hyperkalemia) due to potassium in noni.

Foods That May Interact with Noni
None known

Supplements That May Interact with Noni
None known

NORTHERN PRICKLY ASH

Also known as the toothache tree, this small deciduous aromatic shrub native to eastern North America was a favorite of Native Americans for easing the pain of toothache and rheumatism. The herb's aromatic bitter oil, which contains xanthoxylin, has cleansing, stimulating, diaphoretic, and antirheumatic properties.

Scientific Name
Zanthoxylum americanum

Northern Prickly Ash Is Also Commonly Known As
Prickly ash, toothache tree, yellow wood

Medicinal Parts
Bark, root, root bark, berry

Northern Prickly Ash's Uses

To treat low blood pressure, fever, inflammation, rheumatic disorders, and gastrointestinal ailments

Typical Dose

A typical dose of northern prickly ash in tincture form is approximately 5 ml (1:5 dilution in 45 percent alcohol), taken three times daily.

Possible Side Effects

Northern prickly ash's side effects include nausea, vomiting, hypotension (low blood pressure), allergic reactions, and photosensitivity (skin sensitivity to sunlight).

Drugs That May Interact with Northern Prickly Ash

Taking northern prickly ash with these drugs may increase the risk of bleeding and bruising:
- aminosalicylic acid (Nemasol Sodium, Paser)
- antithrombin III (Thrombate III)
- argatroban
- aspirin (Bufferin, Ecotrin)
- bivalirudin (Angiomax)
- choline magnesium trisalicylate (Trilisate)
- choline salicylate (Teejel)
- dalteparin (Fragmin)
- danaparoid (Orgaran)
- enoxaparin (Lovenox)
- fondaparinux (Arixtra)
- heparin (Hepalean, Hep-Lock)
- lepirudin (Refludan)
- salsalate (Amgesic, Salflex)
- tinzaparin (Innohep)
- warfarin (Coumadin, Jantoven)

Taking northern prickly ash with these drugs may interfere with the absorption of the drug:
- ferric gluconate (Ferrlecit)
- ferrous fumarate (Femiron, Feostat)
- ferrous gluconate (Fergon, Novo-Ferrogluc)
- ferrous sulfate (Feratab, Fer-Iron)
- ferrous sulfate and ascorbic acid (FeroGrad 500, Vitelle Irospan)
- iron-dextran complex (Dexferrum, INFeD)
- polysaccharide-iron complex (Hytinic, Niferex)

Lab Tests That May Be Altered by Northern Prickly Ash

None known

Diseases That May Be Worsened or Triggered by Northern Prickly Ash

May worsen inflammatory or infectious gastrointestinal ailments by irritating the gastrointestinal tract.

Foods That May Interact with Northern Prickly Ash

None known

Supplements That May Interact with Northern Prickly Ash

Increased risk of bleeding when used with herbs and supplements that might affect platelet aggregation. (For a list of herbs and supplements with anticoagulant/antiplatelet effects, see Appendix B.)

NUTMEG

The delicious smell of nutmeg was so revered that it was scattered over the streets of Rome in preparation for the coronation of Emperor Henry VI in

1191. Nutmeg is the seed of the *Myristica fragrans* tree, which takes seven years to bear fruit and can continue producing until its ninetieth year. Traditionally, nutmeg has been used in tiny amounts to relieve nausea, vomiting, flatulence, toothache, and chronic diarrhea and as an aphrodisiac.

Scientific Name
Myristica fragrans

Nutmeg Is Also Commonly Known As
Mace, macis, myristica

Medicinal Parts
Seed, oil from seed

Nutmeg's Uses
To treat diarrhea, dysentery, cramps, vomiting, headaches, fever, impotence, rheumatism, and nerve pain

Typical Dose
A typical internal dose of nutmeg may range from 1 to 3 drops of nutmeg oil taken two to three times a day.

Possible Side Effects
Nutmeg's side effects include nausea, vomiting, spontaneous abortion, and allergic reactions.

Drugs That May Interact with Nutmeg
Taking nutmeg with these drugs may increase the effects of the drug:
- bismuth (Kaopectate, Pepto-Bismol)
- bismuth subsalicylate, metronidazole, and tetracycline (Helidac)
- charcoal (Charcoal Plus DS, EZ-Char)
- difenoxin and atropine (Motofen)
- diphenoxylate and atropine (Lomotil, Lonox)
- haloperidol (Haldol, Novo-Peridol)
- iproniazid (Marsilid)
- lactobacillus (Kala, Probiotica)
- loperamide (Diarr-Eze, Imodium A-D)
- moclobemide (Alti-Moclobemide, Nu-Moclobemide)
- nifuroxazide (Akabar, Diarret)
- octreotide (Sandostatin)
- olanzapine (Zydis, Zyprexa)
- opium tincture
- paregoric
- phenelzine (Nardil)
- prochlorperazine (Compazine, Compro)
- psyllium (Metamucil, Reguloid)
- quetiapine (Seroquel)
- risperidone (Risperdal)
- selegiline (Eldepryl)
- tranylcypromine (Parnate)

Lab Tests That May Be Altered by Nutmeg
None known

Diseases That May Be Worsened or Triggered by Nutmeg
None known

Foods That May Interact with Nutmeg
None known

Supplements That May Interact with Nutmeg
Increased risk of additive toxicity when used with herbs containing safrole, such as basil, camphor, cinnamon, and sassafras.

OAK

Because of its high tannic acid content, oak bark was once an important ingredient used in the tanning of leather. Today it is used in powdered form to treat nosebleeds, in ointment form for hemorrhoids, and as a gargle for sore throats. Also, because of its anti-inflammatory and astringent properties, cold compresses made of oak bark tea are used for treating cuts and burns.

Scientific Name
Quercus robur

Oak Is Also Commonly Known As
Common oak, English oak, oak bark, tanner's bark

Medicinal Parts
Bark, leaf, seed

Oak's Uses
To treat eczema, genital and anal inflammation, gastrointestinal inflammation, diarrhea, cough, varicose veins, and rashes. Germany's Commission E has approved the use of oak to treat diarrhea, inflammation of the mouth and throat, cough, bronchitis, and skin inflammation.

Typical Dose
A typical internal dose is approximately 1 gm of coarsely powdered bark mixed with 150 ml cold water, boiled for 2 minutes, strained and taken as a tea, up to three times a day.

Possible Side Effects
Oak's side effects include nausea, vomiting, anorexia, and allergic reactions.

Drugs That May Interact with Oak
Taking oak with these drugs may cause or increase kidney damage:

- etodolac (Lodine, Utradol)
- ibuprofen (Advil, Motrin)
- indomethacin (Indocin, Novo-Methacin)
- ketoprofen (Orudis, Rhodis)
- ketorolac (Acular, Toradol)
- meloxicam (MOBIC, Mobicox)
- metformin (Glucophage, Riomet)
- methotrexate (Rheumatrex, Trexall)
- miglitol (Glyset)
- morphine hydrochloride
- morphine sulfate (Kadian, MS Contin)
- naproxen (Aleve, Naprosyn)
- nitrofurantoin (Furadantin, Macrobid)
- ofloxacin (Floxin, Ocuflox)
- penicillin (Pfizerpen, Wycillin)
- piroxicam (Feldene, Nu-Pirox)
- propoxyphene (Darvon, Darvon-N)
- rifampin (Rifadin, Rimactane)
- stavudine (Zerit)
- sucralfate (Carafate, Sulcrate)
- tramadol (Ultram)
- valacyclovir (Valtrex)
- valganciclovir (Valcyte)
- vancomycin (Vancocin)
- zidovudine (Novo-AZT, Retrovir)

Taking oak with these drugs may interfere with the absorption of the drug:
- ferric gluconate (Ferrlecit)
- ferrous fumarate (Femiron, Feostat)
- ferrous gluconate (Fergon, Novo-Ferrogluc)
- ferrous sulfate (Feratab, Fer-Iron)
- ferrous sulfate and ascorbic acid (FeroGrad 500, Vitelle Irospan)

- iron-dextran complex (Dexferrum, INFeD)
- morphine hydrochloride
- morphine sulfate (Kadian, MS Contin)
- polysaccharide-iron complex (Hytinic, Niferex)

Lab Tests That May Be Altered by Oak
None known

Diseases That May Be Worsened or Triggered by Oak
None known

Foods That May Interact with Oak
None known

Supplements That May Interact with Oak
- The tannins in oak may cause the alkaloids in certain other herbs to separate and settle, increasing the risk of toxic reactions. (For a list of herbs and other substances high in alkaloids, see Appendix B.)
- May cause the separation and settling out of iron salts when taken with iron supplements.

OATS

A hardy cereal grain, oats are a concentrated source of nutrients that contain more soluble fiber than any other grain. They help to lower cholesterol levels, slow absorption of glucose into the blood, and prolong the feeling of satiety. Oats also have anti-inflammatory properties.

Scientific Name
Avena sativa

Oats Are Also Commonly Known As
Haver, haver-corn, oat bran, oatstraw, wild oats

Medicinal Parts
Fruit or seed

Oats' Uses
To lower cholesterol and treat gout, rheumatism, skin diseases, insomnia, and symptoms of old age

Typical Dose
A typical dose of oats to lower cholesterol is 50 to 100 gm, four times a day.

Possible Side Effects
Oats' side effects include bloating and flatulence.

Drugs That May Interact with Oats
Taking oats (in the form of oat bran) with these drugs may interfere with the absorption and effectiveness of the drug:
- all drugs taken by mouth
- atorvastatin (Lipitor)
- fluvastatin (Lescol)
- lovastatin (Altocor, Mevacor)
- pravastatin (Novo-Pravastatin, Pravachol)
- rosuvastatin (Crestor)
- simvastatin (Apo-Simvastatin, Zocor)

Taking oats with these drugs may reduce the effects of the drug:
- morphine hydrochloride
- morphine sulfate (Kadian, MS Contin)

Lab Tests That May Be Altered by Oats
- Oat bran may lower the results of after-eating blood sugar and insulin tests.
- Oat bran lowers the results of cholesterol tests.

Diseases That May Be Worsened or Triggered by Oats

None known

Foods That May Interact with Oats

None known

Supplements That May Interact with Oats

None known

OLEANDER

A poisonous evergreen shrub with pink, red, or white flowers commonly seen beside southern California freeways, the oleander contains the cardiac glycoside oleandrin, which was once used in medicine. All parts of the oleander plant contain cardiac glycosides, and even roasting a hot dog on an oleander stem can lead to poisoning. However, a nontoxic proprietary extract made from oleander leaves is currently being tested as a treatment for cancer, HIV/AIDS, hepatitis C, and psoriasis.

Scientific Name

Nerium oleander

Oleander Is Also Commonly Known As

Adelfa, laurier rose, rose bay, rose laurel

Medicinal Parts

Leaf

Oleander's Uses

To treat skin disease, scabies, hemorrhoids, heart disease, constipation, menstrual problems, and parasites

Typical Dose

There is no typical dose of oleander.

Possible Side Effects

❶ Oleander's side effects include nausea, vomiting, diarrhea, stupor, cardiac arrhythmia, and allergic reactions. Oleander contains cardiac glycosides, which can help control irregular heartbeat, reduce the backup of blood and fluid in the body, and increase blood flow through the kidneys, helping to excrete sodium and relieve swelling in body tissues. However, a buildup of cardiac glycosides can occur, especially when the herb is combined with certain medications or other herbs that contain cardiac glycosides, causing arrhythmia, abnormally slow heartbeat, heart failure, and even death.

Drugs That May Interact with Oleander

Taking oleander with these drugs may increase the therapeutic and/or adverse effects of the drug:

- betamethasone (Betatrex, Maxivate)
- calcium acetate (PhosLo)
- calcium carbonate (Rolaids Extra Strength, Tums)
- calcium chloride
- calcium citrate (Osteocit)
- calcium glubionate
- calcium gluceptate
- calcium gluconate
- cascara
- cortisone (Cortone)
- deflazacort (Calcort, Dezacor)
- dexamethasone (Decadron, Dexasone)
- docusate (Colace, Ex-Lax Stool Softener)
- docusate and senna (Peri-Colace, Senokot-S)
- hydrocortisone (Cetacort, Locoid)

- lactulose (Constulose, Enulose)
- magnesium citrate (Citro-Mag)
- magnesium hydroxide (Dulcolax Milk of Magnesia, Phillips' Milk of Magnesia)
- magnesium hydroxide and mineral oil (Phillips' M-O)
- magnesium oxide (Mag-Ox 400, Uro-Mag)
- magnesium sulfate (Epsom salts)
- methylprednisolone (Depo-Medrol, Medrol)
- polyethylene glycol-electrolyte solution (Colyte, MiraLax)
- prednisolone (Inflamase Forte, Pred Forte)
- prednisone (Apo-Prednisone, Deltasone)
- psyllium (Metamucil, Reguloid)
- quinidine (Novo-Quinidin, Quinaglute Dura-Tabs)
- sorbitol (Sorbilax)
- triamcinolone (Aristocort, Tri-Nasal)

Taking oleander with this drug may be harmful:
- digitalis (Digitek, Lanoxin)—may increase risk of cardiac glycoside toxicity

Lab Tests That May Be Altered by Oleander
None known

Disease That May Be Worsened or Triggered by Oleander
None known

Foods That May Interact with Oleander
None known

Supplements That May Interact with Oleander
- Increased risk of cardiac glycoside toxicity when used with other herbs that contain cardiac glycosides, such as black hellebore, calotropis, motherwort, and others. (For a list of cardiac glycoside–containing herbs and supplements, see Appendix B.)
- Increased risk of cardiotoxicity due to potassium depletion when taken with cardioactive herbs, such as adonis, digitalis, lily-of-the-valley, and squill. (For a list of cardioactive herbs and supplements, see Appendix B.)
- Increased risk of potassium depletion when used in conjunction with horsetail plant or licorice.
- Increased risk of potassium depletion when used with stimulant laxative herbs, such as black root, cascara sagrada, castor oil, and senna. (For a list of stimulant laxative herbs and supplements, see Appendix B.)
- May increase the therapeutic effects of oleander when taken with calcium supplements.

OLIVE

> The branches of the olive tree were considered a symbol of everlasting power by the Egyptians, and the oil pressed from the fruit of this tree was held in such high esteem that it was used in the mummification of their royalty. Olive oil is used today to treat elevated blood pressure and cholesterol, heart disease, diabetes, migraines, constipation, and numerous other ailments. Olive leaf contains oleuropein acid, a natural antibacterial, antifungal agent that may help bolster the immune system and fight chronic viral and yeast infections.

Scientific Name
Olea europaea

Olive Is Also Commonly Known As
Oleae folium, olivier

Medicinal Parts
Leaf, oil taken from the fruit

Olive's Uses
To treat arteriosclerosis, hypertension, rheumatism, gout, and fever; to enhance immunity and control hyperglycemia

Typical Dose
A typical dose of olive leaf may range from 7 to 8 gm of the dried leaves mixed with 150 ml of boiling water, steeped for 30 minutes and taken as tea. A typical dose of olive oil is 15 to 30 ml, three times a day.

Possible Side Effects
Olive oil's side effects include eye irritation, dermatitis, and allergic reactions.

Drugs That May Interact with Olive
Taking olive (leaf or oil) with these drugs may increase the risk of hypoglycemia (low blood sugar):
- acarbose (Prandase, Precose)
- acetohexamide
- chlorpropamide (Diabinese, Novo-Propamide)
- gliclazide (Diamicron, Novo-Gliclazide)
- glimepiride (Amaryl)
- glipizide (Glucotrol)
- glipizide and metformin (Metaglip)
- gliquidone (Beglynor, Glurenorm)
- glyburide (DiaBeta, Micronase)
- glyburide and metformin (Glucovance)

- insulin (Humulin, Novolin R)
- metformin (Glucophage, Riomet)
- miglitol (Glyset)
- nateglinide (Starlix)
- pioglitazone (Actos)
- repaglinide (GlucoNorm, Prandin)
- rosiglitazone (Avandia)
- rosiglitazone and metformin (Avandamet)
- tolazamide (Tolinase)
- tolbutamide (Apo-Tolbutamide, Tol-Tab)

Lab Tests That May Be Altered by Olive
- Olive leaf may decrease blood glucose levels.
- Olive leaf may decrease serum calcium levels.
- Olive leaf may decrease blood pressure levels.

Diseases That May Be Worsened or Triggered by Olive
- Olive leaf may complicate diabetes treatment by lowering blood sugar too far.
- Olive oil may trigger gallbladder colic.

Foods That May Interact with Olive
None known

Supplements That May Interact with Olive
Olive leaf may increase blood glucose–lowering effects and risk of hypoglycemia (low blood sugar) when used with herbs and supplements that lower glucose levels, such as alpha-lipoic acid, chromium, devil's claw, Panax ginseng, and psyllium. (For a list of herbs and supplements that lower blood glucose levels, see Appendix B.)

ONION

An ancient remedy for wounds, earache, tumors, and numerous other ailments, the onion gets its name from the Latin word *unio*, meaning "one," as the onion plant produces just a single bulb. The onion is rich in powerful sulfur-containing compounds, which may be the reason it helps lower total cholesterol and raise HDL "good" cholesterol, thin the blood, ward off infections, and ease breathing difficulties.

Scientific Name

Allium cepa

Onion Is Also Commonly Known As

Green onion, shallot

Medicinal Parts

Bulb

Onion's Uses

To treat digestive problems, cough, colds, whooping cough, asthma, angina, worm infestation, and bacterial or fungal infections; to improve the gallbladder's performance. Germany's Commission E has approved the use of onion to treat arteriosclerosis, cough, bronchitis, fevers, colds, hypertension, dyspeptic complaints such as heartburn and loss of appetite, tendency to infection, and inflammation of the mouth and throat.

Typical Dose

A typical daily dose is approximately 50 gm of fresh onion or fresh onion juice, or 20 gm of dried onion.

Possible Side Effects

Onion's side effects include gastrointestinal distress and halitosis.

Drugs That May Interact with Onion

Taking onion with these drugs may increase the risk of bleeding or bruising:

- abciximab (ReoPro)
- aspirin (Bufferin, Ecotrin)
- celecoxib (Celebrex)
- enoxaparin (Lovenox)
- etodolac (Lodine, Utradol)
- heparin (Hepalean, Hep-Lock)
- ibuprofen (Advil, Motrin)
- indomethacin (Indocin, Novo-Methacin)
- ketoprofen (Orudis, Rhodis)
- ketorolac (Acular, Toradol)
- ticlopidine (Alti-Ticlopidine, Ticlid)
- urokinase (Abbokinase)
- warfarin (Coumadin, Jantoven)

Taking onion with these drugs may increase the risk of hypoglycemia (low blood sugar):

- acarbose (Prandase, Precose)
- acetohexamide
- chlorpropamide (Diabinese, Novo-Propamide)
- gliclazide (Diamicron, Novo-Gliclazide)
- glimepiride (Amaryl)
- glipizide (Glucotrol)
- glipizide and metformin (Metaglip)
- gliquidone (Beglynor, Glurenorm)
- glyburide (DiaBeta, Micronase)
- glyburide and metformin (Glucovance)
- insulin (Humulin, Novolin R)
- metformin (Glucophage, Riomet)
- miglitol (Glyset)
- nateglinide (Starlix)

- pioglitazone (Actos)
- repaglinide (GlucoNorm, Prandin)
- rosiglitazone (Avandia)
- rosiglitazone and metformin (Avandamet)
- tolazamide (Tolinase)
- tolbutamide (Apo-Tolbutamide, Tol-Tab)

Lab Tests That May Be Altered by Onion
May decrease blood glucose levels.

Diseases That May Be Worsened or Triggered by Onion
None known

Foods That May Interact with Onion
None known

Supplements That May Interact with Onion
Increased risk of bleeding when used with herbs and supplements that might affect platelet aggregation. (For a list of herbs and supplements with anticoagulant/antiplatelet effects, see Appendix B.)

OREGANO

Traditionally a symbol of happiness, oregano takes its name from the Greek words *oros*, meaning "mountain," and *ganos*, meaning "joy," a reference to the spectacular sight of its purplish red flowers splashed across the Mediterranean hillsides. Oregano has antibacterial, antifungal, and antioxidant properties, which is why it is sometimes used as an internal treatment for respiratory and intestinal disorders and as a topical treatment for infection.

Scientific Name
Origanum vulgare

Oregano Is Also Commonly Known As
Mountain mint, origano, wild marjoram, wintersweet

Medicinal Parts
Oil, leaf

Oregano's Uses
To treat respiratory disorders, painful menstruation, rheumatoid arthritis, urinary tract disorders, and cough

Typical Dose
A typical dose of oregano is approximately 1 heaping tsp of dried herb mixed with 250 ml boiling water, steeped for 10 minutes, strained and taken as a tea.

Possible Side Effects
Oregano's side effects include nausea, vomiting, and allergic reactions.

Drugs That May Interact with Oregano
Taking oregano with these drugs may interfere with the absorption of the drug:
- ferrous sulfate (Feratab, Fer-Iron)
- iron-dextran complex (Dexferrum, INFeD)

Lab Tests That May Be Altered by Oregano
None known

Diseases That May Be Worsened or Triggered by Oregano
May trigger reactions in those allergic to basil, lavender, and other members of the Lamiaceae family.

Foods That May Interact with Oregano

None known

Supplements That May Interact with Oregano

None known

PAPAYA

> Papaya, the sweet, tender, pear-shaped fruit of the papaya tree, which is native to Central America, was supposedly called the "fruit of the angels" by Christopher Columbus because it was so delicious. Papaya contains several enzymes that digest protein, including papain and chymopapain, and is used in certain digestive aids. These enzymes have also been shown to decrease inflammation and improve the healing of burns and wounds.

Scientific Name

Carica papaya

Papaya Is Also Commonly Known As

Mamaeire, melon tree, papain, papaw

Medicinal Parts

Leaf

Papaya's Uses

To treat intestinal parasites, various gastrointestinal ailments, hemorrhoids, cough; to improve wound healing

Typical Dose

There is no typical dose of papaya.

Possible Side Effects

Papaya's side effects include allergic reactions.

Drugs That May Interact with Papaya

Taking papaya with these drugs may increase the risk of bleeding or bruising:

- antithrombin III (Thrombate III)
- argatroban
- bivalirudin (Angiomax)
- dalteparin (Fragmin)
- danaparoid (Orgaran)
- enoxaparin (Lovenox)
- fondaparinux (Arixtra)
- heparin (Hepalean, Hep-Lock)
- lepirudin (Refludan)
- tinzaparin (Innohep)
- warfarin (Coumadin, Jantoven)

Lab Tests That May Be Altered by Papaya

May increase plasma international normalized ratio (INR) in those who are also taking warfarin.

Diseases That May Be Worsened or Triggered by Papaya

Papaya may trigger an existing latex allergy.

Foods That May Interact with Papaya

- Those who are sensitive to kiwi or fig may also develop a sensitivity to the papain in papaya.
- Potato protein may inhibit papain's ability to break down protein.

Supplements That May Interact with Papaya

Increased risk of bleeding when used with herbs and supplements that might affect platelet aggregation. (For a list of herbs and supplements with anticoagulant/antiplatelet effects, see Appendix B.)

PARSLEY

Parsley, a Mediterranean native related to celery, has been grown domestically for more than two thousand years. It was considered sacred by the ancient Greeks, who used it to decorate tombs and recognize those who won athletic contests. This lacy little green plant contains several anti-cancer ingredients, including vitamin C, beta-carotene, chlorophyll, coumarins, flavonoids, monoterpenes, and volatile oils.

Scientific Name
Petroselinum crispum

Parsley Is Also Commonly Known As
Garden parsley, petersylinge, rock parsley

Medicinal Parts
Leaf, whole plant, seed

Parsley's Uses
Parsley herb and root are used to treat problems with the gastrointestinal and urinary tracts. Parsley fruit is used to treat menstrual problems and problems with the gastrointestinal and urinary tracts; and to improve digestion. Germany's Commission E has approved the use of parsley herb and root to treat infections of the urinary tract, and kidney and bladder stones.

Typical Dose
A typical daily dose of parsley is approximately 6 gm of the crushed herb and root.

Possible Side Effects
Parsley's side effects include nausea, vomiting, and allergic reactions.

Drugs That May Interact with Parsley
Taking parsley with these drugs may increase the risk of bleeding and bruising:

- abciximab (ReoPro)
- aspirin (Bufferin, Ecotrin)
- celecoxib (Celebrex)
- enoxaparin (Lovenox)
- etodolac (Lodine, Utradol)
- heparin (Hepalean, Hep-Lock)
- ibuprofen (Advil, Motrin)
- indomethacin (Indocin, Novo-Methacin)
- ketoprofen (Orudis, Rhodis)
- ketorolac (Acular, Toradol)

Taking parsley with these drugs may increase the risk of hypotension (low blood pressure):

- acebutolol (Novo-Acebutolol, Sectral)
- amlodipine (Norvasc)
- atenolol (Apo-Atenol, Tenormin)
- benazepril (Lotensin)
- betaxolol (Betoptic S, Kerlone)
- bisoprolol (Monocor, Zebeta)
- bumetanide (Bumex, Burinex)
- candesartan (Atacand)
- captopril (Capoten, Novo-Captopril)
- carteolol (Cartrol, Ocupress)
- carvedilol (Coreg)
- chlorothiazide (Diuril)
- chlorthalidone (Apo-Chlorthalidone, Thalitone)
- clonidine (Catapres, Duraclon)
- diazoxide (Hyperstat, Proglycem)
- diltiazem (Cardizem, Tiazac)
- doxazosin (Alti-Doxazosin, Cardura)
- enalapril (Vasotec)
- eplerenone (Inspra)
- eprosartan (Teveten)

- esmolol (Brevibloc)
- felodipine (Plendil, Renedil)
- fenoldopam (Corlopam)
- fosinopril (Monopril)
- furosemide (Apo-Furosemide, Lasix)
- guanabenz (Wytensin)
- guanadrel (Hylorel)
- guanfacine (Tenex)
- hydralazine (Apresoline, Novo-Hylazin)
- hydrochlorothiazide (Apo-Hydro, Microzide)
- hydrochlorothiazide and triamterene (Dyazide, Maxzide)
- indapamide (Lozol, Nu-Indapamide)
- irbesartan (Avapro)
- isradipine (DynaCirc)
- labetalol (Normodyne, Trandate)
- lisinopril (Prinivil, Zestril)
- losartan (Cozaar)
- mecamylamine (Inversine)
- mefruside (Baycaron)
- methyclothiazide (Aquatensen, Enduron)
- methyldopa (Apo-Methyldopa, Nu-Medopa)
- metolazone (Mykrox, Zaroxolyn)
- metoprolol (Betaloc, Lopressor)
- minoxidil (Loniten, Rogaine)
- moexipril (Univasc)
- nadolol (Apo-Nadol, Corgard)
- nicardipine (Cardene)
- nifedipine (Adalat CC, Procardia)
- nisoldipine (Sular)
- nitroglycerin (Minitran, Nitro-Dur)
- nitroprusside (Nipride, Nitropress)
- olmesartan (Benicar)
- oxprenolol (Slow-Trasicor, Trasicor)
- perindopril erbumine (Aceon, Coversyl)
- phenoxybenzamine (Dibenzyline)

- phentolamine (Regitine, Rogitine)
- pindolol (Apo-Pindol, Novo-Pindol)
- polythiazide (Renese)
- prazosin (Minipress, Nu-Prazo)
- propranolol (Inderal, InnoPran XL)
- quinapril (Accupril)
- ramipril (Altace)
- reserpine
- spironolactone (Aldactone, Novo-Spiroton)
- telmisartan (Micardis)
- terazosin (Alti-Terazosin, Hytrin)
- timolol (Betimol, Timoptic)
- torsemide (Demadex)
- trandolapril (Mavik)
- triamterene (Dyrenium)
- trichlormethiazide (Metatensin, Naqua)
- valsartan (Diovan)
- verapamil (Calan, Isoptin SR)

❶ Taking parsley with these drugs may cause or increase serotonin syndrome (symptoms of which include agitation, rapid heart rate, flushing, heavy sweating, and possibly even death):

- acetaminophen and codeine (Capital and Codeine, Tylenol with Codeine)
- alfentanil (Alfenta)
- aspirin and codeine (Coryphen Codeine)
- belladonna and opium (B&O Supprettes)
- buprenorphine (Buprenex, Subutex)
- buprenorphine and naloxone (Suboxone)
- butorphanol (Apo-Butorphanol, Stadol)
- codeine (Codeine Contin)
- dihydrocodeine, aspirin, and caffeine (Synalgos-DC)
- fentanyl (Actiq, Duragesic)
- hydrocodone and acetaminophen (Vicodin, Zydone)

- hydrocodone and aspirin (Damason-P)
- hydrocodone and ibuprofen (Vicoprofen)
- hydromorphone (Dilaudid, PMS-Hydromorphone)
- levomethadyl acetate hydrochloride
- levorphanol (LevoDromoran)
- meperidine (Demerol, Meperitab)
- meperidine and promethazine
- methadone (Dolophine, Methadose)
- morphine sulfate (Kadian, MS Contin)
- nalbuphine (Nubain)
- opium tincture
- oxycodone (OxyContin, Roxicodone)
- oxycodone and acetaminophen (Endocet, Percocet)
- oxycodone and aspirin (Endodan, Percodan)
- oxymorphone (Numorphan)
- paregoric
- pentazocine (Talwin)
- phenoperidine
- propoxyphene (Darvon, Darvon-N)
- propoxyphene and acetaminophen (Darvocet-N 50, Darvocet-N 100)
- propoxyphene, aspirin, and caffeine (Darvon Compound)
- remifentanil (Ultiva)
- sufentanil (Sufenta)

Taking parsley with these drugs may be harmful:

- lithium (Eskalith, Carbolith)—may lead to dehydration and lithium toxicity
- selegiline (Eldepryl)—may increase the therapeutic and/or adverse effects of the drug

Lab Tests That May Be Altered by Parsley
None known

Diseases That May Be Worsened or Triggered by Parsley
May worsen kidney disease.

Foods That May Interact with Parsley
None known

Supplements That May Interact with Parsley
None known

PASSION FLOWER

A climbing vine native to North, Central, and South America, passion flower is known for its beautiful large, aromatic flowers. The name passion flower dates back to the seventeenth century and refers to the passion of Christ: the flower's twelve petals represent the apostles, and its three stamens represent his wounds. One double-blind study found that 45 drops per day of passion flower extract taken for four weeks was as effective in relieving anxiety as 30 mg per day of oxazepam, a standard antianxiety medication.

Scientific Name
Passiflora incarnata

Passion Flower Is Also Commonly Known As
Apricot vine, Jamaican honeysuckle, maypop, passion vine, passion fruit

Medicinal Parts
Above-ground parts

Passion Flower's Uses
To treat anxiety, hysteria, and nervous gastrointestinal problems; to treat opiate withdrawal. Ger-

many's Commission E has approved the use of passion flower to treat insomnia and nervousness.

Typical Dose

A typical dose of passion flower is approximately 1 tsp of dried herb mixed with 150 ml of boiling water, steeped for 10 minutes, strained and taken as a tea.

Possible Side Effects

Passion flower's side effects include nausea, vomiting, and allergic reactions.

Drugs That May Interact with Passion Flower

Taking passion flower with these drugs may increase the risk of bleeding or bruising:

- abciximab (ReoPro)
- aspirin (Bufferin, Ecotrin)
- celecoxib (Celebrex)
- enoxaparin (Lovenox)
- etodolac (Lodine, Utradol)
- heparin (Hepalean, Hep-Lock)
- ibuprofen (Advil, Motrin)
- indomethacin (Indocin, Novo-Methacin)
- ketoprofen (Orudis, Rhodis)
- ketorolac (Acular, Toradol)
- meloxicam (MOBIC, Mobicox)
- naproxen (Aleve, Naprosyn)
- piroxicam (Feldene, Nu-Pirox)
- rofecoxib (Vioxx)
- ticlopidine (Alti-Ticlopidine, Ticlid)
- urokinase (Abbokinase)
- warfarin (Coumadin, Jantoven)

Taking passion flower with these drugs may increase the risk of excessive sedation and mental depression and impairment:

- acetaminophen and codeine (Capital and Codeine, Tylenol with Codeine)
- alfentanil (Alfenta)
- alprazolam (Apo-Alpraz, Xanax)
- amobarbital (Amytal)
- amobarbital and secobarbital (Tuinal)
- aspirin and codeine (Coryphen Codeine)
- belladonna and opium (B&O Supprettes)
- bromazepam (Apo-Bromazepam, Gen-Bromazepam)
- brotizolam (Lendorm, Sintonal)
- buprenorphine (Buprenex, Subutex)
- buprenorphine and naloxone (Suboxone)
- butabarbital (Butisol Sodium)
- butalbital, acetaminophen, and caffeine (Esgic, Fioricet)
- butalbital, aspirin, and caffeine (Fiorinal)
- butorphanol (Apo-Butorphanol, Stadol)
- chloral hydrate (Aquachloral Supprettes, Somnote)
- chlordiazepoxide (Apo-Chlordiazepoxide, Librium)
- clobazam (Alti-Clobazam, Frisium)
- clonazepam (Klonopin, Rivotril)
- clorazepate (Tranxene, T-Tab)
- codeine (Codeine Contin)
- dexmedetomidine (Precedex)
- diazepam (Apo-Diazepam, Valium)
- dihydrocodeine, aspirin, and caffeine (Synalgos-DC)
- diphenhydramine (Benadryl Allergy, Nytol)
- estazolam (ProSom)
- fentanyl (Actiq, Duragesic)
- flurazepam (Apo-Flurazepam, Dalmane)
- glutethimide
- haloperidol (Haldol, Novo-Peridol)
- hydrocodone and acetaminophen (Vicodin, Zydone)

- hydrocodone and aspirin (Damason-P)
- hydrocodone and ibuprofen (Vicoprofen)
- hydromorphone (Dilaudid, PMS-Hydro-morphone)
- hydroxyzine (Atarax, Vistaril)
- levomethadyl acetate hydrochloride
- levorphanol (LevoDromoran)
- loprazolam (Dormonoct, Havlane)
- lorazepam (Ativan, Nu-Loraz)
- meperidine (Demerol, Meperitab)
- meperidine and promethazine
- mephobarbital (Mebaral)
- methadone (Dolophine, Methadose)
- methohexital (Brevital, Brevital Sodium)
- midazolam (Apo-Midazolam, Versed)
- morphine sulfate (Kadian, MS Contin)
- nalbuphine (Nubain)
- opium tincture
- oxycodone (OxyContin, Roxicodone)
- oxycodone and acetaminophen (Endocet, Percocet)
- oxycodone and aspirin (Endodan, Percodan)
- oxymorphone (Numorphan)
- paregoric
- pentazocine (Talwin)
- pentobarbital (Nembutal)
- phenobarbital (Luminal Sodium, PMS-Phenobarbital)
- phenoperidine
- prazepam
- primidone (Apo-Primidone, Mysoline)
- promethazine (Phenergan)
- propofol (Diprivan)
- propoxyphene (Darvon, Darvon-N)
- propoxyphene and acetaminophen (Darvocet-N 50, Darvocet-N 100)
- propoxyphene, aspirin, and caffeine (Darvon Compound)
- quazepam (Doral)
- remifentanil (Ultiva)
- secobarbital (Seconal)
- sodium oxybate (Xyrem)
- sufentanil (Sufenta)
- s-zopiclone (Lunesta)
- temazepam (Novo-Temazepam, Restoril)
- tetrazepam (Mobiforton, Musapam)
- thiopental (Pentothal)
- triazolam (Apo-Triazo, Halcion)
- zaleplon (Sonata, Stamoc)
- zolpidem (Ambien)
- zopiclone (Alti-Zopiclone, Gen-Zopiclone)

Taking passion flower with this drug may be harmful:

- selegiline (Eldepryl)—may increase the therapeutic and/or adverse effects of the drug

Lab Tests That May Be Altered by Passion Flower
None known

Diseases That May Be Worsened or Triggered by Passion Flower
None known

Foods That May Interact with Passion Flower
None known

Supplements That May Interact with Passion Flower
- Increased risk of bleeding when used with herbs and supplements that might affect platelet aggregation, such as angelica, danshen, garlic, ginger, ginkgo biloba, red clover, turmeric, white willow, and others. (For a list of herbs and supplements with

anticoagulant/antiplatelet effects, see Appendix B.)

- May enhance therapeutic and adverse effects of herbs and supplements that have sedative properties, such as 5-HTP, kava kava, St. John's wort, and valerian. (For a list of herbs and supplements that have sedative properties, see Appendix B.)

Pau D'Arco

> Pau d'arco, the inner bark of an evergreen tree found in South America, is used traditionally as a tea to treat colds, fungal infections, and other conditions. Possessing disease-fighting compounds called naphthoquinones, pau d'arco has been sold in North America as an alternative treatment for cancer, diabetes, yeast infections, and warts.

Scientific Name
Tabebuia impetiginosa

Pau D'Arco Is Also Commonly Known As
Ipe, lapacho, lapacho morado, trumpet bush

Medicinal Parts
Wood, bark

Pau D'Arco's Uses
To treat diarrhea, bladder infections, intestinal parasites, diabetes, asthma, syphilis, boils, and wounds

Typical Dose
A typical daily dose of pau d'arco may range from 1 to 4 gm in capsule form, taken in divided doses.

Possible Side Effects
Pau d'arco's side effects include nausea, vomiting, and allergic reactions.

Drugs That May Interact with Pau D'Arco
Taking pau d'arco with these drugs may increase the risk of bleeding or bruising:

- abciximab (ReoPro)
- aminosalicylic acid (Nemasol Sodium, Paser)
- antithrombin III (Thrombate III)
- argatroban
- aspirin (Bufferin, Ecotrin)
- aspirin and dipyridamole (Aggrenox)
- bivalirudin (Angiomax)
- choline magnesium trisalicylate (Trilisate)
- choline salicylate (Teejel)
- clopidogrel (Plavix)
- dalteparin (Fragmin)
- danaparoid (Orgaran)
- dipyridamole (Novo-Dipiradol, Persantine)
- enoxaparin (Lovenox)
- eptifibatide (Integrillin)
- fondaparinux (Arixtra)
- heparin (Hepalean, Hep-Lock)
- indobufen (Ibustrin)
- lepirudin (Refludan)
- salsalate (Amgesic, Salflex)
- ticlopidine (Alti-Ticlopidine, Ticlid)
- tinzaparin (Innohep)
- tirofiban (Aggrastat)
- warfarin (Coumadin, Jantoven)

Lab Tests That May Be Altered by Pau D'Arco
May increase plasma prothrombin time (PT) and plasma international normalized ratio (INR) in those who are also taking warfarin.

Diseases That May Be Worsened or Triggered by Pau D'Arco

May worsen bleeding disorders.

Foods That May Interact with Pau D'Arco

None known

Supplements That May Interact with Pau D'Arco

Increased risk of bleeding when used with herbs and supplements that might affect platelet aggregation. (For a list of herbs and supplements with anticoagulant/antiplatelet effects, see Appendix B.)

PECTIN

Pectin, a soluble fiber extracted from citrus peels, apples, and sugar beets, forms a gel-like substance in the intestines that can trap fats such as cholesterol, which are then excreted. Pectin is linked to reduced total cholesterol and LDL "bad" levels, which may help protect against atherosclerosis. It has also been found to be helpful in treating diarrhea and lowering high blood glucose levels.

Scientific Name

Pectin

Medicinal Parts

Plant cell walls

Pectin's Uses

To treat diarrhea, elevated cholesterol levels, and elevated blood glucose

Typical Dose

A typical daily dose of pectin to treat diarrhea is approximately 30 ml of 10 percent pectin, taken in combination with kaolin (Kaopectate) or paregoric (Parepectolin).

Possible Side Effects

Pectin's side effects include nausea, vomiting, anorexia, and allergic reactions.

Drugs That May Interact with Pectin

Taking pectin with these drugs may interfere with the action of the drug:

- atorvastatin (Lipitor)
- fluvastatin (Lescol)
- lovastatin (Altocor, Mevacor)
- pravastatin (Novo-Pravastatin, Pravachol)
- rosuvastatin (Crestor)
- simvastatin (Apo-Simvastatin, Zocor)

Taking pectin may interfere with absorption of these drugs:

- all drugs taken orally

Lab Tests That May Be Altered by Pectin

- May decrease serum cholesterol levels.

Diseases That May Be Worsened or Triggered by Pectin

None known

Foods That May Interact with Pectin

May decrease absorption of dietary nutrients.

Supplements That May Interact with Pectin

May significantly decrease absorption of beta-carotene when taken concurrently.

PERILLA

Perilla, an herb from the mint family that is relatively common in East Asian countries, is an excellent vegetable source of omega-3 and omega-6 fatty acids. Recent research suggests that perilla oil may be able to inhibit abnormal blood clotting, alleviate chronic inflammation, and prevent certain types of irregular heartbeat. Japanese dental researchers have also found that perilla seed extract combats streptococci and other bacteria that can cause cavities and periodontal disease.

Scientific Name
Perilla fructescens

Perilla Is Also Commonly Known As
Beefsteak plant, wild coleus

Medicinal Parts
Leaf, seed, oil taken from seed

Perilla's Uses
To treat chills, headache, fever, cough, and shortness of breath

Typical Dose
A typical daily dose of perilla is approximately 10 to 20 gm of oil.

Possible Side Effects
Perilla's side effects include nausea, vomiting, and allergic reactions.

Drugs That May Interact with Perilla
Taking perilla with these drugs may increase the drug's effects:
- beclomethasone (Beconase, Vanceril)
- betamethasone (Celestone, Diprolene)
- budesonide (Entocort, Rhinocort)
- budesonide and formoterol (Symbicort)
- cortisone (Cortone)
- deflazacort (Calcort, Dezacor)
- dexamethasone (Decadron, Dexasone)
- flunisolide (AeroBid, Nasarel)
- fluorometholone (Eflone, Flarex)
- fluticasone (Cutivate, Flonase)
- hydrocortisone (Anusol-HC, Locoid)
- loteprednol (Alrex, Lotemax)
- medrysone (HMS Liquifilm)
- methylprednisolone (DepoMedrol, Medrol)
- prednisolone (Inflamase Forte, Pred Forte)
- prednisone (Apo-Prednisone, Deltasone)
- rimexolone (Vexol)
- triamcinolone (Aristocort, Trinasal)

Lab Tests That May Be Altered by Perilla
None known

Diseases That May Be Worsened or Triggered by Perilla
None known

Foods That May Interact with Perilla
None known

Supplements That May Interact with Perilla
None known

PILL-BEARING SPURGE

> Also known as asthma weed, pill-bearing spurge breaks up mucus and relaxes bronchial spasms, prompting some to use it to treat asthmatic conditions, chronic bronchitis, emphysema, hay fever, and chronic inflammation of the respiratory duct. However, toxic doses of the herb have induced respiratory failure in small animals.

Scientific Name
Euphorbia pilulifera

Pill-Bearing Spurge Is Also Commonly Known As
Asthma weed, catshair, garden spurge, milkweed, snake weed

Medicinal Parts
Whole plant

Pill-Bearing Spurge's Uses
To treat allergies, asthma, bronchitis, colds, diarrhea, sexually transmitted diseases, and snakebite

Typical Dose
A typical dose of pill-bearing spurge may range from 120 to 300 mg in powdered form, taken three times daily.

Possible Side Effects
Pill-bearing spurge's side effects include nausea, vomiting, gastric symptoms, and allergic reactions.

Drugs That May Interact with Pill-Bearing Spurge
Taking pill-bearing spurge with these drugs may interfere with the action of the drug:

- cyclosporine (Neoral, Sandimmune)
- erythromycin (Erythrocin, Staticin)

Lab Tests That May Be Altered by Pill-Bearing Spurge
None known

Diseases That May Be Worsened or Triggered by Pill-Bearing Spurge
May worsen inflammatory or infectious gastrointestinal ailments by irritating the gastrointestinal tract.

Food That May Interact with Pill-Bearing Spurge
None known

Supplements That May Interact with Pill-Bearing Spurge
None known

PINEAPPLE

> Christopher Columbus is credited with "discovering" pineapple on the Caribbean island of Guadeloupe in 1493 and bringing it back to Europe as a rare delicacy. In Colonial America, pineapple was such a luxurious treat, it became the premier symbol of prestige, social class, and hospitality. The pineapple's health benefits center on its rich supply of bromelain, a group of protein-digesting enzymes that reduce inflammation and swelling, aid digestion, and may even have anticancer properties.

Scientific Name
Ananas comosus

Pineapple Is Also Commonly Known As
Ananas, golden rocket

Medicinal Parts
Fruit

Pineapple's Uses
To treat digestive problems, inflammation, asthma, obesity, constipation, and wounds

Typical Dose
A standard dose has not been established.

Possible Side Effects
Pineapple's side effects include diarrhea and allergic reactions.

Drugs That May Interact with Pineapple
Taking pineapple with these drugs may increase the risk of bleeding and bruising:
- alteplase (Activase, Cathflo Activase)
- aminosalicylic acid (Nemasol Sodium, Paser)
- antithrombin III (Thrombate III)
- argatroban
- aspirin (Bufferin, Ecotrin)
- bivalirudin (Angiomax)
- choline magnesium trisalicylate (Trilisate)
- choline salicylate (Teejel)
- dalteparin (Fragmin)
- danaparoid (Orgaran)
- enoxaparin (Lovenox)
- fondaparinux (Arixtra)
- heparin (Hepalean, Hep-Lock)
- lepirudin (Refludan)
- reteplase (Retavase)
- salsalate (Amgesic, Salflex)
- streptokinase (Streptase)
- tenecteplase (TNKase)
- tinzaparin (Innohep)
- urokinase (Abbokinase)
- warfarin (Coumadin, Jantoven)

Taking pineapple with these drugs may interfere with the action of the drug:
- benazepril (Lotensin)
- captopril (Capoten, Novo-Captopril)
- cilazapril (Inhibace)
- delapril (Adecut, Delakete)
- enalapril (Vasotec)
- fosinopril (Monopril)
- imidapril (Novarok, Tanatril)
- lisinopril (Prinivil, Zestril)
- moexipril (Univasc)
- perindopril erbumine (Aceon, Coversyl)
- quinapril (Accupril)
- ramipril (Altace)
- spirapril
- trandolapril (Mavik)

Lab Tests That May Be Altered by Pineapple
None known

Diseases That May Be Worsened or Triggered by Pineapple
None known

Foods That May Interact with Pineapple
None known

Supplements That May Interact with Pineapple
None known

PLEURISY ROOT

> Pleurisy root was first used by Native Americans as an internal remedy for pulmonary infections and an external remedy for wounds. It gets its name from the herb's ability to ease the pain and difficulty in breathing seen in pleurisy, the inflammation of the membrane that surrounds the lungs and lines the rib cage. Pleurisy root is a powerful expectorant and sweat-inducer that is used to treat colds, respiratory problems, and flu.

Scientific Name
Asclepias tuberosa

Pleurisy Root Is Also Commonly Known As
Butterfly weed, Canada root, orange milkweed, swallow-wort, tuber root

Medicinal Parts
Root

Pleurisy Root's Uses
To treat cough, pleurisy, pain, rheumatism, and difficulty in breathing

Typical Dose
There is no typical dose of pleurisy root.

Possible Side Effects
Pleurisy root's side effects include gastrointestinal irritation, nausea, and vomiting. Pleurisy root contains cardiac glycosides, which can help control irregular heartbeat, reduce the backup of blood and fluid in the body, and increase blood flow through the kidneys, helping to excrete sodium and relieve swelling in body tissues. However, a buildup of cardiac glycosides can occur, especially when the herb is combined with certain medications or other herbs that contain cardiac glycosides, causing arrhythmia, abnormally slow heartbeat, heart failure, and even death.

Drugs That May Interact with Pleurisy Root
Taking pleurisy root with this drug may be harmful:
- digitalis (Digitek, Lanoxin)—may increase the risk of cardiac glycoside toxicity

Lab Tests That May Be Altered by Pleurisy Root
None known

Diseases That May Be Worsened or Triggered by Pleurisy Root
May worsen heart disease.

Foods That May Interact with Pleurisy Root
None known

Supplements That May Interact with Pleurisy Root
Increased risk of cardiac glycoside toxicity when used with other herbs that contain cardiac glycosides, such as black hellebore, calotropis, motherwort, and others. (For a list of cardiac glycoside–containing herbs and supplements, see Appendix B.)

POKE

> Poke, also known as pokeweed, is a large, shrubby plant native to eastern North America

that farmers consider a major pest because it is highly toxic to livestock. Although the leaves are poisonous, some people eat poke salad made out of the young poke plants, as the toxins develop as the plant ages. Poke contains potent anti-inflammatory agents, antiviral proteins, and substances that affect cell division.

Scientific Name
Phytolacca americana

Poke Is Also Commonly Known As
American nightshade, American pokeweed, cokan, crowberry, jalap, pigeon berry, poke berry, poke root, pokeweed

Medicinal Parts
Root, berry

Poke's Uses
To treat stomach ailments, rheumatism, tonsillitis, mumps, constipation, and ringworm

Typical Dose
A typical daily dose of poke is approximately 60 to 100 mg as a powder.

Possible Side Effects
❶ Poke's side effects include lowered blood pressure, confusion, blurred vision, and nausea. All parts of the poke plant, except for the aboveground leaves grown in early spring, are considered toxic. Even one poke berry can be toxic to a child; ten berries can be toxic to an adult.

Drugs That May Interact with Poke
Taking poke with these drugs may increase the risk of excessive sedation and mental depression and impairment:

- acetaminophen and codeine (Capital and Codeine, Tylenol with Codeine)
- alfentanil (Alfenta)
- alprazolam (Apo-Alpraz, Xanax)
- amobarbital (Amytal)
- amobarbital and secobarbital (Tuinal)
- aspirin and codeine (Coryphen Codeine)
- belladonna and opium (B&O Supprettes)
- bromazepam (Apo-Bromazepam, Gen-Bromazepam)
- brotizolam (Lendorm, Sintonal)
- buprenorphine (Buprenex, Subutex)
- buprenorphine and naloxone (Suboxone)
- butabarbital (Butisol Sodium)
- butalbital, acetaminophen, and caffeine (Esgic, Fioricet)
- butalbital, aspirin, and caffeine (Fiorinal)
- butorphanol (Apo-Butorphanol, Stadol)
- chloral hydrate (Aquachloral Supprettes, Somnote)
- chlordiazepoxide (Librium, Apo-Chlordiazepoxide)
- clobazam (Alti-Clobazam, Frisium)
- clonazepam (Klonopin, Rivotril)
- clorazepate (Tranxene, T-Tab)
- codeine (Codeine Contin)
- dexmedetomidine (Precedex)
- diazepam (Apo-Diazepam, Valium)
- dihydrocodeine, aspirin, and caffeine (Synalgos-DC)
- diphenhydramine (Benadryl Allergy, Nytol)
- estazolam (ProSom)
- fentanyl (Actiq, Duragesic)
- flurazepam (Apo-Flurazepam, Dalmane)
- glutethimide

- haloperidol (Haldol, Novo-Peridol)
- hydrocodone and acetaminophen (Vicodin, Zydone)
- hydrocodone and aspirin (Damason-P)
- hydrocodone and ibuprofen (Vicoprofen)
- hydromorphone (Dilaudid, PMS-Hydromorphone)
- hydroxyzine (Atarax, Vistaril)
- levomethadyl acetate hydrochloride
- levorphanol (LevoDromoran)
- loprazolam (Dormonoct, Havlane)
- lorazepam (Ativan, Nu-Loraz)
- meperidine (Demerol, Meperitab)
- meperidine and promethazine
- mephobarbital (Mebaral)
- methadone (Dolophine, Methadose)
- methohexital (Brevital, Brevital Sodium)
- midazolam (Apo-Midazolam, Versed)
- morphine sulfate (Kadian, MS Contin)
- nalbuphine (Nubain)
- opium tincture
- oxycodone (OxyContin, Roxicodone)
- oxycodone and acetaminophen (Endocet, Percocet)
- oxycodone and aspirin (Endodan, Percodan)
- oxymorphone (Numorphan)
- paregoric
- pentazocine (Talwin)
- pentobarbital (Nembutal)
- phenobarbital (Luminal Sodium, PMS-Phenobarbital)
- phenoperidine
- prazepam
- primidone (Apo-Primidone, Mysoline)
- promethazine (Phenergan)
- propofol (Diprivan)
- propoxyphene (Darvon, Darvon-N)
- propoxyphene and acetaminophen (Darvocet-N 50, Darvocet-N 100)
- propoxyphene, aspirin, and caffeine (Darvon Compound)
- quazepam (Doral)
- remifentanil (Ultiva)
- secobarbital (Seconal)
- sodium oxybate (Xyrem)
- sufentanil (Sufenta)
- s-zopiclone (Lunesta)
- temazepam (Novo-Temazepam, Restoril)
- tetrazepam (Mobiforton, Musapam)
- thiopental (Pentothal)
- triazolam (Apo-Triazo, Halcion)
- zaleplon (Sonata, Stamoc)
- zolpidem (Ambien)
- zopiclone (Alti-Zopiclone, Gen-Zopiclone)

Lab Tests That May Be Altered by Poke
None known

Diseases That May Be Worsened or Triggered by Poke
None known

Foods That May Interact with Poke
None known

Supplements That May Interact with Poke
None known

POMEGRANATE

Native to Iran and northern India, the pomegranate tree produces a round, leathery fruit that is full of juicy red seeds. Pomegranates are high in polyphenols, particularly the punicalagins, which are found only in pomegranates and have superior free-radical scavenging ability. In 2005, a study published in the *Proceedings of the National Academy of Sciences USA* noted that pomegranate juice may protect against the development of prostate cancer.

Scientific Name
Punica granatum

Pomegranate Is Also Commonly Known As
Delima, granatum, grenadier

Medicinal Parts
Bark, flowers, fruit, fruit peel, root

Pomegranate's Uses
To treat tapeworm, diarrhea, dysentery, sore throat, and hemorrhoids

Typical Dose
A typical dose of pomegranate to treat tapeworms is approximately 60 ml of a decoction made of 1 part pomegranate bark powder mixed with 5 parts water, boiled for 30 minutes, and taken in four doses throughout the day.

Possible Side Effects
Pomegranate's side effects include nausea, vomiting, anorexia, and allergic reactions.

Drugs That May Interact with Pomegranate
Taking pomegranate juice with these drugs may increase the action of the drug:

- benazepril (Lotensin)
- captopril (Capoten, Novo-Captopril)
- cilazapril (Inhibace)
- delapril (Adecut, Delakete)
- enalapril (Vasotec)
- fosinopril (Monopril)
- imidapril (Novarok, Tanatril)
- lisinopril (Prinivil, Zestril)
- moexipril (Univasc)
- perindopril erbumine (Aceon, Coversyl)
- quinapril (Accupril)
- ramipril (Altace)
- spirapril
- trandolapril (Mavik)

Lab Tests That May Be Altered by Pomegranate
None known

Diseases That May Be Worsened or Triggered by Pomegranate
None known

Foods That May Interact with Pomegranate
None known

Supplements That May Interact with Pomegranate

- The tannins in pomegranate may cause the alkaloids in certain other herbs to separate and settle, increasing the risk of toxic reactions. (For a list of herbs and other substances high in alkaloids, see Appendix B.)
- Increased risk of low blood pressure (hypotension) or increased therapeutic effects when used with herbs and supplements with hypotensive activity. (For a list of herbs and supplements with hypotensive activity, see Appendix B.)

POPLAR

Also known as the quaking aspen, this North American tree grows up to a hundred feet in height. An extract of its pale yellow bark was used traditionally to treat intermittent fevers and as a diuretic for urinary infections and gonorrhea. Native Americans made an ointment out of the bark, root, bud, and/or blossoms to treat wounds, burns, and colds.

Scientific Name
Populus species

Poplar Is Also Commonly Known As
Black poplar, European aspen, quaking aspen, white poplar

Medicinal Parts
Bark, leaf, leaf bud

Poplar's Uses
To treat wounds, hemorrhoids, sunburn, frostbite, arthritis, and urinary tract infections. Germany's Commission E has approved the use of poplar to treat wounds, burns, and hemorrhoids.

Typical Dose
A typical daily internal dose is approximately 10 gm of poplar leaves, while an external dose is approximately 5 gm of poplar leaf buds in a semi-solid preparation applied to the skin.

Possible Side Effects
Poplar's side effects include allergic skin reactions, vomiting, and liver toxicity.

Drugs That May Interact with Poplar
Taking poplar with these drugs may increase the risk of bleeding and bruising:
- aminosalicylic acid (Nemasol Sodium, Paser)
- antithrombin III (Thrombate III)
- argatroban
- aspirin (Bufferin, Ecotrin)
- bivalirudin (Angiomax)
- choline magnesium trisalicylate (Trilisate)
- choline salicylate (Teejel)
- dalteparin (Fragmin)
- danaparoid (Orgaran)
- enoxaparin (Lovenox)
- fondaparinux (Arixtra)
- heparin (Hepalean, Hep-Lock)
- lepirudin (Refludan)
- salsalate (Amgesic, Salflex)
- tinzaparin (Innohep)
- warfarin (Coumadin, Jantoven)

Taking poplar with these drugs may interfere with absorption of the drug:
- ferric gluconate (Ferrlecit)
- ferrous fumarate (Femiron, Feostat)
- ferrous gluconate (Fergon, Novo-Ferrogluc)
- ferrous sulfate (Feratab, Fer-Iron)
- ferrous sulfate and ascorbic acid (FeroGrad 500, Vitelle Irospan)
- iron-dextran complex (Dexferrum, INFeD)
- polysaccharide-iron complex (Hytinic, Niferex)

Lab Tests That May Be Altered by Poplar
None known

Diseases That May Be Worsened or Triggered by Poplar
None known

Foods That May Interact with Poplar
None known

Supplements That May Interact with Poplar
None known

POPPY

> Otherwise known as the opium poppy, the pods of the *Papaver somniferum* produce a milky substance that contains opium and the alkaloids morphine, codeine, noscapine, papaverine, and thebaine. Although the plant is illegal in the United States, the seeds (which contain no drugs) are available. The seeds are 44 to 50 percent oil and are a good source of linoleic and oleic acids. In China, poppy seeds are used to treat nausea and vomiting.

Scientific Name
Papaver somniferum

Poppy Is Also Commonly Known As
Garden poppy, mawseed, opium poppy, poppyseed, thebaine poppy

Medicinal Parts
Extract taken from the seed

Poppy's Uses
To treat pain, gallstones, dysentery, cough, and diarrhea; as a sedative

Typical Dose
A typical daily dose of extract of poppy seed has not been established.

Possible Side Effects
Poppy's side effects include constipation, headache, rashes, weakness, and trembling.

Drugs That May Interact with Poppy
Taking poppy with these drugs may increase the risk of excessive sedation and mental depression and impairment:
- acetaminophen and codeine (Capital and Codeine, Tylenol with Codeine)
- alfentanil (Alfenta)
- alprazolam (Apo-Alpraz, Xanax)
- amobarbital (Amytal)
- amobarbital and secobarbital (Tuinal)
- aspirin and codeine (Coryphen Codeine)
- belladonna and opium (B&O Supprettes)
- bromazepam (Apo-Bromazepam, Gen-Bromazepam)
- brotizolam (Lendorm, Sintonal)
- buprenorphine (Buprenex, Subutex)
- buprenorphine and naloxone (Suboxone)
- butabarbital (Butisol Sodium)
- butalbital, acetaminophen, and caffeine (Esgic, Fioricet)
- butalbital, aspirin, and caffeine (Fiorinal)
- butorphanol (Apo-Butorphanol, Stadol)
- chloral hydrate (Aquachloral Supprettes, Somnote)
- chlordiazepoxide (Apo-Chlordiazepoxide, Librium)
- clobazam (Alti-Clobazam, Frisium)
- clonazepam (Klonopin, Rivotril)
- clorazepate (Tranxene, T-Tab)
- codeine (Codeine Contin)
- dexmedetomidine (Precedex)
- diazepam (Apo-Diazepam, Valium)
- dihydrocodeine, aspirin, and caffeine (Synalgos-DC)

- diphenhydramine (Benadryl Allergy, Ny-tol)
- estazolam (ProSom)
- fentanyl (Actiq, Duragesic)
- flurazepam (Apo-Flurazepam, Dalmane)
- glutethimide
- haloperidol (Haldol, Novo-Peridol)
- hydrocodone and acetaminophen (Vicodin, Zydone)
- hydrocodone and aspirin (Damason-P)
- hydrocodone and ibuprofen (Vicoprofen)
- hydromorphone (Dilaudid, PMS-Hydromorphone)
- hydroxyzine (Atarax, Vistaril)
- levomethadyl acetate hydrochloride
- levorphanol (LevoDromoran)
- loprazolam (Dormonoct, Havlane)
- lorazepam (Ativan, Nu-Loraz)
- meperidine (Demerol, Meperitab)
- meperidine and promethazine
- mephobarbital (Mebaral)
- methadone (Dolophine, Methadose)
- methohexital (Brevital, Brevital Sodium)
- midazolam (Apo-Midazolam, Versed)
- morphine sulfate (Kadian, MS Contin)
- nalbuphine (Nubain)
- opium tincture
- oxycodone (OxyContin, Roxicodone)
- oxycodone and acetaminophen (Endocet, Percocet)
- oxycodone and aspirin (Endodan, Percodan)
- oxymorphone (Numorphan)
- paregoric
- pentazocine (Talwin)
- pentobarbital (Nembutal)
- phenobarbital (Luminal Sodium, PMS-Phenobarbital)
- phenoperidine

- prazepam
- primidone (Apo-Primidone, Mysoline)
- promethazine (Phenergan)
- propofol (Diprivan)
- propoxyphene (Darvon, Darvon-N)
- propoxyphene and acetaminophen (Darvocet-N 50, Darvocet-N 100)
- propoxyphene, aspirin, and caffeine (Darvon Compound)
- quazepam (Doral)
- remifentanil (Ultiva)
- secobarbital (Seconal)
- sodium oxybate (Xyrem)
- sufentanil (Sufenta)
- s-zopiclone (Lunesta)
- temazepam (Novo-Temazepam, Restoril)
- tetrazepam (Mobiforton, Musapam)
- thiopental (Pentothal)
- triazolam (Apo-Triazo, Halcion)
- zaleplon (Sonata, Stamoc)
- zolpidem (Ambien)
- zopiclone (Alti-Zopiclone, Gen-Zopiclone)

Lab Tests That May Be Altered by Poppy

May cause a false positive reading on urine tests for heroin and morphine.

Diseases That May Be Worsened or Triggered by Poppy

None known

Foods That May Interact with Poppy

None known

Supplements That May Interact with Poppy

None known

POTASSIUM

Working with sodium and chloride, the mineral potassium helps keep body fluids balanced and properly distributed. Potassium is also needed for the metabolism of protein and carbohydrates, muscle contraction, and the maintenance of proper blood pressure and heart rhythm. A deficiency of potassium may trigger irregular heartbeat, nausea, vomiting, diarrhea, muscle weakness and twitching, and possibly a heart attack.

Typical Dose

The Food and Nutrition Board has set the Adequate Intake (AI) for potassium for men and women ages nineteen and up at 4,700 mg per day.

Possible Side Effects

Large amounts of supplemental potassium can cause muscle fatigue, nausea and vomiting, irregular heartbeat, and heart attack.

Drugs That May Interact with Potassium

Taking potassium with these drugs increases the risk of hyperkalemia (high blood levels of potassium):

- amiloride (Midamor)
- benazepril (Lotensin)
- candesartan (Atacand)
- captopril (Capoten, Novo-Captopril)
- cilazapril (Inhibace)
- delapril (Adecut, Delakete)
- enalapril (Vasotec)
- eprosartan (Teveten)
- fosinopril (Monopril)
- hydrochlorothiazide and triamterene (Dyazide, Maxzide)
- imidapril (Novarok, Tanatril)
- irbesartan (Avapro)
- lisinopril (Prinivil, Zestril)
- losartan (Cozaar)
- moexipril (Univasc)
- olmesartan (Benicar)
- olmesartan and hydrochlorothiazide (Benicar HCT)
- perindopril erbumine (Aceon, Coversyl)
- quinapril (Accupril)
- ramipril (Altace)
- spirapril
- spironolactone (Aldactone, Novo-Spiroton)
- telmisartan (Micardis)
- trandolapril (Mavik)
- triamterene (Dyrenium)
- valsartan (Diovan)

Drugs That May Interfere with the Absorption, Utilization, or Excretion of Potassium

- acetazolamide (Apo-Acetazolamide, Diamox)
- albuterol (Proventil, Ventolin)
- amikacin (Amikin)
- amiloride and hydrochlorothiazide (Nu-Amilzide, Moduret)
- ammonium chloride
- amoxicillin (Amoxil, Novamoxin)
- amphotericin B (Amphocin, Fungizone)
- ampicillin (Omnipen, Totacillin)
- arsenic trioxide (Trisenox)
- aspirin (Bufferin, Ecotrin)
- aspirin and dipyridamole (Aggrenox)
- atenolol and chlorthalidone (Tenoretic)
- basiliximab (Simulect)
- beclomethasone (Beconase, Vanceril)

- betamethasone (Betatrex, Maxivate)
- bisacodyl (Carter's Little Pills, Dulcolax)
- budesonide (Entocort, Rhinocort)
- bumetanide (Bumex, Burinex)
- busulfan (Busulfex, Myleran)
- butalbital, aspirin, and caffeine (Fiorinal)
- candesartan and hydrochlorothiazide (Atacand HCTZ)
- carbenicillin (Geocillin)
- carboplatin (Paraplatin, Paraplatin-AQ)
- carisoprodol and aspirin (Soma Compound)
- carisoprodol, aspirin, and codeine (Soma Compound with Codeine)
- cascara
- caspofungin (Cancidas)
- celecoxib (Celebrex)
- chlorothiazide (Diuril)
- chlorthalidone (Apo-Chlorthalidone, Thalitone)
- choline magnesium trisalicylate (Trilisate)
- choline salicylate (Teejel)
- cidofovir (Vistide)
- cisplatin (Platinol, Platinol-AQ)
- cloxacillin (Cloxapen, Nu-Cloxi)
- colchicine (ratio-Colchicine)
- colchicine and probenecid (ColBenemid)
- cortisone (Cortone)
- cyclophosphamide (Cytoxan, Neosar)
- cyclosporine (Neoral, Sandimmune)
- denileukin diftitox (ONTAK)
- dexamethasone (Decadron, Dexasone)
- dicloxacillin (Dycill, Pathocil)
- diflorasone (Florone, Maxiflor)
- digoxin (Digoxin, Lanoxin)
- digoxin immune fab (Digibind, Digi-Fab)
- disopyramide (Norpace, Rhythmodan)
- enalapril and hydrochlorothiazide (Vaseretic)
- enoxacin (Penetrex)
- epoprostenol (Flolan)
- ethacrynic acid (Edecrin)
- etidronate (Didronel)
- fenofibrate (Apo-Fenofibrate, TriCor)
- fenoldopam (Corlopam)
- ferric gluconate (Ferrlecit)
- fluconazole (Apo-Fluconazole, Diflucan)
- fucytosine (Ancobon)
- fludrocortisone (Florinef)
- flunisolide (AeroBid-M, Nasarel)
- fluticasone (Cutivate, Flonase)
- fondaparinux (Arixtra)
- foscarnet (Foscavir)
- fosphenytoin (Cerebyx)
- furosemide (Apo-Furosemide, Lasix)
- gemfibrozil (Apo-Gemfibrozil, Lopid)
- gemtuzumab ozogamicin (Mylotarg)
- gentamicin (Alcomicin, Gentacidin)
- halobetasol (Ultravate)
- hydralazine (Apresoline, Novo-Hylazin)
- hydralazine and hydrochlorothiazide (Apresazide)
- hydrochlorothiazide (Apo-Hydro, Microzide)
- hydrocodone and aspirin (Azdone, Lortab ASA)
- hydrocortisone (Cetacort, Locoid)
- imatinib (Gleevec)
- inamrinone
- indapamide (Lozol, Nu-Indapamide)
- irbesartan and hydrochlorothiazide (Avalide)
- itraconazole (Sporanox)
- kanamycin (Kantrex)
- leflunomide (Arava)
- levalbuterol (Xopenex)
- levodopa (Dopar, Larodopa)
- levodopa-carbidopa (Nu-Levocarb, Sinemet)

- losartan and hydrochlorothiazide (Hyzaar)
- magnesium oxide (Mag-Ox 400, Uro-Mag)
- mannitol (Osmitrol, Resectisol)
- methazolamide (Apo-Methazolamide, Neptazane)
- methocarbamol and aspirin (Robaxisal)
- methyclothiazide (Aquatensen, Enduron)
- methyldopa and hydrochlorothiazide (Aldoril, PMS-Dopazide)
- methylprednisolone (Depoject Injection, Medrol Oral)
- metolazone (Mykrox, Zaroxolyn)
- mineral oil (Fleet Mineral Oil Enema, Milkinol)
- moexipril and hydrochlorothiazide (Uniretic)
- mometasone furoate (Elocom, Nasonex)
- mycophenolate (CellCept)
- nafcillin (Nafcil Injection, Unipen Oral)
- neomycin (Myciguent, Neo-Fradin)
- ondansetron (Zofran)
- oxaliplatin (Eloxatin)
- oxycodone and aspirin (Oxycodan, Percodan)
- pamidronate (Aredia)
- penicillin G benzathine (Bicillin L-A, Permapen)
- penicillin G benzathine and penicillin G procaine (Bicicillin C-R)
- penicillin G procaine (Pfizerpen-AS, Wycillin)
- penicillin V potassium (Suspen, Truxcillin)
- piperacillin (Pipracil)
- piperacillin and tazobactam sodium (Zosyn)
- plicamycin (Mithracin)
- polythiazide (Renese)
- prazosin and polythiazide (Minizide)
- prednisolone (Inflamase Forte, Pred Forte)
- prednisone (Apo-Prednisone, Deltasone)
- propranolol and hydrochlorothiazide (Inderide)
- salsalate (Amgesic, Salflex)
- sodium bicarbonate (Brioschi, Neut)
- sodium chloride (Nasal Moist, Simply Saline)
- sodium phosphate (Fleet Enema, Fleet Phospho-Soda)
- sodium polystyrene sulfonate (Kayexalate)
- streptomycin
- tacrolimus (Prograf, Protopic)
- telmisartan and hydrochlorothiazide (Micardis HCT, Micardis Plus)
- ticarcillin (Ticar)
- ticarcillin and clavulanate potassium (Timentin)
- tobramycin (Nebcin, Tobrex)
- torsemide (Demadex)
- triamcinolone (Aristocort, Trinasal)
- trichlormethiazide (Metahydrin, Naqua)
- valsartan and hydrochlorothiazide (Diovan HCT)
- voriconazole (VFEND)
- zoledronic Acid (Zometa)

Lab Tests That May Be Altered by Potassium
May reduce blood pressure readings.

Diseases That May Be Worsened or Triggered by Potassium
May worsen gastrointestinal motility ailments (such as irritable bowel syndrome, gastroesophageal reflux disease [GERD], or constipation) if potassium supplements are taken orally.

Foods That May Interact with Potassium
None known

Supplements That May Interact with Potassium
None known

PRICKLY PEAR CACTUS

The succulent fruit of this American desert plant has been used as a food for centuries, and the sap taken from its pads is used to soothe minor cuts, sunburns, or skin irritation. A study published in the *American Journal of Clinical Nutrition* in 2004 noted that consuming fresh prickly pear cactus fruit pulp (which is rich in vitamin C) reduced the oxidation of fats, a process that can contribute to atherosclerosis. Another study, published in the *Archives of Internal Medicine* in 2004, found that an extract of the prickly pear cactus moderately reduced hangover symptoms.

Scientific Name
Opuntia ficus indica

Prickly Pear Cactus Is Also Commonly Known As
Cactus flower, cactus pear fruit, nopol, tuna cardona

Medicinal Parts
Leaf, flower, fruit, stem

Prickly Pear Cactus's Uses
To treat viruses, diabetes, elevated cholesterol, diarrhea, and colitis

Typical Dose
A typical daily dose of prickly pear cactus is approximately 100 to 500 gm of broiled stems.

Possible Side Effects
Prickly pear cactus's side effects include nausea, diarrhea, and headache.

Drugs That May Interact with Prickly Pear Cactus
Taking prickly pear cactus with these drugs may increase the risk of hypoglycemia (low blood sugar):

- acarbose (Prandase, Precose)
- acetohexamide
- chlorpropamide (Diabinese, Novo-Propamide)
- gliclazide (Diamicron, Novo-Gliclazide)
- glimepiride (Amaryl)
- glipizide (Glucotrol)
- glipizide and metformin (Metaglip)
- gliquidone (Beglynor, Glurenorm)
- glyburide (DiaBeta, Micronase)
- glyburide and metformin (Glucovance)
- insulin (Humulin, Novolin R)
- metformin (Glucophage, Riomet)
- miglitol (Glyset)
- nateglinide (Starlix)
- pioglitazone (Actos)
- repaglinide (Prandin, GlucoNorm)
- rosiglitazone (Avandia)
- rosiglitazone and metformin (Avandamet)
- tolazamide (Tolinase)
- tolbutamide (Apo-Tolbutamide, Tol-Tab)

Lab Tests That May Be Altered by Prickly Pear Cactus
- May lower blood sugar levels.
- May lower total cholesterol and LDL "bad" cholesterol levels.

Diseases That May Be Worsened or Triggered by Prickly Pear Cactus
Prickly pear cactus may reduce blood sugar levels too low in people receiving treatment for type 2 diabetes.

Foods That May Interact with Prickly Pear Cactus

None known

Supplements That May Interact with Prickly Pear Cactus

None known

Psyllium, Psyllium Seed

A time-honored treatment for constipation, diarrhea, and elevated cholesterol, psyllium is the active ingredient found in the laxative Metamucil. Within its seed and husk are water-soluble fibers that form a gel in the intestines which increases stool weight, transit time, and the frequency of bowel movements.

Scientific Name

Plantago ovata (psyllium), *Plantago afra* (psyllium seed)

Psyllium Is Also Commonly Known As

Blond psyllium, blood plantago, Indian plantago, spogel

Psyllium Seed Is Also Commonly Known As

Fleaseed, flea work psyllion

Medicinal Parts

Seed, seed husk

Psyllium's Uses

Psyllium is used to treat constipation, hemorrhoids, dysentery, gout, pain, rheumatism, and inflammation of the gastrointestinal tract. Germany's Commission E has approved the use of psyllium to treat diarrhea, constipation, hemorrhoids, and elevated cholesterol, and psyllium seed to treat diarrhea and constipation.

Typical Dose

A typical dose of psyllium may range from 2.0 to 6.0 gm of psyllium powder. A typical daily dose of psyllium seed may range from 12 to 40 gm in divided amounts, always taken with plenty of water.

Possible Side Effects

Psyllium's side effects include flatulence, gastrointestinal distension, and allergic reactions. Psyllium seed's side effects include allergic reactions. If either psyllium or psyllium seed is taken improperly, it may trigger blockages of the esophagus or intestines.

Drugs That May Interact with Psyllium

Taking psyllium or psyllium seed with these drugs may increase the risk of hypoglycemia (low blood sugar):

- acarbose (Prandase, Precose)
- acetohexamide
- chlorpropamide (Diabinese, Novo-Propamide)
- gliclazide (Diamicron, Novo-Gliclazide)
- glimepiride (Amaryl)
- glipizide (Glucotrol)
- glipizide and metformin (Metaglip)
- gliquidone (Beglynor, Glurenorm)
- glyburide (DiaBeta, Micronase)
- glyburide and metformin (Glucovance)
- insulin (Humulin, Novolin R)
- metformin (Glucophage, Riomet)
- miglitol (Glyset)

- nateglinide (Starlix)
- pioglitazone (Actos)
- repaglinide (GlucoNorm, Prandin)
- rosiglitazone (Avandia)
- rosiglitazone and metformin (Avandamet)
- tolazamide (Tolinase)
- tolbutamide (Apo-Tolbutamide, Tol-Tab)

Taking psyllium or psyllium seed with these drugs may interfere with the absorption of the drug:
- all drugs taken orally
- carbamazepine (Carbatrol, Tegretol)
- digitalis (Digitek, Lanoxin)
- warfarin (Coumadin, Jantoven)

Taking psyllium or psyllium seed with these drugs may be harmful:
- lithium (Eskalith, Carbolith)—may decrease drug levels in spite of escalations in dosage

Lab Tests That May Be Altered by Psyllium
- Psyllium and psyllium seed may reduce "after-eating" (postprandial) blood glucose levels.
- Psyllium and psyllium seed may reduce total cholesterol levels, LDL "bad" cholesterol levels, and LDL:HDL ratio.

Diseases That May Be Worsened or Triggered by Psyllium
- Psyllium and psyllium seed may reduce blood sugar levels too low in people with type 2 diabetes.
- Psyllium and psyllium seed may worsen cases of fecal impaction, spastic bowel, or gastrointestinal tract narrowing or obstruction.
- Psyllium and psyllium seed increase risk of

esophageal blockage in people with swallowing disorders.

Foods That May Interact with Psyllium
None known

Supplements That May Interact with Psyllium
- May decrease absorption of iron when taken concurrently with iron supplements.
- May reduce the absorption of calcium, iron, zinc, and vitamin B_{12} from supplements if psyllium seed is taken within a few hours of taking the supplements.

QUASSIA

Quassia is an herbal remedy taken from the bark of the *Picrasma excelsa* tree, native to Jamaica and the Caribbean islands that grows to heights of fifty to one hundred feet. It gets its name from Quassi, an eighteenth-century native of the South American country Surinam (formerly Dutch Guiana), who became well known for successfully treating malignant fevers with the herb. Quassia's active ingredient is *quassin*, an extremely bitter alkaloid used to treat indigestion, loss of appetite, nausea, and worm infestation.

Scientific Name
Picrasma excelsa

Quassia Is Also Commonly Known As
Bitter ash, bitterwood, Jamaica quassia

Medicinal Parts
Trunk wood

Quassia's Uses

To treat heartburn, bloating, loss of appetite, fever, malaria, lice, and worm infestations; as an antiseptic wound treatment

Typical Dose

A typical dose of quassia may range from 0.3 to 0.6 gm of the herb, taken three times daily.

Possible Side Effects

Quassia's side effects include dizziness, headache, and uterine pain.

Drugs That May Interact with Quassia

Taking quassia with these drugs may increase the risk of hypokalemia (low levels of potassium in the blood):

- acetazolamide (Apo-Acetazolamide, Diamox Sequels)
- azosemide (Diat)
- bumetanide (Bumex, Burinex)
- chlorothiazide (Diuril)
- chlorthalidone (Apo-Chlorthalidone, Thalitone)
- ethacrynic acid (Edecrin)
- etozolin (Elkapin)
- furosemide (Apo-Furosemide, Lasix)
- hydrochlorothiazide (Apo-Hydro, Microzide)
- hydroflumethiazide (Diucardin, Saluron)
- indapamide (Lozol, Nu-Indapamide)
- mannitol (Osmitrol, Resectisol)
- mefruside (Baycaron)
- methazolamide (Apo-Methazolamide, Neptazane)
- methyclothiazide (Aquatensen, Enduron)
- metolazone (Mykrox, Zaroxolyn)
- olmesartan and hydrochlorothiazide (Benicar HCT)
- polythiazide (Renese)
- torsemide (Demadex)
- trichlormethiazide (Metatensin, Naqua)
- urea (Amino-Cerv, UltraMide)
- xipamide (Diurexan, Lumitens)

Lab Tests That May Be Altered by Quassia

None known

Diseases That May Be Worsened or Triggered by Quassia

May worsen inflammatory gastrointestinal ailments by irritating the gastrointestinal tract.

Foods That May Interact with Quassia

None known

Supplements That May Interact with Quassia

- Increased risk of cardiac glycoside toxicity when used with other herbs that contain cardiac glycosides, such as black hellebore, calotropis, motherwort, and others. (For a list of cardiac glycoside–containing herbs and supplements, see Appendix B.)
- Increased risk of cardiotoxicity due to potassium depletion when taken with cardioactive herbs, such as adonis, digitalis, lily-of-the-valley, and squill. (For a list of cardioactive herbs and supplements, see Appendix B.)
- Increased risk of potassium depletion when used with other stimulant laxative herbs, such as black root, cascara sagrada, castor oil, and senna. (For a list of stimulant laxative herbs and supplements, see Appendix B.)

QUILLAJA

Taken from the *Quillaja saponaria* tree, a member of the rose family native to Chile, the soapy, slippery quillaja bark has long been used by those living in the Andes as a treatment for respiratory problems. Quillaja contains saponins, "natural detergent compounds" that help to thin mucous secretions in the airways, so the mucus can be more easily expelled through coughing.

Scientific Name
Quillaja saponaria

Quillaja Is Also Commonly Known As
China bark, cullay, Panama bark, quillaia, quillaja bark, soap bark tree

Medicinal Parts
Bark

Quillaja's Uses
To treat cough, dandruff, athlete's foot, and chronic bronchitis and other conditions affecting the respiratory tract

Typical Dose
A typical dose of quillaja is approximately 200 mg of bark, finely chopped and steeped as tea.

Possible Side Effects
Quillaja's side effects include mucous membrane irritation, stomach pain, and diarrhea.

Drugs That May Interact with Quillaja
Taking quillaja with these drugs may increase the risk of hyperglycemia (high blood sugar):

- glipizide and metformin (Metaglip)
- glyburide and metformin (Glucovance)
- metformin (Glucophage, Riomet)

Lab Tests That May Be Altered by Quillaja
None known

Diseases That May Be Worsened or Triggered by Quillaja
May worsen inflammatory gastrointestinal ailments by irritating the gastrointestinal tract.

Foods That May Interact with Quillaja
May decrease mineral absorption of dietary calcium, iron, or zinc when taken concurrently with foods containing these minerals.

Supplements That May Interact with Quillaja
May decrease mineral absorption when taken concurrently with calcium, iron, or zinc supplements.

QUININE

Quinine, an alkaloid extracted from the bark of the South American cinchona tree, was once the treatment of choice for malaria, until it was replaced by more effective synthetic drugs. However, it is still sometimes used to treat resistant malaria, nighttime leg cramps, and fever.

Scientific Name
Cinchona pubescens

Quinine Is Also Commonly Known As
Cinchona, Jesuit's bark, Peruvian bark

Medicinal Parts

Bark

Quinine's Uses

To treat digestive problems, malaria, muscle pain, fever, flu, flatulence, and enlarged spleen. Germany's Commission E has approved the use of quinine to treat loss of appetite and dyspeptic complaints, such as heartburn and bloating.

Typical Dose

A typical daily dose of quinine in the form of cinchona liquid extract may range from 0.6 to 3.0 gm.

Possible Side Effects

Quinine's side effects include itching and eczema.

Drugs That May Interact with Quinine

Taking quinine with these drugs may increase the risk of bleeding and bruising:

- abciximab (ReoPro)
- antithrombin III (Thrombate III)
- argatroban
- aspirin (Bufferin, Ecotrin)
- aspirin and dipyridamole (Aggrenox)
- bivalirudin (Angiomax)
- clopidogrel (Plavix)
- dalteparin (Fragmin)
- danaparoid (Orgaran)
- dipyridamole (Persantine, Novo-Dipiradol)
- enoxaparin (Lovenox)
- eptifibatide (Integrillin)
- fondaparinux (Arixtra)
- heparin (Hepalean, Hep-Lock)
- indobufen (Ibustrin)
- lepirudin (Refludan)
- ticlopidine (Alti-Ticlopidine, Ticlid)
- tinzaparin (Innohep)
- tirofiban (Aggrastat)
- warfarin (Coumadin, Jantoven)

Taking quinine with these drugs may be harmful:

- carbamazepine (Carbatrol, Tegretol)—may increase blood levels of the drug
- quinidine (Novo-Quinidin, Quinaglute Dura-Tabs)—may increase the therapeutic and/or adverse effects of the drug

Lab Tests That May Be Altered by Quinine

None known

Diseases That May Be Worsened or Triggered by Quinine

May worsen gastrointestinal disorders by increasing the risk of bleeding.

Foods That May Interact with Quinine

None known

Supplements That May Interact with Quinine

Increased risk of bleeding when used with herbs and supplements that might affect platelet aggregation. (For a list of herbs and supplements with anticoagulant/antiplatelet effects, see Appendix B.)

RASPBERRY

Native to North America, the raspberry bush is best known for its delicate, hollow red berries, but it's the leaves that are used in herbal medicine. Raspberry leaf tea, which contains tannins and vitamin C, has been traditionally used to ease the nausea associated with pregnancy and to ensure an easy labor, delivery, and postpartum recovery. It is also used to treat the common cold, control diarrhea, ease menstrual cramps, and regulate the menstrual cycle.

Scientific Name
Rubus idaeus

Raspberry Is Also Commonly Known As
Bramble, hindberry, red raspberry

Medicinal Parts
Leaf

Raspberry's Uses
To treat cough, urinary tract infections, and morning sickness

Typical Dose
A typical dose of raspberry leaf is approximately 1.5 gm mixed with 150 ml boiling water, steeped for 5 minutes, strained and taken as a tea.

Possible Side Effects
Raspberry leaf's side effects include allergic reactions.

Drugs That May Interact with Raspberry
Taking raspberry leaf with these drugs may increase the risk of hypoglycemia (low blood sugar):

- acarbose (Prandase, Precose)
- acetohexamide
- chlorpropamide (Diabinese, Novo-Propamide)
- gliclazide (Diamicron, Novo-Gliclazide)
- glimepiride (Amaryl)
- glipizide (Glucotrol)
- glipizide and metformin (Metaglip)
- gliquidone (Beglynor, Glurenorm)
- glyburide (DiaBeta, Micronase)
- glyburide and metformin (Glucovance)
- insulin (Humulin, Novolin R)
- metformin (Glucophage, Riomet)
- miglitol (Glyset)
- nateglinide (Starlix)
- pioglitazone (Actos)
- repaglinide (GlucoNorm, Prandin)
- rosiglitazone (Avandia)
- rosiglitazone and metformin (Avandamet)
- tolazamide (Tolinase)
- tolbutamide (Apo-Tolbutamide, Tol-Tab)

Taking raspberry leaf (in the form of tea) with these drugs may interfere with absorption of the drug:
- ferric gluconate (Ferrlecit)
- ferrous fumarate (Femiron, Feostat)
- ferrous gluconate (Fergon, Novo-Ferrogluc)
- ferrous sulfate (Feratab, Fer-Iron)
- ferrous sulfate and ascorbic acid (FeroGrad 500, Vitelle Irospan)
- glipizide and metformin (Metaglip)
- glyburide and metformin (Glucovance)
- iron-dextran complex (Dexferrum, INFeD)
- metformin (Glucophage, Riomet)
- polysaccharide-iron complex (Hytinic, Niferex)
- rosiglitazone and metformin (Avandamet)

Lab Tests That May Be Altered by Raspberry

None known

Diseases That May Be Worsened or Triggered by Raspberry

This herb may have estrogen-like effects and should not be used by women with estrogen-sensitive breast cancer or other hormone-sensitive conditions.

Foods That May Interact with Raspberry

None known

Supplements That May Interact with Raspberry

- May decrease absorption of minerals due to its high tannin content.
- The tannins in raspberry leaf may cause the alkaloids in certain other herbs to separate and settle, increasing the risk of toxic reactions. (For a list of herbs and other substances high in alkaloids, see Appendix B.)

RAUWOLFIA

Rauwolfia serpentina, a small shrub native to India and Asia, was named *serpentina* because its roots resemble snakes (thus its common name, snakeroot). The dried root of the plant contains many alkaloids, the most important of which are reserpine and rescinnamine, which are used in modern medicine to reduce elevated blood pressure. In traditional Indian medicine, a tea made from rauwolfia root is used to treat hypertension, paranoia and schizophrenia, cholera, and snakebite.

Scientific Name

Rauwolfia serpentina

Rauwolfia Is Also Commonly Known As

Indian snakeroot, snakeroot

Medicinal Parts

Root

Rauwolfia's Uses

To treat liver disease, vomiting, flatulence, insomnia, elevated blood pressure, anxiety, and snakebite. Germany's Commission E has approved the use of rauwolfia to treat elevated blood pressure, nervousness, and insomnia.

Typical Dose

A typical daily dose of rauwolfia is approximately 600 mg.

Possible Side Effects

Rauwolfia's side effects include depression, nasal congestion, drowsiness, and erectile dysfunction.

Drugs That May Interact with Rauwolfia

Taking rauwolfia with these drugs may increase the action of the drug:

- acetophenazine
- amobarbital (Amytal)
- amobarbital and secobarbital (Tuinal)
- aniracetam (Ampamet, Draganon)
- aripiprazole (Abilify)
- benperidol (Anquil, Glianimon)
- bromperidol (Impromen, Tesoprel)
- butabarbital (Butisol Sodium)
- butalbital, acetaminophen, and caffeine (Esgic, Fioricet)

- butalbital, aspirin, and caffeine (Fiorinal)
- chlorpromazine (Largactil, Thorazine)
- clozapine (Clozaril, GenClozapine)
- droperidol (Inapsine)
- flupenthixol (Fluanxol)
- fluphenazine (Prolixin, Modecate)
- haloperidol (Haldol, Novo-Peridol)
- loxapine (Loxitane, Nu-Loxapine)
- mephobarbital (Mebaral)
- mesoridazine (Serentil)
- methohexital (Brevital, Brevital Sodium)
- molindone (Moban)
- olanzapine (Zydis, Zyprexa)
- pentobarbital (Nembutal)
- perphenazine (Apo-Perphenazine, Trilafon)
- phenobarbital (Luminal Sodium, PMS-Phenobarbital)
- pimozide (Orap)
- pipamperone (Dipiperon, Piperonil)
- piracetam (Geram, Piracetam Verla)
- primidone (Apo-Primidone, Mysoline)
- prochlorperazine (Compazine, Compro)
- quetiapine (Seroquel)
- risperidone (Risperdal)
- secobarbital (Seconal)
- thiopental (Pentothal)—used for convulsions
- thioridazine (Mellaril)
- thiothixene (Navane)
- trifluoperazine (Novo-Trifluzine, Stelazine)
- ziprasidone (Geodon)
- zuclopenthixol (Clopixol)

Taking rauwolfia with these drugs may cause excessive sedation and mental depression and impairment:

- acetaminophen and codeine (Capital and Codeine, Tylenol with Codeine)
- alfentanil (Alfenta)
- alprazolam (Apo-Alpraz, Xanax)
- amobarbital (Amytal)
- amobarbital and secobarbital (Tuinal)
- aspirin and codeine (Coryphen Codeine)
- belladonna and opium (B&O Supprettes)
- bromazepam (Apo-Bromazepam, Gen-Bromazepam)
- brotizolam (Lendorm, Sintonal)
- buprenorphine (Buprenex, Subutex)
- buprenorphine and naloxone (Suboxone)
- butabarbital (Butisol Sodium)
- butalbital, acetaminophen, and caffeine (Esgic, Fioricet)
- butalbital, aspirin, and caffeine (Fiorinal)
- butorphanol (Apo-Butorphanol, Stadol)
- chloral hydrate (Aquachloral Supprettes, Somnote)
- chlordiazepoxide (Apo-Chlordiazepoxide, Librium)
- clobazam (Alti-Clobazam, Frisium)
- clonazepam (Klonopin, Rivotril)
- clorazepate (Tranxene, T-Tab)
- codeine (Codeine Contin)
- dexmedetomidine (Precedex)
- diazepam (Apo-Diazepam, Valium)
- dihydrocodeine, aspirin, and caffeine (Synalgos-DC)
- diphenhydramine (Benadryl Allergy, Nytol)
- estazolam (ProSom)
- fentanyl (Actiq, Duragesic)
- flurazepam (Apo-Flurazepam, Dalmane)
- glutethimide
- haloperidol (Haldol, Novo-Peridol)
- hydrocodone and acetaminophen (Vicodin, Zydone)
- hydrocodone and aspirin (Damason-P)

- hydrocodone and ibuprofen (Vicoprofen)
- hydromorphone (Dilaudid, PMS-Hydromorphone)
- hydroxyzine (Atarax, Vistaril)
- levomethadyl acetate hydrochloride
- levorphanol (LevoDromoran)
- loprazolam (Dormonoct, Havlane)
- lorazepam (Ativan, Nu-Loraz)
- meperidine (Demerol, Meperitab)
- meperidine and promethazine
- mephobarbital (Mebaral)
- methadone (Dolophine, Methadose)
- methohexital (Brevital, Brevital Sodium)
- midazolam (Apo-Midazolam, Versed)
- morphine sulfate (Kadian, MS Contin)
- nalbuphine (Nubain)
- opium tincture
- oxycodone (OxyContin, Roxicodone)
- oxycodone and acetaminophen (Endocet, Percocet)
- oxycodone and aspirin (Endodan, Percodan)
- oxymorphone (Numorphan)
- paregoric
- pentazocine (Talwin)
- pentobarbital (Nembutal)
- phenobarbital (Luminal Sodium, PMS-Phenobarbital)
- phenoperidine
- prazepam
- primidone (Apo-Primidone, Mysoline)
- promethazine (Phenergan)
- propofol (Diprivan)
- propoxyphene (Darvon, Darvon-N)
- propoxyphene and acetaminophen (Darvocet-N 50, Darvocet-N 100)
- propoxyphene, aspirin, and caffeine (Darvon Compound)

- quazepam (Doral)
- remifentanil (Ultiva)
- secobarbital (Seconal)
- sodium oxybate (Xyrem)
- sufentanil (Sufenta)
- s-zopiclone (Lunesta)
- temazepam (Novo-Temazepam, Restoril)
- tetrazepam (Mobiforton, Musapam)
- thiopental (Pentothal)
- triazolam (Apo-Triazo, Halcion)
- zaleplon (Sonata, Stamoc)
- zolpidem (Ambien)
- zopiclone (Alti-Zopiclone, Gen-Zopiclone)

Taking rauwolfia with these drugs may increase the risk of hypertension (high blood pressure):
- albuterol (Proventil, Ventolin)
- brimonidine (Alphagan P, PMS-Brimonidine Tartrate)
- dobutamine (Dobutrex)
- dopamine (Intropin)
- dopexamine (Dopacard)
- ephedrine (PretzD)
- iproniazid (Marsilid)
- isoetharine (Beta2, Bronkosol)
- isoproterenol (Isuprel)
- metaproterenol (Alupent)
- metaraminol (Aramine)
- moclobemide (Alti-Moclobemide, Nu-Moclobemide)
- norepinephrine (Levophed)
- phenelzine (Nardil)
- phenylephrine (Neo-Synephrine, Vicks Sinex Nasal Spray)
- pseudoephedrine (Dimetapp Decongestant, Sudafed)
- selegiline (Eldepryl)

- terbutaline (Brethine)
- tranylcypromine (Parnate)

Taking rauwolfia with these drugs may interfere with the blood pressure–raising effects of the drug:
- ephedrine (Pretz-D)
- epinephrine (Adrenalin, EpiPen)
- isoproterenol (Isuprel)
- norepinephrine (Levophed)

Taking rauwolfia with these drugs may reduce the effectiveness of the herb:
- amitriptyline (Elavil, Levate)
- amitriptyline and chlordiazepoxide (Limbitrol)
- amitriptyline and perphenazine (Etrafon, Triavil)
- amoxapine (Asendin)
- clomipramine (Anafranil, Novo-Clopramine)
- desipramine (Alti-Desipramine, Norpramin)
- doxepin (Sinequan, Zonalon)
- imipramine (Apo-Imipramine, Tofranil)
- lofepramine (Feprapax, Gamanil)
- melitracen (Dixeran)
- nortriptyline (Aventyl HCl, Pamelor)
- protriptyline (Vivactil)
- trimipramine (Apo-Trimip, Surmontil)

Taking rauwolfia with these drugs may reduce the effects of the drug and increase the risk of extrapyramidal symptoms (tremors, rigidity, drooling, rolling eyes, and a masklike expression):
- levodopa (Dopar, Larodopa)
- levodopa-carbidopa (Nu-Levocarb, Sinemet)

Taking rauwolfia with these drugs may be harmful:

- digitalis (Digitek, Lanoxin)—may cause severe bradycardia (abnormally slow heart rate)

Lab Tests That May Be Altered by Rauwolfia
- May increase urinary excretion of 5-hydroxyindoleacetic acid (5-HIAA).
- May decrease urinary 17-hydroxycorticosteroid levels.
- May decrease urinary norepinephrine levels.
- May increase or decrease urinary vanillylmandelic acid (VMA) levels.
- May alter results of urinary 17-ketosteroid colorimetric assays.
- May increase urinary excretion of sodium.
- May increase or decrease urinary 4-hydroxy-3-methoxy phenylethylene glycol (HMPG) levels.
- May increase or decrease urinary catecholamine excretion.
- May cause false positive results in urine guaiacols spot test.
- May cause decrease in red blood cells.
- May cause false increase in serum bilirubin.
- May increase serum sodium.
- May increase blood glucose levels.
- May decrease serum gastrin.
- May cause thrombocytopenia and decreased blood platelet counts.
- May increase plasma prolactin levels in those with hypertension.
- May decrease serum thyroxine (T4) levels.
- May cause false negative test results for tyramine.
- May increase gastric analysis and basal nocturnal acid output.
- May decrease blood pressure readings in those with mild to moderate hypertension.

- May cause positive test results for lupus erythematosus (LE) cells.
- May cause positive results on fecal occult blood tests by activating peptic ulcers and causing bleeding.

Diseases That May Be Worsened or Triggered by Rauwolfia

Increased risk of central nervous system depression when used concurrently with alcohol.

Foods That May Interact with Rauwolfia

None known

Supplements That May Interact with Rauwolfia

- Increased risk of angina-like symptoms, arrhythmia, and bradycardia (abnormally slow heart rate) when used with herbs that contain cardiac glycosides, such as black hellebore, calotropis, motherwort, and others. (For a list of cardiac glycoside–containing herbs and supplements, see Appendix B.)
- May decrease ephedrine effects and pressor effects when taken concurrently with ma-huang.

RED CLOVER

Despite its name, the most obvious thing about red clover's appearance is its pink flowers. A perennial that grows wild in North America and Europe, red clover contains substances that, when consumed, can mimic some of the effects of estrogen in the human body. Researchers are currently investigating the herb's ability to soothe menopausal symptoms and possibly aid in combating cancer.

Scientific Name

Trifolium pratense

Red Clover Is Also Commonly Known As

Purple clover, trefoil, wild clover

Medicinal Parts

Flower heads

Red Clover's Uses

To treat respiratory conditions, cough, menopausal symptoms, psoriasis, and eczema

Typical Dose

A typical dose of red clover may range from 1.5 to 3.0 ml of liquid extract (1:1 in 25 percent ethanol), taken three times daily.

Possible Side Effects

Red clover's side effects include an increased risk of bleeding.

Drugs That May Interact with Red Clover

Taking red clover with these drugs may increase the risk of bleeding and bruising:

- abciximab (ReoPro)
- alteplase (Activase, Cathflo Activase)
- antithrombin III (Thrombate III)
- argatroban
- aspirin (Bufferin, Ecotrin)—bleeding
- bivalirudin (Angiomax)
- celecoxib (Celebrex)
- choline magnesium trysalicylate (Trilisate)
- clopidogrel (Plavix)
- dalteparin (Fragmin)
- danaparoid (Orgaran)—bleeding
- diclofenac (Cataflam, Voltaren)

- diflunisal (Apo-Diflunisal, Dolobid)
- dipyridamole (Novo-Dipiradol, Persantine)
- drotrecogin alfa (Xigris)
- enoxaparin (Lovenox)
- etodolac (Lodine, Utradol)
- fenoprofen (Nalfon)
- flurbiprofen (Ansaid, Ocufen)
- fondaparinux (Arixtra)
- heparin (Hepalean, Hep-Lock)
- hydrocodone and aspirin (Damason-P)
- hydrocodone and ibuprofen (Vicoprofen)
- ibritumomab (Zevalin)
- ibuprofen (Advil, Motrin)
- indomethacin (Indocin, Novo-Methacin)
- ketoprofen (Orudis, Rhodis)
- ketorolac (Acular, Toradol)
- lepirudin (Refludan)
- meloxicam (MOBIC, Mobicox)
- nabumetone (Apo-Nabumetone, Relefan)
- nadroparin (Fraxiparine)
- naproxen (Aleve, Naprosyn)
- oxaprozin (Apo-Oxaprozin, Daypro)
- piroxicam (Feldene, Nu-Pirox)
- reteplase (Retavase)
- rofecoxib (Vioxx)
- salsalate (Amgesic, Salflex)
- streptokinase (Streptase)
- sulindac (Clinoril, Nu-Sundac)
- tiaprofenic acid (Dom-Tiaprofenic, Surgam)
- ticlopidine (Alti-Ticlopidine, Ticlid)
- tenecteplase (TNKase)
- tinzaparin (Innohep)
- tolmetin (Tolectin)
- urokinase (Abbokinase)
- valdecoxib (Bextra)
- warfarin (Coumadin, Jantoven)

Taking red clover with these drugs may reduce the effectiveness of the drug or increase side effects:

- cyproterone and ethinyl estradiol (Diane-35)
- estradiol (Climara, Estrace)
- estradiol and norethindrone (Activella, CombiPatch)
- estradiol and testosterone (Climacteron)
- estrogens (conjugated A/synthetic) (Cenestin)
- estrogens (conjugated/equine) (Cenestin, Premarin)
- estrogens (conjugated/equine) and medroxy-progesterone (Premphase, Prempro)
- estrogens (esterified) (Estratab, Menest)
- estrogens (esterified) and methyltestosterone (Estratest, Estratest H.S.)
- estropipate (Ogen, Ortho-Est)
- ethinyl estradiol (Estinyl)
- ethinyl estradiol and desogestrel (Cyclessa, Ortho-Cept)
- ethinyl estradiol and ethynodiol diacetate (Demulen, Zovia)
- ethinyl estradiol and etonogestrel (NuvaRing)
- ethinyl estradiol and levonorgestrel (Alesse, Triphasil)
- ethinyl estradiol and norelgestromin (Evra, Ortho Evra)
- ethinyl estradiol and norethindrone (Brevicon, Ortho-Novum)
- ethinyl estradiol and norgestimate (Cyclen, Ortho Tri-Cyclen)
- ethinyl estradiol and norgestrel (Cryselle, Ovral)
- mestranol and norethindrone (Necon 1/50, Ortho-Novum 1/50)
- progesterone (Crinone, Prometrium)
- tamoxifen (Nolvadex, Tamofen)

Lab Tests That May Be Altered by Red Clover
None known

Diseases That May Be Worsened or Triggered by Red Clover
- May worsen bleeding disorders due to its coumarin content.
- This herb may have estrogen-like effects and should not be used by women with estrogen-sensitive breast cancer or other hormone-sensitive conditions.

Foods That May Interact with Red Clover
None known

Supplements That May Interact with Red Clover
- Increased risk of bleeding when used with herbs and supplements that might affect platelet aggregation. (For a list of herbs and supplements with anticoagulant/antiplatelet effects, see Appendix B.)
- May increase action of herbs and supplements that have estrogenic activity, such as black cohosh, chaste tree berry, and soy. (For a list of herbs and supplements that have estrogenic activity, see Appendix B.)

RED YEAST RICE

Used in China for centuries as both a food and a medicine, red yeast rice is created by the fermenting of *Monascus purpureus* yeast that grows on red rice. Used traditionally to promote blood circulation, soothe upset stomach, and treat hangovers, red yeast rice has been found to contain substances very similar to those found in the statin drugs that lower cholesterol. Researchers from the UCLA School of Medicine found that red yeast rice significantly lowered total cholesterol, LDL "bad" cholesterol, and blood fats within eight weeks.

Scientific Name
Monascus purpureus

Red Yeast Rice Is Also Commonly Known As
Hong qu, red yeast, red rice, xue zhi kang, zhi tai

Medicinal Parts
Rice is fermented with *Monascus purpureus* yeast to make red yeast rice.

Red Yeast Rice's Uses
To treat elevated cholesterol, poor blood circulation, and indigestion

Typical Dose
A typical dose of red yeast rice ranges from 600 to 1,200 mg.

Possible Side Effects
Red yeast rice's side effects include nausea, vomiting, anorexia, allergic reactions, and damage to muscle tissues

Drugs That May Interact with Red Yeast Rice
Taking red yeast rice with these drugs may increase the risk of adverse effects or drug toxicity:
- atorvastatin (Lipitor)
- fluvastatin (Lescol)
- lovastatin (Altocor, Mevacor)

- pravastatin (Novo-Pravastatin, Pravachol)
- rosuvastatin (Crestor)
- simvastatin (Apo-Simvastatin, Zocor)

Taking red yeast rice with these drugs may cause or increase kidney damage:

- etodolac (Lodine, Utradol)
- ibuprofen (Advil, Motrin)
- indomethacin (Indocin, Novo-Methacin)
- ketoprofen (Orudis, Rhodis)
- ketorolac (Acular, Toradol)
- metformin (Glucophage, Riomet)

Lab Tests That May Be Altered by Red Yeast Rice

- May decrease serum cholesterol levels.
- May increase serum creatine kinase levels.
- May increase serum liver transaminase levels.

Diseases That May Be Worsened or Triggered by Red Yeast Rice

May worsen liver or thyroid dysfunction

Foods That May Interact with Red Yeast Rice

- Concomitant use with grapefruit or grapefruit products may increase serum levels of lovastatin (a constituent of red yeast rice) by inhibiting lovastatin's cytochrome P450 metabolism. (See grapefruit section.)
- Absorption of lovastatin (a constituent of red yeast rice) is increased by the presence of food.
- Alcohol may impair liver function in those taking red yeast rice.

Supplements That May Interact with Red Yeast Rice

- Increased risk of liver damage when combined with herbs and supplements that can cause hepatotoxicity (destructive effects on the liver), such as bishop's weed, borage, chaparral, uva ursi, and others. (For a list of herbs and supplements that can cause hepatotoxicity, see Appendix B.)
- Serum levels of red yeast rice and its lovastatin constituent may be decreased by St. John's wort.
- May alter effects of herbs and supplements that have thyroid activity, such as bugleweed and wild thyme. (For a list of herbs and supplements that affect the thyroid, see Appendix B.)
- May increase action of herbs and supplements that lower cholesterol, such as chromium, flaxseed, and psyllium. (For a list of herbs and supplements that lower cholesterol, see Appendix B.)
- May lower coenzyme Q_{10} levels.

REISHI MUSHROOM

The reishi mushroom, which grows wild on decaying stumps and trees in coastal areas of China, is sometimes used by patients with HIV or cancer to stimulate the immune system. Extracts of reishi appear to promote the activity of macrophages (cells that engulf invading organisms). Tested as a treatment for neurasthenia (characterized by nervous exhaustion), reishi mushroom extract produced significant improvement in fatigue and sense of well-being after volunteers used it for eight weeks.

Scientific Name

Ganoderma lucidum

Reishi Mushroom Is Also Commonly Known As

Ling chih, ling zhi, mushroom of spiritual potency, spirit plant

Medicinal Parts

Body and mycelium

Reishi Mushroom's Uses

To treat high blood pressure, high cholesterol, viral infections, asthma, tumors, inflammatory disease, and hepatitis; to strengthen the immune system

Typical Dose

A typical daily dose of reishi mushroom may range from 1.5 to 9.0 gm of crude dried mushroom.

Possible Side Effects

Reishi mushroom's side effects include stomach upset, dryness of mouth and throat, nosebleed, itchiness, and bloody stools.

Drugs That May Interact with Reishi Mushroom

Taking reishi mushroom with these drugs may increase the risk of bleeding or bruising:

- abciximab (ReoPro)
- acemetacin (Acemetacin Heumann, Acemetacin Sandoz)
- antithrombin III (Thrombate III)
- argatroban
- aspirin (Bufferin, Ecotrin)
- aspirin and dipyridamole (Aggrenox)
- bivalirudin (Angiomax)
- celecoxib (Celebrex)
- choline magnesium trisalicylate (Trilisate)
- choline salicylate (Teejel)
- clopidogrel (Plavix)
- dalteparin (Fragmin)
- danaparoid (Orgaran)
- diclofenac (Cataflam, Voltaren)
- diflunisal (Apo-Diflunisal, Dolobid)
- dipyridamole (Novo-Dipiradol, Persantine)
- dipyrone (Analgina, Dinador)
- enoxaparin (Lovenox)
- eptifibatide (Integrillin)
- etodolac (Lodine, Utradol)
- etoricoxib (Arcoxia)
- fenoprofen (Nalfon)
- flurbiprofen (Ansaid, Ocufen)
- fondaparinux (Arixtra)
- heparin (Hepalean, Hep-Lock)
- ibuprofen (Advil, Motrin)
- indobufen (Ibustrin)
- indomethacin (Indocin, Novo-Methacin)
- ketoprofen (Orudis, Rhodis)
- ketorolac (Acular, Toradol)
- lepirudin (Refludan)
- magnesium salicylate (Doan's, Mobidin)
- meclofenamate (Meclomen)
- mefenamic acid (Ponstan, Ponstel)
- meloxicam (MOBIC, Mobicox)
- nabumetone (Apo-Nabumetone, Relafen)
- naproxen (Aleve, Naprosyn)
- niflumic acid (Niflam, Nifluril)
- nimesulide (Areuma, Aulin)
- oxaprozin (Apo-Oxaprozin, Daypro)
- piroxicam (Feldene, Nu-Pirox)
- rofecoxib (Vioxx)
- salasalate (Amgesic, Salflex)
- sulindac (Clinoril, Nu-Sundac)
- tenoxicam (Dolmen, Mobiflex)
- tiaprofenic acid (DomTiaprofenic, Surgam)
- ticlopidine (Alti-Ticlopidine, Ticlid)

- tinzaparin (Innohep)
- tirofiban (Aggrastat)
- tolmetin (Tolectin)
- valdecoxib (Bextra)
- warfarin (Coumadin, Jantoven)

Lab Tests That May Be Altered by Reishi Mushroom
May increase bleeding time due to antiplatelet activity.

Diseases That May Be Worsened or Triggered by Reishi Mushroom
May worsen bleeding disorders.

Foods That May Interact with Reishi Mushroom
None known

Supplements That May Interact with Reishi Mushroom

- Increased risk of bleeding when used with herbs and supplements that might affect platelet aggregation. (For a list of herbs and supplements with anticoagulant/antiplatelet effects, see Appendix B.)
- Increased risk of hypotension or increased therapeutic effects when used with herbs and supplements with hypotensive activity, such as black cohosh, danshen, and Panax ginseng. (For a list of herbs and supplements with hypotensive activity, see Appendix B.)

RIBOFLAVIN

Formerly known as vitamin B_2, riboflavin helps to prevent oxidative damage to body cells, extract energy from food, keep the immune system strong, and manufacture blood cells. A lack of riboflavin can cause the development of cracks at the corners of the mouth, vision problems, and burning and itching of the eyes.

Typical Dose
The Food and Nutrition Board has set the RDA for riboflavin at 1.3 mg per day for men ages nineteen and up and 1.1 mg per day for women ages nineteen and over.

Possible Side Effects
Riboflavin is considered to be very safe, although taking large doses for a long time may interfere with the metabolism of other B vitamins.

Drugs That May Interact with Riboflavin
None known

Drugs That May Interfere with the Absorption, Utilization, or Excretion of Riboflavin

- amikacin (Amikin)
- amitriptyline (Elavil, Vanatrip)
- amoxapine (Asendin)
- amoxicillin (Amoxil, Novamoxin)
- ampicillin (Omnipen, Totacillin)
- azithromycin (Zithromax)
- carbenicillin (Geocillin)
- cefaclor (Ceclor)
- cefadroxil (Duricef)
- cefamandole (Mandol)
- cefazolin (Ancef, Kefzol)
- cefdinir (Omnicef)
- cefditoren (Spectracef)
- cefepime (Maxipime)

- cefonicid (Monocid)
- cefoperazone (Cefobid)
- cefotaxime (Claforan)
- cefotetan (Cefotan)
- cefoxitin (Mefoxin)
- cefpodoxime (Vantin)
- cefprozil (Cefzil)
- ceftazidime (Ceptaz, Fortaz)
- ceftibuten (Cedax)
- ceftizoxime (Cefizox)
- ceftriaxone (Rocephin)
- cefuroxime (Ceftin, Kefurox)
- cephalexin (Biocef, Keftab)
- cephalothin (Ceporacin)
- cephapirin (Cefadyl)
- cepharadine (Velosef)
- chlorpromazine (Thorazine)
- cinoxacin (Cinobac)
- ciprofloxacin (Ciloxan, Cipro)
- clarithromycin (Biaxin, Biaxin XL)
- clomipramine (Anafranil, Novo-Clopramine)
- cloxacillin (Cloxapen, Nu-Cloxi)
- demeclocycline (Declomycin)
- desipramine (Alti-Desipramine, Norpramin)
- dicloxacillin (Dycill, Pathocil)
- dirithromycin (Dynabac)
- doxepin (Sinequan, Zonalon)
- doxorubicin (Adriamycin, Rubex)
- doxorubicin liposomal (Doxil)
- doxycycline (Apo-Doxy, Vibramycin)
- erythromycin (Erythrocin, Staticin)
- fluphenazine (Modecate, Prolixin)
- gatofloxacin (Tequin, Zymar)
- gentamicin (Alcomicin, Gentacidin)
- imipramine (Apo-Imipramine, Tofranil)
- kanamycin (Kantrex)
- levofloxacin (Levaquin, Quixin)

- levonorgestrel (Norplant Implant, Plan B)
- linezolid (Zyvox)
- lomefloxacin (Maxaquin)
- loracarbef (Lorabid)
- meclocycline (Meclan Topical)
- mesoridazine (Serentil)
- metoclopramide (Octamide, Relgan)
- minocycline (Dynacin, Minocin)
- moxifloxacin (Avelox)
- nafcillin (Nafcil Injection, Unipen Oral)
- nalidixic acid (NegGram)
- norethindrone (Aygestin, Micronor)
- norfloxacin (Chibroxin Ophthalmic, Noroxin Oral)
- nortriptyline (Aventyl HCl, Pamelor)
- ofloxacin (Floxin, Ocuflox)
- penicillin G benzathine (Bicillin L-A, Permapen)
- penicillin G benzathine and penicillin G procaine (Bicicillin C-R)
- penicillin G procaine (Pfizerpen-AS, Wycillin)
- pencillin V potassium (Suspen, Truxcillin)
- perphenazine (Apo-Perphenazine, Trilafon)
- piperacillin (Pipracil)
- piperacillin and tazobactam sodium (Zosyn)
- prochlorperazine (Compazine, Compro)
- promethazine (Phenergan)
- protriptyline (Triptil, Vivactil)
- sparfloxacin (Zagam)
- sulfadiazine (Microsulfon)
- sulfisoxazole (Gantrisin)
- tetracycline (Novo-Tetra, Sumycin)
- thiethylperazine (Norzine, Torecan)
- thioridazine (Mellaril)
- ticarcillin (Ticar)
- ticarcillin and clavulanate potassium (Timentin)
- tobramycin (Nebcin, Tobrex)
- trifluoperazine (Novo-Trifluzine, Stelazine)

- trimethoprim (Primsol, Trimpex)
- trimipramine (Apo-Trimip, Surmontil)
- trovafloxacin (Trovan)

Lab Tests That May Be Altered by Riboflavin

- May confound results of diagnostic urine tests that rely on a color change (for example, urine Diagnex blue excretion test, urinalysis based on color reactions or spectrometry) by turning urine bright yellow.
- May confound results of Abbott TDx drugs-of-abuse urine assays if riboflavin is taken in large doses.
- May cause false increase in serum acetoacetate decarboxylase test.
- May cause false increase in urinary catecholamine fluorometric assays.
- May cause false increase in plasma and urine fluorometric urobilinogen tests.

Diseases That May Be Worsened or Triggered by Riboflavin

None known

Foods That May Interact with Riboflavin

Food may increase absorption of riboflavin.

Supplements That May Interact with Riboflavin

May improve uptake of iron in those with anemia who also have a riboflavin deficiency.

ROSE HIPS

Rose hips are the small fruit produced by the rose plant after the blossom falls away. An excellent source of antioxidants, rose hips contain twenty times as much vitamin C as oranges, when compared ounce for ounce. In 2005, Scandinavian researchers looked at the effects of rose hips on osteoarthritis. Ninety-four people with knee or hip osteoarthritis were given either an herbal remedy made from rose hips or a placebo for three months. Compared to placebo, rose hips triggered a reduction in pain, stiffness, and disability, and those who took the herb were able to cut back on their standard medicines.

Scientific Name

Rosa canina

Rose Hip Is Also Commonly Known As

Brier hip, dog rose, hip, hogseed, sweet briar, witches' brier

Medicinal Parts

Fruit

Rose Hips' Uses

To treat rheumatism, gout, scurvy, kidney stones, and colds

Typical Dose

A typical dose of rose hips may range from 1 to 2 gm of powdered herb mixed with 150 ml boiling water, steeped 10 to 15 minutes, then strained and taken as a tea.

Possible Side Effects

Rose hips' side effects include nausea, vomiting, anorexia, diarrhea, and allergic reactions.

Drugs That May Interact with Rose Hips

Taking rose hips with these drugs may be harmful:

- ferrous sulfate (Feratab, Fer-Iron)—may increase iron absorption
- fluphenazine (Modecate, Prolixin)—may reduce blood levels of the drug
- warfarin (Coumadin, Jantoven)—may reduce effectiveness of the drug

Lab Tests That May Be Altered by Rose Hips

- May cause false negative results in stool occult blood tests (guaiac) with intake of 250 mg vitamin C or more per day.
- May cause false decrease in glucose oxidase test (for example, Clinistix) after ingesting more than 500 mg of vitamin C.
- May cause false increase in cupric sulfate test (for example, Clinitest) due to vitamin C in rose hips.
- May cause false increase in liver function tests aspartate aminotransferase (AST), serum glutamic-oxaloacetic transaminase (SGOT), and bilirubin.
- May increase urinary calcium excretion.
- May decrease urinary sodium excretion.
- May cause false increase in serum assay tests for carbamazepine (Tegretol) based on Ames ARIS method.
- May cause false negative results in tests for acetaminophen.

Diseases That May Be Worsened or Triggered by Rose Hips

- May interfere with blood sugar control in diabetes.
- May increase hemochromatosis, thalassemia, or other ailments worsened by increased iron absorption.
- May increase the risk of kidney stone formation and sickle cell crisis.

Foods That May Interact with Rose Hips

Increased absorption of iron from foods due to vitamin C content of rose hips.

Supplements That May Interact with Rose Hips

Increased absorption of iron from supplements due to vitamin C content of rose hips.

ROSEMARY

Because ancient Greeks believed that rosemary strengthened the brain, they wore garlands made from the herb when taking examinations. Rosemary was also thought to prevent fairies from stealing infants, preserve youthfulness, and ensure marital fidelity when included in a bride's bouquet. Today its oil is used to ease headaches, reduce flatulence and stimulate digestion, treat painful menstrual periods, and strengthen the blood vessels.

Scientific Name

Rosmarinus officinalis

Rosemary Is Also Commonly Known As

Compass plant, compass weed, polar plant, rusmari

Medicinal Parts

Leaf, twig tip, above-ground parts, oil taken from the leaf

Rosemary's Uses

To treat rheumatism, headaches, circulation problems, menstrual complaints, poor memory, heartburn, and bloating. Germany's Commission E has approved the use of rosemary to treat dyspeptic complaints such as heartburn and bloating, loss of appetite, rheumatism, and problems with blood pressure.

Typical Dose
A typical daily dose of rosemary may range from 4 to 6 gm of the whole herb.

Possible Side Effects
Rosemary's side effects, when taken internally, include gastrointestinal irritation, vomiting, and coma. When used externally, it may cause contact allergies and photosensitivity.

Drugs That May Interact with Rosemary
Taking rosemary with these drugs may increase skin sensitivity to sunlight:
- bumetanide (Bumex, Burinex)
- celecoxib (Celebrex)
- ciprofloxacin (Ciloxan, Cipro)
- doxycycline (Apo-Doxy, Vibramycin)
- enalapril (Vasotec)
- etodolac (Lodine, Utradol)
- fluphenazine (Modecate, Prolixin)
- fosinopril (Monopril)
- furosemide (Apo-Furosemide, Lasix)
- gatifloxacin (Tequin, Zymar)
- hydrochlorothiazide (Apo-Hydro, Microzide)
- ibuprofen (Advil, Motrin)
- indomethacin (Indocin, Novo-Methacin)
- ketoprofen (Orudis, Rhodis)
- ketorolac (Acular, Toradol)
- lansoprazole (Prevacid)
- levofloxacin (Levaquin, Quixin)
- lisinopril (Prinivil, Zestril)
- loratadine (Alavert, Claritin)
- methotrexate (Rheumatrex, Trexall)
- naproxen (Aleve, Naprosyn)
- nortriptyline (Aventyl HCl, Pamelor)
- ofloxacin (Floxin, Ocuflox)
- omeprazole (Losec, Prilosec)
- phenytoin (Dilantin, Phenytek)
- piroxicam (Feldene, Nu-Pirox)
- prochlorperazine (Compazine, Compro)
- quinapril (Accupril)
- risperidone (Risperdal)
- rofecoxib (Vioxx)
- tetracycline (Novo-Tetra, Sumycin)

Lab Tests That May Be Altered by Rosemary
None known

Diseases That May Be Worsened or Triggered by Rosemary
May worsen seizure activity.

Foods That May Interact with Rosemary
None known

Supplements That May Interact with Rosemary
None known

RUE

This hardy, evergreen shrub native to southern Europe has a strong, disagreeable smell, as indicated by one of its scientific names, *graveolens*, which means "strong smelling." Its other name, *ruta*, is believed to come from the Greek word *reuo*, which means "to set free," because rue seemed to be so effective at banishing dis-

> eases. Rue has stimulating effects on the uterus and has been used as a contraceptive and to induce abortions.

Scientific Name
Ruta graveolens

Rue Is Also Commonly Known As
Bitter herb, common rue, herb-of-grace, herby-grass

Medicinal Parts
Above-ground parts, oil

Rue's Uses
Internally used to treat cramps, diarrhea, intestinal worms, and menstrual distress; as a contraceptive. Topically used to treat skin inflammation, arthritis, earache, toothache, and warts.

Typical Dose
A typical oral dose of rue may range from 0.5 to 1.0 gm of the crushed herb per day. There is no standard topical dosage.

Possible Side Effects
When taken internally, rue's side effects include gastrointestinal distress, fatigue, dizziness, and kidney and liver damage. When used topically, its side effects include skin rash and blisters.

Drugs That May Interact with Rue
Taking rue with these drugs may increase the risk of bleeding or bruising:
- abciximab (ReoPro)
- aspirin (Bufferin, Ecotrin)
- celecoxib (Celebrex)
- enoxaparin (Lovenox)
- heparin (Hepalean, Hep-Lock)
- indomethacin (Indocin, Novo-Methacin)
- etodolac (Lodine, Utradol)
- ibuprofen (Advil, Motrin)
- ketoprofen (Orudis, Rhodis)
- ketorolac (Acular, Toradol)

Taking rue with these drugs may cause or increase kidney damage:
- etodolac (Lodine, Utradol)
- ibuprofen (Advil, Motrin)
- indomethacin (Indocin, Novo-Methacin)
- ketoprofen (Orudis, Rhodis)
- ketorolac (Acular, Toradol)
- metformin (Glucophage, Riomet)

Taking rue with these drugs may increase the risk of hypotension (excessively low blood pressure):
- acebutolol (Novo-Acebutolol, Sectral)
- amlodipine (Norvasc)
- atenolol (Apo-Atenol, Tenormin)
- benazepril (Lotensin)
- betaxolol (Betoptic S, Kerlone)
- bisoprolol (Monocor, Zebeta)
- bumetanide (Bumex, Burinex)
- candesartan (Atacand)
- captopril (Capoten, Novo-Captopril)
- carteolol (Cartrol, Ocupress)
- carvedilol (Coreg)
- chlorothiazide (Diuril)
- chlorthalidone (Apo-Chlorthalidone, Thalitone)
- clonidine (Catapres, Duraclon)
- diazoxide (Hyperstat, Proglycem)

- diltiazem (Cardizem, Tiazac)
- doxazosin (Alti-Doxazosin, Cardura)
- enalapril (Vasotec)
- eplerenone (Inspra)
- eprosartan (Teveten)
- esmolol (Brevibloc)
- felodipine (Plendil, Renedil)
- fenoldopam (Corlopam)
- fosinopril (Monopril)
- furosemide (Apo-Furosemide, Lasix)
- guanabenz (Wytensin)
- guanadrel (Hylorel)
- guanfacine (Tenex)
- hydralazine (Apresoline, Novo-Hylazin)
- hydrochlorothiazide (Apo-Hydro, Microzide)
- hydrochlorothiazide and triamterene (Dyazide, Maxzide)
- indapamide (Lozol, Nu-Indapamide)
- irbesartan (Avapro)
- isradipine (DynaCirc)
- labetalol (Normodyne, Trandate)
- lisinopril (Prinivil, Zestril)
- losartan (Cozaar)
- mecamylamine (Inversine)
- mefruside (Baycaron)
- methyclothiazide (Aquatensen, Enduron)
- methyldopa (Apo-Methyldopa, Nu-Medopa)
- metolazone (Mykrox, Zaroxolyn)
- metoprolol (Betaloc, Lopressor)
- minoxidil (Loniten, Rogaine)
- moexipril (Univasc)
- nadolol (Apo-Nadol, Corgard)
- nicardipine (Cardene)
- nifedipine (Adalat CC, Procardia)
- nisoldipine (Sular)
- nitroglycerin (Minitran, Nitro-Dur)
- nitroprusside (Nipride, Nitropress)
- olmesartan (Benicar)
- oxprenolol (Slow-Trasicor, Trasicor)
- perindopril erbumine (Aceon, Coversyl)
- phenoxybenzamine (Dibenzyline)
- phentolamine (Regitine, Rogitine)
- pindolol (Apo-Pindol, Novo-Pindol)
- polythiazide (Renese)
- prazosin (Minipress, Nu-Prazo)
- propranolol (Inderal, InnoPran XL)
- quinapril (Accupril)
- ramipril (Altace)
- reserpine
- spironolactone (Aldactone, Novo-Spiroton)
- telmisartan (Micardis)
- terazosin (Alti-Terazosin, Hytrin)
- timolol (Betimol, Timoptic)
- torsemide (Demadex)
- trandolapril (Mavik)
- triamterene (Dyrenium)
- trichlormethiazide (Metatensin, Naqua)
- valsartan (Diovan)
- verapamil (Calan, Isoptin SR)

Taking rue with these drugs may be harmful:
- digitalis (Digitek, Lanoxin)—may increase the risk of hypotension (low blood pressure), irregular heartbeat, and slow heartbeat

Lab Tests That May Be Altered by Rue
None known

Diseases That May Be Worsened or Triggered by Rue
- May worsen inflammatory ailments of the gastrointestinal tract.
- May worsen kidney inflammation.

Foods That May Interact with Rue
None known

Supplements That May Interact with Rue
None known

SAFFLOWER

The scientific name for safflower, *Carthamus*, comes from the Arabic word for dye, and in times past the reddish yellow flowers were a necessary ingredient in clothing dye. The flower has also been used for thousands of years in traditional Chinese medicine to dissolve blood clots. Safflower is also used to treat menstrual disorders, tone the uterus after childbirth, and ease joint stiffness and pain. Modern scientific research shows that safflower oil may help prevent heart disease by lowering cholesterol levels.

Scientific Name
Carthamus tinctorius

Safflower Is Also Commonly Known As
American saffron, dyer's saffron, fake saffron, zaffer

Medicinal Parts
Flower, oil taken from seed

Safflower's Uses
Safflower is used to treat constipation, fever, cough, and menstrual irregularities. Safflower oil is used to lower the risk of cardiovascular disease by reducing total LDL ("bad") cholesterol.

Typical Dose
A typical dose of safflower is approximately 3 gm of the dried flowers taken three times daily. There is no standard dose of the oil.

Possible Side Effects
Safflower's side effects include nausea, vomiting, anorexia, and allergic reactions.

Drugs That May Interact with Safflower
Taking safflower with these drugs may increase the risk of bleeding or bruising:

- abciximab (ReoPro)
- aminosalicylic acid (Nemasol Sodium, Paser)
- antithrombin III (Thrombate III)
- argatroban
- aspirin (Bufferin, Ecotrin)
- aspirin and dipyridamole (Aggrenox)
- bivalirudin (Angiomax)
- choline magnesium trisalicylate (Trilisate)
- choline salicylate (Teejel)
- clopidogrel (Plavix)
- dalteparin (Fragmin)
- danaparoid (Orgaran)
- dipyridamole (Novo-Dipiradol, Persantine)
- enoxaparin (Lovenox)
- eptifibatide (Integrillin)
- fondaparinux (Arixtra)
- heparin (Hepalean, Hep-Lock)
- indobufen (Ibustrin)
- lepirudin (Refludan)
- salsalate (Amgesic, Salflex)
- ticlopidine (Alti-Ticlopidine, Ticlid)
- tinzaparin (Innohep)
- tirofiban (Aggrastat)
- warfarin (Coumadin, Jantoven)

Lab Tests That May Be Altered by Safflower

None known

Diseases That May Be Worsened or Triggered by Safflower

May increase the risk of bleeding or bruising in people with bleeding disorders or ulcers.

Foods That May Interact with Safflower

None known

Supplements That May Interact with Safflower

Increased risk of bleeding when used with herbs and supplements that might affect platelet aggregation, such as angelica, danshen, garlic, ginger, ginkgo biloba, red clover, turmeric, white willow, and others. (For a list of herbs and supplements with anticoagulant/antiplatelet effects, see Appendix B.)

SAGE

Sage's scientific name, *Salvia officinalis*, comes from the Latin word *salvare*, which means "to save," and for centuries sage was believed to be a powerful curative herb. Its antioxidant and antibacterial properties have made it a favorite for treating colds, gastrointestinal disorders, diarrhea, sore throat, and gum disease. Sage is also thought to be able to stop the flow of breast milk in nursing mothers and to ease menopausal hot flashes.

Scientific Name

Salvia officinalis

Sage Is Also Commonly Known As

Dalmatian sage, garden sage, Greek sage

Medicinal Parts

Leaf, above-ground parts, oil taken from the leaf

Sage's Uses

To treat flatulence, bloating, loss of appetite, diarrhea, bleeding gums, and laryngitis. Germany's Commission E has approved the use of sage to treat inflammation of the mouth and throat, excessive perspiration, and loss of appetite.

Typical Dose

A typical internal dose of sage may range from 1 to 4 ml of extract (1:1 dilution in 45 percent alcohol), taken three times daily.

Possible Side Effects

Sage's side effects include nausea, vomiting, anorexia, stomatitis, dry mouth, oral irritation, and allergic reactions.

Drugs That May Interact with Sage

Taking sage with these drugs may interfere with the action of the drug:

- acetazolamide (Apo-Acetazolamide, Diamox Sequels)
- amobarbital (Amytal)
- barbexaclone (Maliasin)
- carbamazepine (Carbatrol, Tegretol)
- clonazepam (Klonopin, Rivotril)
- clorazepate (Tranxene, T-Tab)
- diazepam (Apo-Diazepam, Valium)
- ethosuximide (Zarontin)
- felbamate (Felbatol)
- fosphenytoin (Cerebyx)

- gabapentin (Neurontin, Nu-Gabapentin)
- lamotrigine (Lamictal)
- levetiracetam (Keppra)
- lorazepam (Ativan, Nu-Loraz)
- mephobarbital (Mebaral)
- methsuximide (Celontin)
- oxazepam (Novoxapam, Serax)
- oxcarbazepine (Trileptal)
- pentobarbital (Nembutal)
- phenobarbital (Luminal Sodium, PMS-Phenobarbital)
- phenytoin (Dilantin, Phenytek)
- primidone (Apo-Primidone, Mysoline)
- thiopental (Pentothal)
- tiagabine (Gabitril)
- topiramate (Topamax)
- valproic acid (Depacon, Depakote ER)
- vigabatrin (Sabril)
- zonisamide (Zonegran)

Taking sage with these drugs may induce seizures:
- carbamazepine (Carbatrol, Tegretol)
- desipramine (Alti-Desipramine, Norpramin)
- methylphenidate (Concerta, Ritalin)
- nortriptyline (Aventyl HCl, Pamelor)
- olanzapine (Zydis, Zyprexa)
- oxcarbazepine (Trileptal)
- phenytoin (Dilantin, Phenytek)
- prochlorperazine (Compazine, Compro)
- quetiapine (Seroquel)
- tramadol (Ultram)
- venlafaxine (Effexor)

Taking sage with these drugs may disrupt blood sugar control:
- acarbose (Prandase, Precose)
- glipizide (Glucotrol)

- glyburide (DiaBeta, Micronase)
- insulin (Humulin, Novolin R)
- metformin (Glucophage, Riomet)
- miglitol (Glyset)
- pioglitazone (Actos)
- repaglinide (GlucoNorm, Prandin)
- rosiglitazone (Avandia)

Taking sage (in the form of tea) with these drugs may reduce or prevent drug absorption:
- ferric gluconate (Ferrlecit)
- ferrous fumarate (Femiron, Feostat)
- ferrous gluconate (Fergon, Novo-Ferrogluc)
- ferrous sulfate (Feratab, Fer-Iron)
- ferrous sulfate and ascorbic acid (FeroGrad 500, Vitelle Irospan)
- iron-dextran complex (Dexferrum, INFeD)
- polysaccharide-iron complex (Hytinic, Niferex)

Lab Tests That May Be Altered by Sage
May decrease blood glucose levels.

Diseases That May Be Worsened or Triggered by Sage
- May increase already elevated blood pressure.
- May worsen seizure disorders.

Foods That May Interact with Sage
None known

Supplements That May Interact with Sage
- May increase blood glucose–lowering effects and risk of hypoglycemia (low blood sugar) when used with herbs and supplements that lower glucose levels, such as alpha-lipoic acid, chromium, devil's claw, Panax ginseng, and psyllium. (For a list of herbs and supplements that lower blood glucose levels, see Appendix B.)

- May enhance therapeutic and adverse effects of herbs and supplements that have sedative properties, such as 5-HTP, kava kava, St. John's wort, and valerian. (For a list of herbs and supplements that have sedative properties, see Appendix B.)

SARSAPARILLA

A popular flavoring agent for soft drinks in the Caribbean, in the sixteenth century, sarsaparilla was thought to be a cure for syphilis. One variation, *Smilax glabra*, is still used for that purpose today in traditional Chinese medicine. It is used by herbalists as a blood purifier and a treatment for psoriasis and rheumatism.

Scientific Name
Smilax species

Sarsaparilla Is Also Commonly Known As
Jamaican sarsaparilla, Mexican sarsaparilla, salsaparilha, sarsa, smilax

Medicinal Parts
Root and all underground parts

Sarsaparilla's Uses
To treat psoriasis, kidney disease, and rheumatism; as a diuretic

Typical Dose
A typical daily dose of sarsaparilla may range from 0.3 to 1.5 gm of the dried, powdered root.

Possible Side Effects
Sarsaparilla's side effects include nausea and kidney irritation.

Drugs That May Interact with Sarsaparilla
Taking sarsaparilla with this drug may be harmful:
- digitalis (Digitek, Lanoxin)—may increase absorption of the drug

Lab Tests That May Be Altered by Sarsaparilla
None known

Diseases That May Be Worsened or Triggered by Sarsaparilla
None known

Foods That May Interact with Sarsaparilla
None known

Supplements That May Interact with Sarsaparilla
- May increase absorption of digitalis glycoside.
- May affect absorption or elimination of herbs taken concurrently.

SASSAFRAS

Sassafras albidum, a tree from the laurel family native to eastern North America, contains the volatile oil safrole in the bark of its roots. Safrole has a long history of use as a food flavoring and was the basis of root beer. Native Americans also used sassafras infusions to reduce fever, kill parasitic worms, treat colds, and relieve constipation. Dried sassafras leaves were once a popular spice, and early European settlers enjoyed sassafras tea.

> But in 1960, safrole was found to cause liver cancer in rats, and the FDA banned its use.

Scientific Name
Sassafras albidum

Sassafras Is Also Commonly Known As
Ague tree, cinnamon wood, root bark, saloop, sassafrax, saxifras

Medicinal Parts
Root bark, root wood, oil taken from root wood

Sassafras's Uses
To treat disorders of the urinary tract, syphilis, skin ailments, inflammation of the mucous membranes, and rheumatism; as a blood purifier and tonic

Typical Dose
A typical dose of sassafras may range from 2 to 4 ml of liquid extract (1:1 in 25 percent alcohol), taken three times daily, or 1/4 tsp of sassafras powder mixed with 250 ml boiling water, steeped for 15 minutes, strained and taken as a tea.

Possible Side Effects
❶ Sassafras's side effects include hot flashes, hallucinations, elevated blood pressure, stupor, and paralysis. As the safrole in sassafras is considered carcinogenic and the herb is believed to be toxic, experts suggest avoiding this herb altogether.

Drugs That May Interact with Sassafras
Taking sassafras with these drugs may increase the risk of excessive sedation and mental depression and impairment:

- alprazolam (Apo-Alpraz, Xanax)
- amitriptyline (Elavil, Levate)
- amoxapine (Asendin)
- bupropion (Wellbutrin, Zyban)
- buspirone (BuSpar, Nu-Buspirone)
- clonazepam (Klonopin, Rivotril)
- cyclobenzaprine (Flexeril, Novo-Cycloprine)
- desipramine (Alti-Desipramine, Norpramin)
- diazepam (Apo-Diazepam, Valium)
- diphenhydramine (Benadryl Allergy, Nytol)
- doxepin (Sinequan, Zonalon)
- fluoxetine (Prozac, Sarafem)
- fluphenazine (Modecate, Prolixin)
- flurazepam (Apo-Flurazepam, Dalmane)
- imipramine (Apo-Imipramine, Tofranil)
- lorazepam (Ativan, Nu-Loraz)
- metoclopramide (Apo-Metoclop, Reglan)
- midazolam (Apo-Midazolam, Versed)
- morphine hydrochloride
- morphine sulfate (Kadian, MS Contin)
- nefazodone (Serzone)
- nortriptyline (Aventyl HCl, Pamelor)
- olanzapine (Zydis, Zyprexa)
- oxazepam (Novoxapam, Serax)
- oxcarbazepine (Trileptal)
- prochlorperazine (Compazine, Compro)
- propoxyphene (Darvon, Darvon-N)
- quetiapine (Seroquel)
- risperidone (Risperdal)
- temazepam (Novo-Temazepam, Restoril)
- tramadol (Ultram)
- triazolam (Apo-Triazo, Halcion)
- zolpidem (Ambien)

Lab Tests That May Be Altered by Sassafras
May cause false positive results in blood tests for phenytoin when sassafras oil is taken.

Diseases That May Be Worsened or Triggered by Sassafras

May worsen urinary irritation.

Foods That May Interact with Sassafras

None known

Supplements That May Interact with Sassafras

- May enhance therapeutic and adverse effects of herbs and supplements that have sedative properties, such as 5-HTP, kava kava, St. John's wort, and valerian. (For a list of herbs and supplements that have sedative properties, see Appendix B.)
- Increased risk of additive toxicity when used with herbs containing safrole, such as basil, camphor, cinnamon, and nutmeg.

SAW PALMETTO

> Also known as the American dwarf palm tree, saw palmetto produces berries that Native Americans used to treat urinary tract and prostate problems. Studies have shown that saw palmetto decreases the symptoms of enlarged prostate glands, and an extract taken from the oil of the saw palmetto berry is an accepted medical treatment for this condition in Europe. Research is currently under way to determine whether saw palmetto may be able to fight prostate cancer. Saw palmetto has also been used to improve sexual stamina, relieve inflammation, and increase breast size.

Scientific Name

Serenoa repens

Saw Palmetto Is Also Commonly Known As

American dwarf palm tree, cabbage palm, sabal, shrub palmetto

Medicinal Parts

Fruit

Saw Palmetto's Uses

To treat inflammation of the bladder, testicles, urinary tract, and breasts; enlarged prostate; cough; eczema; bedwetting; and low libido. Germany's Commission E has approved the use of saw palmetto to treat irritable bladder and prostate complaints.

Typical Dose

A typical daily dose of saw palmetto may range from 1 to 2 gm of the herb.

Possible Side Effects

Saw palmetto's side effects include headache, nausea, vomiting, abdominal pain, urine retention, impotence, and allergic reactions.

Drugs That May Interact with Saw Palmetto

Taking saw palmetto with these drugs may reduce or prevent drug absorption:

- ferric gluconate (Ferrlecit)
- ferrous fumarate (Femiron, Feostat)
- ferrous gluconate (Fergon, Novo-Ferrogluc)
- ferrous sulfate (Feratab, Fer-Iron)
- ferrous sulfate and ascorbic acid (Fero-Grad 500, Vitelle Irospan)
- iron-dextran complex (Dexferrum, INFeD)
- polysaccharide-iron complex (Hytinic, Niferex)

Taking saw palmetto with these drugs may increase the risk of bleeding and bruising:

- abciximab (ReoPro)
- acemetacin (Acemetacin Heumann, Acemetacin Sandoz)
- antithrombin III (Thrombate III)
- argatroban
- aspirin (Bufferin, Ecotrin)
- aspirin and dipyridamole (Aggrenox)
- bivalirudin (Angiomax)
- celecoxib (Celebrex)
- choline magnesium trisalicylate (Trilisate)
- choline salicylate (Teejel)
- clopidogrel (Plavix)
- dalteparin (Fragmin)
- danaparoid (Orgaran)
- diclofenac (Cataflam, Voltaren)
- diflunisal (Apo-Diflunisal, Dolobid)
- dipyridamole (Novo-Dipiradol, Persantine)
- dipyrone (Analgina, Dinador)
- enoxaparin (Lovenox)
- eptifibatide (Integrillin)
- etodolac (Lodine, Utradol)
- etoricoxib (Arcoxia)
- fenoprofen (Nalfon)
- flurbiprofen (Ansaid, Ocufen)
- fondaparinux (Arixtra)
- heparin (Hepalean, Hep-Lock)
- ibuprofen (Advil, Motrin)
- indobufen (Ibustrin)
- indomethacin (Indocin, Novo-Methacin)
- ketoprofen (Orudis, Rhodis)
- ketorolac (Acular, Toradol)
- lepirudin (Refludan)
- magnesium salicylate (Doan's, Mobidin)
- meclofenamate (Meclomen)
- mefenamic acid (Ponstel, Ponstan)
- meloxicam (MOBIC, Mobicox)
- nabumetone (Apo-Nabumetone, Relafen)
- naproxen (Aleve, Naprosyn)
- niflumic acid (Niflam, Nifluril)
- nimesulide (Areuma, Aulin)
- oxaprozin (Apo-Oxaprozin, Daypro)
- piroxicam (Feldene, Nu-Pirox)
- rofecoxib (Vioxx)
- salsalate (Amgesic, Salflex)
- sulindac (Clinoril, Nu-Sundac)
- tenoxicam (Dolmen, Mobiflex)
- tiaprofenic acid (Dom Tiaprofenic, Surgam)
- ticlopidine (Alti-Ticlopidine, Ticlid)
- tinzaparin (Innohep)
- tirofiban (Aggrastat)
- tolmetin (Tolectin)
- valdecoxib (Bextra)
- warfarin (Coumadin, Jantoven)

Taking saw palmetto with these drugs may increase the action of the drug:
- carvedilol (Coreg)
- labetalol (Normodyne, Trandate)
- prazosin (Minipress, Nu-Prazo)

Lab Tests That May Be Altered by Saw Palmetto
- May increase bleeding time due to antiplatelet activity.
- May cause metabolic changes in semen specimens.

Diseases That May Be Worsened or Triggered by Saw Palmetto
None known

Foods That May Interact with Saw Palmetto
None known

Supplements That May Interact with Saw Palmetto
None known

SCHISANDRA

Schisandra's Chinese name, *wu-wei-zi*, means "five taste fruit," referring to the sweet, salty, hot, sour, and bitter tastes of its tiny red berries. Schisandra is used in traditional Chinese medicine to treat kidney and lung conditions, insomnia, cough, and exhaustion and to increase the body's ability to handle stress. Modern research suggests that the lignans found in the berries (schizandrin, deoxyschizandrin, pregomisin, and gomisins) may have a protective effect on the liver.

Scientific Name
Schisandra chinesis

Schisandra Is Also Commonly Known As
Chinese mock-barberry, gomishi, lemonwood, wu-wei-zi

Medicinal Parts
Fruit

Schisandra's Uses
To treat insomnia, cough, diarrhea, hepatitis, and anxiety

Typical Dose
A typical daily dose of schisandra is up to 6 gm of powder or extract.

Possible Side Effects
Schisandra's side effects include stomach upset and hives.

Drugs That May Interact with Schisandra
Taking schisandra with these drugs may decrease the effectiveness of the drug:

- antithymocyte globulin, equine (Atgam)
- antithymocyte globulin, rabbit (Thymoglobulin)
- azathioprine (Imuran)
- basiliximab (Simulect)
- beclomethasone (Beconase, Vanceril)
- betamethasone (Celestone, Diprolene)
- budesonide (Entocort, Rhinocort)
- budesonide and formoterol (Symbicort)
- cortisone (Cortone)
- cyclosporine (Neoral, Sandimmune)
- daclizumab (Zenapax)
- deflazacort (Calcort, Dezacor)
- dexamethasone (Decadron, Dexasone)
- efalizumab (Raptiva)
- flunisolide (AeroBid, Nasarel)
- fluorometholone (Eflone, Flarex)
- fluticasone (Cutivate, Flonase)
- hydrocortisone (Anusol-HC, Locoid)
- loteprednol (Alrex, Lotemax)
- medrysone (HMS Liquifilm)
- methotrexate (Rheumatrex, Trexall)
- methylprednisolone (DepoMedrol, Medrol)
- muromonab-CD3 (Orthoclone OKT 3)
- mycophenolate (CellCept)
- pimecrolimus (Elidel)
- prednisolone (Inflamase Forte, Pred Forte)
- prednisone (Apo-Prednisone, Deltasone)
- rimexolone (Vexol)
- sirolimus (Rapamune)
- tacrolimus (Prograf, Protopic)
- thalidomide (Thalomid)
- triamcinolone (Aristocort, Trinasal)

Lab Tests That May Be Altered by Schisandra

May decrease results of alanine aminotransferase (ALT) and aspartic acid transaminase (AST) tests.

Diseases That May Be Worsened or Triggered by Schisandra

May worsen gastroesophageal reflux disease (GERD) or peptic ulcer disease.

Foods That May Interact with Schisandra

None known

Supplements That May Interact with Schisandra

None known

SCOPOLIA

Scopolia, which is native to southern Germany, Austria, and southwest Russia, is a creeping woodland plant that grows in moist, rocky beech woods and damp, stony places in hilly areas. Its roots and rhizomes contain the alkaloids hyoscyamine and scopolamine, which have been used to treat chronic diarrhea, dysentery, stomachaches, and manic-depressive states. The dried root is also hypnotic and narcotic and induces a sleep that resembles normal sleep.

Scientific Name

Scopolia carniolica

Scopolia Is Also Commonly Known As

Belladonna scopola, Japanese belladonna, Russian belladonna, scopola

Medicinal Parts

Root, rhizome

Scopolia's Uses

To treat spasms and pain in the gastrointestinal and urinary tracts. Germany's Commission E has approved the use of scopolia to treat gallblader and liver complaints.

Typical Dose

A typical daily dose of scopolia has not been established.

Possible Side Effects

Scopolia's side effects include a decline in sweat secretion causing heat buildup, urinary difficulties, dry mouth, and rapid heartbeat.

Drugs That May Interact with Scopolia

Taking scopolia with these drugs increases the therapeutic and/or adverse effects of the drug:

- amantadine (Endantadine, Symmetrel)
- amitriptyline (Elavil, Levate)
- amitriptyline and chlordiazepoxide (Limbitrol)
- amitriptyline and perphenazine (Etrafon, Triavil)
- amoxapine (Asendin)
- atropine (Isopto Atropine, Sal-Tropine)
- benztropine (Apo-Benztropine, Cogentin)
- clidinium and chlordiazepoxide (Apo-Chlorax, Librax)
- clomipramine (Anafranil, Novo-Clopramine)
- cyclopentolate (Cyclogyl, Cylate)
- desipramine (Alti-Desipramine, Norpramin)
- dicyclomine (Bentyl, Lomine)
- doxepin (Sinequan, Zonalon)

- glycopyrrolate (Robinul, Robinul Forte)
- homatropine (Isopto Homatropine)
- hyoscyamine (Hyosine, Levsin)
- hyoscyamine, atropine, scopolamine, and phenobarbital (Donnatal, Donnatal Extentabs)
- imipramine (Apo-Imipramine, Tofranil)
- ipratropium (Atrovent, Nu-Ipratropium)
- lofepramine (Feprapax, Gamanil)
- melitracen (Dixeran)
- nortriptyline (Aventyl HCl, Pamelor)
- oxitropium (Oxivent, Tersigat)
- prifinium (Padrin, Riabel)
- procyclidine (Kemadrin, Procyclid)
- propantheline (Propanthel)
- protriptyline (Vivactil)
- quinidine (Novo-Quinidin, Quinaglute Dura-Tabs)
- scopolamine (Scopace, Transderm Scop)
- tiotropium (Spiriva)
- tolterodine (Detrol, Detrol LA)
- trihexyphenidyl (Apo-Trihex)
- trimethobenzamide (Tigan)
- trimipramine (Apo-Trimip, Surmontil)

Lab Tests That May Be Altered by Scopolia
None known

Diseases That May Be Worsened or Triggered by Scopolia
- May trigger a rapid heart rate and constipation due to gyoscyaine and scopolamine content.
- May worsen congestive heart failure, gastro-esophageal reflux (GERD), fever, stomach ulcers, gastrointestinal infections, narrow-angle glaucoma, gastrointestinal obstructive disease, ulcerative colitis, and urinary retention due to gyoscyaine and scopolamine content.

Foods That May Interact with Scopolia
None known

Supplements That May Interact with Scopolia
May increase positive and negative effects of herbs and supplements that have anticholinergic effects, such as belladonna, henbane, and jimson weed. (For a list of herbs and supplements that have anticholinergic effects, see Appendix B.)

SCOTCH BROOM

Scotch broom, native to the British Isles, is so named because its long, thin, resilient branches grow close together, making it a good choice for broom-making. With its bright yellow flowers, it is so attractive and visible that the twelfth-century warrior Geoffrey of Anjou thrust a bunch of Scotch broom (also called *Planta genista*) into his helmet so that his troops would be sure to see and follow him. Because of this, Geoffrey received the nickname Plantagenet, which became the family name of a long line of British kings.

Scientific Name
Cytisus scoparius

Scotch Broom Is Also Commonly Known As
Basam, bizzom, broom, Irish tops, scoparium

Medicinal Parts
Flower, above-ground parts

Scotch Broom's Uses

Scotch broom herb is used to treat irregular heartbeat, low blood pressure, postpartum bleeding, heavy menstruation, kidney stones, and snakebite. Scotch broom flower is used to treat rheumatism, gout, and jaundice and to purify the blood. Germany's Commission E has approved the use of Scotch broom herb to treat circulatory problems and excessively low blood pressure.

Typical Dose

A typical dose of Scotch broom herb may range from 1 to 2 gm of the herb or flowers steeped in 150 ml boiling water for 10 minutes, then strained. This infusion is taken three times daily.

Possible Side Effects

Scotch broom flower's side effects include nausea, dizziness, and rapid heart rate. Scotch broom herb's side effects include headache, dizziness, palpitations, and sleepiness.

Drugs That May Interact with Scotch Broom

Taking Scotch broom with these drugs may increase the risk of hypertension (high blood pressure) or hypertensive crisis (a rapid and severe increase in blood pressure that can trigger a heart attack, stroke, and other problems):

- ergotamine (Cafergor, Cafergot)
- levalbuterol (Xopenex)
- iproniazid (Marsilid)
- moclobemide (Alti-Moclobemide, Nu-Moclobemide)
- levothyroxine (Levothroid, Synthroid)
- nortriptyline (Aventyl HCl, Pamelor)
- phenelzine (Nardil)
- pseudoephedrine (Dimetapp Decongestant, Sudafed)
- rizatriptan benzoate (Maxalt)
- selegiline (Eldepryl)
- tranylcypromine (Parnate)
- zolmitriptan (Zomig)

Taking Scotch broom with these drugs may increase the risk of rapid heart rate and/or arrhythmia:

- ephedrine (Pretz-D)
- levalbuterol (Xopenex)
- levothyroxine (Levothroid, Synthroid)

Taking Scotch broom with these drugs may increase the risk of hyperglycemia (high blood sugar):

- metformin (Glucophage, Riomet)
- miglitol (Glyset)
- pioglitazone (Actos)
- repaglinide (GlucoNorm, Prandin)
- rosiglitazone (Avandia)

Taking Scotch broom herb with these drugs may increase the risk of adverse effects:

- haloperidol (Haldol, Novo-Peridol)
- quinidine (Novo-Quinidin, Quinaglute Dura-Tabs)
- pseudoephedrine (Dimetapp Decongestant, Sudafed)
- venlafaxine (Effexor)

Lab Tests That May Be Altered by Scotch Broom

None known

Diseases That May Be Worsened or Triggered by Scotch Broom

May worsen elevated blood pressure and atrioventricular block (A-V block).

Foods That May Interact with Scotch Broom

None known

Supplements That May Interact with Scotch Broom

None known

SCULLCAP

Scullcap gets its name from its flower, which resembles a cap. Almost all of the scientific research on scullcap has been done on the Chinese species (*Scutellaria baicalensis*) as opposed to the American species (*S. laterifolia*). The Chinese version has been found to inhibit bacteria and viruses, lower fever, and reduce blood pressure. In China, it is used to treat fevers, colds, headaches, high blood pressure, insomnia, intestinal problems, and other conditions.

Scientific Name

Scutellaria baicalensis

Scullcap Is Also Commonly Known As

Baikal scullcap, Chinese scullcap, ogon, skullcap, wogon

Medicinal Parts

Root

Scullcap's Uses

To treat jaundice, pelvic inflammation, high blood pressure, fever, headache, irritability, seizures, and other problems

Typical Dose

A typical dose of scullcap may range from 6 to 15 gm of herb.

Possible Side Effects

Scullcap's more common side effects include liver toxicity and fever.

Drugs That May Interact with Scullcap

Taking scullcap with these drugs may increase the risk of excessive sedation and mental depression and impairment:

- acetaminophen and codeine (Capital and Codeine, Tylenol with Codeine)
- alfentanil (Alfenta)
- alprazolam (Apo-Alpraz, Xanax)
- amobarbital (Amytal)
- amobarbital and secobarbital (Tuinal)
- aspirin and codeine (Coryphen Codeine)
- belladonna and opium (B&O Supprettes)
- bromazepam (Apo-Bromazepam, Gen-Bromazepam)
- brotizolam (Lendorm, Sintonal)
- buprenorphine (Buprenex, Subutex)
- buprenorphine and naloxone (Suboxone)
- butabarbital (Butisol Sodium)
- butalbital, acetaminophen, and caffeine (Esgic, Fioricet)
- butalbital, aspirin, and caffeine (Fiorinal)
- butorphanol (Apo-Butorphanol, Stadol)
- chloral hydrate (Aquachloral Supprettes, Somnote)

- chlordiazepoxide (Apo-Chlordiazepoxide, Librium)
- clobazam (Alti-Clobazam, Frisium)
- clonazepam (Klonopin, Rivotril)
- clorazepate (Tranxene, T-Tab)
- codeine (Codeine Contin)
- dexmedetomidine (Precedex)
- diazepam (Apo-Diazepam, Valium)
- dihydrocodeine, aspirin, and caffeine (Synalgos-DC)
- diphenhydramine (Benadryl Allergy, Nytol)
- estazolam (ProSom)
- fentanyl (Actiq, Duragesic)
- flurazepam (Apo-Flurazepam, Dalmane)
- glutethimide
- haloperidol (Haldol, Novo-Peridol)
- hydrocodone and acetaminophen (Vicodin, Zydone)
- hydrocodone and aspirin (Damason-P)
- hydrocodone and ibuprofen (Vicoprofen)
- hydromorphone (Dilaudid, PMS-Hydromorphone)
- hydroxyzine (Atarax, Vistaril)
- levomethadyl acetate hydrochloride
- levorphanol (LevoDromoran)
- loprazolam (Dormonoct, Havlane)
- lorazepam (Ativan, Nu-Loraz)
- meperidine (Demerol, Meperitab)
- meperidine and promethazine
- mephobarbital (Mebaral)
- methadone (Dolophine, Methadose)
- methohexital (Brevital, Brevital Sodium)
- midazolam (Apo-Midazolam, Versed)
- morphine sulfate (Kadian, MS Contin)
- nalbuphine (Nubain)
- opium tincture
- oxycodone (OxyContin, Roxicodone)
- oxycodone and acetaminophen (Endocet, Percocet)
- oxycodone and aspirin (Endodan, Percodan)
- oxymorphone (Numorphan)
- paregoric
- pentazocine (Talwin)
- pentobarbital (Nembutal)
- phenobarbital (Luminal Sodium, PMS-Phenobarbital)
- phenoperidine
- prazepam
- primidone (Apo-Primidone, Mysoline)
- promethazine (Phenergan)
- propofol (Diprivan)
- propoxyphene (Darvon, Darvon-N)
- propoxyphene and acetaminophen (Darvocet-N 50, Darvocet-N 100)
- propoxyphene, aspirin, and caffeine (Darvon Compound)
- quazepam (Doral)
- remifentanil (Ultiva)
- secobarbital (Seconal)
- sodium oxybate (Xyrem)
- sufentanil (Sufenta)
- s-zopiclone (Lunesta)
- temazepam (Novo-Temazepam, Restoril)
- tetrazepam (Mobiforton, Musapam)
- thiopental (Pentothal)
- triazolam (Apo-Triazo, Halcion)
- zaleplon (Sonata, Stamoc)
- zolpidem (Ambien)
- zopiclone (Alti-Zopiclone, Gen-Zopiclone)

Taking scullcap with these drugs may interfere with the action of the drug:
- antithymocyte globulin, equine (Atgam)
- antithymocyte globulin, rabbit (Thymoglobulin)

- azathioprine (Imuran)
- basiliximab (Simulect)
- cyclosporine (Neoral, Sandimmune)
- daclizumab (Zenapax)
- efalizumab (Raptiva)
- methotrexate (Rheumatrex, Trexall)
- muromonab-CD3 (Orthoclone OKT 3)
- mycophenolate (CellCept)
- pimecrolimus (Elidel)
- sirolimus (Rapamune)
- tacrolimus (Prograf, Protopic)
- thalidomide (Thalomid)

Lab Test That May Be Altered by Scullcap

May reduce blood sugar levels and test levels following a meal due to alpha-glucosidase activity.

Diseases That May Be Worsened or Triggered by Scullcap

- May cause blood sugar levels to fall too low in diabetics.
- May worsen spleen or stomach ailments.

Foods That May Interact with Scullcap

None known

Supplements That May Interact with Scullcap

May enhance therapeutic and adverse effects of herbs and supplements that have sedative properties, such as 5-HTP, kava kava, St. John's wort, and valerian. (For a list of herbs and supplements that have sedative properties, see Appendix B.)

SEA BUCKTHORN

The sea buckthorn, which grows throughout Eurasia, is a thorny shrub with a tolerance for salinity that allows it to grow well near the sea. A medicinal oil made from its berries, which are extremely high in vitamin C, is sometimes used to treat cardiac disorders and stomach and intestinal diseases; when applied to the skin, it is used to heal burns, eczema, and radiation injuries. Chinese researchers tested the effects of sea buckthorn extract on fifty people with cirrhosis of the liver, a chronic disease that leaves the liver covered with fibrous tissue. Six months of treatment with sea buckthorn extract reduced fibrosis and improved liver function.

Scientific Name

Hippophae rhamnoides

Sea Buckthorn Is Also Commonly Known As

Argasse, finbar, meerdorn, sallow thorn, seedorn

Medicinal Parts

Berry, oil taken from the seed

Sea Buckthorn's Uses

To treat sunburn, wounds, arthritis, ulcers, and gout

Typical Dose

A typical daily dose of sea buckthorn is approximately 500 to 1,500 mg of seed oil.

Possible Side Effects

No serious side effects have been reported when sea buckthorn is used in the proper dosage and proper way, under a physician's supervision.

Drugs That May Interact with Sea Buckthorn

Taking sea buckthorn with these drugs may increase the risk of bleeding and bruising:

- abciximab (ReoPro)
- antithrombin III (Thrombate III)
- argatroban
- aspirin (Bufferin, Ecotrin)
- aspirin and dipyridamole (Aggrenox)
- bivalirudin (Angiomax)
- clopidogrel (Plavix)
- dalteparin (Fragmin)
- danaparoid (Orgaran)
- dipyridamole (Novo-Dipiradol, Persantine)
- enoxaparin (Lovenox)
- eptifibatide (Integrillin)
- fondaparinux (Arixtra)
- heparin (Hepalean, Hep-Lock)
- indobufen (Ibustrin)
- lepirudin (Refludan)
- ticlopidine (Alti-Ticlopidine, Ticlid)
- tinzaparin (Innohep)
- tirofiban (Aggrastat)
- warfarin (Coumadin, Jantoven)

Lab Tests That May Be Altered by Sea Buckthorn

None known

Diseases That May Be Worsened or Triggered by Sea Buckthorn

None known

Foods That May Interact with Sea Buckthorn

None known

Supplements That May Interact with Sea Buckthorn

Increased risk of bleeding when used with herbs and supplements that might affect platelet aggregation. (For a list of herbs and supplements with anticoagulant/antiplatelet effects, see Appendix B.)

SENEGA

> Native to eastern North America, senega gets its common name, snakeroot, from the twisted, snakelike appearance of its roots. Snakeroot was used by Native Americans to treat snakebite, earaches, toothaches, sore throats, croup, and colds. Today it is mainly used as an expectorant in cough syrups, lozenges, and teas and as a gargle for sore throats.

Scientific Name

Polygala senega

Senega Is Also Commonly Known As

Milkwort, rattlesnake root, seneca snakeroot, seneka, snakeroot

Medicinal Parts

Root

Senega's Uses

To treat snakebite, asthma, bronchitis, and croup

Typical Dose

A typical daily dose of senega is up to 1 gm of dry powdered root, taken three times a day.

Possible Side Effects

Senega's side effects include dizziness, blurred vision, and nausea.

Drugs That May Interact with Senega

Taking senega with these drugs may increase the risk of bleeding or bruising:

- aminosalicylic acid (Nemasol Sodium, Paser)
- antithrombin III (Thrombate III)
- argatroban
- aspirin (Bufferin, Ecotrin)
- bivalirudin (Angiomax)
- choline magnesium trisalicylate (Trilisate)
- choline salicylate (Teejel)
- dalteparin (Fragmin)
- danaparoid (Orgaran)
- enoxaparin (Lovenox)
- fondaparinux (Arixtra)
- heparin (Hepalean, Hep-Lock)
- lepirudin (Refludan)
- salsalate (Amgesic, Salflex)
- tinzaparin (Innohep)
- warfarin (Coumadin, Jantoven)

Taking senega with these drugs may increase the risk of hypoglycemia (low blood sugar):

- acarbose (Prandase, Precose)
- acetohexamide
- chlorpropamide (Diabinese, Novo-Propamide)
- gliclazide (Diamicron, Novo-Gliclazide)
- glimepiride (Amaryl)
- glipizide (Glucotrol)
- glipizide and metformin (Metaglip)
- gliquidone (Beglynor, Glurenorm)
- glyburide (DiaBeta, Micronase)
- glyburide and metformin (Glucovance)
- insulin (Humulin, Novolin R)
- metformin (Glucophage, Riomet)
- miglitol (Glyset)
- nateglinide (Starlix)
- pioglitazone (Actos)
- repaglinide (GlucoNorm, Prandin)

- rosiglitazone (Avandia)
- rosiglitazone and metformin (Avandamet)
- s-zopiclone (Lunesta)
- tolazamide (Tolinase)
- tolbutamide (Apo-Tolbutamide, Tol-Tab)

Taking senega with these drugs may increase the risk of excessive sedation and mental depression and impairment:

- acetaminophen and codeine (Capital and Codeine, Tylenol with Codeine)
- alfentanil (Alfenta)
- alprazolam (Apo-Alpraz, Xanax)
- amobarbital (Amytal)
- amobarbital and secobarbital (Tuinal)
- aspirin and codeine (Coryphen Codeine)
- belladonna and opium (B&O Supprettes)
- bromazepam (Apo-Bromazepam, Gen-Bromazepam)
- brotizolam (Lendorm, Sintonal)
- buprenorphine (Buprenex, Subutex)
- buprenorphine and naloxone (Suboxone)
- butabarbital (Butisol Sodium)
- butalbital, acetaminophen, and caffeine (Esgic, Fioricet)
- butalbital, aspirin, and caffeine (Fiorinal)
- butorphanol (Apo-Butorphanol, Stadol)
- chloral hydrate (Aquachloral Supprettes, Somnote)
- chlordiazepoxide (Apo-Chlordiazepoxide, Librium)
- clobazam (Alti-Clobazam, Frisium)
- clonazepam (Klonopin, Rivotril)
- clorazepate (Tranxene, T-Tab)
- codeine (Codeine Contin)
- dexmedetomidine (Precedex)
- diazepam (Apo-Diazepam, Valium)
- dihydrocodeine, aspirin, and caffeine (Synalgos-DC)

- diphenhydramine (Benadryl Allergy, Nytol)
- estazolam (ProSom)
- fentanyl (Actiq, Duragesic)
- flurazepam (Apo-Flurazepam, Dalmane)
- glutethimide
- haloperidol (Haldol, Novo-Peridol)
- hydrocodone and acetaminophen (Vicodin, Zydone)
- hydrocodone and aspirin (Damason-P)
- hydrocodone and ibuprofen (Vicoprofen)
- hydromorphone (Dilaudid, PMS-Hydromorphone)
- hydroxyzine (Atarax, Vistaril)
- levomethadyl acetate hydrochloride
- levorphanol (LevoDromoran)
- loprazolam (Dormonoct, Havlane)
- lorazepam (Ativan, Nu-Loraz)
- meperidine (Demerol, Meperitab)
- meperidine and promethazine
- mephobarbital (Mebaral)
- methadone (Dolophine, Methadose)
- methohexital (Brevital, Brevital Sodium)
- midazolam (Apo-Midazolam, Versed)
- morphine sulfate (Kadian, MS Contin)
- nalbuphine (Nubain)
- opium tincture
- oxycodone (OxyContin, Roxicodone)
- oxycodone and acetaminophen (Endocet, Percocet)
- oxycodone and aspirin (Endodan, Percodan)
- oxymorphone (Numorphan)
- paregoric
- pentazocine (Talwin)
- pentobarbital (Nembutal)
- phenobarbital (Luminal Sodium, PMS-Phenobarbital)
- phenoperidine
- prazepam

- primidone (Apo-Primidone, Mysoline)
- promethazine (Phenergan)
- propofol (Diprivan)
- propoxyphene (Darvon, Darvon-N)
- propoxyphene and acetaminophen (Darvocet-N 50, Darvocet-N 100)
- propoxyphene, aspirin, and caffeine (Darvon Compound)
- quazepam (Doral)
- remifentanil (Ultiva)
- secobarbital (Seconal)
- sodium oxybate (Xyrem)
- sufentanil (Sufenta)
- temazepam (Novo-Temazepam, Restoril)
- tetrazepam (Mobiforton, Musapam)
- thiopental (Pentothal)
- triazolam (Apo-Triazo, Halcion)
- zaleplon (Sonata, Stamoc)
- zolpidem (Ambien)
- zopiclone (Alti-Zopiclone, Gen-Zopiclone)

Lab Tests That May Be Altered by Senega

None known

Diseases That May Be Worsened or Triggered by Senega

May worsen inflammatory gastrointestinal ailments or ulcers.

Foods That May Interact with Senega

None known

Supplements That May Interact with Senega

None known

SENNA

Native to Eurasia and cultivated in India and the Middle East, senna, a member of the pea family, is valued for the purgative action of its leaves and pods. Both contain substances called anthranoids, which strongly stimulate contractions in the colon and speed elimination. Because senna pods contain about twice as many anthranoids as the leaves, the leaves are considered a safer choice.

Scientific Name

Cassia species

Senna Is Also Commonly Known As

Alexandria senna, India senna, Khartoum senna

Medicinal Parts

Leaf, pod

Senna's Uses

To treat constipation, liver disease, jaundice, anemia, and typhoid fever. Germany's Commission E has approved the use of senna to treat constipation.

Typical Dose

A typical dose of senna may range from 0.1 to 0.2 gm herb mixed with 150 ml hot water, steeped for 10 minutes, strained and taken as a tea.

Possible Side Effects

Senna's side effects include nausea, vomiting, cramping, diarrhea, flatulence, irregular heartbeat, and kidney damage.

Drugs That May Interact with Senna

Taking senna with these drugs may increase the risk of hypokalemia (low levels of potassium in the blood):

- acetazolamide (Apo-Acetazolamide, Diamox Sequels)
- azosemide (Diat)
- bepridil (Vascor)
- bumetanide (Bumex, Burinex)
- chlorothiazide (Diuril)
- chlorthalidone (Apo-Chlorthalidone, Thalitone)
- ethacrynic acid (Edecrin)
- etozolin (Elkapin)
- flecainide (Tambocor)
- furosemide (Apo-Furosemide, Lasix)
- hydrochlorothiazide (Apo-Hydro, Microzide)
- hydroflumethiazide (Diucardin, Saluron)
- indapamide (Lozol, Nu-Indapamide)
- insulin (Humulin, Novolin R)
- mannitol (Osmitrol, Resectisol)
- mefruside (Baycaron)
- methazolamide (Apo-Methazolamide,)
- methyclothiazide (Aquatensen, Enduron)
- methylprednisolone (Depo-Medrol, Medrol)
- metolazone (Mykrox, Zaroxolyn)
- olmesartan and hydrochlorothiazide (Benicar HCT)
- polythiazide (Renese)
- prednisone (Apo-Prednisone, Deltasone)
- sildenafil (Viagra)
- torsemide (Demadex)
- trichlormethiazide (Metatensin, Naqua)
- urea (Amino-Cerv, UltraMide)
- xipamide (Diurexan, Lumitens)

Taking senna with these drugs may increase the risk of arrhythmia (irregular heartbeat):
- acebutolol (Novo-Acebutolol, Sectral)
- adenosine (Adenocard, Adenoscan)
- amiodarone (Cordarone, Pacerone)
- bepridil (Vascor)
- bretylium
- digitalis (Digitek, Lanoxin)
- diltiazem (Cardizem, Tiazac)
- disopyramide (Norpace, Rhythmodan)
- dofetilide (Tikosyn)
- esmolol (Brevibloc)
- flecainide (Tambocor)
- ibutilide (Corvert)
- insulin (Humulin, Novolin R)
- lidocaine (Lidoderm, Xylocaine)
- methylprednisolone (Depo-Medrol, Medrol)
- mexiletine (Mexitil, Novo-Mexiletine)
- moricizine (Ethmozine)
- phenytoin (Dilantin, Phenytek)
- prednisone (Apo-Prednisone, Deltasone)
- procainamide (Procanbid, Pronestyl-SR)
- propafenone (Rhythmol, GenPropafenone)
- propranolol (Inderal, InnoPran XL)
- quinidine (Novo-Quinidin, Quinaglute DuraTabs)
- sildenafil (Viagra)
- sotalol (Betapace, Sorine)
- tocainide (Tonocard)
- verapamil (Calan, Isoptin SR)

Taking senna with these drugs may decrease blood levels of estrogen:
- cyproterone and ethinyl estradiol (Diane-35)
- estradiol (Climara, Estrace)
- estradiol and norethindrone (Activella, CombiPatch)
- estradiol and testosterone (Climacteron)
- estrogens, conjugated A/synthetic (Cenestin)
- estrogens, conjugated/equine (Premarin, Congest)
- estrogens, conjugated/equine, and medroxy-progesterone (Premphase, Prempro)
- estrogens (esterified) (Estratab, Menest)
- estrogens (esterified) and methyltestosterone (Estratest, Estratest H.S.)
- estropipate (Ogen, OrthoEst)
- ethinyl estradiol (Estinyl)
- ethinyl estradiol and desogestrel (Cyclessa, Ortho-Cept)
- ethinyl estradiol and ethynodiol diacetate (Demulen, Zovia)
- ethinyl estradiol and etonogestrel (NuvaRing)
- ethinyl estradiol and levonorgestrel (Alesse, Triphasil)
- ethinyl estradiol and norelgestromin (Evra, Ortho Evra)
- ethinyl estradiol and norethindrone (Brevicon, Ortho-Novum)
- ethinyl estradiol and norgestimate (Cyclen, Ortho Tri-Cyclen)
- ethinyl estradiol and norgestrel (Cryselle, Ovral)
- mestranol and norethindrone (Necon 1/50, Ortho-Novum 1/50)
- polyestradiol

Taking senna with these drugs may increase the drug's therapeutic and adverse effects:
- cascara
- docusate (Colace, Ex-Lax Stool Softener)
- docusate and senna (Peri-Colace, Senokot-S)
- lactulose (Constulose, Enulose)
- magnesium hydroxide (Dulcolax Milk of Magnesia, Phillips' Milk of Magnesia)

- magnesium hydroxide and mineral oil (Phillips' M-O)
- magnesium citrate (Citro-Mag)
- magnesium oxide (Mag-Ox 400, Uro-Mag)
- magnesium sulfate (Epsom salts)
- polyethylene glycolelectrolyte solution (Colyte, MiraLax)
- psyllium (Metamucil, Reguloid)
- sorbitol (Sorbilax)

Lab Tests That May Be Altered by Senna

- May decrease blood levels of estriol.
- May decrease twenty-four-hour urine tests of estriol.
- May reduce serum potassium levels.
- May confound results of diagnostic urine tests that rely on a color change by discoloring urine (pink, red, purple, or orange).

Diseases That May Be Worsened or Triggered by Senna

- May worsen potassium deficiency and electrolyte imbalances.
- May worsen diarrhea or dehydration.
- May worsen gastrointestinal ailments.
- May worsen heart ailments by causing an electrolyte imbalance.

Foods That May Interact with Senna

None known

Supplements That May Interact with Senna

- Increased action of jimson weed in cases of chronic use or abuse of senna.
- Increased risk of potassium depletion when used in conjunction with horsetail plant or licorice.

- Increased risk of potassium depletion when used with other stimulant laxative herbs, such as black root, cascara sagrada, and castor oil. (For a list of stimulant laxative herbs and supplements, see Appendix B.)

SHEPHERD'S PURSE

Shepherd's purse gets its name from its seed pods, which are shaped like purses. Its primary medical use is in stopping bleeding (including nosebleeds and profuse menstruation), but it is also used to treat hemorrhoids, varicose veins, and urinary infections.

Scientific Name

Capsella bursa-pastoris

Shepherd's Purse Is Also Commonly Known As

Blindweed, cocowort, lady's purse, pepper-and-salt, shepherd's heart, St. James' weed

Medicinal Parts

Aerial parts

Shepherd's Purse's Uses

To treat nosebleed, menstrual difficulties, headache, and bladder inflammation. Germany's Commission E has approved the use of shepherd's purse to treat wounds, burns, premenstrual syndrome (PMS), and nosebleed.

Typical Dose

A typical daily dose of shepherd's purse may range from 10 to 15 gm of the herb.

Possible Side Effects

Shepherd's purse's side effects include abnormal thyroid function, abnormal menstruation, and elevated or lowered blood pressure.

Drugs That May Interact with Shepherd's Purse

Taking shepherd's purse with these drugs may be harmful:

- digitalis (Digitek, Lanoxin)—may increase the risk of excessively low blood pressure, irregular heartbeat, and slow heartbeat
- levothyroxine (Levothroid, Synthroid)—may interfere with the action of the drug

Lab Tests That May Be Altered by Shepherd's Purse

None known

Diseases That May Be Worsened or Triggered by Shepherd's Purse

May interfere with therapy for thyroid or heart conditions.

Foods That May Interact with Shepherd's Purse

None known

Supplements That May Interact with Shepherd's Purse

None known

SLIPPERY ELM

Slippery elm, named after its slick, mucilaginous inner bark, was used by Native Americans to treat sore throat, skin ulcers, toothaches, burns, and other ailments. The gummy secretions from the bark were made into antiseptic poultices that were applied to infected wounds, while gargles and mouthwashes were used to coat the throat and soothe the digestive tract.

Scientific Name

Ulmus rubra

Slippery Elm Is Also Commonly Known As

Red elm, sweet elm

Medicinal Parts

Inner rind of bark

Slippery Elm's Uses

To treat ulcers, wounds, gout, and rheumatism

Typical Dose

A typical dose of slippery elm is 4 to 16 ml per day of a decoction (made with ethanol in a 1:8 ratio).

Possible Side Effects

Slippery elm's side effects include inflammation of the skin.

Drugs That May Interact with Slippery Elm

Taking slippery elm with these drugs may reduce or prevent drug absorption:

- ferric gluconate (Ferrlecit)
- ferrous fumarate (Femiron, Feostat)
- ferrous gluconate (Fergon, Novo-Ferrogluc)
- ferrous sulfate (Feratab, Fer-Iron)
- ferrous sulfate and ascorbic acid (Fero-Grad 500, Vitelle Irospan)
- iron-dextran complex (Dexferrum, INFeD)
- polysaccharide-iron complex (Hytinic, Niferex)

Lab Tests That May Be Altered by Slippery Elm

None known

Diseases That May Be Worsened or Triggered by Slippery Elm

None known

Foods That May Interact with Slippery Elm

None known

Supplements That May Interact with Slippery Elm

None known

SOLOMON'S SEAL

Native to Europe, eastern Asia, and North America, Solomon's seal is a common ornamental plant that has been used for thousands of years in herbal medicine. Some say its name came from markings on the rootstock that look like the Star of David, also known as the Seal of Solomon. Others say that the wise King Solomon put his seal of approval on the plant. Still others say it was so named because the root of the plant has the ability to seal up and heal wounds. Often used in the form of a poultice to prevent excessive bruising and to stimulate tissue repair, it is said that Solomon's seal can make bruises or black eyes vanish in one or two nights.

Scientific Name

Polygonatum multiflorum

Solomon's Seal Is Also Commonly Known As

Dropberry, lady's seals, sealroot, sealwort, St. Mary's seal

Medicinal Parts

Rhizome, roots

Solomon's Seal's Uses

To treat respiratory and lung disorders, bruises, hemorrhoids, redness of the skin, finger ulcers, or boils

Typical Dose

There is no typical dose of Solomon's seal.

Possible Side Effects

Solomon's seal's side effects include gastrointestinal irritation.

Drugs That May Interact with Solomon's Seal

Taking Solomon's seal with these drugs may increase the risk of hypoglycemia (low blood sugar):

- acarbose (Prandase, Precose)
- acetohexamide
- chlorpropamide (Diabinese, Novo-Propamide)
- gliclazide (Diamicron, Novo-Gliclazide)
- glimepiride (Amaryl)
- glipizide (Glucotrol)
- glipizide and metformin (Metaglip)
- gliquidone (Beglynor, Glurenorm)
- glyburide (DiaBeta, Micronase)
- glyburide and metformin (Glucovance)
- insulin (Humulin, Novolin R)
- metformin (Glucophage, Riomet)
- miglitol (Glyset)
- nateglinide (Starlix)
- pioglitazone (Actos)
- repaglinide (GlucoNorm, Prandin)
- rosiglitazone (Avandia)
- rosiglitazone and metformin (Avandamet)

- tolazamide (Tolinase)
- tolbutamide (Apo-Tolbutamide, Tol-Tab)

Lab Tests That May Be Altered by Solomon's Seal
None known

Diseases That May Be Worsened or Triggered by Solomon's Seal
None known

Foods That May Interact with Solomon's Seal
None known

Supplements That May Interact with Solomon's Seal

May increase blood glucose–lowering effects and risk of hypoglycemia (low blood sugar) when used with herbs and supplements that lower glucose levels, such as alpha-lipoic acid, chromium, devil's claw, Panax ginseng, and psyllium. (For a list of herbs and supplements that lower blood glucose levels, see Appendix B.)

SORREL

> Sorrel takes its name from the French word *surele*, which means "sour." This acidic herb was often eaten by Egyptians and Romans to counteract an overly rich diet. Pliny the Elder, a noted Roman scientist, wrote that those who carried sorrel on their person were protected from scorpion stings. The fresh or dried leaves of the sorrel plant have astringent, diuretic, and laxative properties, and are also used to treat fevers and scurvy.

Scientific Name
Rumex acetosa

Sorrel Is Also Commonly Known As
Acedera comun, garden sorrel, sorrel dock, sour dock

Medicinal Parts
Leaf, whole herb

Sorrel's Uses
To treat inflammation of the nasal passages and respiratory tract, scurvy, and skin infections

Typical Dose
A typical dose of sorrel is approximately 50 drops of liquid extract (1:4 in 19 percent ethanol) taken three times daily.

Possible Side Effects
Sorrel's side effects include diarrhea and skin inflammation. The oxalic acid in sorrel can damage the digestive tract, heart, lungs, and other parts of the body.

Drugs That May Interact with Sorrel
Taking sorrel with these drugs may increase the effects of the drug:

- acetazolamide (Apo-Acetazolamide, Diamox Sequels)
- amiloride (Midamor)
- azosemide (Diat)
- bumetanide (Bumex, Burinex)
- chlorothiazide (Diuril)
- chlorthalidone (Apo-Chlorthalidone, Thalitone)
- ethacrynic acid (Edecrin)

- etozolin (Elkapin)
- furosemide (Apo-Furosemide, Lasix)
- hydrochlorothiazide (Apo-Hydro, Microzide)
- hydrochlorothiazide and triamterene (Dyazide, Maxzide)
- hydroflumethiazide (Diucardin, Saluron)
- indapamide (Lozol, NuIndapamide)
- mannitol (Osmitrol, Resectisol)
- mefruside (Baycaron)
- methazolamide (Apo-Methazolamide, Neptazane)
- methyclothiazide (Aquatensen, Enduron)
- metolazone (Mykrox, Zaroxolyn)
- olmesartan and hydrochlorothiazide (Benicar HCT)
- polythiazide (Renese)
- spironolactone (Aldactone, Novo-Spiroton)
- torsemide (Demadex)
- triamterene (Dyrenium)
- trichlormethiazide (Metatensin, Naqua)
- urea (Amino-Cerv, UltraMide)
- xipamide (Diurexan, Lumitens)

Lab Tests That May Be Altered by Sorrel
None known

Diseases That May Be Worsened or Triggered by Sorrel
May worsen gastrointestinal ailments by irritating gastrointestinal tract.

Foods That May Interact with Sorrel
May decrease mineral absorption from food when taken with calcium, iron, or zinc.

Supplements That May Interact with Sorrel
- May decrease mineral absorption when taken with calcium, iron, or zinc supplements.

- The tannins in sorrel may cause the alkaloids in certain other herbs to separate and settle, increasing the risk of toxic reactions. (For a list of herbs and other substances that are high in alkaloids, see Appendix B.)

SOYBEAN

> Soy has been used in traditional Chinese medicine for thousands of years and is a mainstay of the Asian diet. Soy contains isoflavones and other health-promoting substances that have long been used to treat fever, headache, lack of appetite, various kinds of liver disease, and "female complaints." The Food and Drug Administration allows food manufacturers to label their soy products as "heart healthy," and the American College of Obstetricians and Gynecologists has put its stamp of approval on soy as an effective method of combating hot flashes.

Scientific Name
Glycine soja

Soybean Is Also Commonly Known As
Diadzein, natto, soja, soy, soy milk, tofu

Medicinal Parts
Bean

Soybean's Uses
To treat elevated cholesterol, nervous conditions, menopausal hot flashes and night sweats, joint pain, and gallbladder ailments

Typical Dose

A typical dose of soybean is up to 50 gm per day of soy protein.

Possible Side Effects

Soybean's side effects include stomach pain, diarrhea, and decreased estrogen levels.

Drugs That May Interact with Soybean

Taking soybean with these drugs may reduce or prevent drug absorption:

- ferric gluconate (Ferrlecit)
- ferrous fumarate (Femiron, Feostat)
- ferrous gluconate (Fergon, Novo-Ferrogluc)
- ferrous sulfate (Feratab, Fer-Iron)
- ferrous sulfate and ascorbic acid (Fero-Grad 500, Vitelle Irospan)
- iron-dextran complex (Dexferrum, INFeD)
- polysaccharide-iron complex (Hytinic, Niferex)

Taking soybean with these drugs may reduce absorption of the drug:

- levothyroxine (Levothroid, Synthroid)
- liothyronine (Cytomel, Triostat)
- liotrix (Thyrolar)

Taking soybean with these drugs may reduce the effectiveness of the drug:

- tamoxifen (Nolvadex, Tamofen)
- warfarin (Coumadin, Jantoven)

Lab Tests That May Be Altered by Soybean

- May decrease parathyroid hormone levels when taken in high amounts by postmenopausal women.
- May increase thyroid-stimulating hormone (TSH) levels, particularly in those with low iodine levels.

Diseases That May Be Worsened or Triggered by Soybean

- People with allergic rhinitis and asthma have a greater than average risk of suffering from soy hull allergy.
- There is some evidence that soy may worsen breast cancer.
- May increase the risk of kidney stones and bladder cancer.

Foods That May Interact with Soybean

Decreased absorption of nonheme (plant-based) iron in foods when soy is taken in the form of soy protein isolate.

Supplements That May Interact with Soybean

None known

SPINACH

Brought to Europe by the Moors in the eighth century when they conquered Spain, in modern times spinach has been shown to guard against cancer, protect eyesight, and reduce the risk of heart disease. Surprisingly, it may also help fight depression, thanks to its folic acid content. In one study, seventy-five depressed, medicated patients enjoyed significant relief from depression when given 200 mcg of folic acid daily (the amount found in less than a cup of cooked spinach).

Scientific Name

Spinacia oleracea

Spinach Is Also Commonly Known As
Spinatblatter

Medicinal Parts
Leaf

Spinach's Uses
To treat gastrointestinal ailments, stimulate the appetite, promote growth in children, and fight fatigue

Typical Dose
There is no typical dose of spinach.

Possible Side Effects
Spinach has no side effects when used as part of a balanced diet under a physician's supervision.

Drugs That May Interact with Spinach
Taking spinach with this drug may be harmful:

- warfarin (Coumadin, Jantoven)—the vitamin K in spinach may reduce the effectiveness of the drug

Lab Tests That May Be Altered by Spinach
May decrease prothrombin time (PT) and plasma international normalized ratio (INR) due to high amounts of vitamin K.

Diseases That May Be Worsened or Triggered by Spinach
May worsen existing kidney damage.

Foods That May Interact with Spinach
May decrease mineral absorption from food when taken with calcium, iron, or zinc.

Supplements That May Interact with Spinach
May decrease mineral absorption when taken with calcium, iron, or zinc supplements.

SQUILL

> Squill is a centuries-old medicine used as a diuretic and a stimulating expectorant for respiratory conditions such as bronchitis and lung disease. In the sixth century B.C., Pythagoras invented oxymel of squill, an expectorant preparation used for coughs. Squill is still used as a stimulating expectorant and diuretic as well as a cardiac tonic that slows and strengthens the pulse.

Scientific Name
Urginea maritima

Squill Is Also Commonly Known As
Indian squill, maritime squill, sea onion, scilla, white squill

Medicinal Parts
Bulb

Squill's Uses
To treat asthma, heart problems, whooping cough, back pain, hemorrhoids, and wounds. Germany's Commission E has approved the use of squill to treat irregular heartbeat, cardiac insufficiency, and nervous heart complaints.

Typical Dose
A typical daily dose of squill (as standardized sea onion powder) is 0.1 to 0.5 gm.

Possible Side Effects

❗ Squill's side effects include irregular heartbeat, anxiety, tremors, nausea, and allergic reactions. Squill contains cardiac glycosides, which can help control irregular heartbeat, reduce the backup of blood and fluid in the body, and increase blood flow through the kidneys, helping to excrete sodium and relieve swelling in body tissues. However, a buildup of cardiac glycosides can occur, especially when the herb is combined with certain medications or other herbs that contain cardiac glycosides, causing arrhythmias, abnormally slow heartbeat, heart failure, and even death.

Drugs That May Interact with Squill

Taking squill with these drugs may increase the risk of arrhythmia (irregular heartbeat):

- albuterol (Proventil, Ventolin)
- brimonidine (Alphagan P, PMS-Brimonidine Tartrate)
- cilostazol (Pletal)
- dobutamine (Dobutrex)
- dopamine (Intropin)
- dopexamine (Dopacard)
- enoximone (Perfan)
- ephedrine (Pretz-D)
- inamrinone
- isoetharine (Beta-2, Bronkosol)
- isoproterenol (Isuprel)
- metaproterenol (Alupent)
- metaraminol (Aramine)
- milrinone (Primacor)
- norepinephrine (Levophed)
- pentoxifylline (Pentoxil, Trental)
- phenylephrine (Neo-Synephrine Extra Strength, Vicks Sinex Nasal Spray)
- pseudoephedrine (Dimetapp Decongestant, Sudafed)
- quinidine (Novo-Quinidin, Quinaglute Dura-Tabs)
- sildenafil (Viagra)
- tadalafil (Cialis)
- terbutaline (Brethine)
- theophylline and guaifenesin (Elixophyllin-GC, Quibron)
- theophylline (Elixophyllin, Uniphyl)
- vardenafil (Levitra)

Taking squill with these drugs may increase the therapeutic and/or adverse effects of the drug:

- beclomethasone (Beconase, Vanceril)
- betamethasone (Celestone, Diprolene)
- budesonide (Entocort, Rhinocort)
- budesonide and formoterol (Symbicort)
- calcium acetate (PhosLo)
- calcium carbonate (Rolaids Extra Strength, Tums)
- calcium chloride
- calcium citrate (Osteocit)
- calcium glubionate
- calcium gluceptate
- calcium gluconate
- cascara
- cortisone (Cortone)
- deflazacort (Calcort, Dezacor)
- dexamethasone (Decadron, Dexasone)
- digitalis (Digitek, Lanoxin)
- docusate (Colace, Ex-Lax Stool Softener)
- docusate and senna (Peri-Colace, Senokot-S)
- flunisolide (AeroBid, Nasarel)
- fluorometholone (Eflone, Flarex)
- fluticasone (Cutivate, Flonase)
- hydrocortisone (Cetacort, Locoid)
- lactulose (Constulose, Enulose)
- magnesium citrate (Citro-Mag)

- magnesium hydroxide (Dulcolax Milk of Magnesia, Phillips' Milk of Magnesia)
- magnesium hydroxide and mineral oil (Phillips' M-O)
- magnesium oxide (Mag-Ox 400, Uro-Mag)
- magnesium sulfate (Epsom salts)
- methylprednisolone (Depo-Medrol, Medrol)
- polyethylene glycol-electrolyte solution (Colyte, MiraLax)
- prednisolone (Inflamase Forte, Pred Forte)
- prednisone (Apo-Prednisone, Deltasone)
- psyllium (Metamucil, Reguloid)
- quinidine (Novo-Quinidin, Quinaglute Dura-Tabs)
- sorbitol (Sorbilax)
- triamcinolone (Aristocort, Trinasal)

Lab Tests That May Be Altered by Squill

May decrease red blood cell concentrations.

Diseases That May Be Worsened or Triggered by Squill

- May worsen inflammatory or infectious gastrointestinal ailments by irritating the gastrointestinal tract.
- May worsen existing cases of low potassium or calcium levels.
- May worsen various heart ailments.

Foods That May Interact with Squill

None known

Supplements That May Interact with Squill

- Increased risk of cardiac glycoside toxicity when used with other herbs that contain cardiac glycosides, such as black hellebore, calotropis, motherwort, and others. (For a list of cardiac glycoside–containing herbs and supplements, see Appendix B.)
- Increased risk of cardiotoxicity due to potassium depletion when taken with cardioactive herbs, such as adonis, digitalis, and lily-of-the-valley. (For a list of cardioactive herbs and supplements, see Appendix B.)
- Increased risk of potassium depletion when used in conjunction with horsetail plant or licorice.
- Increased risk of potassium depletion when used with stimulant laxative herbs, such as black root, cascara sagrada, castor oil, and senna. (For a list of stimulant laxative herbs and supplements, see Appendix B.)

STEVIA

Native to Paraguay, the unassuming little stevia plant has leaves that are approximately thirty times sweeter than sugar, with virtually no calories. The Guarani Indians have chewed these leaves for their sweet taste and have used them to sweeten medicinal teas and the beverage yerba maté. Stevia has recently gained attention as a noncaloric sugar alternative and a sweetener used in food manufacturing, particularly in Japan. It may also have medicinal benefits: An extract of stevia called stevoiside was recently tested in over 150 men and women with mildly elevated blood pressure. After two years' treatment, blood pressure fell significantly in those taking the herbal extract compared to those who had received a placebo.

Scientific Name

Stevia rebaudiana

Stevia Is Also Commonly Known As
Azucacca, sweet herb, sweetleaf, yerba dulce

Medicinal Parts
Leaf

Stevia's Uses
To treat diabetes and low blood pressure; as a contraceptive

Typical Dose
There is no typical dose of stevia.

Possible Side Effects
Stevia's side effects include low blood pressure and reduced heart rate.

Drugs That May Interact with Stevia
Taking stevia with these drugs may increase the risk of hypotension (excessively low blood pressure):

- acebutolol (Novo-Acebutolol, Sectral)
- amlodipine (Norvasc)
- atenolol (Apo-Atenol, Tenormin)
- benazepril (Lotensin)
- betaxolol (Betoptic S, Kerlone)
- bisoprolol (Monocor, Zebeta)
- bumetanide (Bumex, Burinex)
- candesartan (Atacand)
- captopril (Capoten, Novo-Captopril)
- carteolol (Cartrol, Ocupress)
- carvedilol (Coreg)
- chlorothiazide (Diuril)
- chlorthalidone (Apo-Chlorthalidone, Thalitone)
- clonidine (Catapres, Duraclon)
- diazoxide (Hyperstat, Proglycem)
- diltiazem (Cardizem, Tiazac)
- doxazosin (Cardura, Alti-Doxazosin)
- enalapril (Vasotec)
- eplerenone (Inspra)
- eprosartan (Teveten)
- esmolol (Brevibloc)
- felodipine (Plendil, Renedil)
- fenoldopam (Corlopam)
- fosinopril (Monopril)
- furosemide (Apo-Furosemide, Lasix)
- guanabenz (Wytensin)
- guanadrel (Hylorel)
- guanfacine (Tenex)
- hydralazine (Apresoline, Novo-Hylazin)
- hydrochlorothiazide (Apo-Hydro, Microzide)
- hydrochlorothiazide and triamterene (Dyazide, Maxzide)
- indapamide (Lozol, Nu-Indapamide)
- irbesartan (Avapro)
- isradipine (DynaCirc)
- labetalol (Normodyne, Trandate)
- lisinopril (Prinivil, Zestril)
- losartan (Cozaar)
- mecamylamine (Inversine)
- mefruside (Baycaron)
- methyclothiazide (Aquatensen, Enduron)
- methyldopa (Apo-Methyldopa, Nu-Medopa)
- metolazone (Mykrox, Zaroxolyn)
- metoprolol (Betaloc, Lopressor)
- minoxidil (Loniten, Rogaine)
- moexipril (Univasc)
- nadolol (Apo-Nadol, Corgard)
- nicardipine (Cardene)
- nifedipine (Adalat CC, Procardia)
- nisoldipine (Sular)
- nitroglycerin (Minitran, Nitro-Dur)

- nitroprusside (Nipride, Nitropress)
- olmesartan (Benicar)
- oxprenolol (Slow-Trasicor, Trasicor)
- perindopril erbumine (Aceon, Coversyl)
- phenoxybenzamine (Dibenzyline)
- phentolamine (Regitine, Rogitine)
- pindolol (Apo-Pindol, Novo-Pindol)
- polythiazide (Renese)
- prazosin (Minipress, Nu-Prazo)
- propranolol (Inderal, InnoPran XL)
- quinapril (Accupril)
- ramipril (Altace)
- reserpine
- spironolactone (Aldactone, Novo-Spiroton)
- telmisartan (Micardis)
- terazosin (Alti-Terazosin, Hytrin)
- timolol (Betimol, Timoptic)
- torsemide (Demadex)
- trandolapril (Mavik)
- triamterene (Dyrenium)
- trichlormethiazide (Metatensin, Naqua)
- valsartan (Diovan)
- verapamil (Calan, Isoptin SR)

Taking stevia with these drugs may increase the effects of the drug:
- amlodipine (Norvasc)
- bepridil (Vascor)
- diltiazem (Cardizem, Tiazac)
- felodipine (Plendil, Renedil)
- isradipine (DynaCirc)
- lacidipine (Aponil, Caldine)
- lercanidipine (Cardiovasc, Carmen)
- manidipine (Calslot, Iperten)
- nicardipine (Cardene)
- nifedipine (Adalat CC, Procardia)
- nilvadipine

- nimodipine (Nimotop)
- nisoldipine (Sular)
- nitrendipine
- pinaverium (Dicetel)
- verapamil (Calan, Isoptin SR)

Taking stevia with these drugs may increase the risk of hypoglycemia (low blood sugar):
- acarbose (Prandase, Precose)
- acetohexamide
- chlorpropamide (Diabinese, Novo-Propamide)
- gliclazide (Diamicron, Novo-Gliclazide)
- glimepiride (Amaryl)
- glipizide (Glucotrol)
- glipizide and metformin (Metaglip)
- gliquidone (Beglynor, Glurenorm)
- glyburide (DiaBeta, Micronase)
- glyburide and metformin (Glucovance)
- insulin (Humulin, Novolin R)
- metformin (Glucophage, Riomet)
- miglitol (Glyset)
- nateglinide (Starlix)
- pioglitazone (Actos)
- repaglinide (GlucoNorm, Prandin)
- rosiglitazone (Avandia)
- rosiglitazone and metformin (Avandamet)
- tolazamide (Tolinase)
- tolbutamide (Apo-Tolbutamide, Tol-Tab)

Lab Tests That May Be Altered by Stevia
- May decrease blood pressure.
- May decrease blood glucose levels.

Diseases That May Be Worsened or Triggered by Stevia
May lower blood sugar in diabetics and interfere with therapy to control blood sugar.

Foods That May Interact with Stevia
None known

Supplements That May Interact with Stevia
- Increased risk of hypotension or increased therapeutic effects when used with herbs and supplements that may lower blood pressure, such as black cohosh, danshen, and Panax ginseng. (For a list of herbs and supplements with hypotensive activity, see Appendix B.)
- May increase blood glucose–lowering effects and risk of hypoglycemia (low blood sugar) when used with herbs and supplements that lower glucose levels, such as alpha-lipoic acid, chromium, devil's claw, Panax ginseng, and psyllium. (For a list of herbs and supplements that lower blood glucose levels, see Appendix B.)

STINGING NETTLE

This tall, hairy, innocuous-looking weed with tiny greenish white flowers can be found growing along the banks of streams and rivers throughout Europe and the United States. But beware—it causes a nasty sting when you touch it with your bare skin, thanks to the formic acid on the hairs that cover the plant. Used as a medicine in Europe for over two thousand years, teas made from the stems and leaves of the stinging nettle have been used as diuretics, as treatments for prostate problems, and to stop bleeding.

Scientific Name
Urtica dioica

Stinging Nettle Is Also Commonly Known As
Common nettle, nettle, ortie, small nettle

Medicinal Parts
Flowering plant, root

Stinging Nettle's Uses
To treat infections of the urinary tract and kidney; bladder stones, prostatitis, rheumatism, and gout. Germany's Commission E has approved the use of stinging nettle flowering plant to treat rheumatism, urinary tract infections, and bladder and kidney stones, and the use of stinging nettle root to treat irritable bladder and prostate problems.

Typical Dose
A typical daily dose of stinging nettle may range from 8 to 12 gm of the flowering plant or 4 to 6 gm of the root.

Possible Side Effects
Stinging nettle's side effects include gastric irritation and allergic reactions.

Drugs That May Interact with Stinging Nettle
Taking stinging nettle plant with these drugs may increase the risk of excessive sedation and mental depression and impairment:
- acetaminophen and codeine (Capital and Codeine, Tylenol with Codeine)
- alfentanil (Alfenta)
- alprazolam (Apo-Alpraz, Xanax)
- amitriptyline (Elavil, Levate)
- amobarbital (Amytal)
- amobarbital and secobarbital (Tuinal)
- amoxapine (Asendin)
- aspirin and codeine (Coryphen Codeine)

- belladonna and opium (B&O Supprettes)
- bromazepam (Apo-Bromazepam, Gen-Bromazepam)
- brotizolam (Lendorm, Sintonal)
- buprenorphine (Buprenex, Subutex)
- buprenorphine and naloxone (Suboxone)
- bupropion (Wellbutrin, Zyban)
- buspirone (BuSpar, Nu-Buspirone)
- butabarbital (Butisol Sodium)
- butalbital, acetaminophen, and caffeine (Esgic, Fioricet)
- butalbital, aspirin, and caffeine (Fiorinal)
- butorphanol (Apo-Butorphanol, Stadol)
- carbamazepine (Carbatrol, Tegretol)
- chloral hydrate (Aquachloral Supprettes, Somnote)
- chlordiazepoxide (Apo-Chlordiazepoxide, Librium)
- clobazam (Alti-Clobazam, Frisium)
- clonazepam (Klonopin, Rivotril)
- clorazepate (Tranxene, T-Tab)
- codeine (Codeine Contin)
- cyclobenzaprine (Flexeril, Novo-Cycloprine)
- desipramine (Alti-Desipramine, Norpramin)
- dexmedetomidine (Precedex)
- diazepam (Apo-Diazepam, Valium)
- dihydrocodeine, aspirin, and caffeine (Synalgos-DC)
- diphenhydramine (Benadryl Allergy, Nytol)
- doxepin (Sinequan, Zonalon)
- estazolam (ProSom)
- fentanyl (Actiq, Duragesic)
- fluoxetine (Prozac, Sarafem)
- fluphenazine (Prolixin, Modecate)
- flurazepam (Apo-Flurazepam, Dalmane)
- fosphenytoin (Cerebyx)
- glutethimide
- haloperidol (Haldol, Novo-Peridol)
- hydrocodone and acetaminophen (Vicodin, Zydone)
- hydrocodone and aspirin (Damason-P)
- hydrocodone and ibuprofen (Vicoprofen)
- hydromorphone (Dilaudid, PMS-Hydromorphone)
- hydroxyzine (Atarax, Vistaril)
- imipramine (Apo-Imipramine, Tofranil)
- levetiracetam (Keppra)
- levomethadyl acetate hydrochloride
- levorphanol (LevoDromoran)
- loprazolam (Dormonoct, Havlane)
- lorazepam (Ativan, Nu-Loraz)
- meperidine (Demerol, Meperitab)
- meperidine and promethazine
- mephobarbital (Mebaral)
- methadone (Dolophine, Methadose)
- methohexital (Brevital, Brevital Sodium)
- metoclopramide (Apo-Metoclop, Reglan)
- midazolam (Apo-Midazolam, Versed)
- morphine hydrochloride
- morphine sulfate (Kadian, MS Contin)
- nalbuphine (Nubain)
- nefazodone (Serzone)
- nortriptyline (Aventyl HCl, Pamelor)
- olanzapine (Zydis, Zyprexa)
- opium tincture
- oxazepam (Novoxapam, Serax)
- oxcarbazepine (Trileptal)
- oxycodone (OxyContin, Roxicodone)
- oxycodone and acetaminophen (Endocet, Percocet)
- oxycodone and aspirin (Endodan, Percodan)
- oxymorphone (Numorphan)
- paregoric
- pentazocine (Talwin)
- pentobarbital (Nembutal)

- phenobarbital (Luminal Sodium, PMS-Phenobarbital)
- phenoperidine
- phenytoin (Dilantin, Phenytek)
- prazepam
- primidone (Apo-Primidone, Mysoline)
- prochlorperazine (Compazine, Compro)
- promethazine (Phenergan)
- propofol (Diprivan)
- propoxyphene (Darvon, Darvon-N)
- propoxyphene and acetaminophen (Darvocet-N 50, Darvocet-N 100)
- propoxyphene, aspirin, and caffeine (Darvon Compound)
- quazepam (Doral)
- quetiapine (Seroquel)
- remifentanil (Ultiva)
- risperidone (Risperdal)
- secobarbital (Seconal)
- sodium oxybate (Xyrem)
- sufentanil (Sufenta)
- s-zopiclone (Lunesta)
- temazepam (Novo-Temazepam, Restoril)
- tetrazepam (Mobiforton, Musapam)
- thiopental (Pentothal)
- tramadol (Ultram)
- triazolam (Apo-Triazo, Halcion)
- zaleplon (Sonata, Stamoc)
- zolpidem (Ambien)
- zopiclone (Alti-Zopiclone, Gen-Zopiclone)

Taking stinging nettle plant with these drugs may interfere with the action of the drug:

- abciximab (ReoPro)
- antithrombin III (Thrombate III)
- argatroban
- aspirin (Bufferin, Ecotrin)

- aspirin and dipyridamole (Aggrenox)
- bivalirudin (Angiomax)
- carbamazepine (Carbatro, Tegretol)
- clopidogrel (Plavix)
- dalteparin (Fragmin)
- danaparoid (Orgaran)
- dipyridamole (NovoDipiradol, Persantine)
- enoxaparin (Lovenox)
- eptifibatide (Integrillin)
- fondaparinux (Arixtra)
- fosphenytoin (Cerebyx)
- heparin (Hepalean, Hep-Lock)
- indobufen (Ibustrin)
- lepirudin (Refludan)
- levetiracetam (Keppra)
- phenytoin (Dilantin, Phenytek)
- ticlopidine (Alti-Ticlopidine, Ticlid)
- tinzaparin (Innohep)
- tirofiban (Aggrastat)
- warfarin (Coumadin, Jantoven)

Taking stinging nettle with these drugs may increase the diuretic effects of the drug:

- acetazolamide (Apo-Acetazolamide, Diamox Sequels)
- amiloride (Midamor)
- azosemide (Diat)
- bumetanide (Bumex, Burinex)
- chlorothiazide (Diuril)
- chlorthalidone (Apo-Chlorthalidone, Thalitone)
- ethacrynic acid (Edecrin)
- etozolin (Elkapin)
- furosemide (Apo-Furosemide, Lasix)
- hydrochlorothiazide (Apo-Hydro, Microzide)
- hydrochlorothiazide and triamterene (Dyazide, Maxzide)

- hydroflumethiazide (Diucardin, Saluron)
- indapamide (Lozol, Nu-Indapamide)
- mannitol (Osmitrol, Resectisol)
- mefruside (Baycaron)
- methazolamide (Apo-Methazolamide, Neptazane)
- methyclothiazide (Aquatensen, Enduron)
- metolazone (Mykrox, Zaroxolyn)
- olmesartan and hydrochlorothiazide (Benicar HCT)
- polythiazide (Renese)
- spironolactone (Aldactone, Novo-Spiroton)
- torsemide (Demadex)
- triamterene (Dyrenium)
- trichlormethiazide (Metatensin, Naqua)
- urea (Amino-Cerv, UltraMide)
- xipamide (Diurexan, Lumitens)

Taking stinging nettle plant with these drugs may reduce or prevent drug absorption:
- ferric gluconate (Ferrlecit)
- ferrous fumarate (Femiron, Feostat)
- ferrous gluconate (Fergon, Novo-Ferrogluc)
- ferrous sulfate (Feratab, Fer-Iron)
- ferrous sulfate and ascorbic acid (FeroGrad 500, Vitelle Irospan)
- iron-dextran complex (Dexferrum, INFeD)
- polysaccharide-iron complex (Hytinic, Niferex)

Taking stinging nettle plant with this drug may be harmful:
- lithium (Carbolith, Eskalith)—may increase the risk of dehydration and lithium toxicity

Lab Tests That May Be Altered by Stinging Nettle
None known

Diseases That May Be Worsened or Triggered by Stinging Nettle
May worsen congestive heart failure or kidney dysfunction.

Foods That May Interact with Stinging Nettle
None known

Supplements That May Interact with Stinging Nettle
When taken in excessive amounts, may increase the risk of clotting in those using anticoagulants due to vitamin K content, especially if taken with other vitamin K–rich herbs, such as alfalfa and parsley. (For a list of herbs and supplements that contain vitamin K, see Appendix B.)

ST. JOHN'S WORT

Named for St. John, the patron saint of nurses, this herb in medieval times was believed to be such a powerful healer that if people put a cutting of it under their pillows on St. John's Eve, St. John himself would appear in their dreams and ward off death for another year. The herb's scientific name, *Hypericum*, comes from the Greek word meaning "over an apparition," referring to the herb's purported ability to make evil spirits fly away with just one whiff of its pungent odor.

Scientific Name
Hypericum perforatum

St. John's Wort Is Also Commonly Known As
Amber, goatweed, hardhay, klamath weed, tipton weed

Medicinal Parts
Flower, bud, whole plant

St. John's Wort's Uses
To treat depression, anxiety, worm infestation, asthma, gout, rheumatism, and burns. Germany's Commission E has approved the use of St. John's wort to treat anxiety, depressive moods, blunt injuries, inflammation of the skin, wounds, and burns.

Typical Dose
A typical dose of St. John's wort in tablet/capsule form is approximately 300 mg Hypericum extract (standardized to 0.3 percent hypericin) taken three times daily.

Possible Side Effects
St. John's wort's side effects include dizziness, fatigue, restlessness, insomnia, constipation, and photosensitivity.

Drugs That May Interact with St. John's Wort
Taking St. John's wort with these drugs may increase the risk of bleeding or bruising:
- antithrombin III (Thrombate III)
- argatroban
- bivalirudin (Angiomax)
- dalteparin (Fragmin)
- danaparoid (Orgaran)
- enoxaparin (Lovenox)
- fondaparinux (Arixtra)
- heparin (Hepalean, Hep-Lock)
- lepirudin (Refludan)
- tinzaparin (Innohep)
- warfarin (Coumadin, Jantoven)

Taking St. John's wort with these drugs may increase the risk of hypoglycemia (low blood sugar):
- acarbose (Prandase, Precose)
- acetohexamide
- chlorpropamide (Diabinese, Novo-Propamide)
- gliclazide (Diamicron, Novo-Gliclazide)
- glimepiride (Amaryl)
- glipizide (Glucotrol)
- glipizide and metformin (Metaglip)
- gliquidone (Beglynor, Glurenorm)
- glyburide (DiaBeta, Micronase)
- glyburide and metformin (Glucovance)
- insulin (Humulin, Novolin R)
- metformin (Glucophage, Riomet)
- miglitol (Glyset)
- nateglinide (Starlix)
- pioglitazone (Actos)
- repaglinide (GlucoNorm, Prandin)
- rosiglitazone (Avandia)
- rosiglitazone and metformin (Avandamet)
- tolazamide (Tolinase)
- tolbutamide (Apo-Tolbutamide, Tol-Tab)

Taking St. John's wort with these drugs may interfere with the effectiveness of the drug:
- acebutolol (Novo-Acebutolol, Sectral)
- alprazolam (Apo-Alpraz, Xanax)
- amlodipine (Norvasc)
- amobarbital (Amytal)
- amobarbital and secobarbital (Tuinal)
- amprenavir (Agenerase)
- antithymocyte globulin, equine (Atgam)
- antithymocyte globulin, rabbit (Thymoglobulin)

- atenolol (Apo-Atenol, Tenormin)
- atorvastatin (Lipitor)
- azathioprine (Imuran)
- basiliximab (Simulect)
- befunolol (Bentos, Betaclar)
- bepridil (Vascor)
- betaxolol (Betoptic S, Kerlone)
- bisoprolol (Monocor, Zebeta)
- bromazepam (Apo-Bromazepam, Gen-Bromazepam)
- brotizolam (Lendorm, Sintonal)
- butabarbital (Butisol Sodium)
- butalbital, acetaminophen, and caffeine (Esgic, Fioricet)
- butalbital, aspirin, and caffeine (Fiorinal)
- carteolol (Cartrol, Ocupress)
- carvedilol (Coreg)
- celiprolol
- chlordiazepoxide (Apo-Chlordiazepoxide, Librium)
- chlorzoxazone (Strifon Forte)
- clobazam (Alti-Clobazam, Frisium)
- clonazepam (Klonopin, Rivotril)
- clorazepate (Tranxene, T-Tab)
- clozapine (Clozaril, Gen-Clozapine)
- cyclophosphamide (Cytoxan, Neosar)
- cyclosporine (Neoral, Sandimmune)
- cyproterone and ethinyl estradiol (Diane-35)
- daclizumab (Zenapax)
- delavirdine (Rescriptor)
- diazepam (Apo-Diazepam, Valium)
- diltiazem (Cardizem, Tiazac)
- efalizumab (Raptiva)
- efavirenz (Sustiva)
- esmolol (Brevibloc)
- estazolam (ProSom)
- estradiol (Climara, Estrace)
- estradiol and medroxyprogesterone (Lunelle)
- estradiol and norethindrone (Activella, CombiPatch)
- estradiol and testosterone (Climacteron)
- estrogens (conjugated A/synthetic) (Cenestin)
- estrogens (conjugated/equine) (Congest, Premarin)
- estrogens (conjugated/equine) and medroxyprogesterone (Premphase, Prempro)
- estrogens (esterified) (Estratab, Menest)
- estrogens (esterified) and methyltestosterone (Estratest, Estratest H.S.)
- estropipate (Ogen, OrthoEst)
- ethinyl estradiol (Estinyl)
- ethinyl estradiol and desogestrel (Cyclessa, Ortho-Cept)
- ethinyl estradiol and drospirenone (Yasmin)
- ethinyl estradiol and ethynodiol diacetate (Demulen, Zovia)
- ethinyl estradiol and etonogestrel (NuvaRing)
- ethinyl estradiol and levonorgestrel (Alesse, Triphasil)
- ethinyl estradiol and norelgestromin (Evra, Ortho Evra)
- ethinyl estradiol and norethindrone (Brevicon, Ortho-Novum)
- ethinyl estradiol and norgestimate (Cyclen, Ortho Tri-Cyclen)
- ethinyl estradiol and norgestrel (Cryselle, Ovral)
- etoposide (Toposar, VePesid)
- felodipine (Plendil, Renedil)
- flurazepam (Apo-Flurazepam, Dalmane)
- fluvastatin (Lescol)
- imatinib (Gleevec)
- indinavir (Crixivan)
- irinotican (Camptosar)
- isradipine (DynaCirc)

- labetalol (Normodyne, Trandate)
- lacidipine (Aponil, Caldine)
- lercanidipine (Cardiovasc, Carmen)
- levobetaxolol (Betaxon)
- levobunolol (Betagan, Novo-Levobunolol)
- levonorgestrel
- lopinavir and ritonavir (Kaletra)
- loprazolam (Dormonoct, Havlane)
- lorazepam (Ativan, Nu-Loraz)
- lovastatin (Altocor, Mevacor)
- manidipine (Calslot, Iperten)
- medroxyprogesterone (Depo-Provera, Provera)
- mephobarbital (Mebaral)
- mestranol and norethindrone (Necon 1/50, Ortho-Novum 1/50)
- methohexital (Brevital, Brevital Sodium)
- methotrexate (Rheumatrex, Trexall)
- metipranolol (OptiPranolol)
- metoprolol (Betaloc, Lopressor)
- midazolam (Apo-Midazolam, Versed)
- muromonab-CD3 (Orthoclone OKT 3)
- mycophenolate (CellCept)
- nadolol (Apo-Nadol, Corgard)
- nelfinavir (Viracept)
- nevirapine (Viramune)
- nicardipine (Cardene)
- nifedipine (Adalat CC, Procardia)
- nilvadipine
- nimodipine (Nimotop)
- nisoldipine (Sular)
- nitrendipine
- norgestrel (Ovrette)
- oxazepam (Novoxapam, Serax)
- oxprenolol (Slow-Trasicor, Trasicor)
- paclitaxel (Onzol, Taxol)
- pentobarbital (Nembutal)
- phenobarbital (Luminal Sodium, PMS-Phenobarbital)
- phenytoin (Dilantin, Phenytek)
- pimecrolimus (Elidel)
- pinaverium (Dicetel)
- pindolol (Apo-Pindol, Novo-Pindol)
- polyestradiol
- pravastatin (Novo-Pravastatin, Pravachol)
- prazepam
- primidone (Apo-Primidone, Mysoline)
- propranolol (Inderal, InnoPran XL)
- quazepam (Doral)
- reserpine
- ritonavir (Norvir)
- rosuvastatin (Crestor)
- saquinavir (Fortovase, Invirase)
- secobarbital (Seconal)
- simvastatin (Apo-Simvastatin, Zocor)
- sirolimus (Rapamune)
- sotalol (Betapace, Sorine)
- tacrolimus (Prograf, Protopic)
- tamoxifen (Nolvadex, Tamofen)
- temazepam (Novo-Temazepam, Restoril)
- tetrazepam (Mobiforton, Musapam)
- thalidomide (Thalomid)
- theophylline (Elixophyllin, Uniphyl)
- thiopental (Pentothal)
- timolol (Betimol, Timoptic)
- triazolam (Apo-Triazo, Halcion)
- verapamil (Calan, Isoptin SR)

Taking St. John's wort with these drugs may interfere with absorption of the drug:
- ferric gluconate (Ferrlecit)
- ferrous fumarate (Femiron, Feostat)
- ferrous gluconate (Fergon, Novo-Ferrogluc)
- ferrous sulfate (Feratab, Fer-Iron)

- ferrous sulfate and ascorbic acid (FeroGrad 500, Vitelle Irospan)
- iron-dextran complex (Dexferrum, INFeD)
- polysaccharide-iron complex (Hytinic, Niferex)

❶ Taking St. John's wort with these drugs may cause or increase serotonin syndrome (symptoms of which include agitation, rapid heart rate, flushing, heavy sweating, and possibly even death):
- amitriptyline (Elavil, Levate)
- amitriptyline and chlordiazepoxide (Limbitrol)
- amitriptyline and perphenazine (Etrafor, Triavil)
- amoxapine (Asendin)
- buspirone (BuSpar, Nu-Buspirone)
- citalopram (Celexa)
- clomipramine (Anafranil, Novo-Clopramine)
- desipramine (Alti-Desipramine, Norpramin)
- dextroamphetamine (Dexedrine, Dextrostat)
- dextroamphetamine and amphetamine (Adderall, Adderall XR)
- doxepin (Sinequan, Zonalon)
- fluoxetine (Prozac, Sarafem)
- fluvoxamine (Alti-Fluvoxamine, Luvox)
- imipramine (Apo-Imipramine, Tofranil)
- iproniazid (Marsilid)
- lofepramine (Feprapax, Gamanil)
- melitracen (Dixeran)
- methamphetamine (Desoxyn)
- moclobemide (Alti-Moclobemide, Nu-Moclo-bemide)
- nefazodone (Serzone)
- nortriptyline (Aventyl HCl, Pamelor)
- paroxetine (Paxil)
- phenelzine (Nardil)
- protriptyline (Vivactil)
- s-citalopram (Lexapro)
- selegiline (Eldepryl)
- sertraline (Apo-Sertraline, Zoloft)
- tranylcypromine (Parnate)
- trazodone (Desyrel, Novo-Trazodone)
- trimipramine (Apo-Trimip, Surmontil)
- venlafaxine (Effexor)

Taking St. John's wort with these drugs may increase the therapeutic and/or adverse effects of the drug:
- almotriptan (Axert)
- eletriptan (Relpax)
- frovatriptan (Frova)

Taking St. John's wort with these drugs may increase skin sensitivity to sunlight:
- acemetacin (Acemetacin Heumann, Acemetacin Sandoz)
- acetohexamide
- aminolevulinic acid (Levulan Kerastick)
- aspirin (Bufferin, Ecotrin)
- azosemide (Diat)
- benazepril (Lotensin)
- bumetanide (Bumex, Burinex)
- captopril (Capoten, Novo-Captopril)
- celecoxib (Celebrex)
- chlorothiazide (Diuril)
- chlorpropamide (Diabinese, Novo-Propamide)
- choline magnesium trisalicylate (Trilisate)
- choline salicylate (Teejel)
- cilazapril (Inhibace)
- delapril (Adecut, Delakete)
- demeclocycline (Declomycin)
- diclofenac (Cataflam, Voltaren)
- diflunisal (Apo-Diflunisal, Dolobid)
- dipyrone (Analgina, Dinador)
- doxycycline (Apo-Doxy, Vibramycin)

- enalapril (Vasotec)
- erythromycin and sulfisoxazole (Eryzole, Pediazole)
- ethacrynic acid (Edecrin)
- etodolac (Lodine, Utradol)
- etoricoxib (Arcoxia)
- etozolin (Elkapin)
- fenoprofen (Nalfon)
- flurbiprofen (Ansaid, Ocufen)
- fosinopril (Monopril)
- furosemide (Apo-Furosemide, Lasix)
- glimepiride (Amaryl)
- glipizide (Glucotrol)
- glyburide (DiaBeta, Micronase)
- hydrochlorothiazide (Apo-Hydro, Microzide)
- hydrochlorothiazide and triamterene (Dyazide, Maxzide)
- hydroflumethiazide (Diucardin, Saluron)
- ibuprofen (Advil, Motrin)
- imidapril (Novarok, Tanatril)
- indomethacin (Indocin, Novo-Methacin)
- ketoprofen (Orudis, Rhodis)
- ketorolac (Acular, Toradol)
- lisinopril (Prinivil, Zestril)
- magnesium salicylate (Doan's, Mobidin)
- meclofenamate (Meclomen)
- mefenamic acid (Ponstan, Ponstel)
- meloxicam (MOBIC, Mobicox)
- methyclothiazide (Aquatensen, Enduron)
- minocycline (Dynacin, Minocin)
- moexipril (Univasc)
- nabumetone (Apo-Nabumetone, Relafen)
- naproxen (Aleve, Naprosyn)
- niflumic acid (Niflam, Nifluril)
- nimesulide (Areuma, Aulin)
- olmesartan and hydrochlorothiazide (Benicar HCT)
- oxaprozin (Apo-Oxaprozin, Daypro)
- oxytetracycline (Terramycin, Terramycin IM)
- perindopril erbumine (Aceon, Coversyl)
- piroxicam (Feldene, Nu-Pirox)
- polythiazide (Renese)
- quinapril (Accupril)
- ramipril (Altace)
- rofecoxib (Vioxx)
- salsalate (Amgesic, Salflex)
- spirapril
- sulfacetamide (Bleph-10, Klaron)
- sulfadiazine (Microsulfon)
- sulfamethoxazole and trimethoprim (Bactrim, Septra)
- sulfisoxazole (Gantrisin)
- sulfur and sulfacetamide (Nocosyn, Rosanil)
- sulindac (Clinoril, Nu-Sundac)
- tenoxicam (Dolmen, Mobiflex)
- tetracycline (Novo-Tetra, Sumycin)
- tiaprofenic acid (DomTiaprofenic, Surgam)
- tolazamide (Tolinase)
- tolbutamide (Apo-Tolbutamide, Tol-Tab)
- tolmetin (Tolectin)
- torsemide (Demadex)
- trandolapril (Mavik)
- trichlormethiazide (Metatensin, Naqua)
- valdecoxib (Bextra)
- xipamide (Diurexan, Lumitens)

Taking St. John's wort with these drugs may reduce blood levels of the drug:
- amiodarone (Cordarone, Pacerone)
- digitalis (Digitek, Lanoxin)
- methadone (Dolophine, Methadose)

Taking St. John's wort with these drugs may be harmful:

- acitretin (Soriatane)—may increase the risk of unplanned pregnancy and birth defects
- carbamazepine (Carbatrol, Tegretrol)—may alter blood levels of the drug
- loperamide (Diarr-EZ, Imodium A-D)—may increase the risk of confusion, agitation, disorientation, and other symptoms of delirium

Lab Tests That May Be Altered by St. John's Wort
- May increase levels of growth hormone (somatotropin, GH).
- May decrease levels of serum prolactin.
- May decrease levels of theophylline.
- May decrease levels of serum iron.
- May decrease levels of digitalis.
- May decrease prothrombin time (PT) and plasma international normalized ratio (INR) in those who are also taking warfarin.
- May increase thyroid-stimulating hormone (TSH) levels.

Diseases That May Be Worsened or Triggered by St. John's Wort
- May trigger psychosis in those with Alzheimer's disease or schizophrenia.
- May trigger mania or hypomania in those with bipolar disorder.
- May trigger hypomania in those with major depression.

Foods That May Interact with St. John's Wort
Because of possible monoamine oxidase inhibiting (MAOI) action of St. John's wort, limit intake of foods high in tyramine, such as aged cheese, red wine, bananas, aged or cured meat, and yeast-containing products.

Supplements That May Interact with St. John's Wort
- May decrease therapeutic effects of digitalis.
- May increase positive and negative effects of herbs and supplements that have serotonergic properties, such as 5-hydroxytryptophan (5-HTP) and S-adenosylmethionine (SAMe). (For a list of herbs and supplements that have serotonergic properties, see Appendix B.)

STONE ROOT

A strong diuretic, stone root is used in the prevention and treatment of stones and gravel in the urinary system and gallbladder. Stone root is also used to improve the structure and function of the veins, and many healers recommend it for varicose veins, hemorrhoids, and anal fissures. Contrary to its name, it's not just the root but also the flowers and leaves of the plant that are effective and used in herbal remedies.

Scientific Name
Collinsonia canadensis

Stone Root Is Also Commonly Known As
Archangel, Canadian horsemint, hardhack, horse-weed, knob root, rock-weed

Medicinal Parts
Roots, rhizome

Stone Root's Uses
To treat gastrointestinal disorders, bladder inflammation, and kidney stones

Typical Dose

A typical dose of stone root may range from 1 to 4 ml of liquid extract (1:1).

Possible Side Effects

Stone root's side effects include gastrointestinal irritation, nausea, dizziness, and painful urination.

Drugs That May Interact with Stone Root

Taking stone root with these drugs may increase the diuretic effects of the drug:

- acetazolamide (Apo-Acetazolamide, Diamox Sequels)
- amiloride (Midamor)
- azosemide (Diat)
- bumetanide (Bumex, Burinex)
- chlorothiazide (Diuril)
- chlorthalidone (Apo-Chlorthalidone, Thalitone)
- ethacrynic acid (Edecrin)
- etozolin (Elkapin)
- furosemide (Apo-Furosemide, Lasix)
- hydrochlorothiazide (Apo-Hydro, Microzide)
- hydrochlorothiazide and triamterene (Dyazide, Maxzide)
- hydroflumethiazide (Diucardin, Saluron)
- indapamide (Lozol, Nu-Indapamide)
- mannitol (Osmitrol, Resectisol)
- mefruside (Baycaron)
- methazolamide (Apo-Methazolamide, Neptazane)
- methyclothiazide (Aquatensen, Enduron)
- metolazone (Mykrox, Zaroxolyn)
- olmesartan and hydrochlorothiazide (Benicar HCT)
- polythiazide (Renese)
- spironolactone (Aldactone, Novo-Spiroton)
- torsemide (Demadex)
- triamterene (Dyrenium)
- trichlormethiazide (Metatensin, Naqua)
- urea (Amino-Cerv, UltraMide)
- xipamide (Diurexan, Lumitens)

Lab Tests That May Be Altered by Stone Root

None known

Diseases That May Be Worsened or Triggered by Stone Root

None known

Foods That May Interact with Stone Root

None known

Supplements That May Interact with Stone Root

May enhance the effects of herbs and supplements that have diuretic properties, such as agrimony, celery, shepherd's purse, and yarrow. (For a list of herbs that have diuretic properties, see Appendix B.)

STROPHANTHUS

The seeds of the woody, climbing *Strophanthus hispidus* plant, originating in tropical Africa, contain a thick liquid used by natives to poison the tips of their arrows. Animals could rarely run more than a hundred yards after being wounded by one of these poisoned arrows, although their flesh supposedly could be eaten "without bad effect." Strophantin, a cardiac glycoside isolated from strophanthus seeds in 1885, was once used medically to treat weak hearts, although more sophisticated medicines have since taken its place.

Scientific Name
Strophanthus gratus, Strophanthus kombe

Strophanthus Is Also Commonly Known As
Kombé, kombé seed, strophanthi granti semen, strophanthus seeds

Medicinal Parts
Seed

Strophanthus's Uses
To treat cardiac insufficiency, arteriosclerosis, and elevated blood pressure

Typical Dose
A typical daily dose of strophanthus seeds is approximately 1.5 gm of tincture (made from 1 part of coarsely ground strophanthus seed powder stabilized with 10 parts of 70 percent ethanol).

Possible Side Effects
Strophanthus's side effects include nausea, vomiting, headache, stupor, and irregular heartbeat. Strophanthus contains cardiac glycosides, which can help control irregular heartbeat, reduce the backup of blood and fluid in the body, and increase blood flow through the kidneys, helping to excrete sodium and relieve swelling in body tissues. However, a buildup of cardiac glycosides can occur, especially when the herb is combined with certain medications or other herbs that contain cardiac glycosides, causing arrhythmias, abnormally slow heartbeat, heart failure, and even death.

Drugs That May Interact with Strophanthus
Taking strophanthus with these drugs may increase the therapeutic and/or adverse effects of the drug:

- betamethasone (Betatrex, Maxivate)
- calcium acetate (PhosLo)
- calcium carbonate (Rolaids Extra Strength, Tums)
- calcium chloride
- calcium citrate (Osteocit)
- calcium glubionate
- calcium gluceptate
- calcium gluconate
- cascara
- cortisone (Cortone)
- deflazacort (Calcort, Dezacor)
- dexamethasone (Decadron, Dexasone)
- digitalis (Digitek, Lanoxin)
- docusate (Colace, Ex-Lax Stool Softener)
- docusate and Senna (Peri-Colace, Senokot-S)
- hydrocortisone (Cetacort, Locoid)
- lactulose (Constulose, Enulose)
- magnesium citrate (Citro-Mag)
- magnesium hydroxide (Dulcolax Milk of Magnesia, Phillips' Milk of Magnesia)
- magnesium hydroxide and mineral oil (Phillips' M-O)
- magnesium oxide (Mag-Ox 400, Uro-Mag)
- magnesium sulfate (Epsom salts)
- methylprednisolone (Depo-Medrol, Medrol)
- polyethylene glycol-electrolyte solution (Colyte, MiraLax)
- prednisolone (Inflamase Forte, Pred Forte)
- prednisone (Apo-Prednisone, Deltasone)
- psyllium (Metamucil, Reguloid)
- quinidine (Novo-Quinidin, Quinaglute Dura-Tabs)
- quinine (Quinine-Odan)
- sorbitol (Sorbilax)
- triamcinolone (Aristocort, Trinasal)

Taking strophanthus with these drugs may cause depletion of electrolytes, increasing the risk of herb toxicity:

- beclomethasone (Beconase, Vanceril)
- betamethasone (Celestone, Diprolene)
- budesonide (Entocort, Rhinocort)
- budesonide and Formoterol (Symbicort)
- cortisone (Cortone)
- deflazacort (Calcort, Dezacor)
- dexamethasone (Decadron, Dexasone)
- flunisolide (AeroBid, Nasarel)
- fluorometholone (Eflone, Flarex)
- fluticasone (Cutivate, Flonase)
- hydrocortisone (Anusol-HC, Locoid)
- loteprednol (Alrex, Lotemax)
- medrysone (HMS Liquifilm)
- methylprednisolone (DepoMedrol, Medrol)
- prednisolone (Inflamase Forte, Pred Forte)
- prednisone (Apo-Prednisone, Deltasone)
- rimexolone (Vexol)
- triamcinolone (Aristocort, Trinasal)

Lab Tests That May Be Altered by Strophanthus
None known

Diseases That May Be Worsened or Triggered by Strophanthus
May trigger irregular heartbeat.

Foods That May Interact with Strophanthus
None known

Supplements That May Interact with Strophanthus
- Increased risk of cardiac glycoside toxicity when used with other herbs that contain cardiac glycosides, such as black hellebore, calotropis, motherwort, and others. (For a list

of cardiac glycoside–containing herbs and supplements, see Appendix B.)
- Strophanthus seed toxicity can be increased through the use of herbs containing anthraquinone, such as aloe, cascara sagrada, and senna. (For a list of herbs containing anthraquinone, see Appendix B.)
- Increased risk of toxicity when taken with quinine.
- Increased risk of toxicity when taken with mahuang.
- May increase adverse side effects of strophanthus when taken with licorice.

SWAMP MILKWEED

Named *Asclepias* for the Greek god of healing, and *incarnata*, which means "flesh," for the flesh color of its flowers, swamp milkweed grows in moist, marshy environments. Its stems and leaves produce a milky, bitter juice. Traditionally used as a cure for lung and digestive ailments, the active ingredients in this "milk" are chemicals called cardenolides, which are cardiac glycosides. When a caterpillar feasts on milkweed, its body becomes replete with cardenolides, making it poisonous to most predators even after it has turned into a butterfly.

Scientific Name
Asclepias incarnata

Swamp Milkweed Is Also Commonly Known As
Rose-colored silkweed, swamp silkweed

Medicinal Parts
Rhizome, root

Swamp Milkweed's Uses
To treat digestive disorders

Typical Dose
There is no typical dose of swamp milkweed.

Possible Side Effects
Swamp milkweed's side effects include nausea and vomiting. Swamp milkweed contains cardiac glycosides, which can help control irregular heartbeat, reduce the backup of blood and fluid in the body, and increase blood flow through the kidneys, helping to excrete sodium and relieve swelling in body tissues. However, a buildup of cardiac glycosides can occur, especially when the herb is combined with certain medications or other herbs that contain cardiac glycosides, causing arrhythmias, abnormally slow heartbeat, heart failure, and even death.

Drugs That May Interact with Swamp Milkweed
Taking swamp milkweed with this drug may be harmful:
- digitalis (Digitek, Lanoxin)—may increase adverse effects of the drug

Lab Tests That May Be Altered by Swamp Milkweed
None known

Diseases That May Be Worsened or Triggered by Swamp Milkweed
May worsen heart disease due to cardiac glycosides in the herb.

Foods That May Interact with Swamp Milkweed
None known

Supplements That May Interact with Swamp Milkweed
- Increased risk of cardiac glycoside toxicity when used with other herbs that contain cardiac glycosides, such as black hellebore, calotropis, motherwort, and others. (For a list of cardiac glycoside–containing herbs and supplements, see Appendix B.)
- Increased risk of cardiotoxicity due to potassium depletion when taken with cardioactive herbs, such as adonis, digitalis, lily-of-the-valley, and squill. (For a list of cardioactive herbs and supplements, see Appendix B.)
- Increased risk of potassium depletion when used in conjunction with horsetail plant or licorice.
- Increased risk of potassium depletion when used with stimulant laxative herbs, such as black root, cascara sagrada, castor oil, and senna. (For a list of stimulant laxative herbs and supplements, see Appendix B.)

SWEET CLOVER

Sweet clover, found throughout much of North America, produces sweet, vanilla-scented yellow blooms on spikelike stalks. It contains small amounts of coumarin, an ingredient in prescription blood thinners, and has been used to improve blood circulation, heal wounds, and treat varicose veins and hemorrhoids.

Scientific Name
Melilotus officinalis

Sweet Clover Is Also Commonly Known As
Common melilot, field melilot, hay flower, king's clover, sweet lucerne, yellow sweet clover

Medicinal Part
Flowering herb

Sweet Clover's Uses
To treat problems arising from poor circulation in the legs, including pain, night cramps, swelling, hemorrhoids, and itching; as a diuretic. Germany's Commission E has approved the use of sweet clover to treat vein problems, hemorrhoids, and blunt injuries.

Typical Dose
A typical daily dose of sweet clover in the form of tea may range from 1 to 2 tsp of the herb steeped in 150 ml of boiling water for 5 to 10 minutes, taken two to three times a day.

Possible Side Effects
Sweet clover's side effects include headache, stupor, and transitory liver damage.

Drugs That May Interact with Sweet Clover
Taking sweet clover with these drugs may increase the risk of bleeding or bruising:
- abciximab (ReoPro)
- antithrombin III (Thrombate III)
- argatroban
- aspirin (Bufferin, Ecotrin)
- aspirin and dipyridamole (Aggrenox)
- bivalirudin (Angiomax)
- celecoxib (Celebrex)
- clopidogrel (Plavix)
- dalteparin (Fragmin)
- danaparoid (Orgaran)
- dipyridamole (Novo-Dipiradol, Persantine)
- enoxaparin (Lovenox)—bleeding
- eptifibatide (Integrillin)
- etodolac (Lodine, Utradol)—bleeding
- fondaparinux (Arixtra)
- heparin (Hepalean, Hep-Lock)
- ibuprofen (Advil, Motrin)
- indobufen (Ibustrin)
- indomethacin (Indocin, Novo-Methacin)
- ketoprofen (Orudis, Rhodis)
- ketorolac (Acular, Toradol)
- lepirudin (Refludan)
- ticlopidine (Alti-Ticlopidine, Ticlid)
- tinzaparin (Innohep)
- tirofiban (Aggrastat)
- warfarin (Coumadin, Jantoven)

Lab Tests That May Be Altered by Sweet Clover
May increase results of liver enzyme tests.

Diseases That May Be Worsened or Triggered by Sweet Clover
None known

Foods That May Interact with Sweet Clover
None known

Supplements That May Interact with Sweet Clover
Increased risk of bleeding when used with herbs and supplements that might affect platelet aggregation. (For a list of herbs and supplements with anticoagulant/antiplatelet effects, see Appendix B.)

SWEET ORANGE

> The orange, the most commonly grown tree fruit in the world, is thought to have originated in China, India, and perhaps southeast Asia, been transported to the Mediterranean by the fifteenth century, and taken to the New World by the mid-sixteenth century. Excellent sources of vitamin C, oranges also contain flavonoids that increase the body's resistance to carcinogens, allergens, and viruses while strengthening collagen (the protein that provides structure for the body's tissues).

Scientific Name
Citrus sinensis

Sweet Orange Is Also Commonly Known As
China orange, citrus dulcis, orange

Medicinal Parts
Peel of the fruit, oil taken from the peel, fruit juice

Sweet Orange's Uses
To treat lack of appetite and stomach complaints

Typical Dose
A typical daily dose of sweet orange is approximately 750 ml of juice or 10 to 15 grams of dry peel.

Possible Side Effects
Sweet orange's side effects include colic when the peel is taken in large amounts.

Drugs That May Interact with Sweet Orange
Taking sweet orange in the form of juice with these drugs may reduce or prevent absorption of the drug:

- celiprolol (Celicard)
- fexofenadine (Allegra)
- ivermectin (Stromectol)

Lab Tests That May Be Altered by Sweet Orange
None known

Diseases That May Be Worsened or Triggered by Sweet Orange
None known

Foods That May Interact with Sweet Orange
None known

Supplements That May Interact with Sweet Orange
None known

SWEET VERNAL GRASS

> Native to Europe, parts of Asia, and North Africa, this aromatic grass, which contains coumarin (a blood thinner) and benzoic acid (which gives it its newly mown hay aroma), is a potent allergen for many hay fever sufferers. However, a traditional remedy for an attack of hay fever is a tincture of sweet vernal grass made with spirit of wine (rectified ethyl alcohol), which is poured into the palm of the hand and sniffed heartily into the nose.

Scientific Name
Anthoxanthum odoratum

Sweet Vernal Grass Is Also Commonly Known As
Spring grass

Medicinal Parts

Whole plant

Sweet Vernal Grass's Uses

To treat nausea, headaches, insomnia, and urinary tract infections

Typical Dose

There is no typical dose of sweet vernal grass.

Possible Side Effects

Sweet vernal grass's side effects include headache and dizziness.

Drugs That May Interact with Sweet Vernal Grass

Taking sweet vernal grass with these drugs may increase the risk of bleeding or bruising:

- abciximab (ReoPro)
- antithrombin III (Thrombate III)
- argatroban
- aspirin (Bufferin, Ecotrin)
- aspirin and dipyridamole (Aggrenox)
- bivalirudin (Angiomax)
- clopidogrel (Plavix)
- dalteparin (Fragmin)
- danaparoid (Orgaran)
- dipyridamole (Novo-Dipiradol, Persantine)
- enoxaparin (Lovenox)
- eptifibatide (Integrillin)
- fondaparinux (Arixtra)
- heparin (Hepalean, Hep-Lock)
- indobufen (Ibustrin)
- lepirudin (Refludan)
- ticlopidine (Alti-Ticlopidine, Ticlid)
- tinzaparin (Innohep)
- tirofiban (Aggrastat)
- warfarin (Coumadin, Jantoven)

Lab Tests That May Be Altered by Sweet Vernal Grass

None known

Diseases That May Be Worsened or Triggered by Sweet Vernal Grass

None known

Foods That May Interact with Sweet Vernal Grass

None known

Supplements That May Interact with Sweet Vernal Grass

Increased risk of bleeding when used with herbs and supplements that might affect platelet aggregation. (For a list of herbs and supplements with anticoagulant/antiplatelet effects, see Appendix B.)

TAMARIND

The massive tamarind tree, native to tropical Africa but widely grown in India, produces a curved brown bean pod containing a sticky pulp surrounding several seeds. The tamarind pulp has a sweet, sour, fruity aroma and taste; it is high in acid and sugar and rich in vitamin B and calcium. These flavors make tamarind a much-valued ingredient in many Asian and Latin American dishes. Tamarind pulp is also used as a mild laxative, digestive, antiseptic, and fever-reducer. It also has a reputation for enhancing a woman's sexual enjoyment.

Scientific Name

Tamarindus indica

Tamarind Is Also Commonly Known As
Imlee

Medicinal Parts
Fruit pulp, seed

Tamarind's Uses
To treat constipation, fever, hemorrhoids, and liver ailments

Typical Dose
A typical daily dose of tamarind is up to 50 gm of tamarind paste, made from the fruit.

Possible Side Effects
No adverse effects have been reported with the proper use of tamarind under a physician's supervision.

Drugs That May Interact with Tamarind
Taking tamarind with this drug may be harmful:
- ibuprofen (Advil, Motrin)—may increase absorption and blood levels of the drug

Lab Tests That May Be Altered by Tamarind
None known

Diseases That May Be Worsened or Triggered by Tamarind
None known

Foods That May Interact with Tamarind
None known

Supplements That May Interact with Tamarind
None known

THIAMIN

Thiamin, formerly known as vitamin B_1, plays a role in the health of every cell in the body by assisting in the breakdown and conversion of carbohydrate, fat, and protein into energy. A lack of thiamin can cause enlargement and slowing of the heart, depression, confusion, and other problems. The classic thiamin deficiency disease, beriberi, can cause irritability, loss of appetite, weakness, poor coordination, tingling sensations throughout the body, and pain in the calves.

Typical Dose
The Food and Nutrition Board has set the RDA for thiamin at 1.2 mg per day for men ages nineteen and up and 1.1 mg per day for women ages nineteen and over.

Possible Side Effects
There are no known toxic effects from consuming up to 200 mg per day of supplemental thiamin, although excessive amounts of this vitamin may interfere with the absorption of other B vitamins.

Drugs That May Interact with Thiamin
None known

Drugs That May Interfere with the Absorption, Utilization, or Excretion of Thiamin
- amikacin (Amikin)
- amoxicillin (Amoxil, Novamoxin)
- ampicillin (Omnipen, Totacillin)
- azithromycin (Zithromax)
- bumetanide (Bumex, Burinex)
- carbenicillin (Geocillin)

- cefaclor (Ceclor)
- cefadroxil (Duricef)
- cefamandole (Mandol)
- cefazolin (Ancef, Kefzol)
- cefdinir (Omnicef)
- cefditoren (Spectracef)
- cefepime (Maxipime)
- cefonicid (Monocid)
- cefoperazone (Cefobid)
- cefotaxime (Claforan)
- cefotetan (Cefotan)
- cefoxitin (Mefoxin)
- cefpodoxime (Vantin)
- cefprozil (Cefzil)
- ceftazidime (Ceptaz, Fortaz)
- ceftibuten (Cedax)
- ceftizoxime (Cefizox)
- ceftriaxone (Rocephin)
- cefuroxime (Ceftin, Kefurox)
- cephalexin (Biocef, Keftab)
- cephalothin (Ceporacin)
- cephapirin (Cefadyl)
- cepharadine (Velosef)
- cimetidine (Nu-Cimet, Tagamet)
- cinoxacin (Cinobac)
- ciprofloxacin (Ciloxan, Cipro)
- clarithromycin (Biaxin, Biaxin XL)
- cloxacillin (Cloxapen, Nu-Cloxi)
- demeclocycline (Declomycin)
- dicloxacillin (Dycill, Pathocil)
- digitalis (Digitek, Lanoxin)
- dirithromycin (Dynabac)
- doxycycline (Apo-Doxy, Vibramycin)
- erythromycin (Erythrocin, Staticin)
- ethacrynic acid (Edecrin)
- famotidine (Apo-Famotidine, Pepcid)
- fluorouracil (Adrucil, Efudex)
- fosphenytoin (Cerebyx)
- furosemide (Apo-Furosemide, Lasix)
- gatofloxacin (Tequin, Zymar)
- gentamicin (Alcomicin, Gentacidin)
- kanamycin (Kantrex)
- lansoprazole (Prevacid)
- levofloxacin (Levaquin, Quixin)
- linezolid (Zyvox)
- lomefloxacin (Maxaquin)
- loracarbef (Lorabid)
- meclocycline (Meclan Topical)
- minocycline (Dynacin, Minocin)
- moxifloxacin (Avelox)
- nafcillin (Nafcil Injection, Unipen Oral)
- nalidixic acid (NegGram)
- nizatidine (Apo-Nizatidine, Axid)
- norfloxacin (Chibroxin Ophthalmic, Noroxin Oral)
- ofloxacin (Floxin, Ocuflox)
- omeprazole (Losec, Prilosec)
- pantoprazole (Pantoloc, Protonix)
- penicillin G benzathine (Bicillin L-A, Permapen)
- penicillin G benzathine and penicillin G procaine (Bicicillin C-R)
- penicillin G procaine (Pfizerpen-AS, Wycillin)
- penicillin V potassium (Suspen, Truxcillin)
- phenytoin (Dilantin, Phenytek)
- piperacillin (Pipracil)
- piperacillin and tazobactam sodium (Zosyn)
- rabeprazole (Aciphex, Pariet)
- ranitidine (Alti-Ranitidine, Zantac)
- sparfloxacin (Zagam)
- sulfadiazine (Microsulfon)
- sulfisoxazole (Gantrisin)
- tetracycline (Novo-Tetra, Sumycin)
- theophylline (Elixophyllin, Uniphyl)

- ticarcillin (Ticar)
- ticarcillin and clavulanate potassium (Timentin)
- tobramycin (Nebcin, Tobrex)
- torsemide (Demadex)
- trimethoprim (Primsol, Trimpex)
- trovafloxacin (Trovan)
- zonisamide (Zonegran)

Lab Tests That May Be Altered by Thiamin
None known

Diseases That May Be Worsened or Triggered by Thiamin
None known

Foods That May Interact with Thiamin
Coffee (regular and decaffeinated), tea, shellfish, and raw freshwater fish can deactivate thiamin.

Supplements That May Interact with Thiamin
Areca (betel) nut and horsetail can deactivate thiamin.

THUNDER GOD VINE

> This flowering, woody shrub has been used by traditional Chinese doctors for over four hundred years to treat rheumatoid arthritis, eczema, leprosy, and other ailments. Extracts of the root of the thunder god vine have been used to suppress inflammation and quiet the immune system, which is most likely why it may be helpful in treating rheumatoid arthritis and other autoimmune diseases.

Scientific Name
Tripterygium wilfordii

Thunder God Vine Is Also Commonly Known As
Huang-t'eng ken, lei-kung t'eng, threewingnut, yellow vine

Medicinal Parts
Leaf, root

Thunder God Vine's Uses
To treat rheumatoid arthritis, multiple sclerosis, abscesses, inflammation, and excessively heavy menstrual periods

Typical Dose
A typical dose of thunder god vine extract for the treatment of rheumatoid arthritis may range from 180 to 570 mg per day.

Possible Side Effects
Thunder god vine's side effects include gastrointestinal irritation, diarrhea, hair loss, menstrual changes, and headache.

Drugs That May Interact with Thunder God Vine
Taking thunder god vine with these drugs may cause or increase kidney damage:
- etodolac (Lodine, Utradol)
- ibuprofen (Advil, Motrin)
- indomethacin (Indocin, Novo-Methacin)
- ketoprofen (Orudis, Rhodis)
- ketorolac (Acular, Toradol)
- metformin (Glucophage, Riomet)

Lab Tests That May Be Altered by Thunder God Vine
None known

Diseases That May Be Worsened or Triggered by Thunder God Vine

May contribute to osteoporosis.

Foods That May Interact with Thunder God Vine

None known

Supplements That May Interact with Thunder God Vine

None known

TONKA BEAN

The tall tropical South American tonka tree produces pulpy, egg-shaped pods that contain fragrant black, almond-shaped seeds (beans) used primarily for flavoring. The tonka beans contain coumarin, an anticoagulant that has a delicious vanilla-like aroma. Because of this, the beans have been used to scent tobacco and snuff, to flavor castor oil, and as a vanilla substitute. In traditional Suriname medicine, a decoction made of tonka beans boiled with sugar was considered an effective treatment for the common cold.

Scientific Name

Dipteryx odorata

Tonka Bean Is Also Commonly Known As

Cumaru, Dutch tonka, English tonka, tonka seed, tonquin bean

Medicinal Parts

Seed

Tonka Bean's Uses

To treat cramps, nausea, cough, spasms, tuberculosis, earache, mouth ulcers, and sore throat; as an aphrodisiac

Typical Dose

There is no typical dose of tonka beans.

Possible Side Effects

Tonka bean's side effects include nausea, vomiting, diarrhea, insomnia, and dizziness.

Drugs That May Interact with Tonka Bean

Taking tonka beans with these drugs may increase the risk of bleeding or bruising:

- antithrombin III (Thrombate III)
- aminosalicylic acid (Nemasol Sodium, Paser)
- aspirin (Bufferin, Ecotrin)
- choline magnesium trisalicylate (Trilisate)
- choline salicylate (Teejel)
- salsalate (Amgesic, Salflex)
- argatroban
- bivalirudin (Angiomax)
- dalteparin (Fragmin)
- danaparoid (Orgaran)
- enoxaparin (Lovenox)
- fondaparinux (Arixtra)
- heparin (Hepalean, Hep-Lock)
- lepirudin (Refludan)
- tinzaparin (Innohep)
- warfarin (Coumadin, Jantoven)

Lab Tests That May Be Altered by Tonka Bean

None known

Diseases That May Be Worsened or Triggered by Tonka Bean

May cause liver toxicity due to the coumarin in tonka bean.

Foods That May Interact with Tonka Bean

None known

Supplements That May Interact with Tonka Bean

None known

TURMERIC

A broad-leafed shrub grown in India and parts of Asia, turmeric has long been used in traditional Indian Ayurvedic medicine and Chinese medicine. Research has suggested that the curcumin in turmeric can combat bacteria, reduce inflammation, quell indigestion, guard against gallbladder disease, and possibly even inhibit HIV, treat Alzheimer's disease, and destroy certain cancer cells.

Scientific Name

Curcuma domestica

Turmeric Is Also Commonly Known As

Curcuma, curcumin, Indian saffron, nisha, turmeric root

Medicinal Parts

Rhizome

Turmeric's Uses

To treat diarrhea, bronchitis, leprosy, headaches, loss of appetite, heartburn, colic, bruising, and wounds; to prevent Alzheimer's disease. Germany's Commission E has approved the use of turmeric to treat loss of appetite and dyspeptic complaints, such as heartburn and bloating.

Typical Dose

A typical daily dose of turmeric for dyspepsia is approximately 1.5 to 3 gm of the herb, taken in three divided doses.

Possible Side Effects

Turmeric's side effects include nausea and diarrhea.

Drugs That May Interact with Turmeric

Taking turmeric with these drugs may increase the risk of bleeding or bruising:

- abciximab (ReoPro)
- acemetacin (Acemetacin Heumann, Acemetacin Sandoz)
- alteplase (Activase, Cathflo Activase)
- antithrombin III (Thrombate III)
- argatroban
- aspirin (Bufferin, Ecotrin)
- aspirin and dipyridamole (Aggrenox)
- bivalirudin (Angiomax)
- celecoxib (Celebrex)
- choline magnesium trisalicylate (Trilisate)
- choline salicylate (Teejel)
- clopidogrel (Plavix)
- dalteparin (Fragmin)
- danaparoid (Orgaran)
- diclofenac (Cataflam, Voltaren)
- diflunisal (Apo-Diflunisal, Dolobid)
- dipyridamole (Novo-Dipiradol, Persantine)
- dipyrone (Analgina, Dinador)
- enoxaparin (Lovenox)

- eptifibatide (Integrillin)
- etodolac (Lodine, Utradol)
- etoricoxib (Arcoxia)
- fenoprofen (Nalfon)
- flurbiprofen (Ansaid, Ocufen)
- fondaparinux (Arixtra)
- heparin (Hepalean, Hep-Lock)
- ibuprofen (Advil, Motrin)
- indobufen (Ibustrin)—bleeding
- indomethacin (Indocin, Novo-Methacin)
- ketoprofen (Orudis, Rhodis)
- ketorolac (Acular, Toradol)
- lepirudin (Refludan)
- magnesium salicylate (Doan's, Mobidin)
- meclofenamate (Meclomen)
- mefenamic acid (Ponstan, Ponstel)
- meloxicam (MOBIC, Mobicox)
- nabumetone (Apo-Nabumetone, Relafen)
- nadroparin (Fraxiparine)
- naproxen (Aleve, Naprosyn)
- niflumic acid (Niflam, Nifluril)
- nimesulide (Areuma, Aulin)
- oxaprozin (Apo-Oxaprozin, Daypro)
- piroxicam (Feldene, NuPirox)
- reteplase (Retavase)
- rofecoxib (Vioxx)
- salsalate (Amgesic, Salflex)
- streptokinase (Streptase)
- sulindac (Clinoril, NuSundac)
- tenecteplase (TNKase)
- tenoxicam (Dolmen, Mobiflex)
- tiaprofenic acid (DomTiaprofenic, Surgam)
- ticlopidine (Alti-Ticlopidine, Ticlid)
- tinzaparin (Innohep)
- tirofiban (Aggrastat)
- tolmetin (Tolectin)
- urokinase (Abbokinase)

- valdecoxib (Bextra)
- warfarin (Coumadin, Jantoven)

Taking turmeric with these drugs may decrease the effectiveness of the drug:

- antithymocyte globulin (equine) (Atgam)
- antithymocyte globulin (rabbit) (Thymoglobulin)
- azathioprine (Imuran)
- basiliximab (Simulect)
- cyclosporine (Neoral, Sandimmune)
- daclizumab (Zenapax)
- efalizumab (Raptiva)
- methotrexate (Rheumatrex, Trexall)
- muromonab-CD3 (Orthoclone OKT 3)
- mycophenolate (CellCept)
- pimecrolimus (Elidel)
- sirolimus (Rapamune)
- tacrolimus (Prograf, Protopic)
- thalidomide (Thalomid)

Lab Tests That May Be Altered by Turmeric
None known

Diseases That May Be Worsened or Triggered by Turmeric
May cause gallbladder contractions.

Foods That May Interact with Turmeric
None known

Supplements That May Interact with Turmeric
Increased risk of bleeding when used with herbs and supplements that might affect platelet aggregation.

UVA URSI

> This perennial plant produces red berries that look like cranberries but are not as tasty. Yet bears don't seem to mind; they eat large amounts of the uva ursi berries whenever they can find them, which is why one of this herb's common names is bearberry. Test-tube studies indicate that the herb can combat *Candida albicans, Escherichia coli, Staphylococcus aureus*, and other bacteria that cause urinary tract infections, yeast infections, and other common ailments.

Scientific Name

Arctostaphylos uva ursi

Uva Ursi Is Also Commonly Known As

Arberry, bearberry, bear's grape, mountain cranberry, rockberry, upland cranberry

Medicinal Parts

Leaf

Uva Ursi's Uses

To treat urinary problems, constipation, and bronchitis. Germany's Commission E has approved the use of uva ursi to treat urinary tract infections.

Typical Dose

A typical daily dose of uva ursi is 10 gm of finely cut or powdered herb.

Possible Side Effects

Uva ursi's side effects include nausea, vomiting, and liver damage.

Drugs That May Interact with Uva Ursi

Taking uva ursi with these drugs may interfere with the action of the drug:

- azosemide (Diat)
- benazepril (Lotensin)
- bumetanide (Bumex, Burinex)
- chlorothiazide (Diuril)
- ethacrynic acid (Edecrin)
- etozolin (Elkapin)
- furosemide (Apo-Furosemide, Lasix)
- hydrochlorothiazide (Apo-Hydro, Microzide)
- hydrochlorothiazide and triamterene (Dyazide, Maxzide)
- hydroflumethiazide (Diucardin, Saluron)
- methyclothiazide (Aquatensen, Enduron)
- olmesartan and hydrochlorothiazide (Benicar HCT)
- polythiazide (Renese)
- torsemide (Demadex)
- trichlormethiazide (Metatensin, Naqua)
- xipamide (Diurexan, Lumitens)

Taking uva ursi with these drugs may reduce or prevent absorption of the drug:
- ferric gluconate (Ferrlecit)
- ferrous fumarate (Femiron, Feostat)
- ferrous gluconate (Fergon, Novo-Ferrogluc)
- ferrous sulfate (Feratab, Fer-Iron)
- ferrous sulfate and ascorbic acid (Fero-Grad 500, Vitelle Irospan)
- iron-dextran complex (Dexferrum, INFeD)
- polysaccharide-iron complex (Hytinic, Niferex)

Taking uva ursi with these drugs may increase the therapeutic and/or adverse effects of the drug:
- acemetacin (Acemetacin Heumann, Acemetacin Sandoz)
- aspirin (Bufferin, Ecotrin)

- celecoxib (Celebrex)
- choline magnesium trisalicylate (Trilisate)
- choline salicylate (Teejel)
- diclofenac (Cataflam, Voltaren)
- diflunisal (Apo-Diflunisal, Dolobid)
- dipyrone (Analgina, Dinador)
- etodolac (Lodine, Utradol)
- etoricoxib (Arcoxia)
- fenoprofen (Nalfon)
- flurbiprofen (Ansaid, Ocufen)
- ibuprofen (Advil, Motrin)
- indomethacin (Indocin, Novo-Methacin)
- ketoprofen (Orudis, Rhodis)
- ketorolac (Acular, Toradol)
- magnesium salicylate (Doan's, Mobidin)
- meclofenamate (Meclomen)
- mefenamic acid (Ponstan, Ponstel)
- meloxicam (MOBIC, Mobicox)
- nabumetone (Apo-Nabumetone, Relafen)
- naproxen (Aleve, Naprosyn)
- niflumic acid (Niflam, Nifluril)
- nimesulide (Areuma, Aulin)
- oxaprozin (Apo-Oxaprozin, Daypro)
- piroxicam (Feldene, Nu-Pirox)
- rofecoxib (Vioxx)
- salsalate (Amgesic, Salflex)
- sulindac (Clinoril, Nu-Sundac)
- tenoxicam (Dolmen, Mobiflex)
- tiaprofenic acid (DomTiaprofenic, Surgam)
- tolmetin (Tolectin)
- valdecoxib (Bextra)

Taking uva ursi with these drugs may increase the risk of hypokalemia (low levels of potassium in the blood):

- acetazolamide (Apo-Acetazolamide, Diamox Sequels)
- azosemide (Diat)
- bumetanide (Bumex, Burinex)
- chlorothiazide (Diuril)
- chlorthalidone (Apo-Chlorthalidone, Thalitone)
- ethacrynic acid (Edecrin)
- etozolin (Elkapin)
- furosemide (Apo-Furosemide, Lasix)
- hydrochlorothiazide (Apo-Hydro, Microzide)
- hydroflumethiazide (Diucardin, Saluron)
- indapamide (Lozol, Nu-Indapamide)
- mannitol (Osmitrol, Resectisol)
- mefruside (Baycaron)
- methazolamide (Apo-Methazolamide, Neptazane)
- methyclothiazide (Aquatensen, Enduron)
- metolazone (Mykrox, Zaroxolyn)
- olmesartan and hydrochlorothiazide (Benicar HCT)
- polythiazide (Renese)
- torsemide (Demadex)
- trichlormethiazide (Metatensin, Naqua)
- urea (Amino-Cerv, UltraMide)
- xipamide (Diurexan, Lumitens)

Taking uva ursi with these drugs may be harmful:

- etodolac (Lodine, Utradol)—may cause or increase liver damage

Lab Tests That May Be Altered by Uva Ursi

May confound results of diagnostic urine tests that rely on a color change by discoloring urine a greenish brown.

Diseases That May Be Worsened or Triggered by Uva Ursi

May worsen gastrointestinal ailments by irritating the gastrointestinal tract.

Foods That May Interact with Uva Ursi

None known

Supplements That May Interact with Uva Ursi

None known

UZARA

Uzara, a three-foot-high perennial native to South Africa, has large leaves that exude a milky sap when crushed. The dried roots of the plant contain uzarin, a cardioglycoside that acts much like digitalis, strengthening the contractions of the heart and keeping the heartbeat steady. In South Africa, uzara is a traditional remedy for diarrhea and dysentery.

Scientific Name

Xysmalobium undulatum

Uzara Is Also Commonly Known As

Uzarae radix

Medicinal Parts

Root

Uzara's Uses

To treat diarrhea. Germany's Commission E has approved the use of uzara to treat diarrhea.

Typical Dose

A typical daily dose of uzara may range from 45 to 90 mg of the total glycosides calculated as uzarin.

Possible Side Effects

Uzara contains cardiac glycosides, which can help control irregular heartbeat, reduce the backup of blood and fluid in the body, and increase blood flow through the kidneys, helping to excrete sodium and relieve swelling in body tissues. However, a buildup of cardiac glycosides can occur, especially when the herb is combined with certain medications or other herbs that contain cardiac glycosides, causing arrhythmias, abnormally slow heartbeat, heart failure, and even death.

Drugs That May Interact with Uzara

Taking uzara with this drug may increase the risk of hypokalemia (low levels of potassium in the blood) and/or cardiac glycoside toxicity:

- acetazolamide (Apo-Acetazolamide, Diamox Sequels)
- azithromycin (Zithromax)
- azosemide (Diat)
- bumetanide (Bumex, Burinex)
- cascara
- chlorothiazide (Diuril)
- chlorthalidone (Apo-Chlorthalidone, Thalitone)
- clarithromycin (Biaxin, Biaxin XL)
- demeclocycline (Declomycin)
- digitalis (Digitek, Lanoxin)
- dirithromycin (Dynabac)
- docusate and senna (Peri-Colace, Senokot-S)
- doxycycline (Apo-Doxy, Vibramycin)
- erythromycin (Erythrocin, Staticin)
- ethacrynic acid (Edecrin)
- etozolin (Elkapin)
- furosemide (Apo-Furosemide, Lasix)
- hydrochlorothiazide (Apo-Hydro, Microzide)
- hydroflumethiazide (Diucardin, Saluron)
- indapamide (Lozol, Nu-Indapamide)

- josamycin (Iosalide, Josamy)
- mannitol (Osmitrol, Resectisol)
- mefruside (Baycaron)
- methazolamide (Apo-Methazolamide, Neptazane)
- methyclothiazide (Aquatensen, Enduron)
- metolazone (Mykrox, Zaroxolyn)
- midecamycin (Macropen, Midecin)
- minocycline (Dynacin, Minocin)
- olmesartan and hydrochlorothiazide (Benicar HCT)
- oxytetracycline (Terramycin, Terramycin IM)
- polythiazide (Renese)
- quinine (Quinine-Odan)
- roxithromycin (Claramid, Roxibeta)
- spiramycin (Rovamycine)
- tetracycline (Novo-Tetra, Sumycin)
- torsemide (Demadex)
- trichlormethiazide (Metatensin, Naqua)
- troleandomycin (Tao)
- urea (Amino-Cerv, UltraMide)
- xipamide (Diurexan, Lumitens)

Lab Tests That May Be Altered by Uzara
None known

Diseases That May Be Worsened or Triggered by Uzara
None known

Foods That May Interact with Uzara
None known

Supplements That May Interact with Uzara
- Increased risk of cardiac glycoside toxicity when used with other herbs that contain cardiac glycosides, such as black hellebore, calotropis, motherwort, and others. (For a list of cardiac glycoside–containing herbs and supplements, see Appendix B.)
- Increased risk of cardiotoxicity due to potassium depletion when taken with cardioactive herbs, such as adonis, digitalis, lily-of-the-valley, and squill. (For a list of cardioactive herbs and supplements, see Appendix B.)
- Increased risk of potassium depletion when used in conjunction with horsetail plant or licorice.
- Increased risk of potassium depletion when used with stimulant laxative herbs, such as black root, cascara sagrada, castor oil, and senna. (For a list of stimulant laxative herbs and supplements, see Appendix B.)

VALERIAN

Sometimes called herbal Valium because of its ability to relieve anxiety and insomnia, valerian is an ancient herb used in China, Greece, and other parts of the world. Valerian was recommended by the Greek physician Dioscorides for a great many conditions, including liver problems, urinary tract disorders, nausea, and indigestion. Today it is one of the world's most popular herbs and the most widely used sedative in Europe.

Scientific Name
Valeriana officinalis

Valerian Is Also Commonly Known As
All-heal, amantilla, baldrian, Belgium valerian, garden heliotrope, tagara

Medicinal Parts
Root and other underground parts

Valerian's Uses
To treat stress, anxiety, hysteria, insomnia, menopausal symptoms, and lack of concentration. Germany's Commission E has approved the use of valerian to treat insomnia caused by anxiety as well as restlessness.

Typical Dose
A typical dose of valerian in extract form may range from 400 to 900 mg, taken two hours before bedtime.

Possible Side Effects
Valerian's side effects include insomnia, nausea, heart palpitations, and headache.

Drugs That May Interact with Valerian
❶ Taking valerian with these drugs may cause or increase serotonin syndrome (symptoms of which include agitation, rapid heart rate, flushing, heavy sweating, and possibly even death):
- desipramine (Alti-Desipramine, Norpramin)
- doxepin (Sinequan, Zonalon)
- fluvoxamine (Alti-Fluvoxamine, Luvox)
- imipramine (Apo-Imipramine, Tofranil)
- nefazodone (Serzone)
- nortriptyline (Aventyl HCl, Pamelor)
- pramipexole (Mirapex)
- protriptyline (Vivactil)
- trazodone (Desyrel, Novo-Trazodone)
- venlafaxine (Effexor)

Taking valerian with these drugs may increase the risk of bleeding or bruising:

- abciximab (ReoPro)
- alteplase (Activase, Cathflo Activase)
- antithrombin III (Thrombate III)
- argatroban
- aspirin (Bufferin, Ecotrin)
- aspirin and dipyridamole (Aggrenox)
- bivalirudin (Angiomax)
- clopidogrel (Plavix)
- dalteparin (Fragmin)
- danaparoid (Orgaran)
- dipyridamole (Novo-Dipiradol, Persantine)
- enoxaparin (Lovenox)
- eptifibatide (Integrillin)
- fondaparinux (Arixtra)
- heparin (Hepalean, Hep-Lock)
- indobufen (Ibustrin)
- lepirudin (Refludan)
- nadroparin (Fraxiparine)
- reteplase (Retavase)
- streptokinase (Streptase)
- tenecteplase (TNKase)
- ticlopidine (Alti-Ticlopidine, Ticlid)
- tinzaparin (Innohep)
- tirofiban (Aggrastat)
- urokinase (Abbokinase)
- warfarin (Coumadin, Jantoven)

Taking valerian with these drugs may reduce or prevent drug absorption:
- ferric gluconate (Ferrlecit)
- ferrous fumarate (Femiron, Feostat)
- ferrous gluconate (Fergon, Novo-Ferrogluc)
- ferrous sulfate (Feratab, Fer-Iron)
- ferrous sulfate and ascorbic acid (Fero-Grad 500, Vitelle Irospan)
- iron-dextran complex (Dexferrum, INFeD)
- polysaccharide-iron complex (Hytinic, Niferex)

Taking valerian with these drugs may hinder the therapeutic effects of the drug:

- iproniazid (Marsilid)
- moclobemide (Alti-Moclobemide, Nu-Moclobemide)
- phenelzine (Nardil)
- phenytoin (Dilantin, Phenytek)
- selegiline (Eldepryl)
- tranylcypromine (Parnate)
- warfarin (Coumadin, Jantoven)

Taking valerian with these drugs may increase the risk of excessive sedation and mental depression and impairment:

- acetaminophen and codeine (Capital and Codeine, Tylenol with Codeine)
- alfentanil (Alfenta)
- alprazolam (Apo-Alpraz, Xanax)
- allopurinol (Aloprim, Zyloprim)
- amitriptyline (Elavil, Levate)
- amobarbital (Amytal)
- amobarbital and secobarbital (Tuinal)
- amoxapine (Asendin)
- aripiprazole (Abilify)
- aspirin and codeine (Coryphen Codeine)
- baclofen (Lioresal, Nu-Baclo)
- belladonna and opium (B&O Supprettes)
- bromazepam (Apo-Bromazepam, Gen-Bromazepam)
- brotizolam (Lendorm, Sintonal)
- buprenorphine (Buprenex, Subutex)
- buprenorphine and naloxone (Suboxone)
- bupropion (Wellbutrin, Zyban)
- butabarbital (Butisol Sodium)
- butalbital, acetaminophen, and caffeine (Esgic, Fioricet)
- butalbital, aspirin, and caffeine (Fiorinal)
- butorphanol (Apo-Butorphanol, Stadol)
- carbamazepine (Carbatrol, Tegretol)
- chloral hydrate (Aquachloral Supprettes, Somnote)
- chlordiazepoxide (Apo-Chlordiazepoxide, Librium)
- chlorpromazine (Thorazine)
- citalopram (Celexa)
- clobazam (Alti-Clobazam, Frisium)
- clomipramine (Anafranil, Novo-Clopramine)
- clonazepam (Klonopin, Rivotril)
- clonidine (Catapres, Duraclon)
- clorazepate (Tranxene, T-Tab)
- clozapine (Clozaril, Gen-Clozapine)
- codeine (Codeine Contin)
- cyclobenzaprine (Flexeril, Novo-Cycloprine)
- dantrolene (Dantrium)
- desipramine (Alti-Desipramine, Norpramin)
- dexmedetomidine (Precedex)
- diazepam (Apo-Diazepam, Valium)
- dihydrocodeine, aspirin, and caffeine (Synalgos-DC)
- diphenhydramine (Benadryl Allergy, Nytol)
- doxepin (Sinequan, Zonalon)
- doxylamine and pyridoxine (Diclectin)
- estazolam (ProSom)
- fentanyl (Actiq, Duragesic)
- fexofenadine (Allegra)
- fluoxetine (Prozac, Sarafem)
- fluphenazine (Prolixin, Modecate)
- flurazepam (Apo-Flurazepam, Dalmane)
- fluvoxamine (Alti-Fluvoxamine, Luvox)
- gabapentin (Neurontin, Nu-Gabapentin)
- glutethimide
- haloperidol (Haldol, Novo-Peridol)
- hydrocodone and acetaminophen (Vicodin, Zydone)

- hydrocodone and aspirin (Damason-P)
- hydrocodone and ibuprofen (Vicoprofen)
- hydromorphone (Dilaudid, PMS-Hydromorphone)
- hydroxyzine (Atarax, Vistaril)
- imipramine (Apo-Imipramine, Tofranil)
- levomethadyl acetate hydrochloride
- levorphanol (LevoDromoran)
- loprazolam (Dormonoct, Havlane)
- lorazepam (Ativan, Nu-Loraz)
- meperidine (Demerol, Meperitab)
- meperidine and promethazine
- mephobarbital (Mebaral)
- meprobamate (Miltown, Movo-Mepro)
- mesoridazine (Serentil)
- methadone (Dolophine, Methadose)
- methocarbamol (Robaxin)
- methohexital (Brevital, Brevital Sodium)
- methotrimeprazine (Nozain, Novo-Meprazine)
- metoclopramide (Apo-Metoclop, Reglan)
- midazolam (Apo-Midazolam, Versed)
- mirtazapine (Remeron)
- molindone (Moban)
- morphine hydrochloride
- morphine sulfate (Kadian, MS Contin)
- nalbuphine (Nubain)
- nefazodone (Serzone)
- nortriptyline (Aventyl HCl, Pamelor)
- olanzapine (Zydis, Zyprexa)
- opium tincture
- oxazepam (Novoxapam, Serax)
- oxcarbazepine (Trileptal)
- oxycodone (OxyContin, Roxicodone)
- oxycodone and acetaminophen (Endocet, Percocet)
- oxycodone and aspirin (Endodan, Percodan)
- oxymorphone (Numorphan)

- paclitaxel (Onxol, Taxol)
- paregoric
- paroxetine (Paxil)
- pentazocine (Talwin)
- pentobarbital (Nembutal)
- perphenazine (Apo-Perphenazine, Trilafon)
- phenobarbital (Luminal Sodium, PMS-Phenobarbital)
- phenoperidine
- phenytoin (Dilantin, Phenytek)
- pizotifen (Sandomigran)
- pramipexole (Mirapex)
- prazepam
- primidone (Apo-Primidone, Mysoline)
- prochlorperazine (Compazine, Compro)
- promethazine (Phenergan)
- propofol (Diprivan)
- propoxyphene (Darvon, Darvon-N)
- propoxyphene and acetaminophen (Darvocet-N 50, Darvocet-N 100)
- propoxyphene, aspirin, and caffeine (Darvon Compound)
- protriptyline (Vivactil)
- quazepam (Doral)
- quetiapine (Seroquel)
- remifentanil (Ultiva)
- risperidone (Risperdal)
- ropinirole (Requip)
- s-citalopram (Lexapro)
- secobarbital (Seconal)
- sertraline (Apo-Sertraline, Zoloft)
- sodium oxybate (Xyrem)
- sufentanil (Sufenta)
- s-zopiclone (Lunesta)
- temazepam (Novo-Temazepam, Restoril)
- tetrazepam (Mobiforton, Musapam)
- thiethylperazine (Torecan)

- thiopental (Pentothal)
- thioridazine (Mellaril)
- thiothixene (Navane)
- tiagabine (Gabitril)
- tizanidine (Zanaflex)
- tolcapone (Tasmar)
- tramadol (Ultram)
- trazodone (Desyrel, Novo-Trazodone)
- triazolam (Apo-Triazo, Halcion)
- trifluoperazine (Novo-Trifluzine, Stelazine)
- trimipramine (Apo-Trimip, Surmontil)
- venlafaxine (Effexor)
- vigabatrin (Sabril)
- zaleplon (Sonata, Starnoc)
- ziprasidone (Geodon)
- zolpidem (Ambien)
- zopiclone (Alti-Zopiclone, Gen-Zopiclone)
- zuclopenthixol (Clopixol)

Taking valerian with this drug may be harmful:
- loperamide (Diarr-Eze, Imodium A-D)—may increase the risk of confusion, agitation, and other symptoms of delirium

Lab Tests That May Be Altered by Valerian
May increase results of liver function tests including aspartic acid transaminase (AST), alanine aminotransferase (ALT), total bilirubin, and urine bilirubin.

Diseases That May Be Worsened or Triggered by Valerian
None known

Foods That May Interact with Valerian
Increased risk of drowsiness and impaired motor skills when combined with alcohol.

Supplements That May Interact with Valerian
May enhance therapeutic and adverse effects of herbs and supplements that have sedative properties, such as 5-HTP, kava kava, and St. John's wort. (For a list of herbs and supplements that have sedative properties, see Appendix B.)

VITAMIN A

Vitamin A is not a single vitamin; it is the name given to a group of related substances, including retinol and retinal. Vitamin A is vital for night vision, a strong immune system, proper bone growth, the health of the skin, and maintenance of the linings of the intestinal, respiratory, and urinary tracts. A lack of vitamin A can cause blindness, increased susceptibility to infections, loss of appetite, poor bone and tooth formation, and impaired growth.

Typical Dose
The Food and Nutrition Board has set the RDA for vitamin A at 3,000 IU per day for men ages nineteen and up and 2,330 IU per day for women ages nineteen and older.

Possible Side Effects
Excessive amounts of vitamin A can cause nausea, vomiting, lack of appetite, hair loss, pain in the bones and joints, weakness, and irritability.

Drugs That May Interact with Vitamin A
Taking vitamin A with these drugs may increase the risk of vitamin A toxicity (symptoms of which include increased intracranial—inside the skull—

pressure, drowsiness, irritability, headache, nausea, and generalized weakness):

- acitretin (Soriatane)
- alitretinoin (Panretin)
- bexarotene (Targretin)
- fluocinolone, hydroquinone, and tretinoin (Tri-Luma)
- isotretinoin (Accutane, Caravis)
- mequinol and tretinoin (Solagé)
- tretinoin, oral (Vesanoid)

Taking vitamin A with these drugs may increase the risk of benign intracranial hypertension (a disorder that leads to pressure in the brain, vision loss, and headaches, not related to a tumor):

- demeclocycline (Declomycin)
- doxycycline (Apo-Doxy, Vibramycin)
- minocycline (Dynacin, Minocin)
- oxytetracycline (Terramycin, Terramycin IM)
- tetracycline (Novo-Tetra, Sumycin)

Taking vitamin A with this drug may be harmful:

- warfarin (Coumadin, Jantoven)—may increase the risk of bleeding or bruising when large doses of vitamin A are taken

Drugs That May Interfere with the Absorption, Utilization, or Excretion of Vitamin A

- aluminum hydroxide (AlternaGel, Alu-Cap)
- aluminum hydroxide and magnesium carbonate (Gaviscon Liquid)
- aluminum hydroxide and magnesium hydroxide (Maalox, Mylanta)
- aluminum hydroxide, magnesium hydroxide, and simethicone (Mylanta Liquid)
- aluminum hydroxide and magnesium trisilicate (Gaviscon Tablet)

- beclomethasone (Beconase, Vanceril)
- betamethasone (Betatrex, Maxivate)
- budesonide (Entocort, Rhinocort)
- cholestyramine (Prevalite, Questran)
- colesevelam (WelChol)
- colestipol (Colestid)
- cortisone (Cortone)
- dexamethasone (Decadron, Dexasone)
- flunisolide (AeroBid-M, Nasarel)
- fluticasone (Cutivate, Flonase)
- hydrocortisone (Cetacort, Locoid)
- methylprednisolone (Depoject Injection, Medrol Oral)
- mineral oil (Fleet Mineral Oil Enema, Milkinol)
- mometasone furoate (Elocom, Nasonex)
- neomycin (Myciguent, Neo-Fradin)
- orlistat (Xenical)
- prednisolone (Inflamase Forte, Pred Forte)
- prednisone (Apo-Prednisone, Deltasone)
- sucralfate (Carafate, Sulcrate)
- triamcinolone (Aristocort, Trinasal)

Lab Tests That May Be Altered by Vitamin A

- May improve hemoglobin levels in those with low serum levels of retinal plus anemia.
- May cause false increase in bilirubin tests (using Ehrlich's reagent).

Diseases That May Be Worsened or Triggered by Vitamin A

May increase the risk of liver toxicity if taken by those with existing liver disease.

Foods That May Interact with Vitamin A

Vitamin A absorption may be increased when taken with a high-fat meal.

Supplements That May Interact with Vitamin A
None known

VITAMIN B$_6$

> Vitamin B$_6$, also known as pyridoxine, is a group of related substances that help the body extract energy from food; manufacture proteins, hemoglobin, serotonin, and gamma-amminobutyeric acid (GABA); and ensure that the nervous system functions properly. A lack of vitamin B$_6$ causes confusion, depression, skin inflammation, and a weakened immune system.

Typical Dose
The Food and Nutrition Board has set the RDA for vitamin B$_6$ at 1.3 mg per day for males ages nineteen to fifty and 1.7 mg for males ages fifty and up; for women the numbers are 1.3 mg per day for those ages nineteen to fifty and 1.5 mg for those over fifty.

Possible Side Effects
Taking in too much vitamin B$_6$ via supplements can damage the nerves in the extremities.

Drugs That May Interact with Vitamin B$_6$
Taking vitamin B$_6$ with these drugs may reduce blood levels of the drug:
- fosphenytoin (Cerebyx)
- phenobarbital (Luminal Sodium, PMS-Phenobarbital)
- phenytoin (Dilantin, Phenytek)

Taking vitamin B$_6$ with these drugs may be harmful:
- amiodarone (Cordarone, Pacerone)—may increase skin sensitivity to sunlight
- levodopa (Dopar, Larodopa)—may interfere with the therapeutic effects of the drug
- levodopa-carbidopa (Nu-Levocarb, Sinemet)—may interfere with therapeutic effects of the drug
- theophylline (Elixophyllin, Theochron)—may increase the risk of seizures induced by theophylline

Drugs That May Interfere with the Absorption, Utilization, or Excretion of Vitamin B$_6$
- amikacin (Amikin)
- amoxicillin (Amoxil, Novamoxin)
- ampicillin (Omnipen, Totacillin)
- azithromycin (Zithromax)
- beclomethasone (Beconase, Vanceril)
- betamethasone (Betatrex, Maxivate)
- budesonide (Entocort, Rhinocort)
- bumetanide (Bumex, Burinex)
- carbenicillin (Geocillin)
- cefaclor (Ceclor)
- cefadroxil (Duricef)
- cefamandole (Mandol)
- cefazolin (Ancef, Kefzol)
- cefdinir (Omnicef)
- cefditoren (Spectracef)
- cefepime (Maxipime)
- cefonicid (Monocid)
- cefoperazone (Cefobid)
- cefotaxime (Claforan)
- cefotetan (Cefotan)
- cefoxitin (Mefoxin)
- cefpodoxime (Vantin)
- cefprozil (Cefzil)

- ceftazidime (Ceptaz, Fortaz)
- ceftibuten (Cedax)
- ceftizoxime (Cefizox)
- ceftriaxone (Rocephin)
- cefuroxime (Ceftin, Kefurox)
- cephalexin (Biocef, Keftab)
- cephalothin (Ceporacin)
- cephapirin (Cefadyl)
- cepharadine (Velosef)
- cinoxacin (Cinobac)
- ciprofloxacin (Ciloxan, Cipro)
- clarithromycin (Biaxin, Biaxin XL)
- cloxacillin (Cloxapen, Nu-Cloxi)
- cortisone (Cortone)
- cycloserine (Seromycin Pulvules)
- demeclocycline (Declomycin)
- dexamethasone (Decadron, Dexasone)
- dicloxacillin (Dycill, Pathocil)
- dirithromycin (Dynabac)
- doxycycline (Apo-Doxy, Vibramycin)
- enalapril and hydrochlorothiazide (Vaseretic)
- enoxacin (Penetrex)
- erythromycin (Erythrocin, Staticin)
- ethacrynic acid (Edecrin)
- fluorouracil (Adrucil, Efudex)
- flunisolide (AeroBid-M, Nasarel)
- fluticasone (Cutivate, Flonase)
- furosemide (Apo-Furosemide, Lasix)
- gatofloxacin (Tequin, Zymar)
- gentamicin (Alcomicin, Gentacidin)
- hydralazine (Apresoline, Novo-Hylazin)
- hydralazine and hydrochlorothiazide (Apresazide)
- hydrochlorothiazide and triamterene (Dyazide, Maxzide)
- hydrocortisone (Cetacort, Locoid)
- isoniazid (Laniazid Oral, PMS-Isoniazid)
- kanamycin (Kantrex)
- levofloxacin (Levaquin, Quixin)
- levonorgestrel (Norplant Implant, Plan B)
- linezolid (Zyvox)
- lomefloxacin (Maxaquin)
- loracarbef (Lorabid)
- meclocycline (Meclan Topical)
- methyldopa and hydrochlorothiazide (Aldoril, PMS-Dopazide)
- methylprednisolone (Depoject Injection, Medrol Oral)
- minocycline (Dynacin, Minocin)
- mometasone furoate (Elocom, Nasonex)
- moxifloxacin (Avelox)
- nafcillin (Nafcil Injection, Unipen Oral)
- nalidixic acid (NegGram)
- neomycin (Myciguent, Neo-Fradin)
- norethindrone (Aygestin, Micronor)
- norfloxacin (Chibroxin Ophthalmic, Noroxin Oral)
- ofloxacin (Floxin, Ocuflox)
- penicillamine (Cuprimine, Depen)
- penicillin G benzathine (Bicillin L-A, Permapen)
- penicillin G benzathine and penicillin G procaine (Bicillin C-R)
- penicillin G procaine (Pfizerpen-AS, Wycillin)
- penicillin V potassium (Suspen, Truxcillin)
- phenelzine (Nardil)
- phenobarbital (Luminal Sodium, PMS-Phenobarbital)
- piperacillin (Pipracil)
- piperacillin and tazobactam sodium (Zosyn)
- prednisolone (Inflamase Forte, Pred Forte)
- prednisone (Apo-Prednisone, Deltasone)
- primidone (Mysoline, Sertan)
- raloxifene (Evista)
- rifampin and isoniazid (Rifamate)

- sparfloxacin (Zagam)
- sulfadiazine (Microsulfon)
- sulfasalazine (Azulfidine, Salazopyrin)
- sulfisoxazole (Gantrisin)
- tetracycline (Novo-Tetra, Sumycin)
- theophylline (Elixophyllin, Uniphyl)
- ticarcillin (Ticar)
- ticarcillin and clavulanate potassium (Timentin)
- tobramycin (Nebcin, Tobrex)
- torsemide (Demadex)
- triamcinolone (Aristocort, Trinasal)
- trimethoprim (Primsol, Trimpex)
- trovafloxacin (Trovan)

Lab Tests That May Be Altered by Vitamin B$_6$

May cause a false positive result in the spot test with Ehrlich's reagent.

Diseases That May Be Worsened or Triggered by Vitamin B$_6$

None known

Foods That May Interact with Vitamin B$_6$

None known

Supplements That May Interact with Vitamin B$_6$

None known

VITAMIN B$_{12}$

Back in the 1940s, researchers were looking for a cure for pernicious anemia, a disease that causes weakness, rapid heart rate, bruising and bleeding, and in some cases death. The researchers found that eating liver cured the disease. Eventually they were able to isolate the substance in liver that did the trick, naming it vitamin B$_{12}$. A mild B$_{12}$ deficiency can cause fever, loss of appetite, weight loss, weakness, and numbness and tingling in the extremities. A more serious shortage can cause the fatal pernicious anemia.

Typical Dose

The Food and Nutrition Board has set the Adequate Intake (AI) for vitamin B$_{12}$ at 2.4 mcg per day for adult men and women.

Possible Side Effects

According to the National Academy of Sciences' Institute of Medicine, "no adverse effects have been associated with excess vitamin B$_{12}$ intake from food and supplements in healthy individuals."

Drugs That May Interact with Vitamin B$_{12}$

None known

Drugs That May Interfere with the Absorption, Utilization, or Excretion of Vitamin B$_{12}$

- amikacin (Amikin)
- aminosalicylic acid (Nemasol Sodium, Paser)
- amoxicillin (Amoxil, Novamoxin)
- ampicillin (Omnipen, Totacillin)
- azithromycin (Zithromax)
- carbenicillin (Geocillin)
- cefaclor (Ceclor)
- cefadroxil (Duricef)
- cefamandole (Mandol)
- cefazolin (Ancef, Kefzol)
- cefdinir (Omnicef)
- cefditoren (Spectracef)

- cefepime (Maxipime)
- cefonicid (Monocid)
- cefoperazone (Cefobid)
- cefotaxime (Claforan)
- cefotetan (Cefotan)
- cefoxitin (Mefoxin)
- cefpodoxime (Vantin)
- cefprozil (Cefzil)
- ceftazidime (Ceptaz, Fortaz)
- ceftibuten (Cedax)
- ceftizoxime (Cefizox)
- ceftriaxone (Rocephin)
- cefuroxime (Ceftin, Kefurox)
- cephalexin (Biocef, Keftab)
- cephalothin (Ceporacin)
- cephapirin (Cefadyl)
- cepharadine (Velosef)
- chloramphenicol (Diochloram, Pentamycetin)
- cholestyramine (Prevalite, Questran)
- cimetidine (Nu-Cimet, Tagamet)
- cinoxacin (Cinobac)
- ciprofloxacin (Ciloxan, Cipro)
- clarithromycin (Biaxin, Biaxin XL)
- clofibrate (Atromid-S, Novo-Fibrate)
- cloxacillin (Cloxapen, Nu-Cloxi)
- colchicine (ratio-Colchicine)
- colchicine and probenecid (ColBenemid)
- colesevelam (WelChol)
- colestipol (Colestid)
- cycloserine (Seromycin Pulvules)
- delavirdine (Rescriptor)
- demeclocycline (Declomycin)
- dicloxacillin (Dycill, Pathocil)
- didanosine (Videx, Videx EC)
- dirithromycin (Dynabac)
- doxycycline (Apo-Doxy, Vibramycin)
- erythromycin (Erythrocin, Staticin)
- esomeprazole (Nexium)
- famotidine (Apo-Famotidine, Pepcid)
- fosphenytoin (Cerebyx)
- gatofloxacin (Tequin, Zymar)
- gentamicin (Alcomicin, Gentacidin)
- glyburide and metformin (Glucovance)
- isoniazid (Laniazid Oral, PMS-Isoniazid)
- kanamycin (Kantrex)
- lamivudine (Epivir, Heptovir)
- lansoprazole (Prevacid)
- levofloxacin (Levaquin, Quixin)
- levonorgestrel (Norplant Implant, Plan B)
- linezolid (Zyvox)
- lomefloxacin (Maxaquin)
- loracarbef (Lorabid)
- meclocycline (Meclan Topical)
- metformin (Glucophage, Riomet)
- methotrexate (Folex PFS, Rheumatrex)
- methyldopa (Apo-Methyldopa, Nu-Medopa)
- minocycline (Dynacin, Minocin)
- moxifloxacin (Avelox)
- nafcillin (Nafcil Injection, Unipen Oral)
- nalidixic acid (NegGram)
- neomycin (Myciguent, Neo-Fradin)
- nevirapine (Viramune)
- nitrous oxide
- nizatidine (Apo-Nizatidine, Axid)
- norethindrone (Aygestin, Micronor)
- norfloxacin (Chibroxin Ophthalmic, Noroxin Oral)
- ofloxacin (Floxin, Ocuflox)
- omeprazole (Losec, Prilosec)
- pantoprazole (Pantoloc, Protonix)
- penicillin G benzathine (Bicillin L-A, Permapen)
- penicillin G benzathine and penicillin G procaine (Bicillin C-R)
- penicillin G procaine (Pfizerpen-AS, Wycillin)

- penicillin V potassium (Suspen, Truxcillin)
- phenobarbital (Luminal Sodium, PMS-Phenobarbital)
- phenytoin (Dilantin, Phenytek)
- piperacillin (Pipracil)
- piperacillin and tazobactam sodium (Zosyn)
- potassium Chloride (Apo-K, Micro-K)
- primidone (Mysoline, Sertan)
- rabeprazole (Aciphex, Pariet)
- ranitidine (Alti-Ranitidine, Zantac)
- sparfloxacin (Zagam)
- stavudine (Zerit)
- sulfadiazine (Microsulfon)
- sulfasalazine (Azulfidine, Salazopyrin)
- sulfisoxazole (Gantrisin)
- tetracycline (Novo-Tetra, Sumycin)
- ticarcillin (Ticar)
- ticarcillin and clavulanate potassium (Timentin)
- tobramycin (Nebcin, Tobrex)
- trimethoprim (Primsol, Trimpex)
- trovafloxacin (Trovan)
- valproic acid (Depacon, Depakote ER)
- zalcitabine (Hivid)
- zidovudine (Novo-AZT, Retrovir)
- zidovudine and lamivudine (Combivir)
- zidovudine, lamivudine, and abacavir (Trizivir)

Lab Tests That May Be Altered by Vitamin B$_{12}$

May cause false positive results in test for intrinsic factor antibodies.

Diseases That May Be Worsened or Triggered by Vitamin B$_{12}$

May worsen the optic nerve disease known as Leber's disease.

Foods That May Interact with Vitamin B$_{12}$

Absorption of vitamin B$_{12}$ can be decreased through excessive intake of alcohol for more than two weeks.

Supplements That May Interact with Vitamin B$_{12}$

- Vitamin B$_{12}$ deficiency can be masked by intake of folic acid (especially when folic acid is taken in large doses).
- Absorption of vitamin B$_{12}$ can be decreased through use of potassium supplements (particularly potassium chloride) in some people.
- Vitamin C supplements may destroy dietary vitamin B$_{12}$, although iron and nitrates may block this action.

VITAMIN C

Vitamin C, also known as ascorbic acid, helps the body manufacture and repair blood vessels, skin, muscles, teeth, bones, collagen, tendons, ligaments, hormones, and neurotransmitters. A noted free-radical fighter and antioxidant, vitamin C also helps to metabolize fats. A lack of vitamin C can cause anemia, spontaneous bruising, loose teeth, swollen and bleeding gums, and impaired immunity.

Typical Dose

The Food and Nutrition Board has set the RDA for vitamin C at 90 mg per day for adult men and 75 mg per day for adult women.

Possible Side Effects

Excessive amounts of vitamin C can damage the heart and may trigger oxalate kidney stones and a buildup of iron in the body.

Drugs That May Interact with Vitamin C

Taking vitamin C with these drugs may increase drug levels in the body and the risk of adverse effects:

- acetaminophen (Tylenol, Genapap)
- cyproterone and ethinyl estradiol (Diane-35)
- estradiol (Climara, Estrace)
- estradiol and norethindrone (Activella, CombiPatch)
- estradiol and testosterone (Climacteron)
- ethinyl estradiol (Estinyl)
- ethinyl estradiol and desogestrel (Cyclessa, Ortho-Cept)
- ethinyl estradiol and ethynodiol diacetate (Demulen, Zovia)
- ethinyl estradiol and etonogestrel (NuvaRing)
- ethinyl estradiol and levonorgestrel (Alesse, Triphasil)
- ethinyl estradiol and norelgestromin (Evra, Ortho Evra)
- ethinyl estradiol and norethindrone (Brevicon, Ortho-Novum)
- ethinyl estradiol and norgestimate (Cyclen, Ortho Tri-Cyclen)
- ethinyl estradiol and norgestrel (Cryselle, Ovral)

Taking vitamin C with these drugs may reduce drug levels in the body:

- amprenavir (Agenerase)
- fluphenazine (Modecate, Prolixin)
- indinavir (Crixivan)
- lopinavir and ritonavir (Kaletra)
- nelfinavir (Viracept)
- ritonavir (Norvir)
- saquinavir (Fortovase, Invirase)

Taking vitamin C with this drug may be harmful:

- heparin (Hepalean, Hep-Lock)—may reduce the effectiveness of the drug
- warfarin (Coumadin, Jantoven)—may interfere with the action of the drug

Drugs That May Interfere with the Absorption, Utilization, or Excretion of Vitamin C

- aspirin (Bufferin, Ecotrin)
- aspirin and dipyridamole (Aggrenox)
- beclomethasone (Beconase, Vanceril)
- betamethasone (Betatrex, Maxivate)
- budesonide (Entocort, Rhinocort)
- bumetanide (Bumex, Burinex)
- butalbital, aspirin, and caffeine (Fiorinal)
- carisoprodol and aspirin (Soma Compound)
- carisoprodol, aspirin, and codeine (Soma Compound with Codeine)
- choline magnesium trisalicylate (Trilisate)
- choline salicylate (Teejel)
- cortisone (Cortone)
- demeclocycline (Declomycin)
- dexamethasone (Decadron, Dexasone)
- diflorasone (Florone, Maxiflor)
- doxycycline (Apo-Doxy, Vibramycin)
- ethacrynic acid (Edecrin)
- flunisolide (AeroBid-M, Nasarel)
- fluticasone (Cutivate, Flonase)
- furosemide (Apo-Furosemide, Lasix)
- halobetasol (Ultravate)
- hydrocodone and aspirin (Azdone, Lortab ASA)
- hydrocortisone (Cetacort, Locoid)

- levonorgestrel (Norplant Implant, Plan B)
- methocarbamol and aspirin (Robaxisal)
- ethylprednisolone (Depoject Injection, Medrol Oral)
- minocycline (Dynacin, Minocin)
- mometasone furoate (Elocom, Nasonex)
- norethindrone (Aygestin, Micronor)
- oxycodone and aspirin (Oxycodan, Percodan)
- prednisolone (Inflamase Forte, Pred Forte)
- prednisone (Apo-Prednisone, Deltasone)
- tetracycline (Novo-Tetra, Sumycin)
- torsemide (Demadex)
- triamcinolone (Aristocort, Trinasal)

Lab Tests That May Be Altered by Vitamin C

- May cause false negative results in stool occult blood tests (guaiac) with intake of 250 mg vitamin C or more per day.
- May cause false decrease in glucose oxidase test (for example, Clinistix) after ingesting more than 500 mg of vitamin C.
- May cause false increase in cupric sulfate test (for example, Clinitest) due to vitamin C in rose hips.
- May cause false increase in liver function tests AST (aspartate aminotransferase), SGOT (serum glutamic-oxaloacetic transaminase), and bilirubin.
- May increase urinary calcium excretion.
- May decrease urinary sodium excretion.
- May cause false increase in serum assay tests for carbamazepine (Tegretol) based on Ames ARIS method.
- May cause false negative results in tests for acetaminophen.
- May cause false decrease in tests for lactic dehydrogenase (LDH).
- May increase iron status results.
- May lower HDL-2 levels when taken in combination with beta-carotene, vitamin E, and selenium.
- May decrease serum uric acid concentrations.
- May cause false decrease in vitamin B_{12} levels.

Diseases That May Be Worsened or Triggered by Vitamin C

- May encourage the formation of oxalate kidney stones.
- May trigger sickle cell crisis.

Foods That May Interact with Vitamin C

None known

Supplements That May Interact with Vitamin C

- Increased absorption of iron from supplements when taken concurrently with vitamin C.
- Vitamin C may increase serum concentration of vitamin E, while E may increase the serum concentration of C.

VITAMIN D

Vitamin D, which serves as both a vitamin and a hormone, aids in the absorption of dietary calcium; works with other vitamins, minerals, and hormones to build bones; and helps ward off the thinning and hollowing of the bones known as osteoporosis. A lack of vitamin D can cause a softening of the bones called osteomalacia in adults, and rickets in children.

Typical Dose

The Food and Nutrition Board has set the Adequate Intake (AI) for vitamin D at 200 IU per day for men and women ages nineteen to fifty; 400 IU per day for men and women ages fifty-one to sixty-nine; and 600 IU per day for men and women ages seventy years and older.

Possible Side Effects

Excessive amounts of vitamin D can lead to nausea, vomiting, weight loss, weakness, irregular heartbeat, confusion, and other mental changes.

Drugs That May Interact with Vitamin D

Taking vitamin D with these drugs may increase the risk of hypercalcemia (high blood levels of calcium) in those who have hyperparathyroidism:

- chlorothiazide (Diuril)
- hydrochlorothiazide (Apo-Hydro, Microzide)
- hydrochlorothiazide and triamterene (Dyazide, Maxzide)
- hydroflumethiazide (Diucardin, Saluron)
- methyclothiazide (Aquatensen, Enduron)
- olmesartan and hydrochlorothiazide (Benicar HCT)
- polythiazide (Renese)
- trichlormethiazide (Metatensin, Naqua)
- xipamide (Diurexan, Lumitens)

Drugs That May Interfere with the Absorption, Utilization, or Excretion of Vitamin D

- aluminum hydroxide (AlternaGel, Alu-Cap)
- aluminum hydroxide and magnesium carbonate (Gaviscon Liquid)
- aluminum hydroxide and magnesium hydroxide (Maalox, Mylanta)
- aluminum hydroxide, magnesium hydroxide, and simethicone (Mylanta Liquid)
- aluminum hydroxide and magnesium trisilicate (Gaviscon Tablet)

- beclomethasone (Beconase, Vanceril)
- betamethasone (Betatrex, Maxivate)
- budesonide (Entocort, Rhinocort)
- butabarbital (Butisol Sodium)
- butalbital, acetaminophen, and caffeine (Esgic, Fioricet)
- butalbital, aspirin, and caffeine (Fiorinal)
- carbamazepine (Carbatrol, Tegretol)
- cascara
- cholestyramine (Prevalite, Questran)
- cimetidine (Nu-Cimet, Tagamet)
- colesevelam (WelChol)
- colestipol (Colestid)
- cortisone (Cortone)
- dexamethasone (Decadron, Dexasone)
- diflorasone (Florone, Maxiflor)
- ethosuximide (Zarontin)
- ethotoin (Peganone)
- famotidine (Apo-Famotidine, Pepcid)
- flunisolide (AeroBid-M, Nasarel)
- fluticasone (Cutivate, Flonase)
- fosphenytoin (Cerebyx)
- halobetasol (Ultravate)
- heparin (Hepalean, Hep-Lock)
- hydrochlorothiazide (Apo-Hydro, Microzide)
- hydrocortisone (Cetacort, Locoid)
- isoniazid (Laniazid Oral, PMS-Isoniazid)
- magnesium hydroxide (Dulcolax Milk of Magnesia, Phillips' Milk of Magnesia)
- mephenytoin (Mesantoin)
- methsuximide (Celontin)
- methylprednisolone (Depoject Injection, Medrol Oral)
- mineral oil (Fleet Mineral Oil Enema, Milkinol)
- mometasone furoate (Elocom, Nasonex)
- neomycin (Myciguent, Neo-Fradin)
- nizatidine (Apo-Nizatidine, Axid)

- orlistat (Xenical)
- oxcarbazepine (Trileptal)
- phenobarbital (Luminal Sodium, PMS-Phenobarbital)
- phenytoin (Dilantin, Phenytek)
- prednisolone (Inflamase Forte, Pred Forte)
- prednisone (Apo-Prednisone, Deltasone)
- primidone (Mysoline, Sertan)
- ranitidine (Alti-Ranitidine, Zantac)
- rifabutin (Mycobutin)
- rifampin (Rifadin, Rimactane)
- rifampin and Isoniazid (Rifamate)
- rifapentine (Priftin)
- sevelamer (Renagel)
- sucralfate (Carafate, Sulcrate)
- triamcinolone (Aristocort, Trinasal)
- valproic acid (Depacon, Depakote ER)

Lab Tests That May Be Altered by Vitamin D

None known

Diseases That May Be Worsened or Triggered by Vitamin D

May cause or increase hypercalcemia (excessive levels of calcium in the blood), which may lead to kidney stones, calcified tissues, or other problems.

Foods That May Interact with Vitamin D

May increase absorption of calcium and calcium levels.

Supplements That May Interact with Vitamin D

None known

VITAMIN E

Vitamin E is a group of eight different substances, each with different structures and properties. This vitamin "family" has powerful antioxidant properties that protect the body from the free-radical damage that can cause cancer, heart disease, and other degenerative diseases. A lack of vitamin E may lead to destruction of red blood cells, infertility, and damage to the muscles and nerves.

First discovered when scientists found that a certain food-related substance had to be present if laboratory animals were to bear young, vitamin E was given the scientific name *tocopherol,* which means "to bring forth children."

Typical Dose

The Food and Nutrition Board has set the RDA for vitamin E at 22 IU per day for adult men and women.

Possible Side Effects

The RDA for vitamin E was set at 22 IU per day because greater amounts of E can "thin" the blood and increase the risk of unnecessary bleeding and bruising. Excessive amounts of vitamin E may also decrease thyroid hormone levels while increasing levels of blood fats (triglycerides).

Drugs That May Interact with Vitamin E

Taking vitamin E with these drugs may increase the risk of bleeding or bruising:
- abciximab (ReoPro)
- antithrombin III (Thrombate III)
- argatroban
- aspirin (Bufferin, Ecotrin)
- aspirin and dipyridamole (Aggrenox)

- bivalirudin (Angiomax)
- clopidogrel (Plavix)
- dalteparin (Fragmin)
- danaparoid (Orgaran)
- dipyridamole (Novo-Dipiradol, Persantine)
- enoxaparin (Lovenox)
- eptifibatide (Integrillin)
- fondaparinux (Arixtra)
- heparin (Hepalean, Hep-Lock)
- indobufen (Ibustrin)
- lepirudin (Refludan)
- ticlopidine (Alti-Ticlopidine, Ticlid)
- tinzaparin (Innohep)
- tirofiban (Aggrastat)
- warfarin (Coumadin, Jantoven)

Drugs That May Interfere with the Absorption, Utilization, or Excretion of Vitamin E

- cholestyramine (Prevalite, Questran)
- clofibrate (Atromid-S, Novo-Fibrate)
- colesevelam (WelChol)
- colestipol (Colestid)
- fenofibrate (Apo-Fenofibrate, TriCor)
- gemfibrozil (Apo-Gemfibrozil, Lopid)
- mineral oil (Fleet Mineral Oil Enema, Milkinol)
- neomycin (Myciguent, Neo-Fradin)
- orlistat (Xenical)
- sevelamer (Renagel)
- simvastatin (Apo-Simvastatin, Zocor)
- sucralfate (Carafate, Sulcrate)

Lab Tests That May Be Altered by Vitamin E

May increase plasma prothrombin time (PT) and plasma international normalized ratio (INR) in those who are also taking warfarin or other anti-coagulant medications, especially in the presence of a vitamin K deficiency.

Diseases That May Be Worsened or Triggered by Vitamin E

- May worsen bleeding disorders or diseases involving bleeding, such as bleeding ulcers.
- May worsen retinitis pigmentosa when vitamin E is taken in synthetic form.

Foods That May Interact with Vitamin E

Vitamin E absorption may be increased when taken with a high-fat meal.

Supplements That May Interact with Vitamin E

- Increased risk of bleeding when used with herbs and supplements that might affect platelet aggregation. (For a list of herbs and supplements with anticoagulant/antiplatelet effect, see Appendix B.)
- May lower HDL-2 (high-density lipoprotein-2) levels when taken in combination with beta-carotene, vitamin C, and selenium.
- Vitamin E requirements may increase in response to high intake of omega-6 fatty acids.
- May promote absorption and utilization of vitamin A, reduce symptoms of hypervitaminosis A, and increase storage of vitamin A in the liver.

VITAMIN K

In the early 1900s, a Danish researcher discovered that a certain factor in the fatty parts of food helped in the clotting of blood. He named it the koagulation vitamin, although today we simply call it vitamin K. A lack of vitamin K can cause bleeding and may contribute to osteoporosis.

Typical Dose

The Food and Nutrition Board has set the Adequate Intake for vitamin K at 120 mcg per day for men above the age of nineteen and 90 mcg per day for women above the age of nineteen.

Possible Side Effects

According to the Food and Nutrition Board, "No adverse effects associated with vitamin K consumption from food or supplements have been reported in humans or animals." Despite the lack of known serious side effects, be sure to check with your physician if you are taking medications such as blood thinners that could be affected by the vitamin.

Drugs That May Interact with Vitamin K

Taking vitamin K may interfere with the action of the drug:

- warfarin (Coumadin, Jantoven)

Drugs That May Interfere with the Absorption, Utilization, or Excretion of Vitamin K

- amikacin (Amikin)
- amoxicillin (Amoxil, Novamoxin)
- ampicillin (Omnipen, Totacillin)
- azithromycin (Zithromax)
- beclomethasone (Beconase, Vanceril)
- betamethasone (Betatrex, Maxivate)
- budesonide (Entocort, Rhinocort)
- butabarbital (Butisol Sodium)
- butalbital, acetaminophen, and caffeine (Esgic, Fioricet)
- butalbital, aspirin, and caffeine (Fiorinal)
- carbenicillin (Geocillin)
- cefaclor (Ceclor)
- cefadroxil (Duricef)
- cefamandole (Mandol)
- cefazolin (Ancef, Kefzol)
- cefdinir (Omnicef)
- cefditoren (Spectracef)
- cefepime (Maxipime)
- cefonicid (Monocid)
- cefoperazone (Cefobid)
- cefotaxime (Claforan)
- cefotetan (Cefotan)
- cefoxitin (Mefoxin)
- cefpodoxime (Vantin)
- cefprozil (Cefzil)
- ceftazidime (Ceptaz, Fortaz)
- ceftibuten (Cedax)
- ceftizoxime (Cefizox)
- ceftriaxone (Rocephin)
- cefuroxime (Ceftin, Kefurox)
- cephalexin (Biocef, Keftab)
- cephalothin (Ceporacin)
- cephapirin (Cefadyl)
- cepharadine (Velosef)
- cholestyramine (Prevalite, Questran)
- cinoxacin (Cinobac)
- ciprofloxacin (Ciloxan, Cipro)
- clarithromycin (Biaxin, Biaxin XL)
- clindamycin (Cleocin, Dalacin C)
- cloxacillin (Cloxapen, Nu-Cloxi)
- colesevelam (WelChol)
- colestipol (Colestid)
- cortisone (Cortone)
- demeclocycline (Declomycin)
- dexamethasone (Decadron, Dexasone)
- dicloxacillin (Dycill, Pathocil)
- dirithromycin (Dynabac)
- doxycycline (Apo-Doxy, Vibramycin)
- erythromycin (Erythrocin, Staticin)
- ethosuximide (Zarontin)

- flunisolide (AeroBid-M, Nasarel)
- fluticasone (Cutivate, Flonase)
- fosphenytoin (Cerebyx)
- gatofloxacin (Tequin, Zymar)
- gentamicin (Alcomicin, Gentacidin)
- griseofulvin (Fulvicin-U/F, Grifulvin V)
- kanamycin (Kantrex)
- levofloxacin (Levaquin, Quixin)
- linezolid (Zyvox)
- lomefloxacin (Maxaquin)
- loracarbef (Lorabid)
- meclocycline (Meclan Topical)
- methsuximide (Celontin)
- methylprednisolone (Depoject Injection, Medrol Oral)
- metronidazole (Flagyl, Noritate)
- mineral oil (Fleet Mineral Oil Enema, Milkinol)
- minocycline (Dynacin, Minocin)
- mometasone furoate (Elocom, Nasonex)
- moxifloxacin (Avelox)
- nafcillin (Nafcil Injection, Unipen Oral)
- nalidixic acid (NegGram)
- neomycin (Myciguent, Neo-Fradin)
- norfloxacin (Chibroxin Ophthalmic, Noroxin Oral)
- ofloxacin (Floxin, Ocuflox)
- orlistat (Xenical)
- penicillin G benzathine (Bicillin L-A, Permapen)
- penicillin G benzathine and penicillin G procaine (Bicillin C-R)
- penicillin G procaine (Pfizerpen-AS, Wycillin)
- penicillin V potassium (Suspen, Truxcillin)
- phenobarbital (Luminal Sodium, PMS-Pheno-barbital)
- phenytoin (Dilantin, Phenytek)
- piperacillin (Pipracil)
- piperacillin and tazobactam sodium (Zosyn)

- prednisolone (Inflamase Forte, Pred Forte)
- prednisone (Apo-Prednisone, Deltasone)
- primidone (Mysoline, Sertan)
- sevelamer (Renagel)
- sparfloxacin (Zagam)
- sucralfate (Carafate, Sulcrate)
- sulfadiazine (Microsulfon)
- sulfisoxazole (Gantrisin)
- tetracycline (Novo-Tetra, Sumycin)
- ticarcillin (Ticar)
- ticarcillin and clavulanate potassium (Timentin)
- tobramycin (Nebcin, Tobrex)
- triamcinolone (Aristocort, Trinasal)
- trimethoprim (Primsol, Trimpex)
- trovafloxacin (Trovan)

Lab Tests That May Be Altered by Vitamin K

- May increase urinary calcium excretion.
- May increase urinary hemoglobin levels.
- May decrease urinary hydroxyproline levels.
- May increase urinary porphyrins.
- May increase urinary protein levels.
- May increase urinary urobilinogen.
- May cause false increase in urinary 17-hydroxy-corticosteroids.
- May increase serum bilirubin levels in those with G-6-PD deficiency.
- May decrease blood erythrocyte levels.
- May decrease hematocrit levels.
- May decrease blood hemoglobin levels.
- May decrease levels of leukocytes and platelets.
- May decrease prothrombin time (PT).

Diseases That May Be Worsened or Triggered by Vitamin K

None known

Foods That May Interact with Vitamin K
None known

Supplements That May Interact with Vitamin K

- May increase the risk of clotting in those using anticoagulants, especially if taken with vitamin K–rich herbs such as alfalfa and parsley. (For a list of herbs and supplements that contain vitamin K, see Appendix B.)
- May increase risk of clotting in those using anticoagulants, especially if taken with coenzyme Q_{10}.
- Taking more than 800 IU of vitamin E per day can decrease the clotting effects of vitamin K and increase the risk of bleeding in those taking warfarin or other anticoagulants, especially in the presence of a vitamin K deficiency.

WAHOO

Wahoo is a small, thin shrub, native to the central eastern parts of the United States and Canada, that produces small red fruits that look like strawberries. Traditionally used as a laxative, wahoo is one of the major liver herbs and is used to relieve liver congestion, stimulate the free flow of bile, and aid in the digestive process.

Scientific Name
Euonymus species

Wahoo Is Also Commonly Known As
Arrowwood, bitter ash, fish wood, Indian arrowroot, spindle tree, strawberry tree

Medicinal Parts
Trunk, root bark, fruit

Wahoo's Uses
To treat indigestion and constipation, stimulate the production of bile, and as a tonic

Typical Dose
There is no typical dose of wahoo, which is considered too dangerous for use.

Possible Side Effects
❶ Wahoo is poisonous. Side effects may include severe gastrointestinal distress, bloody diarrhea, circulatory problems, and stupor progressing to unconsciousness. Wahoo contains cardiac glycosides, which can help control irregular heartbeat, reduce the backup of blood and fluid in the body, and increase blood flow through the kidneys, helping to excrete sodium and relieve swelling in body tissues. However, a buildup of cardiac glycosides can occur, especially when the herb is combined with certain medications or other herbs that contain cardiac glycosides, causing arrhythmias, abnormally slow heartbeat, heart failure, and even death.

Drugs That May Interact with Wahoo
Taking wahoo with these drugs may increase the risk of hypokalemia (low levels of potassium in the blood) and/or cardiac glycoside toxicity:

- acetazolamide (Apo-Acetazolamide, Diamox Sequels)
- azithromycin (Zithromax)
- azosemide (Diat)
- bumetanide (Bumex, Burinex)
- cascara

- chlorothiazide (Diuril)
- chlorthalidone (Apo-Chlorthalidone, Thalitone)
- clarithromycin (Biaxin, Biaxin XL)
- demeclocycline (Declomycin)
- digitalis (Digitek, Lanoxin)
- dirithromycin (Dynabac)
- docusate and senna (Peri-Colace, Senokot-S)
- doxycycline (Apo-Doxy, Vibramycin)
- erythromycin (Erythrocin, Staticin)
- ethacrynic acid (Edecrin)
- etozolin (Elkapin)
- furosemide (Apo-Furosemide, Lasix)
- hydrochlorothiazide (Apo-Hydro, Microzide)
- hydroflumethiazide (Diucardin, Saluron)
- indapamide (Lozol, Nu-Indapamide)
- josamycin (Iosalide, Josamy)
- mannitol (Osmitrol, Resectisol)
- mefruside (Baycaron)
- methazolamide (Apo-Methazolamide, Neptazane)
- methyclothiazide (Aquatensen, Enduron)
- metolazone (Mykrox, Zaroxolyn)
- midecamycin (Macropen, Midecin)
- minocycline (Dynacin, Minocin)
- olmesartan and hydrochlorothiazide (Benicar HCT)
- oxytetracycline (Terramycin, Terramycin IM)
- polythiazide (Renese)
- quinine (Quinine-Odan)
- roxithromycin (Claramid, Roxibeta)
- spiramycin (Rovamycine)
- tetracycline (Novo-Tetra, Sumycin)
- torsemide (Demadex)
- trichlormethiazide (Metatensin, Naqua)
- troleandomycin (Tao)

- urea (Amino-Cerv, UltraMide)
- xipamide (Diurexan, Lumitens)

Lab Tests That May Be Altered by Wahoo
None known

Diseases That May Be Worsened or Triggered by Wahoo
May worsen inflammatory gastrointestinal ailments by increasing stomach secretions.

Foods That May Interact with Wahoo
None known

Supplements That May Interact with Wahoo
- Increased risk of cardiac glycoside toxicity when used with other herbs that contain cardiac glycosides, such as black hellebore, calotropis, motherwort, and others. (For a list of cardiac glycoside–containing herbs and supplements, see Appendix B.)
- Increased risk of cardiotoxicity due to potassium depletion when taken with cardioactive herbs, such as adonis, digitalis, lily-of-the-valley, and squill. (For a list of cardioactive herbs and supplements, see Appendix B.)
- Increased risk of potassium depletion when used in conjunction with horsetail plant or licorice.
- Increased risk of potassium depletion when used with other stimulant laxative herbs, such as black root, cascara sagrada, castor oil, and senna. (For a list of stimulant laxative herbs and supplements, see Appendix B.)

WALLFLOWER

An old English favorite, the fragrant golden wall-flower grows all over southern Europe and is often found clinging to cliffs and climbing up walls. In the past, wallflower was used mainly as a diuretic, to promote onset of the menstrual cycle, and to stimulate the action of the heart, in much the same way as digitalis. However, because it is toxic, wallflower is seldom used today.

Scientific Name

Cheiranthus cheiri

Wallflower Is Also Commonly Known As

Beeflower, gillyflower, keiri, wallstock-gillofer

Medicinal Parts

Flower, seed, above-ground parts

Wallflower's Uses

To treat constipation, liver and gallbladder diseases, and encourage menstruation

Typical Dose

A typical dose of wallflower is made by mixing 2 to 3 gm of the herb with 100 ml of very hot water, steeping for 10 minutes, straining, and taking three to four cups of this tea per day.

Possible Side Effects

❶ Wallflower's side effects include poisoning when administered intravenously or through injection. Wallflower contains cardiac glycosides, which can help control irregular heartbeat, reduce the backup of blood and fluid in the body, and increase blood flow through the kidneys, helping to excrete sodium and relieve swelling in body tissues. However, a buildup of cardiac glycosides can occur, especially when the herb is combined with certain medications or other herbs that contain cardiac glycosides, causing arrhythmias, abnormally slow heartbeat, heart failure, and even death.

Drugs That May Interact with Wallflower

Taking wallflower with these drugs may enhance the therapeutic effects of the herb:

- calcium acetate (PhosLo)
- calcium carbonate (Rolaids Extra Strength, Tums)
- calcium chloride
- calcium citrate (Osteocit)
- calcium glubionate
- calcium gluceptate
- calcium gluconate

Taking wallflower with these drugs may increase the risk of cardiac glycoside toxicity:

- acetazolamide (Apo-Acetazolamide, Diamox Sequels)
- azosemide (Diat)
- beclomethasone (Beconase, Vanceril)
- betamethasone (Celestone, Diprolene)
- budesonide (Entocort, Rhinocort)
- budesonide and Formoterol (Symbicort)
- bumetanide (Bumex, Burinex)
- cascara
- chlorothiazide (Diuril)
- chlorthalidone (Apo-Chlorthalidone, Thalitone)
- cortisone (Cortone)
- deflazacort (Calcort, Dezacor)

- dexamethasone (Decadron, Dexasone)
- digitalis (Digitek, Lanoxin)
- docusate and senna (Peri-Colace, Senokot-S)
- ethacrynic acid (Edecrin)
- etozolin (Elkapin)
- flunisolide (AeroBid, Nasarel)
- fluorometholone (Eflone, Flarex)
- fluticasone (Cutivate, Flonase)
- furosemide (Apo-Furosemide, Lasix)
- hydrochlorothiazide (Apo-Hydro, Microzide)
- hydrocortisone (Anusol-HC, Locoid)
- hydroflumethiazide (Diucardin, Saluron)
- indapamide (Lozol, Nu-Indapamide)
- mannitol (Osmitrol, Resectisol)
- mefruside (Baycaron)
- methazolamide (Apo-Methazolamide, Neptazane)
- methyclothiazide (Aquatensen, Enduron)
- methylprednisolone (DepoMedrol, Medrol)
- metolazone (Mykrox, Zaroxolyn)
- olmesartan and hydrochlorothiazide (Benicar HCT)
- polythiazide (Renese)
- prednisolone (Inflamase Forte, Pred Forte)
- prednisone (Apo-Prednisone, Deltasone)
- quinidine (Novo-Quinidin, Quinaglute Dura-Tabs)
- quinine (Quinine-Odan)
- torsemide (Demadex)
- triamcinolone (Aristocort, Trinasal)
- trichlormethiazide (Metatensin, Naqua)
- urea (Amino-Cerv, UltraMide)
- xipamide (Diurexan, Lumitens)

Lab Tests That May Be Altered by Wallflower
None known

Diseases That May Be Worsened or Triggered by Wallflower
May trigger irregular heartbeat.

Foods That May Interact with Wallflower
None known

Supplements That May Interact with Wallflower
- Increased risk of cardiac glycoside toxicity when used with other herbs that contain cardiac glycosides, such as black hellebore, calotropis, motherwort, and others. (For a list of cardiac glycoside–containing herbs and supplements, see Appendix B.)
- Increased risk of cardiotoxicity due to potassium depletion when taken with cardioactive herbs, such as adonis, digitalis, lily-of-the-valley, and squill. (For a list of cardioactive herbs and supplements, see Appendix B.)
- Increased risk of potassium depletion when used in conjunction with horsetail plant or licorice.
- Increased risk of potassium depletion when used with other stimulant laxative herbs, such as black root, cascara sagrada, castor oil, and senna. (For a list of stimulant laxative herbs and supplements, see Appendix B.)
- Increased risk of toxicity when taken with quinine.
- Increased risk of toxicity when taken with ma-huang.

WATERCRESS

The Latin name for watercress, *Nasturtium*, comes from the words *nasus tortus* ("twisted nose"), because of the herb's hot, peppery taste. The spicy taste is due to a compound called phenylethylisothiocyanate (PEITC), which has been shown to have powerful anticancer properties. Watercress is a stimulant and expectorant and has long been used as a treatment for coughs and bronchitis. It is also used as a diuretic, to promote digestion, and, in poultice form, to ease the pain of arthritis and gout.

Scientific Name
Nasturtium officinale

Watercress Is Also Commonly Known As
Berro, cresson au poulet, Indian cress, nasturtii herba, scurvy grass, tall nasturtium

Medicinal Parts
Entire flowering plant

Watercress's Uses
To treat cough, bronchitis, flu, scurvy, and goiter; to improve digestion and stimulate appetite. Germany's Commission E has approved the use of watercress to treat cough and bronchitis.

Typical Dose
A typical daily dose of watercress may range from 4 to 6 gm of the dried herb.

Possible Side Effects
Watercress's side effects include gastrointestinal irritation.

Drugs That May Interact with Watercress
Taking watercress with these drugs may be harmful:

- acetaminophen (Tylenol, Genapap)—may increase the risk of adverse effects of the drug, especially liver damage
- chlorzoxazone (Strifion Forte)—may increase the therapeutic and adverse effects of the drug
- warfarin (Coumadin, Jantoven)—may interfere with the action of the drug

Lab Tests That May Be Altered by Watercress
May decrease plasma prothrombin time (PT) and plasma international normalized ratio (INR) due to vitamin K content.

Diseases That May Be Worsened or Triggered by Watercress
May worsen ulcers or inflammatory kidney disease.

Foods That May Interact with Watercress
None known

Supplements That May Interact with Watercress
None known

WHITE WILLOW

Long before aspirin was found in every medicine chest, people with headaches or other painful conditions reached for the bark of the white willow tree. Known as nature's aspirin, white willow bark contains salicin, a chemical cousin of the popular pain reliever. Like aspirin, salicin quells pain, fever, and inflammation but does not keep the blood thin and help protect against heart attacks.

Scientific Name
Salix species

White Willow Is Also Commonly Known As
Cartkins willow, European willow, pussywillow, withe withy

Medicinal Parts
Bark

White Willow's Uses
To treat rheumatism, gout, diarrhea, gastrointestinal distress, and diseases involving fever, headaches, and pain related to inflammation. Germany's Commission E has approved the use of white willow to treat pain and rheumatism.

Typical Dose
A typical daily dose of white willow may range from 6 to 12 gm of the herb (corresponding to 60 to 120 mg total salicin).

Possible Side Effects
White willow's side effects include gastrointestinal distress.

Drugs That May Interact with White Willow
Taking white willow with these drugs may increase the risk of bleeding or bruising:
- abciximab (ReoPro)
- acemetacin (Acemetacin Heumann, Acemetacin Sandoz)
- alteplase (Activase, Cathflo Activase)
- aminosalicylic acid (Nemasol Sodium, Paser)
- antithrombin III (Thrombate III)
- argatroban
- aspirin (Bufferin, Ecotrin)
- aspirin and dipyridamole (Aggrenox)
- bivalirudin (Angiomax)
- celecoxib (Celebrex)
- choline magnesium trisalicylate (Trilisate)
- choline salicylate (Teejel)
- clopidogrel (Plavix)
- dalteparin (Fragmin)
- danaparoid (Orgaran)
- diclofenac (Cataflam, Voltaren)
- diflunisal (Apo-Diflunisal, Dolobid)
- dipyridamole (Novo-Dipiradol, Persantine)
- dipyrone (Analgina, Dinador)
- enoxaparin (Lovenox)
- eptifibatide (Integrillin)
- etodolac (Lodine, Utradol)
- etoricoxib (Arcoxia)
- fenoprofen (Nalfon)
- flurbiprofen (Ansaid, Ocufen)
- fondaparinux (Arixtra)
- heparin (Hepalean, Hep-Lock)
- ibuprofen (Advil, Motrin)
- indobufen (Ibustrin)
- indomethacin (Indocin, Novo-Methacin)
- ketoprofen (Orudis, Rhodis)
- ketorolac (Acular, Toradol)
- lepirudin (Refludan)
- magnesium salicylate (Doan's, Mobidin)
- meclofenamate (Meclomen)
- mefenamic acid (Ponstan, Ponstel)
- meloxicam (MOBIC, Mobicox)
- nabumetone (Apo-Nabumetone, Relafen)
- nadroparin (Fraxiparine)
- naproxen (Aleve, Naprosyn)
- niflumic acid (Niflam, Nifluril)
- nimesulide (Areuma, Aulin)
- oxaprozin (Apo-Oxaprozin, Daypro)
- piroxicam (Feldene, Nu-Pirox)

- reteplase (Retavase)
- rofecoxib (Vioxx)
- salsalate (Amgesic, Salflex)
- streptokinase (Streptase)
- sulindac (Clinoril, Nu-Sundac)
- tenecteplase (TNKase)
- tenoxicam (Dolmen, Mobiflex)
- tiaprofenic acid (DomTiaprofenic, Surgam)
- ticlopidine (Alti-Ticlopidine, Ticlid)
- tinzaparin (Innohep)
- tirofiban (Aggrastat)
- tolmetin (Tolectin)
- urokinase (Abbokinase)
- valdecoxib (Bextra)
- warfarin (Coumadin, Jantoven)

Taking white willow with these drugs may be harmful:

- benazepril (Lotensin)—may increase the risk of hypertension (high blood pressure)

Lab Tests That May Be Altered by White Willow
None known

Diseases That May Be Worsened or Triggered by White Willow

- May trigger allergic reactions in those allergic to aspirin or salicylates.
- May worsen ulcers, asthma, diabetes, and hemophilia.

Foods That May Interact with White Willow
None known

Supplements That May Interact with White Willow

- Increased risk of bleeding when used with herbs and supplements that might affect platelet

aggregation. (For a list of herbs and supplements with anticoagulant/antiplatelet effects, see Appendix B.)

- May increase beneficial and/or adverse effects of salicylate-containing herbs, such as aspen bark, sweet birch, and poplar.
- The tannins in white willow may cause the alkaloids in certain other herbs to separate and settle, increasing the risk of toxic reactions. (For a list of herbs and other substances high in alkaloids, see Appendix B.)

WILD CARROT

Also known as Queen Anne's lace, wild carrot, with its large, umbrella-shaped clusters of white flowers and small, pale carrotlike root, is a very common weed in the southeastern United States. Wild carrot is thought to be descended from carrots that somehow "escaped" from the gardens of early North American settlers. Juice taken from the root has long been used as a diuretic, while the seeds have been eaten to calm indigestion and flatulence.

Scientific Name
Daucus carota

Wild Carrot Is Also Commonly Known As
Bee's nest, bird's nest, carrot, Queen Anne's lace

Medicinal Parts
Root

Wild Carrot's Uses

To treat gout, indigestion, and heart disease; as a nerve tonic and aphrodisiac

Typical Dose

There is no typical dose of wild carrot.

Possible Side Effects

Wild carrot's side effects include lowered blood pressure, drowsiness, nausea, and allergic reactions (through skin contact).

Drugs That May Interact with Wild Carrot

Taking wild carrot with these drugs may increase skin sensitivity to sunlight:

- bumetanide (Bumex, Burinex)
- celecoxib (Celebrex)
- ciprofloxacin (Cipro, Ciloxan)
- doxycycline (Apo-Doxy, Vibramycin)
- enalapril (Vasotec)
- etodolac (Lodine, Utradol)
- fluphenazine (Modecate, Prolixin)
- fosinopril (Monopril)
- furosemide (Apo-Furosemide, Lasix)
- gatifloxacin (Tequin, Zymar)
- hydrochlorothiazide (Apo-Hydro, Microzide)
- ibuprofen (Advil, Motrin)
- indomethacin (Indocin, Novo-Methacin)
- ketoprofen (Orudis, Rhodis)
- ketorolac (Acular, Toradol)
- lansoprazole (Prevacid)
- levofloxacin (Levaquin, Quixin)
- lisinopril (Prinivil, Zestril)
- loratadine (Alavert, Claritin)
- methotrexate (Rheumatrex, Trexall)
- naproxen (Aleve, Naprosyn)
- nortriptyline (Aventyl HCl, Pamelor)
- ofloxacin (Floxin, Ocuflox)
- omeprazole (Losec, Prilosec)
- phenytoin (Dilantin, Phenytek)
- piroxicam (Feldene, Nu-Pirox)
- prochlorperazine (Compazine, Compro)
- quinapril (Accupril)
- risperidone (Risperdal)
- rofecoxib (Vioxx)
- tetracycline (Novo-Tetra, Sumycin)

Taking wild carrot with these drugs may increase the risk of hypotension (excessively low blood pressure):

- acebutolol (Novo-Acebutolol, Sectral)
- acetazolamide (Apo-Acetazolamide, Diamox Sequels)
- amiloride (Midamor)
- amlodipine (Norvasc)
- atenolol (Apo-Atenol, Tenormin)
- azosemide (Diat)
- benazepril (Lotensin)
- betaxolol (Betoptic S, Kerlone)
- bisoprolol (Monocor, Zebeta)
- bumetanide (Bumex, Burinex)
- candesartan (Atacand)
- captopril (Capoten, Novo-Captopril)
- carteolol (Cartrol, Ocupress)
- carvedilol (Coreg)
- chlorothiazide (Diuril)
- chlorthalidone (Apo-Chlorthalidone, Thalitone)
- clonidine (Catapres, Duraclon)
- diazoxide (Hyperstat, Proglycem)
- diltiazem (Cardizem, Tiazac)
- doxazosin (Alti-Doxazosin, Cardura)
- eplerenone (Inspra)
- eprosartan (Teveten)
- esmolol (Brevibloc)

- ethacrynic acid (Edecrin)
- etozolin (Elkapin)
- felodipine (Plendil, Renedil)
- fenoldopam (Corlopam)
- fosinopril (Monopril)
- furosemide (Apo-Furosemide, Lasix)
- guanabenz (Wytensin)
- guanadrel (Hylorel)
- guanfacine (Tenex)
- hydralazine (Apresoline, Novo-Hylazin)
- hydrochlorothiazide (Apo-Hydro, Microzide)
- hydrochlorothiazide and triamterene (Dyazide, Maxzide)
- hydroflumethiazide (Diucardin, Saluron)
- indapamide (Lozol, Nu-Indapamide)
- irbesartan (Avapro)
- isradipine (DynaCirc)
- labetalol (Normodyne, Trandate)
- lisinopril (Prinivil, Zestril)
- losartan (Cozaar)
- mannitol (Osmitrol, Resectisol)
- mecamylamine (Inversine)
- mefruside (Baycaron)
- methazolamide (Apo-Methazolamide, Nepta-zane)
- methyclothiazide (Aquatensen, Enduron)
- methyldopa (Apo-Methyldopa, Nu-Medopa)
- metolazone (Mykrox, Zaroxolyn)
- metoprolol (Betaloc, Lopressor)
- minoxidil (Loniten, Rogaine)
- moexipril (Univasc)
- nadolol (Apo-Nadol, Corgard)
- nicardipine (Cardene)
- nifedipine (Adalat CC, Procardia)
- nisoldipine (Sular)
- nitroglycerin (Minitran, Nitro-Dur)
- nitroprusside (Nipride, Nitropress)

- olmesartan (Benicar)
- olmesartan and hydrochlorothiazide (Benicar HCT)
- oxprenolol (Slow-Trasicor, Trasicor)
- perindopril erbumine (Aceon, Coversyl)
- phenoxybenzamine (Dibenzyline)
- phentolamine (Regitine, Rogitine)
- pindolol (Apo-Pindol, Novo-Pindol)
- polythiazide (Renese)
- prazosin (Minipress, Nu-Prazo)
- propranolol (Inderal, InnoPran XL)
- quinapril (Accupril)
- ramipril (Altace)
- reserpine
- spironolactone (Aldactone, Novo-Spiroton)
- telmisartan (Micardis)
- terazosin (Alti-Terazosin, Hytrin)
- timolol (Betimol, Timoptic)
- torsemide (Demadex)
- trandolapril (Mavik)
- triamterene (Dyrenium)
- trichlormethiazide (Metatensin, Naqua)
- urea (Amino-Cerv, UltraMide)
- valsartan (Diovan)
- verapamil (Calan, Isoptin SR)
- xipamide (Diurexan, Lumitens)

Taking wild carrot with these drugs may increase the risk of excessive sedation and mental depression and impairment:

- acetaminophen and codeine (Capital and Codeine, Tylenol with Codeine)
- alfentanil (Alfenta)
- alprazolam (Apo-Alpraz, Xanax)
- amobarbital (Amytal)
- amobarbital and secobarbital (Tuinal)
- aspirin and codeine (Coryphen Codeine)

- belladonna and opium (B&O Supprettes)
- bromazepam (Apo-Bromazepam, Gen-Bromazepam)
- brotizolam (Lendorm, Sintonal)
- buprenorphine (Buprenex, Subutex)
- buprenorphine and naloxone (Suboxone)
- butabarbital (Butisol Sodium)
- butalbital, acetaminophen, and caffeine (Esgic, Fioricet)
- butalbital, aspirin, and caffeine (Fiorinal)
- butorphanol (Apo-Butorphanol, Stadol)
- chloral hydrate (Aquachloral Supprettes, Somnote)
- chlordiazepoxide (Apo-Chlordiazepoxide, Librium)
- clobazam (Alti-Clobazam, Frisium)
- clonazepam (Klonopin, Rivotril)
- clorazepate (Tranxene, T-Tab)
- codeine (Codeine Contin)
- dexmedetomidine (Precedex)
- diazepam (Apo-Diazepam, Valium)
- dihydrocodeine, aspirin, and caffeine (Synalgos-DC)
- diphenhydramine (Benadryl Allergy, Nytol)
- estazolam (ProSom)
- fentanyl (Actiq, Duragesic)
- flurazepam (Apo-Flurazepam, Dalmane)
- glutethimide
- haloperidol (Haldol, Novo-Peridol)
- hydrocodone and acetaminophen (Vicodin, Zydone)
- hydrocodone and aspirin (Damason-P)
- hydrocodone and ibuprofen (Vicoprofen)
- hydromorphone (Dilaudid, PMS-Hydromorphone)
- hydroxyzine (Atarax, Vistaril)
- levomethadyl acetate hydrochloride
- levorphanol (LevoDromoran)
- loprazolam (Dormonoct, Havlane)
- lorazepam (Ativan, Nu-Loraz)
- meperidine (Demerol, Meperitab)
- meperidine and promethazine
- mephobarbital (Mebaral)
- methadone (Dolophine, Methadose)
- methohexital (Brevital, Brevital Sodium)
- midazolam (Apo-Midazolam, Versed)
- morphine sulfate (Kadian, MS Contin)
- nalbuphine (Nubain)
- opium tincture
- oxycodone (OxyContin, Roxicodone)
- oxycodone and acetaminophen (Endocet, Percocet)
- oxycodone and aspirin (Endodan, Percodan)
- oxymorphone (Numorphan)
- paregoric
- pentazocine (Talwin)
- pentobarbital (Nembutal)
- phenobarbital (Luminal Sodium, PMS-Phenobarbital)
- phenoperidine
- prazepam
- primidone (Apo-Primidone, Mysoline)
- promethazine (Phenergan)
- propofol (Diprivan)
- propoxyphene (Darvon, Darvon-N)
- propoxyphene and acetaminophen (Darvocet-N 50, Darvocet-N 100)
- propoxyphene, aspirin, and caffeine (Darvon Compound)
- quazepam (Doral)
- remifentanil (Ultiva)
- secobarbital (Seconal)
- sodium oxybate (Xyrem)
- sufentanil (Sufenta)

- s-zopiclone (Lunesta)
- temazepam (Novo-Temazepam, Restoril)
- tetrazepam (Mobiforton, Musapam)
- thiopental (Pentothal)
- triazolam (Apo-Triazo, Halcion)
- zaleplon (Sonata, Stamoc)
- zolpidem (Ambien)
- zopiclone (Alti-Zopiclone, Gen-Zopiclone)

Taking wild carrot with these drugs may increase the risk of cardiac glycoside toxicity:
- digitalis (Digitek, Lanoxin)

Lab Tests That May Be Altered by Wild Carrot
None known

Diseases That May Be Worsened or Triggered by Wild Carrot
May worsen existing kidney irritation or inflammation.

Foods That May Interact with Wild Carrot
None known

Supplements That May Interact with Wild Carrot
May enhance therapeutic and adverse effects of herbs and supplements that have sedative properties, such as 5-HTP, kava kava, St. John's wort, and valerian. (For a list of herbs and supplements that have sedative properties, see Appendix B.)

WILD CHERRY

The wild cherry tree, which grows mostly in North America and Canada, is also known as the black cherry, because the bark of older trees is so dark it is nearly black. The bark of the young trees contains prussic acid, a substance that calms the coughing reflex. Wild cherry was used by Native Americans to treat respiratory complaints and by early North American settlers as a cough syrup and poultice. It is still used today as a cough suppressant in certain cough medicines and lozenges.

Scientific Name
Prunus serotina

Wild Cherry Is Also Commonly Known As
Black choke, choke cherry, rum cherry, wild black cherry

Medicinal Parts
Bark

Wild Cherry's Uses
To treat cough, whooping cough, diarrhea, and bronchitis

Typical Dose
A typical daily dose of wild cherry has not been established.

Possible Side Effects
Wild cherry's side effects include headache, constipation, and ulcers.

Drugs That May Interact with Wild Cherry

Taking wild cherry with these drugs may increase blood levels of the drug:

- alprazolam (Apo-Alpraz, Xanax)
- amlodipine (Norvasc)
- atorvastatin (Lipitor)
- bepridil (Vascor)
- bromazepam (Apo-Bromazepam, Gen-Bromazepam)
- brotizolam (Lendorm, Sintonal)
- buspirone (BuSpar, Nu-Buspirone)
- chlordiazepoxide (Apo-Chlordiazepoxide, Librium)
- clobazam (Alti-Clobazam, Frisium)
- clonazepam (Klonopin, Rivotril)
- clorazepate (Tranxene, T-Tab)
- cyclosporine (Neoral, Sandimmune)
- cyproterone and ethinyl estradiol (Diane-35)
- diazepam (Apo-Diazepam, Valium)
- diltiazem (Cardizem, Tiazac)
- estazolam (ProSom)
- estradiol (Climara, Estrace)
- estradiol and norethindrone (Activella, CombiPatch)
- estradiol and testosterone (Climacteron)
- estrogens, conjugated A/synthetic (Cenestin)
- estrogens, conjugated/equine (Congest, Premarin)
- estrogens, conjugated/equine, and medroxyprogesterone (Premphase, Prempro)
- estrogens (esterified) (Estratab, Menest)
- estrogens (esterified) and methyltestosterone (Estratest, Estratest H.S.)
- estropipate (Ogen, OrthoEst)
- ethinyl estradiol (Estinyl)
- ethinyl estradiol and desogestrel (Cyclessa, Ortho-Cept)
- ethinyl estradiol and ethynodiol diacetate (Demulen, Zovia)
- ethinyl estradiol and etonogestrel (NuvaRing)
- ethinyl estradiol and levonorgestrel (Alesse, Triphasil)
- ethinyl estradiol and norelgestromin (Evra, Ortho Evra)
- ethinyl estradiol and norethindrone (Brevicon, Ortho-Novum)
- ethinyl estradiol and norgestimate (Cyclen, Ortho Tri-Cyclen)
- ethinyl estradiol and norgestrel (Cryselle, Ovral)
- felodipine (Plendil, Renedil)
- fexofenadine (Allegra)
- fluconazole (Apo-Fluconazole, Diflucan)
- flurazepam (Apo-Flurazepam, Dalmane)
- fluvastatin (Lescol)
- isradipine (DynaCirc)
- itraconazole (Sporanox)
- ketoconazole (Apo-Ketoconazole, Nizoral)
- lacidipine (Aponil, Caldine)
- lercanidipine (Cardiovasc, Carmen)
- loprazolam (Dormonoct, Havlane)
- lorazepam (Ativan, Nu-Loraz)
- lovastatin (Altocor, Mevacor)
- manidipine (Calslot, Iperten)
- mestranol and norethindrone (Necon 1/50, Ortho-Novum 1/50)
- midazolam (Apo-Midazolam, Versed)
- nicardipine (Cardene)
- nifedipine (Adalat CC, Procardia)
- nilvadipine
- nimodipine (Nimotop)
- nisoldipine (Sular)
- nitrendipine
- pinaverium (Dicetel)
- polyestradiol

- pravastatin (Novo-Pravastatin, Pravachol)
- prazepam
- quazepam (Doral)
- rosuvastatin (Crestor)
- simvastatin (Apo-Simvastatin, Zocor)
- temazepam (Novo-Temazepam, Restoril)
- tetrazepam (Mobiforton, Musapam)
- triazolam (Apo-Triazo, Halcion)
- verapamil (Calan, Isoptin SR)
- voriconazole (VFEND)

Lab Tests That May Be Altered by Wild Cherry
None known

Diseases That May Be Worsened or Triggered by Wild Cherry
None known

Foods That May Interact with Wild Cherry
None known

Supplements That May Interact with Wild Cherry
None known

WILD LETTUCE

Related to garden lettuce, this wild variation contains a milky substance referred to as lettuce opium, because it has some properties similar to the opium taken from poppies. Used as a sedative, wild lettuce reportedly eases restlessness, anxiety, and insomnia and has been used in place of opium in cough preparations.

Scientific Name
Lactuca virosa

Wild Lettuce Is Also Commonly Known As
Acrid lettuce, bitter lettuce, green endive, lactucarium, lettuce opium, poison lettuce

Medicinal Parts
Leaves, latex (milky fluid in leaves)

Wild Lettuce's Uses
To treat diseases of the urinary tract, asthma, whooping cough, painful menses, and nymphomania

Typical Dose
A typical dose of wild lettuce may range from 0.5 to 3.0 gm of the dried leaves.

Possible Side Effects
Wild lettuce's side effects include sweating, dizziness, rapid heartbeat, and ringing in the ears.

Drugs That May Interact with Wild Lettuce
Taking wild lettuce with these drugs may increase the therapeutic and/or adverse effects of the drug:
- acetaminophen and codeine (Capital and Codeine, Tylenol with Codeine)
- alfentanil (Alfenta)
- alprazolam (Apo-Alpraz, Xanax)
- amobarbital (Amytal)
- amobarbital and secobarbital (Tuinal)
- aspirin and codeine (Coryphen Codeine)
- belladonna and opium (B&O Supprettes)
- bromazepam (Apo-Bromazepam, Gen-Bromazepam)
- brotizolam (Lendorm, Sintonal)
- buprenorphine (Buprenex, Subutex)
- buprenorphine and naloxone (Suboxone)
- butabarbital (Butisol Sodium)

- butalbital, acetaminophen, and caffeine (Esgic, Fioricet)
- butalbital, aspirin, and caffeine (Fiorinal)
- butorphanol (Apo-Butorphanol, Stadol)
- chloral hydrate (Aquachloral Supprettes, Somnote)
- chlordiazepoxide (Apo-Chlordiazepoxide, Librium)
- clobazam (Alti-Clobazam, Frisium)
- clonazepam (Klonopin, Rivotril)
- clorazepate (Tranxene, T-Tab)
- codeine (Codeine Contin)
- dexmedetomidine (Precedex)
- diazepam (Apo-Diazepam, Valium)
- dihydrocodeine, aspirin, and caffeine (Synalgos-DC)
- diphenhydramine (Benadryl Allergy, Nytol)
- estazolam (ProSom)
- fentanyl (Actiq, Duragesic)
- flurazepam (Apo-Flurazepam, Dalmane)
- glutethimide
- haloperidol (Haldol, Novo-Peridol)
- hydrocodone and acetaminophen (Vicodin, Zydone)
- hydrocodone and aspirin (Damason-P)
- hydrocodone and ibuprofen (Vicoprofen)
- hydromorphone (Dilaudid, PMS-Hydromorphone)
- hydroxyzine (Atarax, Vistaril)
- levomethadyl acetate hydrochloride
- levorphanol (Levo-Dromoran)
- loprazolam (Dormonoct, Havlane)
- lorazepam (Ativan, Nu-Loraz)
- meperidine (Demerol, Meperitab)
- meperidine and promethazine
- mephobarbital (Mebaral)
- methadone (Dolophine, Methadose)
- methohexital (Brevital, Brevital Sodium)
- midazolam (Apo-Midazolam, Versed)
- morphine sulfate (Kadian, MS Contin)
- nalbuphine (Nubain)
- opium tincture
- oxycodone (OxyContin, Roxicodone)
- oxycodone and acetaminophen (Endocet, Percocet)
- oxycodone and aspirin (Endodan, Percodan)
- oxymorphone (Numorphan)
- paregoric
- pentazocine (Talwin)
- pentobarbital (Nembutal)
- phenobarbital (Luminal Sodium, PMS-Phenobarbital)
- phenoperidine
- prazepam
- primidone (Apo-Primidone, Mysoline)
- promethazine (Phenergan)
- propofol (Diprivan)
- propoxyphene (Darvon, Darvon-N)
- propoxyphene and acetaminophen (Darvocet-N 50, Darvocet-N 100)
- propoxyphene, aspirin, and caffeine (Darvon Compound)
- quazepam (Doral)
- remifentanil (Ultiva)
- secobarbital (Seconal)
- sodium oxybate (Xyrem)
- sufentanil (Sufenta)
- s-zopiclone (Lunesta)
- temazepam (Novo-Temazepam, Restoril)
- tetrazepam (Mobiforton, Musapam)
- thiopental (Pentothal)
- triazolam (Apo-Triazo, Halcion)
- zaleplon (Sonata, Stamoc)
- zolpidem (Ambien)
- zopiclone (Alti-Zopiclone, Gen-Zopiclone)

Lab Tests That May Be Altered by Wild Lettuce
None known

Diseases That May Be Worsened or Triggered by Wild Lettuce
May worsen cases of benign prostatic hyperplasia (BPH) and narrow-angle glaucoma, due to hyoscyamine content.

Foods That May Interact with Wild Lettuce
None known

Supplements That May Interact with Wild Lettuce
- Increased risk of bleeding when used with herbs and supplements that might affect platelet aggregation. (For a list of herbs and supplements with anticoagulant/antiplatelet effects, see Appendix B.)
- May enhance therapeutic and adverse effects of herbs and supplements that have sedative properties, such as 5-HTP, kava kava, St. John's wort, and valerian. (For a list of herbs and supplements that have sedative properties, see Appendix B.)

WILD YAM

> The rootlike parts of wild yams contain diosgenin, a steroidlike substance that, until 1970, was the sole source of hormone used in the manufacture of birth control pills. Today wild yam continues to be the most popular source of natural progesterone, a common remedy for menopausal symptoms. Wild yam is also used to treat cramps, menstrual problems, and rheumatic conditions.

Scientific Name
Dioscorea villosa

Wild Yam Is Also Commonly Known As
China root, colic root, Mexican wild yam, rheumatism root, yuma

Medicinal Parts
Rhizome, root

Wild Yam's Uses
To treat menstrual problems, rheumatic conditions, and gallbladder colic

Typical Dose
There is no typical dose of wild yam.

Possible Side Effects
Wild yam's side effects include menstrual changes, headache, and allergic reactions.

Drugs That May Interact with Wild Yam
Taking wild yam with these drugs may increase the estrogenic effect of the drug:
- cyproterone and ethinyl estradiol (Diane-35)
- estradiol (Climara, Estrace)
- estradiol and norethindrone (Activella, CombiPatch)
- estradiol and testosterone (Climacteron)
- estrogens (conjugated A/synthetic) (Cenestin)
- estrogens (conjugated/equine) (Congest, Premarin)
- estrogens (conjugated/equine) and medroxyprogesterone (Premphase, Prempro)
- estrogens (esterified) (Estratab, Menest)
- estrogens (esterified) and methyltestosterone (Estratest, Estratest H.S.)
- estropipate (Ogen, Ortho-Est)

- ethinyl estradiol (Estinyl)
- ethinyl estradiol and desogestrel (Cyclessa, Ortho-Cept)
- ethinyl estradiol and ethynodiol diacetate (Demulen, Zovia)
- ethinyl estradiol and etonogestrel (NuvaRing)
- ethinyl estradiol and levonorgestrel (Alesse, Triphasil)
- ethinyl estradiol and norelgestromin (Evra, Ortho Evra)
- ethinyl estradiol and norethindrone (Brevicon, Ortho-Novum)
- ethinyl estradiol and norgestimate (Cyclen, Ortho Tri-Cyclen)
- ethinyl estradiol and norgestrel (Cryselle, Ovral)
- mestranol and norethindrone (Necon 1/50, Ortho-Novum 1/50)
- polyestradiol

Taking wild yam with these drugs may decrease the anti-inflammatory effect of the drug:
- celecoxib (Celebrex)
- etodolac (Lodine, Utradol)
- ibuprofen (Advil, Motrin)
- indomethacin (Indocin, Novo-Methacin)
- ketoprofen (Orudis, Rhodis)
- ketorolac (Acular, Toradol)
- piroxicam, (Feldene, Nu-Pirox)
- rofecoxib (Vioxx)

Lab Tests That May Be Altered by Wild Yam
None known

Diseases That May Be Worsened or Triggered by Wild Yam
This herb may have estrogen-like effects and should not be used by women with estrogen-sensitive breast cancer or other hormone-sensitive conditions.

Foods That May Interact with Wild Yam
None known

Supplements That May Interact with Wild Yam
None known

WINTERGREEN

Sometimes referred to as the little tea in the woods, this aromatic evergreen shrub produces bright red berries that provide wintergreen flavoring, used in teas, candies, and breath mints. Wintergreen leaves contain salicylates, the pain-relieving ingredient in aspirin, which is most likely the reason they have been considered useful in treating nerve ailments, arthritis, and menstrual pain.

Scientific Name
Gaultheria procumbens

Wintergreen Is Also Commonly Known As
Canada tea, checkerberry, deerberry, hillberry, mountain tea, spiceberry, teaberry

Medicinal Parts
Leaf, fruit, oil taken from leaf

Wintergreen's Uses
To treat sciatica and other nerve ailments, menstrual problems, rheumatoid arthritis, asthma, and pleurisy

Typical Dose
There is no standard dosage of wintergreen.

Possible Side Effects

Wintergreen's side effects include lack of appetite, lethargy, and gastrointestinal irritation.

Drugs That May Interact with Wintergreen

Taking wintergreen with these drugs may cause or increase kidney damage:

- etodolac (Lodine, Utradol)
- ibuprofen (Advil, Motrin)
- indomethacin (Indocin, Novo-Methacin)
- ketoprofen (Orudis, Rhodis)
- ketorolac (Acular, Toradol)
- meloxicam (MOBIC, Mobicox)
- metformin (Glucophage, Riomet)
- methotrexate (Rheumatrex, Trexall)
- miglitol (Glyset)
- morphine hydrochloride
- morphine sulfate (Kadian, MS Contin)
- naproxen (Aleve, Naprosyn)
- nitrofurantoin (Furadantin, Macrobid)
- ofloxacin (Floxin, Ocuflox)
- penicillin (Pfizerpen, Wycillin)
- piroxicam (Feldene, Nu-Pirox)
- propoxyphene (Darvon, Darvon-N)
- rifampin (Rifadin, Rimactane)
- stavudine (Zerit)
- sucralfate (Carafate, Sulcrate)
- tramadol (Ultram)
- valacyclovir (Valtrex)
- valganciclovir (Valcyte)
- vancomycin (Vancocin)
- zidovudine (Novo-AZT, Retrovir)

Taking wintergreen with these drugs may increase the risk of bleeding or bruising:

- aminosalicylic acid (Nemasol Sodium, Paser)
- antithrombin III (Thrombate III)
- argatroban
- aspirin (Bufferin, Ecotrin)
- bivalirudin (Angiomax)
- choline magnesium trisalicylate (Trilisate)
- choline salicylate (Teejel)
- dalteparin (Fragmin)
- danaparoid (Orgaran)
- enoxaparin (Lovenox)
- fondaparinux (Arixtra)
- heparin (Hepalean, Hep-Lock)
- lepirudin (Refludan)
- salsalate (Amgesic, Salflex)
- tinzaparin (Innohep)
- warfarin (Coumadin, Jantoven)

Lab Tests That May Be Altered by Wintergreen

None known

Diseases That May Be Worsened or Triggered by Wintergreen

- May worsen gastrointestinal irritation or inflammatory diseases.
- Wintergreen oil may trigger salicylate allergies or other allergic reactions.

Foods That May Interact with Wintergreen

None known

Supplements That May Interact with Wintergreen

None known

WITCH HAZEL

Although it sounds like something brewed on Halloween, the "witch" part of "witch hazel" actually

continued

comes from the Old English word *wice*, meaning "weak." This refers to the pliability and easy breakage of the branches of the *Hamamelis virginiana* shrub, from which witch hazel is derived. "Hazel" refers to the color of the shrub, golden brown mixed with green. Witch hazel, a steam distillate of freshly picked twigs combined with alcohol, is prized for its soothing, anti-inflammatory properties and is used for treating cuts, scrapes, bruises, hemorrhoids, and varicose veins.

Scientific Name
Hamamelis virginiana

Witch Hazel Is Also Commonly Known As
Hamamelis, snapping hazel, spotted alder, striped alder, tobacco wood, winterbloom

Medicinal Parts
Bark, leaf, twigs

Witch Hazel's Uses
To treat wounds, diarrhea, hemorrhoids, and menstrual complaints. Germany's Commission E has approved the topical use of witch hazel bark and leaf to treat hemorrhoids, skin inflammation, problems with veins, and wounds and burns. It has approved the use of witch hazel leaf for treating inflammation of the mouth and throat.

Typical Dose
A typical dose of witch hazel leaf may range from 2 to 3 gm of the herb in 150 ml of water as a gargle solution.

Possible Side Effects
❶ Witch hazel should not be taken internally, as it may cause nausea, vomiting, constipation, and possible liver damage. When used topically, witch hazel may cause allergic reactions.

Drugs That May Interact with Witch Hazel
Taking witch hazel internally with these drugs may increase the risk of hypertension (high blood pressure):

- ephedrine (Pretz-D)
- ergotamine (Cafergor, Cafergot)
- rizatriptan benzoate (Maxalt)
- zolmitriptan (Zomig)

Taking witch hazel internally with these drugs may reduce or prevent absorption of the drug:

- ferric gluconate (Ferrlecit)
- ferrus fumarate (Femiron, Feostat)
- ferrous gluconate (Fergon, Novo-Ferrogluc)
- ferrous sulfate (Feratab, Fer-Iron)
- ferrous sulfate and ascorbic acid (FeroGrad 500, Vitelle Irospan)
- iron-dextran complex (Dexferrum, INFeD)
- polysaccharide-iron complex (Hytinic, Niferex)

Lab Tests That May Be Altered by Witch Hazel
None known

Diseases That May Be Worsened or Triggered by Witch Hazel
Gastrointestinal disturbances may be caused or worsened and liver damage may occur with long-term internal administration of witch hazel.

Foods That May Interact with Witch Hazel
None known

Supplements That May Interact with Witch Hazel
None known

WOOD BETONY

The name "betony" is said to come from the Celtic words *bew*, meaning "head," and *ton*, meaning "good," suggesting that it's good for complaints in the head. And indeed, wood betony has been used for centuries to treat headaches, migraines, and seizures. Also, since it contains high amounts of tannin, wood betony is an effective astringent, anti-inflammatory, and antidiarrheal. One of its chemical components, stachydrine, is used to lower high blood pressure.

Scientific Name
Betonica officinalis

Wood Betony Is Also Commonly Known As
Betony, bishopswort, hedge nettles

Medicinal Parts
Flowering herb, leaf

Wood Betony's Uses
To treat asthma, bronchitis, anxiety, diarrhea, gout, and heartburn; as a sedative

Typical Dose
A typical daily dose of wood betony may range from 1 to 2 gm of the powdered herb, divided into three doses.

Possible Side Effects
Wood betony's side effects include gastrointestinal irritation.

Drugs That May Interact with Wood Betony
Taking wood betony with these drugs may increase the risk of hypotension (excessively low blood pressure):

- acebutolol (Novo-Acebutolol, Sectral)
- amlodipine (Norvasc)
- atenolol (Apo-Atenol, Tenormin)
- benazepril (Lotensin)
- betaxolol (Betoptic S, Kerlone)
- bisoprolol (Monocor, Zebeta)
- bumetanide (Bumex, Burinex)
- candesartan (Atacand)
- captopril (Capoten, Novo-Captopril)
- carteolol (Cartrol, Ocupress)
- carvedilol (Coreg)
- chlorothiazide (Diuril)
- chlorthalidone (Apo-Chlorthalidone, Thalitone)
- clonidine (Catapres, Duraclon)
- diazoxide (Hyperstat, Proglycem)
- diltiazem (Cardizem, Tiazac)
- doxazosin (Alti-Doxazosin, Cardura)
- enalapril (Vasotec)
- eplerenone (Inspra)
- eprosartan (Teveten)
- esmolol (Brevibloc)
- felodipine (Plendil, Renedil)
- fenoldopam (Corlopam)
- fosinopril (Monopril)
- furosemide (Apo-Furosemide, Lasix)
- guanabenz (Wytensin)
- guanadrel (Hylorel)
- guanfacine (Tenex)
- hydralazine (Apresoline, Novo-Hylazin)
- hydrochlorothiazide (Apo-Hydro, Microzide)
- hydrochlorothiazide and triamterene (Dyazide, Maxzide)
- indapamide (Lozol, Nu-Indapamide)
- irbesartan (Avapro)
- isradipine (DynaCirc)

- labetalol (Normodyne, Trandate)
- lisinopril (Prinivil, Zestril)
- losartan (Cozaar)
- mecamylamine (Inversine)
- mefruside (Baycaron)
- methyclothiazide (Aquatensen, Enduron)
- methyldopa (Apo-Methyldopa, Nu-Medopa)
- metolazone (Mykrox, Zaroxolyn)
- metoprolol (Betaloc, Lopressor)
- minoxidil (Loniten, Rogaine)
- moexipril (Univasc)
- nadolol (Apo-Nadol, Corgard)
- nicardipine (Cardene)
- nifedipine (Adalat CC, Procardia)
- nisoldipine (Sular)
- nitroglycerin (Minitran, Nitro-Dur)
- nitroprusside (Nipride, Nitropress)
- olmesartan (Benicar)
- oxprenolol (Slow-Trasicor, Trasicor)
- perindopril erbumine (Aceon, Coversyl)
- phenoxybenzamine (Dibenzyline)
- phentolamine (Regitine, Rogitine)
- pindolol (Apo-Pindol, Novo-Pindol)
- polythiazide (Renese)
- prazosin (Minipress, Nu-Prazo)
- propranolol (Inderal, InnoPran XL)
- quinapril (Accupril)
- ramipril (Altace)
- reserpine
- spironolactone (Aldactone, Novo-Spiroton)
- telmisartan (Micardis)
- terazosin (Alti-Terazosin, Hytrin)
- timolol (Betimol, Timoptic)
- torsemide (Demadex)
- trandolapril (Mavik)
- triamterene (Dyrenium)
- trichlormethiazide (Metatensin, Naqua)

- valsartan (Diovan)
- verapamil (Calan, Isoptin SR)

Lab Tests That May Be Altered by Wood Betony
None known

Diseases That May Be Worsened or Triggered by Wood Betony
None known

Foods That May Interact with Wood Betony
None known

Supplements That May Interact with Wood Betony
The tannins in wood betony may cause the alkaloids in certain other herbs to separate and settle, increasing the risk of toxic reactions. (For a list of herbs and other substances high in alkaloids, see Appendix B.)

WORMSEED

Also known as Eurasian wormwood, this desert plant produces a substance called santonin, which is extracted from its dried, unopened flowerheads. Wormseed is used as a rapid treatment for roundworms and threadworms, although it does not appear to affect tapeworms.

Scientific Name
Artemisia cina

Wormseed Is Also Commonly Known As
Eurasian wormwood, levant, santonica, sea wormwood

Medicinal Parts

Flower bud

Wormseed's Uses

To treat worm infestation and fever

Typical Dose

A typical daily dose of wormseed has not been established.

Possible Side Effects

Wormseed's side effects include muscle twitching, stupor, and kidney irritation.

Drugs That May Interact with Wormseed

Taking wormseed with these anticonvulsant drugs may increase the risk of seizures:

- acetazolamide (Apo-Acetazolamide, Diamox Sequels)
- amobarbital (Amytal)
- barbexaclone (Maliasin)
- carbamazepine (Carbatrol, Tegretol)
- clonazepam (Klonopin, Rivotril)
- clorazepate (Tranxene, T-Tab)
- diazepam (Apo-Diazepam, Valium)
- ethosuximide (Zarontin)
- felbamate (Felbatol)
- fosphenytoin (Cerebyx)
- gabapentin (Neurontin, Nu-Gabapentin)
- lamotrigine (Lamictal)
- levetiracetam (Keppra)
- lorazepam (Ativan, Nu-Loraz)
- mephobarbital (Mebaral)
- methsuximide (Celontin)
- oxazepam (Novoxapam, Serax)
- oxcarbazepine (Trileptal)
- pentobarbital (Nembutal)
- phenobarbital (Luminal Sodium, PMS-Phenobarbital)
- phenytoin (Dilantin, Phenytek)
- primidone (Apo-Primidone, Mysoline)
- thiopental (Pentothal)
- tiagabine (Gabitril)
- topiramate (Topamax)
- valproic acid (Depacon, Depakote ER)
- vigabatrin (Sabril)
- zonisamide (Zonegran)

Lab Tests That May Be Altered by Wormseed

None known

Diseases That May Be Worsened or Triggered by Wormseed

None known

Foods That May Interact with Wormseed

None known

Supplements That May Interact with Wormseed

None known

WORMWOOD

A bitter tonic once used to expel intestinal worms, wormwood was poured into the ink used by medieval scholars to repel bookworms and other book-destroying creatures. Wormwood was the main flavoring in the 136-proof alcoholic beverage called absinthe, a drink now banned in the United States. Today wormwood is primarily used to stimulate the appetite, digestive juices, peristalsis (the movement of substances through the colon), and the action of the liver and gallbladder.

Scientific Name
Artemisia absinthium

Wormwood Is Also Commonly Known As
Absinthe, green ginger

Medicinal Parts
Shoot, leaf

Wormwood's Uses
To treat worm infestation, bloating, liver ailments, loss of appetite, and anemia. Germany's Commission E has approved the use of wormwood to treat dyspeptic complaints, such as heartburn, bloating, and loss of appetite.

Typical Dose
A typical dose of wormwood is 1 to 2 ml of liquid extract taken three times daily.

Possible Side Effects
Wormwood's side effects include vomiting, dizziness, and headache.

Drugs That May Interact with Wormwood
Taking wormwood with these drugs may reduce the seizure threshold:
- amitriptyline (Elavil, Levate)
- amoxapine (Asendin)
- bupropion (Wellbutrin, Zyban)
- carbamazepine (Carbatrol, Tegretol)
- ciprofloxacin (Ciloxan, Cipro)
- desipramine (Alti-Desipramine, Norpramin)
- doxepin (Sinequan, Zonalon)
- fosphenytoin (Cerebyx)
- ganciclovir (Cytovene, Vitrasert)
- imipramine (Apo-Imipramine, Tofranil)
- levetiracetam (Keppra)
- methylphenidate (Concerta, Ritalin)
- metoclopramide (Apo-Metoclop, Reglan)
- metronidazole (Flagyl, Noritate)
- moxifloxacin (Avelox, Vigamox)
- nortriptyline (Aventyl HCl, Pamelor)
- ofloxacin (Floxin, Ocuflox)
- olanzapine (Zydix, Zyprexa)
- oxcarbazepine (Trileptal)
- phenobarbital (Luminal Sodium, PMS-Phenobarbital)
- phenytoin (Dilantin, Phenytek)
- prochlorperazine (Compazine, Compro)
- quetiapine (Seroquel)
- tramadol (Ultram)
- venlafaxine (Effexor)

Taking wormwood with these drugs may interfere with absorption of the drug:
- ferric gluconate (Ferrlecit)
- ferrous fumarate (Femiron, Feostat)
- ferrous gluconate (Fergon, Novo-Ferrogluc)
- ferrous sulfate (Feratab, Fer-Iron)
- ferrous sulfate and ascorbic acid (Fero-Grad 500, Vitelle Irospan)
- iron-dextran complex (Dexferrum, INFeD)
- polysaccharide-iron complex (Hytinic, Niferex)

Lab Tests That May Be Altered by Wormwood
None known

Diseases That May Be Worsened or Triggered by Wormwood
May worsen ulcers by irritating the gastrointestinal tract.

Foods That May Interact with Wormwood
None known

Supplements That May Interact with Wormwood

Increased risk of thujone toxicity when taken with herbs containing thujone, such as oak moss, Oriental arborvitae, sage, tansy, and tree moss.

YARROW

A major healing herb during medieval times, yarrow was carried in pouches by doctors and common people alike as a sort of first-aid kit to treat wounds and ward off infections. Yarrow is used today to treat problems with the gastrointestinal, respiratory, urinary, and reproductive tracts.

Scientific Name

Achillea millefolium

Yarrow Is Also Commonly Known As

Bloodwort, carpenter's weed, milfoil, nose bleed, old man's pepper

Medicinal Parts

Flower, above-ground parts

Yarrow's Uses

To treat mild spasms of the gastrointestinal tract, loss of appetite, wounds, uterine/pelvic complaints, and bleeding hemorrhoids. Germany's Commission E has approved the use of yarrow to treat gastrointestinal discomfort and complaints, loss of appetite, and female abdominal complaints.

Typical Dose

A typical dose of yarrow is approximately 2 gm of finely cut herb mixed with 150 ml boiling water, steeped for 10 to 15 minutes, strained and taken as a tea three to four times daily between meals.

Possible Side Effects

Yarrow's side effects include drowsiness, uterine stimulation, and contact dermatitis.

Drugs That May Interact with Yarrow

Taking yarrow with these drugs may interfere with the absorption of the drug:

- ferric gluconate (Ferrlecit)
- ferrous fumarate (Femiron, Feostat)
- ferrous gluconate (Fergon, Novo-Ferrogluc)
- ferrous sulfate (Feratab, Fer-Iron)
- ferrous sulfate and ascorbic acid (Fero-Grad 500, Vitelle Irospan)
- iron-dextran complex (Dexferrum, INFeD)
- polysaccharide-iron complex (Hytinic, Niferex)

Taking yarrow with these drugs may disrupt blood sugar control:

- acarbose (Prandase, Precose)
- glipizide (Glucotrol)
- glyburide (DiaBeta, Micronase)
- insulin (Humulin, Novolin R)
- metformin (Glucophage, Riomet)
- miglitol (Glyset)
- pioglitazone (Actos)
- repaglinide (GlucoNorm, Prandin)
- rosiglitazone (Avandia)

Taking yarrow with these drugs may increase the risk of hypotension (excessively low blood pressure):

- acebutolol (Novo-Acebutolol, Sectral)
- amlodipine (Norvasc)
- atenolol (Apo-Atenol, Tenormin)
- benazepril (Lotensin)
- betaxolol (Betoptic S, Kerlone)
- bisoprolol (Monocor, Zebeta)
- bumetanide (Bumex, Burinex)
- candesartan (Atacand)
- captopril (Capoten, Novo-Captopril)
- carteolol (Cartrol, Ocupress)
- carvedilol (Coreg)
- chlorothiazide (Diuril)
- chlorthalidone (Apo-Chlorthalidone, Thalitone)
- clonidine (Catapres, Duraclon)
- diazoxide (Hyperstat, Proglycem)
- diltiazem (Cardizem, Tiazac)
- doxazosin (Alti-Doxazosin, Cardura)
- enalapril (Vasotec)
- eplerenone (Inspra)
- eprosartan (Teveten)
- esmolol (Brevibloc)
- felodipine (Plendil, Renedil)
- fenoldopam (Corlopam)
- fosinopril (Monopril)
- furosemide (Apo-Furosemide, Lasix)
- guanabenz (Wytensin)
- guanadrel (Hylorel)
- guanfacine (Tenex)
- hydralazine (Apresoline, Novo-Hylazin)
- hydrochlorothiazide (Apo-Hydro, Microzide)
- hydrochlorothiazide and triamterene (Dyazide, Maxzide)
- indapamide (Lozol, Nu-Indapamide)
- irbesartan (Avapro)
- isradipine (DynaCirc)
- labetalol (Normodyne, Trandate)
- lisinopril (Prinivil, Zestril)
- losartan (Cozaar)
- mecamylamine (Inversine)
- mefruside (Baycaron)
- methyclothiazide (Aquatensen, Enduron)
- methyldopa (Apo-Methyldopa, Nu-Medopa)
- metolazone (Mykrox, Zaroxolyn)
- metoprolol (Betaloc, Lopressor)
- minoxidil (Loniten, Rogaine)
- moexipril (Univasc)
- nadolol (Apo-Nadol, Corgard)
- nicardipine (Cardene)
- nifedipine (Adalat CC, Procardia)
- nisoldipine (Sular)
- nitroglycerin (Minitran, Nitro-Dur)
- nitroprusside (Nipride, Nitropress)
- olmesartan (Benicar)
- oxprenolol (Slow-Trasicor, Trasicor)
- perindopril erbumine (Aceon, Coversyl)
- phenoxybenzamine (Dibenzyline)
- phentolamine (Regitine, Rogitine)
- pindolol (Apo-Pindol, Novo-Pindol)
- polythiazide (Renese)
- prazosin (Minipress, Nu-Prazo)
- propranolol (Inderal, InnoPran XL)
- quinapril (Accupril)
- ramipril (Altace)
- reserpine
- spironolactone (Aldactone, Novo-Spiroton)
- telmisartan (Micardis)
- terazosin (Alti-Terazosin, Hytrin)
- timolol (Betimol, Timoptic)
- torsemide (Demadex)
- trandolapril (Mavik)
- triamterene (Dyrenium)
- trichlormethiazide (Metatensin, Naqua)
- valsartan (Diovan)
- verapamil (Calan, Isoptin SR)

Taking yarrow with these drugs may increase the risk of bleeding or bruising:

- abciximab (ReoPro)
- aminosalicylic acid (Nemasol Sodium, Paser)
- antithrombin III (Thrombate III)
- argatroban
- aspirin (Bufferin, Ecotrin)
- aspirin and dipyridamole (Aggrenox)
- bivalirudin (Angiomax)
- choline magnesium trisalicylate (Trilisate)
- choline salicylate (Teejel)
- clopidogrel (Plavix)
- dalteparin (Fragmin)
- danaparoid (Orgaran)
- dipyridamole (Novo-Dipiradol, Persantine)
- enoxaparin (Lovenox)
- eptifibatide (Integrillin)
- fondaparinux (Arixtra)
- heparin (Hepalean, Hep-Lock)
- indobufen (Ibustrin)
- lepirudin (Refludan)
- salsalate (Amgesic, Salflex)
- ticlopidine (Alti-Ticlopidine, Ticlid)
- tinzaparin (Innohep)
- tirofiban (Aggrastat)
- warfarin (Coumadin, Jantoven)

Taking yarrow with these drugs may increase the risk of excessive sedation and mental depression and impairment:

- acetaminophen and codeine (Capital and Codeine, Tylenol with Codeine)
- alfentanil (Alfenta)
- alprazolam (Apo-Alpraz, Xanax)
- amobarbital (Amytal)
- amobarbital and secobarbital (Tuinal)
- aspirin and codeine (Coryphen Codeine)

- belladonna and opium (B&O Supprettes)
- bromazepam (Apo-Bromazepam, Gen-Bromazepam)
- brotizolam (Lendorm, Sintonal)
- buprenorphine (Buprenex, Subutex)
- buprenorphine and naloxone (Suboxone)
- butabarbital (Butisol Sodium)
- butalbital, acetaminophen, and caffeine (Esgic, Fioricet)
- butalbital, aspirin, and caffeine (Fiorinal)
- butorphanol (Apo-Butorphanol, Stadol)
- chloral hydrate (Aquachloral Supprettes, Somnote)
- chlordiazepoxide (Apo-Chlordiazepoxide, Librium)
- clobazam (Alti-Clobazam, Frisium)
- clonazepam (Klonopin, Rivotril)
- clorazepate (Tranxene, T-Tab)
- codeine (Codeine Contin)
- dexmedetomidine (Precedex)
- diazepam (Apo-Diazepam, Valium)
- dihydrocodeine, aspirin, and caffeine (Synalgos-DC)
- diphenhydramine (Benadryl Allergy, Nytol)
- estazolam (ProSom)
- fentanyl (Actiq, Duragesic)
- flurazepam (Apo-Flurazepam, Dalmane)
- glutethimide
- haloperidol (Haldol, Novo-Peridol)
- hydrocodone and acetaminophen (Vicodin, Zydone)
- hydrocodone and aspirin (Damason-P)
- hydrocodone and ibuprofen (Vicoprofen)
- hydromorphone (Dilaudid, PMS-Hydromorphone)
- hydroxyzine (Atarax, Vistaril)
- levomethadyl acetate hydrochloride

- levorphanol (LevoDromoran)
- loprazolam (Dormonoct, Havlane)
- lorazepam (Ativan, Nu-Loraz)
- meperidine (Demerol, Meperitab)
- meperidine and promethazine
- mephobarbital (Mebaral)
- methadone (Dolophine, Methadose)
- methohexital (Brevital, Brevital Sodium)
- midazolam (Apo-Midazolam, Versed)
- morphine sulfate (Kadian, MS Contin)
- nalbuphine (Nubain)
- opium tincture
- oxycodone (OxyContin, Roxicodone)
- oxycodone and acetaminophen (Endocet, Percocet)
- oxycodone and aspirin (Endodan, Percodan)
- oxymorphone (Numorphan)
- paregoric
- pentazocine (Talwin)
- pentobarbital (Nembutal)
- phenobarbital (Luminal Sodium, PMS-Phenobarbital)
- phenoperidine
- prazepam
- primidone (Apo-Primidone, Mysoline)
- promethazine (Phenergan)
- propofol (Diprivan)
- propoxyphene (Darvon, Darvon-N)
- propoxyphene and acetaminophen (Darvocet-N 50, Darvocet-N 100)
- propoxyphene, aspirin, and caffeine (Darvon Compound)
- quazepam (Doral)
- remifentanil (Ultiva)
- secobarbital (Seconal)
- sufentanil (Sufenta)

- s-zopiclone (Lunesta)
- temazepam (Novo-Temazepam, Restoril)
- tetrazepam (Mobiforton, Musapam)
- thiopental (Pentothal)
- triazolam (Apo-Triazo, Halcion)
- zaleplon (Sonata, Stamoc)
- zolpidem (Ambien)
- zopiclone (Alti-Zopiclone, Gen-Zopiclone)

Taking yarrow with this drug may be harmful:
- sucralfate (Carafate, Sulcrate)—may interfere with the action of the drug

Lab Tests That May Be Altered by Yarrow
None known

Diseases That May Be Worsened or Triggered by Yarrow
None known

Foods That May Interact with Yarrow
None known

Supplements That May Interact with Yarrow
Increased risk of thujone toxicity when taken with herbs containing thujone, such as oak moss, Oriental arborvitae, sage, tansy, and tree moss.

YELLOW DOCK

Native to Europe and Africa, yellow dock, a member of the buckwheat family, gets its scientific name *rumex* from the Latin word for "lance," and *crispus* from the Latin word for "curly," referring to the lancelike, curly shape of the leaf. Yellow dock is one of the chief ingredients of essiac, an anticancer folk remedy. Today we know that yellow dock is a source of emodin and rhein, two phytochemicals shown to exert antitumor activity in laboratory animals.

Scientific Name
Rumex crispus

Yellow Dock Is Also Commonly Known As
Curled dock, garden patience, hualtata, narrow dock, sour dock

Medicinal Parts
Root

Yellow Dock's Uses
To treat sore throat, fever, psoriasis, and inflammation of the nasal passages; to purify the blood

Typical Dose
A typical daily dose of yellow dock may range from 2.5 to 5.0 mg of the dried root.

Possible Side Effects
Yellow dock's side effects include mucous membrane irritation, nausea, vomiting, and allergic reactions.

Drugs That May Interact with Yellow Dock
Taking yellow dock with these drugs may reduce or prevent drug absorption:
- ferric gluconate (Ferrlecit)
- ferrous fumarate (Femiron, Feostat)
- ferrous gluconate (Fergon, Novo-Ferrogluc)
- ferrous sulfate (Feratab, Fer-Iron)
- ferrous sulfate and ascorbic acid (FeroGrad 500, Vitelle Irospan)
- iron-dextran complex (Dexferrum, INFeD)
- polysaccharide-iron complex (Hytinic, Niferex)

Taking yellow dock with these drugs may increase the risk of hypokalemia (low levels of potassium in the blood):
- acetazolamide (Apo-Acetazolamide, Diamox Sequels)
- azosemide (Diat)
- bumetanide (Bumex, Burinex)
- chlorothiazide (Diuril)
- chlorthalidone (Apo-Chlorthalidone, Thalitone)
- digitalis (Digitek, Lanoxin)
- ethacrynic acid (Edecrin)
- etozolin (Elkapin)
- furosemide (Apo-Furosemide, Lasix)
- hydrochlorothiazide (Apo-Hydro, Microzide)
- hydroflumethiazide (Diucardin, Saluron)
- indapamide (Lozol, Nu-Indapamide)
- mannitol (Osmitrol, Resectisol)
- mefruside (Baycaron)
- methazolamide (Apo-Methazolamide, Neptazane)
- methyclothiazide (Aquatensen, Enduron)
- metolazone (Mykrox, Zaroxolyn)
- olmesartan and hydrochlorothiazide (Benicar HCT)
- polythiazide (Renese)
- torsemide (Demadex)
- trichlormethiazide (Metatensin, Naqua)
- urea (Amino-Cerv, UltraMide)
- xipamide (Diurexan, Lumitens)

Taking yellow dock with this drug may be harmful:

- digitalis (Digitek, Lanoxin)—may increase risk of drug toxicity

Lab Tests That May Be Altered by Yellow Dock

- May decrease serum potassium levels.
- May confound results of diagnostic urine tests that rely on a color change by discoloring urine (pink, red, purple, or orange).

Diseases That May Be Worsened or Triggered by Yellow Dock

- May worsen bleeding disorders.
- May worsen kidney damage.

Foods That May Interact with Yellow Dock

May decrease mineral absorption when taken with dietary calcium, iron, or zinc.

Supplements That May Interact with Yellow Dock

- May decrease mineral absorption when taken with calcium, iron, or zinc supplements.
- Increased risk of cardiac glycoside toxicity when used with other herbs that contain cardiac glycosides, such as black hellebore, calotropis, motherwort, and others. (For a list of cardiac glycoside–containing herbs and supplements, see Appendix B.)
- Increased risk of potassium depletion when used with other stimulant laxative herbs, such as black root, cascara sagrada, castor oil, and senna. (For a list of stimulant laxative herbs and supplements, see Appendix B.)

YELLOW GENTIAN

Yellow gentian is named for Gentius, the first-century B.C. king of Illyria, who is credited with discovering the herb's medicinal properties. Yellow gentian contains the extremely bitter glycoside amarogentin, which is said to promote digestion, ease gastrointestinal inflammation, and lessen fevers. An anti-inflammatory, antifungal agent, yellow gentian is thought to help lower fevers and help control blood sugar.

Scientific Name

Gentiana lutea

Yellow Gentian Is Also Commonly Known As

Bitter root, bitterwort, English gentian, gentian, gentian root

Medicinal Parts

Underground parts

Yellow Gentian's Uses

To treat loss of appetite, flatulence, and heartburn. Germany's Commission E has approved the use of yellow gentian to treat loss of appetite, flatulence, and dyspeptic complaints, such as heartburn and bloating.

Typical Dose

A typical dose of yellow gentian is approximately 1 gm of the root.

Possible Side Effects

Yellow gentian's side effects include gastrointestinal distress.

Drugs That May Interact with Yellow Gentian

Taking yellow gentian with these drugs may interfere with the action of the drug:

- aluminum hydroxide (AlternaGel, AluCap)
- aluminum hydroxide and magnesium carbonate (Gaviscon Extra Strength, Gaviscon Liquid)
- aluminum hydroxide and magnesium hydroxide (Maalox, Rulox)
- aluminum hydroxide and magnesium trisilicate (Gaviscon Tablet)
- aluminum hydroxide, magnesium hydroxide, and simethicone (Maalox, Mylanta Liquid)
- calcium carbonate (Rolaids Extra Strength, Tums)
- calcium carbonate and magnesium hydroxide (Mylanta Gelcaps, Rolaids Extra Strength)
- cimetidine (Nu-Cimet, Tagamet)
- esomeprazole (Nexium)
- famotidine (Apo-Famotidine, Pepcid)
- famotidine, calcium carbonate, and magnesium hydroxide (Pepcid Complete)
- lansoprazole (Prevacid)
- magaldrate and simethicone (Riopan Plus, Riopan Plus Double Strength)
- magnesium hydroxide (Dulcolax Milk of Magnesia, Phillips' Milk of Magnesia)
- magnesium oxide (Mag-Ox 400, Uro-Mag)
- magnesium sulfate (Epsom salts)
- nizatidine (Axid, PMS-Nizatidine)
- omeprazole (Losec, Prilosec)
- pantoprazole (Pantoloc, Protonix)
- rabeprazole (Aciphex, Pariet)
- ranitidine (Alti-Ranitidine, Zantac)
- sodium bicarbonate (Brioschi, Neut)

Lab Tests That May Be Altered by Yellow Gentian

None known

Diseases That May Be Worsened or Triggered by Yellow Gentian

May worsen cases of ulcers or other stomach ailments.

Foods That May Interact with Yellow Gentian

None known

Supplements That May Interact with Yellow Gentian

None known

YEW

This forty- to fifty-foot-tall tree with its wide-spreading branches was considered sacred by the Druids, who built their temples nearby. Later, early Christians followed suit, and these trees are still associated with places of worship. The yew's extremely hard, water-resistant wood was once in great demand for making longbows. Yew also has important medicinal uses, as it contains an anticancer substance called taxol, which has been refined to produce a drug used for breast cancer.

Scientific Name

Taxus baccata

Yew Is Also Commonly Known As

Chinwood, common yew, English yew, European yew

Medicinal Parts

Leaves, branches, twig tips

Yew's Uses

To treat epilepsy, worm infestation, diphtheria, rheumatism, and liver ailments

Typical Dose

There is no typical dose of yew.

Possible Side Effects

Yew's side effects include lowered blood pressure, irregular heartbeat, nausea, vomiting, allergic reactions, and joint and muscle pain.

Drugs That May Interact with Yew

Taking yew with these drugs may interfere with the action of the drug:

- omeprazole (Losec, Prilosec)
- pantoprazole (Pantoloc, Protonix)
- ranitidine (Alti-Ranitidine, Zantac)
- sucralfate (Carafate, Sulcrate)

Taking yew with these drugs may worsen the drug's side effects and/or interfere with the drug's action:

- docetaxel (Taxotere)
- paclitaxel (Onxol, Taxol)
- tamoxifen (Nolvadex, Tamofen)

Taking yew with these drugs may be harmful:

- ketoconazole (Apo-Ketoconazole, Nizoral)—may interfere with metabolism of the drug
- sucralfate (Carafate, Sulcrate)—may interfere with the action of the drug

Lab Tests That May Be Altered by Yew

None known

Diseases That May Be Worsened or Triggered by Yew

None known

Foods That May Interact with Yew

None known

Supplements That May Interact with Yew

None known

YOHIMBE

Taken from the bark of a West African tree, yohimbe was traditionally used as an aphrodisiac and a hallucinogen. Today, it is most often taken for impotence, exhaustion, elevated blood pressure, and nerve damage related to diabetes. It's believed that yohimbe helps with impotence by improving blood flow to the penis and increasing excitement of the nerves in the genital area.

Scientific Name

Pausinystalia yohimbe

Yohimbe Is Also Commonly Known As

Johimbi, yohimbe bark, yohimbehe, yohimbine

Medicinal Parts

Bark

Yohimbe's Uses

Treatment of erectile dysfunction, low blood pressure, exhaustion, and angina; as an aphrodisiac

Typical Dose

A typical dose of yohimbe for male erectile dysfunction is approximately 5.4 mg in tablet form, taken three times daily.

Possible Side Effects

Yohimbe's side effects include rapid heart rate, nausea, increased blood pressure, and anxiety.

Drugs That May Interact with Yohimbe

Taking yohimbe with these drugs may increase stimulation of the central nervous system:

- albuterol (Proventil, Ventolin)
- ephedrine (Pretz-D)
- fenoterol (Berotec)
- isoproterenol (Isuprel)
- levalbuterol (Xopenex)
- methylphenidate (Concerta, Ritalin)
- modafinil (Alertec, Provigil)
- naloxone (Narcan)
- naltrexone (ReVia)
- phenylephrine (Mydfrin, Vicks Sinex Nasal Spray)
- terbutaline (Brethine)
- valacyclovir (Valtrex)
- venlafaxine (Effexor)

Taking yohimbe with these drugs may cause or increase the risk of serotonin syndrome (symptoms of which include agitation, rapid heart rate, flushing, heavy sweating, and possibly even death):

- amitriptyline (Elavil, Levate)
- amoxapine (Asendin)
- citalopram (Celexa)
- desipramine (Alti-Desipramine, Norpramin)
- doxepin (Sinequan, Zonalon)
- imipramine (Apo-Imipramine, Tofranil)
- nortriptyline (Aventyl HCl, Pamelor)
- paroxetine (Paxil)
- sertraline (Apo-Sertraline, Zoloft)

Taking yohimbe with these drugs may cause or increase kidney damage:

- etodolac (Lodine, Utradol)
- ibuprofen (Advil, Motrin)
- indomethacin (Indocin, Novo-Methacin)
- ketoprofen (Orudis, Rhodis)
- ketorolac (Acular, Toradol)
- meloxicam (MOBIC, Mobicox)
- metformin (Glucophage, Riomet)
- methotrexate (Rheumatrex, Trexall)
- miglitol (Glyset)
- morphine hydrochloride
- morphine sulfate (Kadian, MS Contin)
- naproxen (Aleve, Naprosyn)
- nitrofurantoin (Furadantin, Macrobid)
- ofloxacin (Floxin, Ocuflox)
- penicillin (Pfizerpen, Wycillin)
- piroxicam (Feldene, Nu-Pirox)
- propoxyphene (Darvon, Darvon-N)
- rifampin (Rifadin, Rimactane)
- stavudine (Zerit)
- sucralfate (Carafate, Sulcrate)
- tramadol (Ultram)
- valacyclovir (Valtrex)
- valganciclovir (Valcyte)
- vancomycin (Vancocin)
- zidovudine (Novo-AZT, Retrovir)

Taking yohimbe with these drugs may increase the therapeutic and/or adverse effects of the drug:

- iproniazid (Marsilid)
- moclobemide (Alti-Moclobemide, Nu-Moclobemide)
- morphine sulfate (Kadian, MS Contin)
- phenelzine (Nardil)
- selegiline (Eldepryl)
- tranylcypromine (Parnate)

Taking yohimbe with these drugs may interfere with blood pressure control:

- acebutolol (Novo-Acebutolol, Sectral)
- acetazolamide (Apo-Acetazolamide, Diamox Sequels)
- amiloride (Midamor)
- amitriptyline (Elavil, Levate)
- amitriptyline and chlordiazepoxide (Limbitrol)
- amitriptyline and perphenazine (Etrafon, Triavil)
- amlodipine (Norvasc)
- amoxapine (Asendin)
- atenolol (Apo-Atenol, Tenormin)
- azosemide (Diat)
- befunolol (Bentos, Betaclar)
- benazepril (Lotensin)
- bepridil (Vascor)
- betaxolol (Betoptic S, Kerlone)
- bisoprolol (Monocor, Zebeta)
- bumetanide (Bumex, Burinex)
- candesartan (Atacand)
- captopril (Capoten, Novo-Captopril)
- carteolol (Cartrol, Ocupress)
- carvedilol (Coreg)
- celiprolol
- chlorothiazide (Diuril)
- chlorthalidone (Apo-Chlorthalidone, Thalitone)
- cilazapril (Inhibace)
- clomipramine (Anafranil, Novo-Clopramine)
- delapril (Adecut, Delakete)
- desipramine (Alti-Desipramine, Norpramin)
- diltiazem (Cardizem, Tiazac)
- doxazosin (Alti-Doxazosin, Cardura)
- doxepin (Sinequan, Zonalon)
- enalapril (Vasotec)
- ephedrine (Pretz-D)
- eprosartan (Teveten)
- esmolol (Brevibloc)
- ethacrynic acid (Edecrin)
- etozolin (Elkapin)
- felodipine (Plendil, Renedil)
- fosfomycin (Monurol)
- fosinopril (Monopril)
- furosemide (Apo-Furosemide, Lasix)
- guanabenz (Wytensin)
- guanadrel (Hylorel)
- guanfacine (Tenex)
- hydralazine (Apresoline, Novo-Hylazin)
- hydrochlorothiazide (Apo-Hydro, Microzide)
- hydrochlorothiazide and triamterene (Dyazide, Maxzide)
- hydroflumethiazide (Diucardin, Saluron)
- imidapril (Novarok, Tanatril)
- imipramine (Apo-Imipramine, Tofranil)
- indapamide (Lozol, Nu-Indapamide)
- irbesartan (Avapro)
- isradipine (DynaCirc)
- labetalol (Normodyne, Trandate)
- lacidipine (Aponil, Caldine)
- lercanidipine (Cardiovasc, Carmen)
- levalbuterol (Xopenex)
- levobetaxolol (Betaxon)
- levobunolol (Betagan, Novo-Levobunolol)
- levothyroxine (Levothroid, Synthroid)
- lisinopril (Prinivil, Zestril)
- lofepramine (Feprapax, Gamanil)
- losartan (Cozaar)
- manidipine (Calslot, Iperten)
- mannitol (Osmitrol, Resectisol)
- mefruside (Baycaron)
- melitracen (Dixeran)
- methazolamide (Apo-Methazolamide, Neptazane)

- methyclothiazide (Aquatensen, Enduron)
- methyldopa (Apo-Methyldopa, Nu-Medopa)
- methylphenidate (Concerta, Ritalin)
- metipranolol (OptiPranolol)
- metolazone (Mykrox, Zaroxolyn)
- metoprolol (Betaloc, Lopressor)
- moclobemide (Alti-Moclobemide, Nu-Moclobemide)
- modafinil (Alertec, Provigil)
- moexipril (Univasc)
- nadolol (Apo-Nadol, Corgard)
- nicardipine (Cardene)
- nifedipine (Adalat CC, Procardia)
- nilvadipine
- nimodipine (Nimotop)
- nisoldipine (Sular)
- nitrendipine
- nortriptyline (Aventyl HCl, Pamelor)
- olmesartan (Benicar)
- olmesartan and hydrochlorothiazide (Benicar HCT)
- oxprenolol (Slow-Trasicor, Trasicor)
- perindopril erbumine (Aceon, Coversyl)
- pinaverium (Dicetel)
- pindolol (Apo-Pindol, Novo-Pindol)
- polythiazide (Renese)
- prazosin (Minipress, Nu-Prazo)
- propranolol (Inderal, InnoPran XL)
- protriptyline (Vivactil)
- pseudoephedrine (Dimetapp Decongestant, Sudafed)
- quinapril (Accupril)
- ramipril (Altace)
- sotalol (Betapace, Sorine)
- spirapril
- spironolactone (Aldactone, Novo-Spiroton)
- telmisartan (Micardis)
- terazosin (Hytrin, Novo-Terazosin)

- timolol (Betimol, Timoptic)
- torsemide (Demadex)
- trandolapril (Mavik)
- tranylcypromine (Parnate)
- triamterene (Dyrenium)
- trichlormethiazide (Metatensin, Naqua)
- trimipramine (Apo-Trimin, Surmontil)
- urea (Amino-Cerv, UltraMide)
- valsartan (Diovan)
- verapamil (Calan, Isoptin SR)
- xipamide (Diurexan, Lumitens)

Taking yohimbe with these drugs may interfere with the action of the drug:
- alprazolam (Apo-Alpraz, Xanax)
- chlorpromazine (Largactil, Thorazine)
- clonidine (Catapres, Duraclon)
- fluphenazine (Modecate, Prolixin)
- guanabenz (Wytensin)
- mesoridazine (Serentil)
- oxazepam (Novoxapam, Serax)
- perphenazine (Apo-Perphenazine, Trilafon)
- prochlorperazine (Compazine, Compro)
- promethazine (Phenergan)
- reserpine
- thiethylperazine (Torecan)
- thioridazine (Mellaril)
- thiothixene (Navane)
- trifluoperazine (Novo-Trifluzine, Stelazine)

Taking yohimbe with these drugs may worsen bipolar disorder:
- carbamazepine (Carbatrol, Tegretol)
- lithium (Carbolith, Eskalith)

Taking yohimbe with these drugs may be harmful:

- prochlorperazine (Compazine, Compro)—may increase risk of abnormally low blood pressure, rapid heartbeat, and dizziness
- sibutramine (Meridia)—may increase the risk of adverse cardiovascular effects
- valproic acid (Depacon, Depakote ER)—may increase the risk of manic episodes

Lab Tests That May Be Altered by Yohimbe
None known

Diseases That May Be Worsened or Triggered by Yohimbe
- May worsen heart disease due to its constituent yohimbine.
- May worsen anxiety and posttraumatic stress disorder (PTSD), cause maniclike behavior in those with bipolar depression, trigger suicidal thoughts in those with endogenous depression, and cause an increase in psychoses in those with schizophrenia.
- May push blood sugar too low in those with diabetes taking oral antidiabetes medicines or insulin.
- May cause blood pressure to rise or fall.

Foods That May Interact with Yohimbe
- May increase central nervous system stimulation when taken with caffeine-containing foods and drinks. (For a list of caffeine-containing herbs, foods, and supplements, see Appendix B.)
- May cause increased blood pressure when taken with foods that have a high tyramine content (for example, red wine, beer, aged cheese, liver, fermented meats).
- Increased risk of hypertensive crisis when taken with large amounts of vasopressor-containing foods, such as chocolate, coffee, cola, tea, and overripe fava beans.

Supplements That May Interact with Yohimbe
- Increased risk of hypertensive crisis when taken with large amounts of herbs and supplements containing caffeine, such as cola nut, guarana, or maté. (For a list of caffeine-containing herbs, foods, and supplements, see Appendix B.)
- Increased risk of hypertensive crisis when taken with large amounts of ma-huang.
- Additive therapeutic and adverse effects when taken with herbs that have monoamine oxidase inhibiting (MAOI) potential, such as ginkgo biloba and St. John's wort. (For a list of herbs and supplements that have MAOI potential, see Appendix B.)

ZINC

This mineral participates in well over a hundred enzyme reactions that help metabolize carbohydrates, synthesize proteins, and transport carbon dioxide. Zinc is also necessary for growth and development, and helps insulin to maintain normal blood sugar levels. A zinc deficiency can cause delayed sexual maturity, poor growth and development, impotence, loss of hair, decreased appetite, diarrhea, and poor wound healing.

Typical Dose
The Food and Nutrition Board has set the RDA for zinc at 11 mg per day for men ages nineteen and up and 8 mg per day for women ages nineteen and up.

Possible Side Effects

Excessive amounts of zinc can lower HDL "good" cholesterol and damage the immune system.

Drugs That May Interact with Zinc

Taking zinc with these drugs may reduce absorption and blood levels of the drug:

- cinoxacin (Cinobac)
- ciprofloxacin (Ciloxan, Cipro)
- demeclocycline (Declomycin)
- doxycycline (Apo-Doxy, Vibramycin)
- gatifloxacin (Tequin, Zymar)
- gemifloxacin (Factive)
- levofloxacin (Levaquin, Quixin)
- lomefloxacin (Maxaquin)
- minocycline (Dynacin, Minocin)
- moxifloxacin (Avelox, Vigamox)
- nalidixic acid (NegGram)
- norfloxacin (Apo-Norflox, Noroxin)
- ofloxacin (Floxin, Ocuflox)
- oxytetracycline (Terramycin, Terramycin IM)
- pefloxacin (Peflacine, Perflox)
- sparfloxacin (Zagam)
- tetracycline (Novo-Tetra, Sumycin)
- trovafloxacin

Drugs That May Interfere with the Absorption, Utilization, or Excretion of Zinc

- aluminum hydroxide (AlternaGel, Alu-Cap)
- aluminum hydroxide and magnesium carbonate (Gaviscon Liquid)
- aluminum hydroxide and magnesium hydroxide (Maalox, Mylanta)
- aluminum hydroxide, magnesium hydroxide, and simethicone (Mylanta Liquid)
- aluminum hydroxide and magnesium trisilicate (Gaviscon Tablet)

- amiloride and hydrochlorothiazide (Moduret, Nu-Amilzide)
- aspirin (Bufferin, Ecotrin)
- aspirin and dipyridamole (Aggrenox)
- atenolol and chlorthalidone (Tenoretic)
- beclomethasone (Beconase, Vanceril)
- benazepril (Lotensin)
- betamethasone (Betatrex, Maxivate)
- budesonide (Entocort, Rhinocort)
- bumetanide (Bumex, Burinex)
- candesartan and hydrochlorothiazide (Atacand HCT)
- captopril (Capoten, Novo-Captopril)
- chlorothiazide (Diuril)
- chlorthalidone (Apo-Chlorthalidone, Thalitone)
- cholestyramine (Prevalite, Questran)
- cimetidine (Nu-Cimet, Tagamet)
- ciprofloxacin (Ciloxan, Cipro)
- cortisone (Cortone)
- delavirdine (Rescriptor)
- demeclocycline (Declomycin)
- dexamethasone (Decadron, Dexasone)
- didanosine (Videx, Videx EC)
- diflorasone (Florone, Maxiflor)
- doxycycline (Apo-Doxy, Vibramycin)
- enalapril (Vasotec)
- enalapril and felodipine (Lexxel)
- enalapril and hydrochlorothiazide (Vaseretic)
- enoxacin (Penetrex)
- ethacrynic acid (Edecrin)
- ethambutol (Myambutol)
- famotidine (Apo-Famotidine, Pepcid)
- flunisolide (AeroBid-M, Nasarel)
- fluticasone (Cutivate, Flonase)
- fosinopril (Monopril)
- furosemide (Apo-Furosemide, Lasix)

- gatofloxacin (Tequin, Zymar)
- halobetasol (Ultravate)
- hydralazine (Apresoline, Novo-Hylazin)
- hydralazine and hydrochlorothiazide (Apresazide)
- hydrochlorothiazide (Apo-Hydro, Microzide)
- hydrochlorothiazide and spironolactone (Aldactazide, Novo-Spirozine)
- hydrochlorothiazide and triamterene (Dyazide, Maxzide)
- hydrocortisone (Cetacort, Locoid)
- indapamide (Lozol, Nu-Indapamide)
- irbesartan and hydrochlorothiazide (Avalide)
- lamivudine (Epivir, Heptovir)
- lansoprazole (Prevacid)
- levofloxacin (Levaquin, Quixin)
- levonorgestrel (Norplant Implant, Plan B)
- lisinopril (Prinivil, Zestril)
- lomefloxacin (Maxaquin)
- losartan and hydrochlorothiazide (Hyzaar)
- magnesium hydroxide (Dulcolax Milk of Magnesia, Phillips' Milk of Magnesia)
- methyclothiazide (Aquatensen, Enduron)
- methyldopa and hydrochlorothiazide (Aldoril, PMS-Dopazide)
- methylprednisolone (Depoject Injection, Medrol Oral)
- metolazone (Mykrox, Zaroxolyn)
- minocycline (Dynacin, Minocin)
- moexipril (Univasc)
- moexipril and hydrochlorothiazide (Uniretic)
- mometasone furoate (Elocom, Nasonex)
- moxifloxacin (Avelox)
- nevirapine (Viramune)
- nizatidine (Apo-Nizatidine, Axid)
- norethindrone (Aygestin, Micronor)
- norfloxacin (Chibroxin Ophthalmic, Noroxin Oral)
- ofloxacin (Floxin, Ocuflox)
- omeprazole (Losec, Prilosec)
- penicillamine (Cuprimine, Depen)
- perindopril erbumine (Aceon, Coversyl)
- polythiazide (Renese)
- prazosin and polythiazide (Minizide)
- prednisolone (Inflamase Forte, Pred Forte)
- prednisone (Apo-Prednisone, Deltasone)
- propranolol and hydrochlorothiazide (Inderide)
- quinapril (Accupril)
- rabeprazole (Aciphex, Pariet)
- ramipril (Altace)
- ranitidine (Alti-Ranitidine, Zantac)
- sparfloxacin (Zagam)
- stavudine (Zerit)
- telmisartan and hydrochlorothiazide (Micardis HCT, Micardis Plus)
- tetracycline (Novo-Tetra, Sumycin)
- torsemide (Demadex)
- trandolapril (Mavik)
- trandolapril and verapamil (Tarka)
- triamcinolone (Aristocort, Trinasal)
- triamterene (Dyrenium)
- trichlormethiazide (Metahydrin, Naqua)
- trovafloxacin (Trovan)
- alsartan and hydrochlorothiazide (Diovan HCT)
- zalcitabine (Hivid)
- zidovudine (Novo-AZT, Retrovir)
- zidovudine and lamivudine (Combivir)
- zidovudine, lamivudine, and abacavir (Trizivir)

Lab Tests That May Be Altered by Zinc

- Taking supplemental zinc (50 mg per day) may increase hemoglobin A1C (HbgA1c) tests in those with type 1 diabetes.

- Taking supplemental zinc may reduce HDL "good" cholesterol levels.
- Taking supplemental zinc may increase LDL:HDL cholesterol ratio.

Diseases That May Be Worsened or Triggered by Zinc

None known

Foods That May Interact with Zinc

- Zinc absorption may be decreased by the phytic acid found in unrefined grain products.

- Zinc absorption may be decreased by a vegetarian diet.

Supplements That May Interact with Zinc

- Absorption of dietary and supplemental copper may be decreased when taken concurrently with zinc.
- Nonheme (nonmeat) iron may decrease absorption of dietary and supplemental zinc.
- Zinc absorption may be decreased by phytic acid supplements (IP-6).

Chapter Three

Medicines That Interact with Herbs

If you're taking a medicine, you can look through this alphabetical list of drugs to see which herbs or nutrients it may interact with. Remember that the interaction can take different forms. The herbs or nutrients may strengthen or weaken a medicine's actions, or the medicine may interfere with the herb or nutrient's absorption or action in the body. After finding your medicine in this chapter, look back at the individual herbs and nutrients listed to see what the specific interactions may be. If you know the brand name of a medicine but not the generic name, see Appendix C.

All oral medicines black walnut, buckthorn, butternut, carrageen, cascara sagrada, castor oil plant, guar gum, marshmallow, oats, pectin, psyllium, psyllium seed

Abacavir (Ziagen) bitter melon, boneset, butterbur, chaparral, colt's foot, comfrey, echinacea, fenugreek, maté

Abciximab (ReoPro) ajava seeds, allspice, andrographis, angelica, anise, arnica, asa foetida, astrag-alus, bilberry, bishop's weed, bladderwrack, bog bean, boldo, borage, borage seed oil, bromelain, buchu, carrageen, cat's claw, cayenne, clove, danshen, deer's tongue, devil's claw, dong quai, English hawthorn, evening primrose oil, fenugreek, feverfew, garlic, ginger, ginkgo biloba, ginseng (American), ginseng (Panax), ginseng (Siberian), grape seed, green tea, horse chestnut, kava kava, licorice, lovage, meadowsweet, onion, parsley, passion flower, pau d'arco, quinine, red clover, reishi mushroom, rue, safflower, saw palmetto, sea buckthorn, stinging nettle, sweet clover, sweet vernal grass, turmeric, valerian, vitamin E, white willow, yarrow

Acarbose (Prandase, Precose) agrimony, aloe, avaram, banaba, barley, basil, bilberry, bitter melon, black tea, bladderwrack, blue cohosh, boneset, buchu, bugleweed, burdock, butterbur, caffeine, chanca piedra, chaparral, Chinese cucumber root, cinnamon, cocoa, coffee, cola nut, colt's foot, comfrey, coriander, country mallow, cumin, damiana, dandelion, devil's claw, echinacea, ethanol, eucalyptus, fenugreek, flax, garlic, ginger, ginkgo biloba, ginseng (American), ginseng (Panax), ginseng (Siberian), glucomannan, goat's rue, gotu kola, green tea, guar gum, gymnema, horehound, horse chestnut, kudzu, laurel, licorice, Madagascar periwinkle, ma-huang, maitake mushroom, marshmallow, maté, milk thistle, myrrh, niacin, olive, onion, prickly pear cactus, psyllium, psyllium seed, raspberry, sage, senega, Solomon's seal, stevia, St. John's wort, yarrow

Acebutolol (Novo-Acebutolol, Sectral) aloe, andrographis, arnica, asa foetida, bishop's weed, black cohosh, blue cohosh, buckthorn, butterbur, carrageen, cascara sagrada, cat's claw, catechu, devil's claw, dong quai, European mistletoe, fumitory, kelp, khat, kudzu, licorice, lily-of-the-valley, ma-huang, motherwort, parsley, rue, senna, stevia, St. John's wort, wild carrot, wood betony, yarrow, yohimbe

Acemetacin (Acemetacin Heumann, Acemetacin Sandoz) bog bean, feverfew, garlic, ginkgo biloba, gossypol, niacin, reishi mushroom, saw palmetto, St. John's wort, turmeric, uva ursi, white willow

Acetaminophen (Genapap, Tylenol) bitter melon, boneset, cabbage, chaparral, colt's foot, comfrey, echinacea, ethanol, fenugreek, maté, vitamin C, watercress

Acetaminophen and codeine (Capital and Codeine, Tylenol with Codeine) ashwagandha, bitter almond, California poppy, corkwood, elecampane, English lavender, ethanol, kava kava, maté, parsley, passion flower, poke, poppy, rauwolfia, scullcap, senega, stinging nettle, valerian, wild carrot, wild lettuce, yarrow

Acetaminophen, chlorpheniramine, and pseudoephedrine (Children's Tylenol Plus Cold, Sinutab Sinus Allergy Maximum Strength) belladonna, corkwood, English lavender, henbane, khat

Acetaminophen, dextromethorphan, and pseudoephedrine (Alka-Seltzer Plus Flu Liqui-Gels, Sudafed Severe Cold) belladonna, corkwood, English lavender, henbane, khat

Acetazolamide (Apo-Acetazolamide, Diamox Sequels) apple cider vinegar, birch, bishop's weed, black root, bladderwrack, blue flag, buckthorn, butternut, calotropis, cascara sagrada, castor oil plant, cedar leaf, colocynth, corn silk, cowslip, cucumber, dandelion, digitalis, evening primrose oil, fo-ti, frangula, gamboge, ginkgo biloba, gossypol, horsetail, Indian hemp, jalap, licorice, lily-of-the-valley, magnesium, ma-huang, manna, maté, mayapple, potassium, quassia, sage, senna, sorrel, stinging nettle, stone root, uva ursi, uzara, wahoo, wallflower, wild carrot, wormseed, yellow dock, yohimbe

Acetohexamide agrimony, aloe, avaram, banaba, barley, basil, bilberry, bitter melon, black tea, bladderwrack, blue cohosh, buchu, bugleweed, burdock, caffeine, chanca piedra, Chinese cucumber root, cinnamon, cocoa, coffee, cola nut, coriander, country mallow, cumin, damiana, dandelion, devil's claw, eucalyptus, fenugreek, flax, garlic, ginger, ginseng (American), ginseng (Panax), ginseng (Siberian), glucomannan, goat's rue, gotu kola, green tea, guar gum, gymnema, horehound, horse chestnut, kudzu, laurel, licorice, Madagascar periwinkle, ma-huang, maitake mushroom, marshmallow, myrrh, niacin, olive, onion, prickly pear cactus, psyllium, psyllium seed, raspberry, senega, Solomon's seal, stevia, St. John's wort

Acetophenazine cowhage, ethanol, rauwolfia

Acetylcholine (Miochol-E) areca nut, Chinese club moss, iboga

Acipimox (Acipimox, Olbetam) gotu kola

Acitretin (Soriatane) ethanol, St. John's wort, vitamin A

Acrivastine and pseudoephedrine (Semprex-D) belladonna, corkwood, English lavender, henbane, khat

Acyclovir (Alti-Acyclovir, Zovirax) echinacea

Adenosine (Adenocard, Adenoscan) aloe, buckthorn, cascara sagrada, fumitory, khat, kudzu, licorice, senna

Aithromycin (Zithromax) biotin

Albendazole (Albenza) ginseng (Panax)

Albuterol (Proventil, Ventolin) black tea, caffeine, cocoa, coffee, cola nut, digitalis, fever bark, green tea, Indian squill, ma-huang, potassium, rauwolfia, squill, yohimbe

Aldesleukin (Proleukin) astragalus, ethanol

Alendronate (Fosamax, Novo-Alendronate) black tea, caffeine, calcium, cocoa, coffee, cola nut, green tea, iron, magnesium

Alfentanil (Alfenta) ashwagandha, bitter almond, California poppy, corkwood, elecampane, English lavender, ethanol, kava kava, maté, parsley, passion flower, poke, poppy, rauwolfia, scullcap, senega, stinging nettle, valerian, wild carrot, wild lettuce, yarrow

Alitretinoin (Panretin) vitamin A

Allopurinol (Aloprim, Zyloprim) bitter melon, boneset, butterbur, chaparral, colt's foot, comfrey, echinacea, fenugreek, kava kava, maté, valerian

Almotriptan (Axert) St. John's wort

Alprazolam (Apo-Alpraz, Xanax) ashwagandha, bitter almond, California poppy, catnip, cowslip, danshen, elecampane, ethanol, German chamomile, goldenseal, gotu kola, guarana, kava kava, lemon balm, linden, maté, nerve root, passion flower, poke, poppy, rauwolfia, sassafras, scullcap, senega, stinging nettle, St. John's wort, valerian, wild carrot, wild cherry, wild lettuce, yarrow, yohimbe

Alprostadil (Caverject, Muse) ethanol

Alteplase (Activase, Cathflo Activase) angelica, arnica, astragalus, bilberry, bladderwrack, borage, cat's claw, cayenne, clove, dong quai, evening primrose oil, feverfew, garlic, ginger, ginkgo biloba, ginseng (American), ginseng (Panax), ginseng (Siberian), green tea, horse chestnut, kava kava, licorice, pineapple, red clover, turmeric, valerian, white willow

Aluminum hydroxide (AlternaGel, Alu-Cap) aletris, angelica, birthwort, black mustard, blessed thistle, buckthorn, calamus, calcium, colombo, cubeb, dandelion, devil's claw, folic acid, ginger, iron, lesser galangal, magnesium, ma-huang, vitamin A, vitamin D, yellow gentian, zinc

Aluminum hydroxide and magnesium carbonate (Gaviscon Extra Strength, Gaviscon Liquid) aletris, angelica, birthwort, black mustard, blessed thistle, buckthorn, calamus, calcium, colombo, cubeb, dandelion, devil's claw, folic acid, ginger, iron, lesser galangal, magnesium, ma-huang, vitamin A, vitamin D, yellow gentian, zinc

Aluminum hydroxide and magnesium hydroxide (Maalox, Mylanta, Rulox) aletris, angelica, birthwort, black mustard, blessed thistle, buckthorn, calamus, calcium, colombo, cubeb, dandelion, devil's claw, folic acid, ginger, lesser galangal, iron, magnesium, ma-huang, vitamin A, vitamin D, yellow gentian, zinc

Aluminum hydroxide and magnesium trisilicate (Gaviscon Tablet) aletris, angelica, birthwort, black mustard, blessed thistle, buckthorn, calamus, calcium, colombo, cubeb, dandelion, devil's claw, folic acid, ginger, iron, lesser galangal, magnesium, ma-huang, vitamin A, vitamin D, yellow gentian, zinc

Aluminum hydroxide, magnesium hydroxide, and simethicone (Maalox, Mylanta Liquid) aletris, angelica, birthwort, black mustard, blessed thistle, buckthorn, calamus, calcium, colombo, cubeb, dandelion, devil's claw, folic acid, ginger, iron, lesser galangal, magnesium, ma-huang, vitamin A, vitamin D, yellow gentian, zinc

Amantadine (Symmetrel) angel's trumpet, belladonna, chaste tree berry, ethanol, henbane, jimson weed, kava kava, scopolia

Amifostine (Ethyol) calcium

Amikacin (Amikin) biotin, calcium, magnesium, niacin, potassium, riboflavin, thiamin, vitamin B_6, vitamin B_{12}, vitamin K

Amiloride (Midamor) birch, bishop's weed, bladderwrack, calcium, cowslip, cucumber, dandelion, folic acid, maté, noni, potassium, sorrel, stinging nettle, stone root, wild carrot, yohimbe

Amiloride plus hydrochlorothiazide (Moduret, Nu-Amilzide) magnesium, potassium, zinc

Aminolevulinic acid (Levulan Kerastick) St. John's wort

Aminosalicylic acid (Nemasol Sodium, Paser) cayenne, folic acid, heartsease, horse chestnut, lovage, lungwort, northern prickly ash, pau d'arco, pineapple, poplar, safflower, senega, tonka bean, vitamin, B_{12} white willow, wintergreen, yarrow

Amiodarone (Cordarone, Pacerone) aloe, buckthorn, cascara sagrada, dong quai, English hawthorn, fumitory, khat, kudzu, licorice, senna, St. John's wort, vitamin B_6

Amitriptyline (Elavil, Levate) angel's trumpet, belladonna, black tea, butterbur, catnip, coffee, corkwood, ergot, ethanol, fennel, ginkgo biloba, goldenseal, henbane, jimson weed, kava kava, lemon balm, ma-huang, marijuana, nerve root, rauwolfia, riboflavin, sassafras, scopolia, stinging nettle, St. John's wort, valerian, wormwood, yohimbe

Amitriptyline and chlordiazepoxide (Limbitrol) angel's trumpet, belladonna, black tea, coffee, corkwood, ergot, ethanol, henbane, jimson weed, ma-huang, marijuana, rauwolfia, scopolia, St. John's wort, yohimbe

Amitriptyline and perphenazine (Triavil, Etrafon) angel's trumpet, belladonna, black tea, coffee, corkwood, ergot, ethanol, henbane, jimson weed, ma-huang, marijuana, rauwolfia, scopolia, St. John's wort, yohimbe

Amlodipine (Norvasc) andrographis, arnica, asa foetida, bishop's weed, black cohosh, blue cohosh, calcium, carrageen, cat's claw, catechu, devil's claw, English hawthorn, European mistletoe, garlic, grapefruit, kelp, khat, licorice, lily-of-the-valley, magnesium, ma-huang, niacin, parsley, rue, stevia, St. John's wort, wild carrot, wild cherry, wood betony, yarrow, yohimbe

Ammonium chloride potassium

Amobarbital (Amytal) ashwagandha, bitter almond, California poppy, cedar leaf, cedarwood oil, cowslip, elecampane, English lavender, ethanol, eucalyptus, evening primrose oil, German chamomile, ginkgo biloba, hops, kava kava, lemon balm, marijuana, maté, passion flower, poke, poppy, rauwolfia, sage, scullcap, senega, stinging nettle, St. John's wort, valerian, wild carrot, wild lettuce, wormseed, yarrow

Amobarbital and secobarbital (Tuinal) ashwagandha, bitter almond, California poppy, cedarwood oil, elecampane, ethanol, eucalyptus, hops, kava kava, lemon balm, marijuana, maté, passion flower, poke, poppy, rauwolfia, scullcap, senega, stinging nettle, St. John's wort, valerian, wild carrot, wild lettuce, yarrow

Amorolfine (Loceryl, Locetar) gossypol

Amoxapine (Asendin) angel's trumpet, belladonna, black tea, catnip, coffee, corkwood, ergot, ethanol, fennel, ginkgo biloba, goldenseal, jimson weed, kava kava, lemon balm, ma-huang, marijuana, nerve root, rauwolfia, riboflavin, sassafras, scopolia, stinging nettle, St. John's wort, valerian, wormwood, yohimbe

Amoxicillin (Amoxil, Novamoxin) biotin, niacin, potassium, riboflavin, thiamin, vitamin B_6, vitamin B_{12}, vitamin K

Amphotericin B (Amphocin, Fungizone) calcium, gossypol, magnesium, potassium

Amphotericin B cholesteryl sulfate complex (Amphotec) gossypol

Amphotericin B lipid complex (Abelcet) gossypol

Amphotericin B liposomal (AmBisome) gossypol

Ampicillin (Omnipen, Totacillin) biotin, niacin, potassium, riboflavin, thiamin, vitamin B_6, vitamin B_{12}, vitamin K

Amprenavir (Agenerase) echinacea, garlic, marijuana, St. John's wort, vitamin C

Anastrozole (Arimidex) black cohosh, dong quai

Aniracetam (Ampamet, Draganon) cowhage, rauwolfia

Antithrombin III (Thrombate III) ajava seeds, alfalfa, allspice, andrographis, angelica, arnica, asa foetida, astragalus, bilberry, bishop's weed, bladderwrack, bog bean, boldo, borage, borage seed oil, bromelain, buchu, carrageen, cat's claw, cayenne, clove, danshen, deer's tongue, dong quai, evening primrose oil, feverfew, garlic, German chamomile, ginger, ginkgo biloba, ginseng (American), ginseng (Panax), ginseng (Siberian), green tea, horse chestnut, kava kava, kelp, licorice, lovage, lungwort, meadowsweet, motherwort, northern prickly ash, papaya, pau d'arco, pineapple, poplar, quinine, red clover, reishi mushroom, safflower, saw palmetto, sea buckthorn, senega, stinging nettle, St. John's wort, sweet clover, sweet vernal grass, tonka bean, turmeric, valerian, vitamin E, white willow, wintergreen, yarrow

Antithymocyte globulin (equine) (Atgam) andrographis, ashwagandha, astragalus, cat's claw, echinacea, larch, maitake mushroom, schisandra, scullcap, St. John's wort, turmeric

Antithymocyte globulin (rabbit) (Thymoglobulin) andrographis, ashwagandha, astragalus, cat's claw, echinacea, larch, maitake mushroom, schisandra, scullcap, St. John's wort, turmeric

Argatroban ajava seeds, alfalfa, allspice, andrographis, angelica, arnica, asa foetida, astragalus, bilberry, bishop's weed, bladderwrack, bog bean, boldo, borage, borage seed oil, bromelain, buchu, carrageen, cat's claw, cayenne, clove, danshen, deer's tongue, dong quai, evening primrose oil, feverfew, garlic, German chamomile, ginger, ginkgo biloba, ginseng (American), ginseng (Panax), ginseng (Siberian), green tea, horse chestnut, kava kava, kelp, licorice, lovage, lungwort, meadowsweet, motherwort, northern prickly ash, papaya, pau d'arco, pineapple, poplar, quinine, red clover, reishi mushroom, safflower, saw palmetto, sea buckthorn, senega, stinging nettle, St. John's wort, sweet clover, sweet vernal grass, tonka bean, turmeric, valerian, vitamin E, white willow, wintergreen, yarrow

Aripiprazole (Abilify) cowhage, gotu kola, kava kava, rauwolfia, valerian

Arsenic trioxide (Trisenox) calcium, magnesium, potassium

Aspirin (Bufferin, Ecotrin) ajava seeds, allspice, andrographis, angelica, anise, arnica, asa foetida, astragalus, bilberry, bishop's weed, bladderwrack, bog bean, boldo, borage, borage seed oil, bromelain, buchu, calcium, carrageen, cat's claw, cayenne, Cherokee rosehip, clove, danshen, deer's tongue, devil's claw, dong quai, English hawthorn, evening primrose oil, fenugreek, feverfew, folic acid, garlic, German chamomile, ginger, ginkgo biloba, ginseng (American), ginseng (Panax), ginseng (Siberian), gossypol, grape seed, green tea, heartsease, horse chestnut, iron, kava kava, licorice, lovage, lungwort, meadowsweet, niacin, northern prickly ash, onion, parsley, passion flower, pau d'arco, pineapple, poplar, potassium, quinine, red clove, reishi mushroom, rue, safflower, saw palmetto, sea buckthorn, senega, stinging nettle, St. John's wort, sweet clover, sweet vernal grass, tonka bean, turmeric, uva ursi, valerian, vitamin C, vitamin E, white willow, wintergreen, yarrow, zinc

Aspirin and codeine (Coryphen Codeine) ashwagandha, bitter almond, calcium, California poppy, corkwood, elecampane, English lavender, ethanol, kava kava, maté, parsley, passion flower, poke, poppy, rauwolfia, scullcap, senega, stinging nettle, valerian, wild carrot, wild lettuce, yarrow

Aspirin and dipyridamole (Aggrenox) ajava seeds, allspice, andrographis, angelica, arnica, asa foetida, astragalus, bilberry, bishop's weed, bladderwrack, bog bean, boldo, borage, borage seed oil, bromelain, buchu, calcium, carrageen, cat's claw, cayenne, clove, danshen, deer's tongue, dong quai, English hawthorn, evening primrose oil, feverfew, folic acid, garlic, ginger, ginkgo biloba, ginseng (American), ginseng (Panax), ginseng (Siberian), horse chestnut, iron, kava kava, licorice, lovage, pau d'arco, potassium, quinine, reishi mushroom, safflower, saw palmetto, sea buckthorn, stinging nettle, sweet clover, sweet vernal grass, turmeric, valerian, vitamin C, vitamin E, white willow, yarrow, zinc

Aspirin and meprobamate (Equagesic, 292 MEP) cowslip

Aspirin and pravastatin (Pravigard PAC) gotu kola

Atenolol (Apo-Atenol, Tenormin) andrographis, arnica, asa foetida, bishop's weed, black cohosh, blue cohosh, butterbur, calcium, carrageen, cat's claw, catechu, devil's claw, dong quai, European mistletoe, fumitory, garlic, ginger, goldenseal, kelp, khat, licorice, lily-of-the-valley, ma-huang, motherwort, parsley, rue, stevia, St. John's wort, wild carrot, wood betony, yarrow, yohimbe

Atenolol plus chlorthalidone (Tenoretic) magnesium, potassium, zinc

Atorvastatin (Lipitor) bitter melon, boneset, butterbur, chaparral, colt's foot, comfrey, echinacea, fenugreek, gotu kola, grapefruit, kava kava, maté, niacin, oats, pectin, red yeast rice, St. John's wort, wild cherry

Atracurium (Tracrium) magnesium

Atropine (Isopto Atropine, Sal-Tropine) angel's trumpet, areca nut, black root, butterbur, calabar bean, catechu, Chinese club moss, iboga, jimson weed, mandrake, scopolia

Azatadine (Optimine) belladonna, corkwood, English lavender, henbane, khat

Azatadine and pseudoephedrine (Rynatan Tablet, Trinalin) belladonna, corkwood, English lavender, henbane, khat

Azathioprine (Imuran) alfalfa, andrographis, ashwagandha, astragalus, cat's claw, echinacea, larch, maitake mushroom, schisandra, scullcap, St. John's wort, turmeric

Azelastine (Astelin, Optivar) belladonna, corkwood, English lavender, ethanol, henbane, khat

Azithromycin (Zithromax) niacin, riboflavin, thiamin, uzara, vitamin B_6, vitamin B_{12}, vitamin K, wahoo

Azosemide (Diat), aloe, apple cider vinegar, birch, bishop's weed, black root, bladderwrack, blue flag, buckthorn, butternut, calotropis, cascara sagrada, castor oil plant, colocynth, corn silk, cowslip, cucumber, dandelion, digitalis, fo-ti, frangula, gamboge, gossypol, horsetail, Indian hemp, jalap, licorice, lily-of-the-valley, manna, maté, mayapple, quassia, senna, sorrel, stinging nettle, St. John's wort, stone root, uva ursi, uzara, wahoo, wallflower, wild carrot, yellow dock, yohimbe

Baclofen (Lioresal, Nu-Baclo) gotu kola, valerian

Balsalazide (Colazal) folic acid

Barbexaclone (Maliasin) cedar leaf, evening primrose oil, ginkgo biloba, sage, wormseed

Basiliximab (Simulect) andrographis, ashwagandha, astragalus, calcium, cat's claw, echinacea, larch, maitake mushroom, potassium, schisandra, scullcap, St. John's wort, turmeric

Beclomethasone (Beconase, Vanceril) adonis, aloe, andrographis, ashwagandha, astragalus, buckthorn, butternut, calcium, cascara sagrada, castor oil plant, frangula, Indian squill, larch, licorice, magnesium, ma-huang, perilla, potassium, schisandra, squill, strophanthus, vitamin A, vitamin B_6, vitamin C, vitamin D, vitamin K, wallflower, zinc

Befunolol (Bentos, Betaclar) butterbur, fumitory, khat, lily-of-the-valley, motherwort, St. John's wort, yohimbe

Belladonna and opium (B&O Supprettes) angel's trumpet, ashwagandha, bitter almond, California poppy, corkwood, elecampane, English lavender, ethanol, kava kava, maté, mayapple, parsley, passion flower, poke, poppy, rauwolfia, scullcap, senega, stinging nettle, valerian, wild carrot, wild lettuce, yarrow

Belladonna, phenobarbital, and ergotamine (Bellamine S, Bel-Tabs) angel's trumpet, country mallow, ergot, mayapple

Benazepril (Lotensin) andrographis, arnica, asa foetida, bishop's weed, black cohosh, blue cohosh, carrageen, cat's claw, catechu, cayenne, dandelion, devil's claw, dong quai, European mistletoe, garlic, ginger, goldenseal, kelp, khat, licorice, ma-huang, parsley, pineapple, pomegranate, potassium, rue, stevia, St. John's wort, uva ursi, white willow, wild carrot, wood betony, yarrow, yohimbe, zinc

Benperidol (Anquil, Glianimon) cowhage, rauwolfia

Benztropine (Apo-Benztropine, Cogentin) angel's trumpet, areca nut, butterbur, calabar bean, catechu, Chinese club moss, ethanol, iboga, jimson weed, mandrake, scopolia

Bepridil (Vascor) aloe, bishop's weed, calcium, cascara sagrada, cat's claw, chicory, Chinese rhubarb, dong quai, English hawthorn, garlic, ginger, grapefruit, guarana, khat, lily-of-the-valley, magnesium, niacin, senna, stevia, St. John's wort, wild cherry, yohimbe

Betamethasone (Betatrex, Maxivate) adonis, aloe, andrographis, ashwagandha, astragalus, buckthorn, butternut, calcium, cascara sagrada, castor oil plant, cat's claw, echinacea, folic acid, frangula, Indian squill, larch, licorice, lily-of-the-valley, magnesium, ma-huang, oleander, perilla, potassium, schisandra, squill, strophanthus, vitamin A, vitamin B_6, vitamin C, vitamin D, vitamin K, wallflower, zinc

Betaxolol (Betoptic S, Kerlone) andrographis, arnica, asa foetida, bishop's weed, black cohosh, blue cohosh, butterbur, carrageen, cat's claw, catechu, devil's claw, dong quai, European mistletoe, fumitory, garlic, kelp, khat, licorice, lily-of-the-valley, ma-huang, motherwort, parsley, rue, stevia, St. John's wort, wild carrot, wood betony, yarrow, yohimbe

Bethanechol (Duvoid, Urecholine) areca nut, Chinese club moss, iboga

Bexarotene (Targretin) dong quai, vitamin A

Bezafibrate (Bezalip, PMS-Bezafibrate) gotu kola

Bifonazole (Amycor, Canesten) gossypol

Bisacodyl (Carter's Little Pills, Dulcolax) calcium, potassium

Bismuth (Kaopectate, Pepto-Bismol) nutmeg

Bismuth subcitrate (DE-NOL) calcium

Bismuth subsalicylate, metronidazole, and tetracycline (Helidac) nutmeg

Bisoprolol (Monocor, Zebeta) andrographis, arnica, asa foetida, bishop's weed, black cohosh, blue cohosh, butterbur, carrageen, cat's claw, catechu, devil's claw, dong quai, European mistletoe, fumitory, garlic, kelp, khat, licorice, lily-of-the-valley, ma-huang, motherwort, parsley, rue, stevia, St. John's wort, wild carrot, wood betony, yarrow, yohimbe

Bivalirudin (Angiomax) ajava seeds, alfalfa, allspice, andrographis, angelica, arnica, asa foetida, astragalus, bilberry, bishop's weed, bladderwrack, bog bean, boldo, borage, borage seed oil, bromelain, buchu, carrageen, cat's claw, cayenne, clove, danshen, deer's tongue, dong quai, evening primrose oil, feverfew, garlic, German chamomile, ginger, ginkgo biloba, ginseng (American), ginseng (Panax), ginseng (Siberian), green tea, horse chestnut, kava kava, kelp, licorice, lovage, lungwort, meadowsweet, motherwort, northern prickly ash, papaya, pau d'arco, pineapple, poplar, quinine, red clover, reishi mushroom, safflower, saw palmetto, sea buckthorn, senega, stinging nettle, St. John's wort, sweet clover, sweet vernal grass, tonka bean, turmeric, valerian, vitamin E, white willow, wintergreen, yarrow

Botulinum toxin type A (Botox, Botox Cosmetic) magnesium

Botulinum toxin type B (Myobloc) magnesium

Bretylium aloe, buckthorn, cascara sagrada, English hawthorn, fumitory, khat, kudzu, licorice, senna

Brimonidine (Alphagan P, PMS-Brimonidine Tartrate) digitalis, fever bark, Indian squill, mahuang, rauwolfia, squill

Bromazepam (Apo-Bromazepam, Gen-Bromazepam) ashwagandha, bitter almond, California poppy, elecampane, ethanol, German chamomile, gotu kola, kava kava, maté, passion flower, poke, poppy, rauwolfia, scullcap, senega, stinging nettle, St. John's wort, valerian, wild carrot, wild cherry, wild lettuce, yarrow

Bromocriptine (Apo-Bromocriptine, Parlodel) chaste tree berry, country mallow, ergot, kava kava

Bromperidol (Impromen, Tesoprel) cowhage, rauwolfia

Brompheniramine and pseudoephedrine (Children's Dimetapp Elixir Cold & Allergy, Lodrane) belladonna, corkwood, English lavender, henbane, khat

Brotizolam (Lendorm, Sintonal) ashwagandha, bitter almond, California poppy, elecampane, ethanol, German chamomile, kava kava, maté, passion flower, poke, poppy, rauwolfia, scullcap, senega, stinging nettle, St. John's wort, valerian, wild carrot, wild cherry, wild lettuce, yarrow

Budesonide (Entocort, Rhinocort) adonis, aloe, andrographis, ashwagandha, astragalus, buckthorn, butternut, calcium, cascara sagrada, castor oil plant, folic acid, frangula, Indian squill, larch, licorice, magnesium, ma-huang, perilla, potassium, schisandra, squill, strophanthus, vitamin A, vitamin B_6, vitamin C, vitamin D, vitamin K, wallflower, zinc

Budesonide and formoterol (Symbicort) adonis, aloe, andrographis, ashwagandha, astragalus, buckthorn, butternut, cascara sagrada, castor oil plant, frangula, Indian squill, larch, licorice, mahuang, perilla, schisandra, squill, strophanthus, wallflower

Bumetanide (Bumex) agrimony, aloe, andrographis, apple cider vinegar, arnica, artichoke, asa foetida, birch, bishop's weed, black cohosh, black root, bladderwrack, blue cohosh, blue flag, buckthorn, butternut, calcium, calotropis, carrageen, cascara sagrada, castor oil plant, cat's claw, catechu, celery, colocynth, coriander, corn silk, cowslip, cucumber, dandelion, devil's claw, digitalis, dong quai, European mistletoe, fennel, fo-ti, frangula, gamboge, garlic, goldenseal, gossypol, horsetail, Indian hemp, jalap, kelp, khat, licorice, lily-of-the-valley, lovage, magnesium, ma-huang, manna, maté, mayapple, motherwort, parsley, potassium, quassia, rosemary, rue, senna, sorrel, stevia, stinging nettle, St. John's wort, stone root, thiamin, uva ursi, uzara, vitamin B_6, vitamin C, wahoo, wallflower, wild carrot, wood betony, yarrow, yellow dock, yohimbe, zinc

Buprenorphine (Buprenex, Subutex) ashwagandha, bitter almond, California poppy, corkwood, elecampane, English lavender, ethanol, gotu kola, kava kava, maté, parsley, passion flower, poke, poppy, rauwolfia, scullcap, senega, stinging nettle, valerian, wild carrot, wild lettuce, yarrow

Buprenorphine and naloxone (Suboxone) ashwagandha, bitter almond, California poppy, corkwood, elecampane, English lavender, ethanol, kava kava, maté, parsley, passion flower, poke, poppy, rauwolfia, scullcap, senega, stinging nettle, valerian, wild carrot, wild lettuce, yarrow

Bupropion (Wellbutrin, Zyban) catnip, ergot, fennel, ginkgo biloba, goldenseal, gotu kola, kava kava, lemon balm, nerve root, sassafras, stinging nettle, valerian, wormwood

Buspirone (BuSpar, Nu-Buspirone) catnip, cowslip, goldenseal, gotu kola, grapefruit, kava kava, lemon balm, nerve root, sassafras, stinging nettle, St. John's wort, wild cherry

Busulfan (Busulfex, Myleran) magnesium, potassium

Butabarbital (Butisol Sodium) ashwagandha, bitter almond, calcium, California poppy, cedarwood oil, cowslip, elecampane, English lavender, ethanol, eucalyptus, folic acid, German chamomile, gotu kola, hops, kava kava, lemon balm, marijuana, maté, passion flower, poke, poppy, rauwolfia, scullcap, senega, stinging nettle, St. John's wort, valerian, vitamin D, vitamin K, wild carrot, wild lettuce, yarrow

Butalbital, acetaminophen, and caffeine (Esgic, Fioricet) ashwagandha, bitter almond, calcium, California poppy, cedarwood oil, elecampane, ethanol, eucalyptus, folic acid, hops, kava kava, lemon balm, marijuana, maté, passion flower, poke, poppy, rauwolfia, scullcap, senega, stinging nettle, St. John's wort, valerian, vitamin D, vitamin K, wild carrot, wild lettuce, yarrow

Butalbital, aspirin, and caffeine (Fiorinal) ashwagandha, bitter almond, calcium, California poppy, cedarwood oil, elecampane, ethanol, eucalyptus, folic acid, hops, iron, kava kava, lemon balm, marijuana, maté, passion flower, poke, poppy, potassium, rauwolfia, scullcap, senega, stinging nettle, St. John's wort, valerian, vitamin C, vitamin D, vitamin K, wild carrot, wild lettuce, yarrow

Butenafine (Lotrimin Ultra, Mentax) gossypol

Butoconazole (Gynazole-1, Mycelex-3) gossypol

Butorphanol (Apo-Butorphanol, Stadol) ashwagandha, bitter almond, California poppy, corkwood, elecampane, English lavender, ethanol, gotu kola, kava kava, maté, parsley, passion flower, poke, poppy, rauwolfia, scullcap, senega, stinging nettle, valerian, wild carrot, wild lettuce, yarrow

Cabergoline (Dostinex) country mallow, ergot

Caffeine-containing drugs (such as Alka-Seltzer Morning Relief Tablets, Cafergot, Excedrin Extra-Strength) horsetail

Calcium acetate (PhosLo) adonis, lily-of-the-valley, oleander, squill, strophanthus, wallflower

Calcium carbonate (Mylanta Children, Tums) adonis, angelica, birthwort, black mustard, blessed thistle, buckthorn, calamus, colombo, cubeb, dandelion, devil's claw, ginger, iron, lesser galangal, lily-of-the-valley, ma-huang, oleander, squill, strophanthus, wallflower, yellow gentian

Calcium carbonate and magnesium hydroxide (Mylanta Gelcaps, Rolaids Extra Strength) aletris, angelica, birthwort, black mustard, blessed thistle, buckthorn, calamus, colombo, cubeb, dandelion, devil's claw, ginger, lesser galangal, ma-huang, yellow gentian

Calcium chloride adonis, lily-of-the-valley, magnesium, oleander, squill, strophanthus, wallflower

Calcium citrate (Osteocit) adonis, lily-of-the-valley, oleander, squill, strophanthus, wallflower

Calcium glubionate adonis, lily-of-the-valley, oleander, squill, strophanthus, wallflower

Calcium gluceptate adonis, lily-of-the-valley, oleander, squill, strophanthus, wallflower

Calcium gluconate adonis, lily-of-the-valley, oleander, squill, strophanthus, wallflower

Candesartan (Atacand) andrographis, arnica, asa foetida, bishop's weed, black cohosh, blue cohosh, carrageen, cat's claw, catechu, devil's claw, dong quai, European mistletoe, garlic, kelp, khat, licorice, ma-huang, parsley, potassium, rue, stevia, wild carrot, wood betony, yarrow, yohimbe

Candesartan plus hydrochlorothiazide (Atacand HCT) magnesium, potassium, zinc

Captopril (Capoten, Novo-Captopril) andrographis, arnica, asa foetida, bishop's weed, black cohosh, blue cohosh, carrageen, cat's claw, catechu, cayenne, devil's claw, dong quai, European mistletoe, garlic, ginger, goldenseal, kelp, khat, licorice, ma-huang, parsley, pineapple, pomegranate, potassium, rue, stevia, St. John's wort, wild carrot, wood betony, yarrow, yohimbe, zinc

Carbachol (Carbastat, Isopto Carbachol) areca nut, Chinese club moss, iboga

Carbamazepine (Carbatrol, Tegretol) avaram, calcium, cedar leaf, English plantain, evening primrose oil, fennel, folic acid, ginkgo biloba, gotu kola, grapefruit, hyssop, kava kava, psyllium, psyllium seed, quinine, sage, stinging nettle, St. John's wort, valerian, vitamin D, wormseed, wormwood, yohimbe

Carbenicillin (Geocillin) biotin, niacin, potassium, riboflavin, thiamin, vitamin B_6, vitamin B_{12}, vitamin K

Carbidopa (Lodsoyn) chaste tree berry, kava kava

Carbinoxamine (Histex CT, Histex PD) belladonna, corkwood, English lavender, henbane, khat

Carbinoxamine and pseudoephedrine (Rondec Drops, Sildec) belladonna, corkwood, English lavender, henbane, khat

Carbinoxamine, pseudoephedrine, and dextromethorphan (Rondec-DM Drops, Tussafed) belladonna, corkwood, English lavender, henbane, khat

Carbocysteine (Mucopront, Rhinatiol) black cohosh, dong quai

Carboplatin (Paraplatin, Paraplatin-AQ) calcium, magnesium, potassium

Carisoprodol plus aspirin (Soma Compound) folic acid, iron, potassium, vitamin C

Carisoprodol plus aspirin plus codeine (Soma Compound with Codeine) folic acid, iron, potassium, vitamin C

Carpipramine (Defecton, Prazinil) cowslip

Carteolol (Cartrol, Ocupress) andrographis, arnica, asa foetida, bishop's weed, black cohosh, blue cohosh, butterbur, carrageen, cat's claw, catechu, devil's claw, dong quai, European mistletoe, fumitory, garlic, kelp, khat, licorice, lily-of-the-valley, ma-huang, motherwort, parsley, rue, stevia, St. John's wort, wild carrot, wood betony, yarrow, yohimbe

Carvedilol (Coreg) andrographis, arnica, asa foetida, bishop's weed, black cohosh, blue cohosh, butterbur, carrageen, cat's claw, catechu, devil's claw, dong quai, European mistletoe, fumitory, garlic, ginger, goldenseal, grapefruit, kelp, khat, licorice, lily-of-the-valley, ma-huang, motherwort, parsley, rue, saw palmetto, stevia, St. John's wort, wild carrot, wood betony, yarrow, yohimbe

Cascara adonis, butternut, calcium, calotropis, cascara sagrada, castor oil plant, frangula, gamboge, Indian squill, licorice, lily-of-the-valley, oleander, potassium, senna, squill, strophanthus, uzara, vitamin D, wahoo, wallflower

Caspofungin (Cancidas) gossypol, potassium

Cefaclor (Ceclor) biotin, niacin, riboflavin, thiamin, vitamin B_6, vitamin B_{12}, vitamin K

Cefadroxil (Duricef) biotin, niacin, riboflavin, thiamin, vitamin B_6, vitamin B_{12}, vitamin K

Cefamandole (Mandol) ethanol, niacin, riboflavin, thiamin, vitamin B_6, vitamin B_{12}, vitamin K

Cefazolin (Ancef, Kefzol) biotin, niacin, riboflavin, thiamin, vitamin B_6, vitamin B_{12}, vitamin K

Cefdinir (Omnicef) biotin, niacin, riboflavin, thiamin, vitamin B_6, vitamin B_{12}, vitamin K

Cefditoren (Spectracef) biotin, niacin, riboflavin, thiamin, vitamin B_6, vitamin B_{12}, vitamin K

Cefepime (Maxipime) biotin, niacin, riboflavin, thiamin, vitamin B_6, vitamin B_{12}, vitamin K

Cefonicid (Monocid) biotin, niacin, riboflavin, thiamin, vitamin B_6, vitamin B_{12}, vitamin K

Cefoperazone (Cefobid) biotin, niacin, riboflavin, thiamin, vitamin B_6, vitamin B_{12}, vitamin K

Cefotaxime (Claforan) biotin, niacin, riboflavin, thiamin, vitamin B_6, vitamin B_{12}, vitamin K

Cefotetan (Cefotan) ethanol, niacin, riboflavin, thiamin, vitamin B_6, vitamin B_{12}, vitamin K

Cefoxitin (Mefoxin) biotin, niacin, riboflavin, thiamin, vitamin B_6, vitamin B_{12}, vitamin K

Cefpodoxime (Vantin) biotin, calcium, niacin, riboflavin, thiamin, vitamin B_6, vitamin B_{12}, vitamin K

Cefprozil (Cefzil) biotin, niacin, riboflavin, thiamin, vitamin B_6, vitamin B_{12}, vitamin K

Ceftazidime (Ceptaz, Fortaz) biotin, niacin, riboflavin, thiamin, vitamin B_6, vitamin B_{12}, vitamin K

Ceftibuten (Cedax) biotin, niacin, riboflavin, thiamin, vitamin B_6, vitamin B_{12}, vitamin K

Ceftizoxime (Cefizox) biotin, niacin, riboflavin, thiamin, vitamin B_6, vitamin B_{12}, vitamin K

Ceftriaxone (Rocephin) biotin, niacin, riboflavin, thiamin, vitamin B_6, vitamin B_{12}, vitamin K

Cefuroxime (Ceftin, Kefurox) biotin, niacin, riboflavin, thiamin, vitamin B_6, vitamin B_{12}, vitamin K

Celecoxib (Celebrex) angelica, anise, arnica, bitter melon, bog bean, boneset, bromelain, butterbur, chaparral, clove, coffee, cola nut, colt's foot, comfrey, coriander, danshen, devil's claw, dong quai, echinacea, fennel, fenugreek, feverfew, folic acid, garlic, German chamomile, ginger, ginkgo biloba, gossypol, horse chestnut, licorice, lovage, maté, meadowsweet, motherwort, niacin, onion, parsley, passion flower, potassium, red clover, reishi mushroom, rosemary, rue, saw palmetto, St. John's wort, sweet clover, turmeric, uva ursi, white willow, wild carrot, wild yam

Celiprolol butterbur, fumitory, khat, lily-of-the-valley, motherwort, St. John's wort, sweet orange, yohimbe

Cephalexin (Biocef, Keftab) biotin, niacin, riboflavin, thiamin, vitamin B_6, vitamin B_{12}, vitamin K

Cephalothin (Ceporacin) biotin, niacin, riboflavin, thiamin, vitamin B_6, vitamin B_{12}, vitamin K

Cephapirin (Cefadyl) biotin, niacin, riboflavin, thiamin, vitamin B_6, vitamin B_{12}, vitamin K

Cepharadine (Velosef) biotin, niacin, riboflavin, thiamin, vitamin B_6, vitamin B_{12}, vitamin K

Cetirizine (Reactine, Zyrtec) belladonna, corkwood, English lavender, henbane, khat

Cevimeline (Evoxac) areca nut, Chinese club moss, iboga

Chloral hydrate (Aquachloral Supprettes, Somnote) ashwagandha, bitter almond, California poppy, cowslip, elecampane, English lavender, ethanol, German chamomile, gotu kola, kava kava, maté, passion flower, poke, poppy, rauwolfia, scullcap, senega, stinging nettle, valerian, wild carrot, wild lettuce, yarrow

Chloramphenicol (Diochloram, Pentamycetin) folic acid, vitamin B_{12}

Chlordiazepoxide (Apo-Chlordiazepoxide, Librium) ashwagandha, bitter almond, California poppy, cowslip, elecampane, English lavender, ethanol, German chamomile, gotu kola, kava kava, maté, passion flower, poke, poppy, rauwolfia, scullcap, senega, stinging nettle, St. John's wort, valerian, wild carrot, wild cherry, wild lettuce, yarrow

Chloroquine (Aralen) ethanol

Chlorothiazide (Diuril) aloe, andrographis, apple cider vinegar, arnica, asa foetida, birch, bishop's weed, black cohosh, black root, bladderwrack, blue cohosh, blue flag, buckthorn, butternut, calcium, calotropis, carrageen, cascara sagrada, castor oil plant, cat's claw, catechu, colocynth, corn silk, cowslip, cucumber, dandelion, devil's claw, digitalis, European mistletoe, fo-ti, frangula, gamboge, ginkgo biloba, gossypol, horsetail, Indian hemp, jalap, kelp, khat, licorice, lily-of-the-valley, magnesium, ma-huang, manna, maté, mayapple, parsley, potassium, quassia, rue, senna, sorrel, stevia, stinging nettle, St. John's wort, stone root, uva ursi, uzara, vitamin D, wahoo, wallflower, wild carrot, wood betony, yarrow, yellow dock, yohimbe, zinc

Chlorpheniramine and acetaminophen (Coricidin HBP Cold and Flu) belladonna, corkwood, English lavender, henbane, khat

Chlorpheniramine and phenylephrine (Histatab Plus, Rynatan) belladonna, corkwood, English lavender, henbane, khat

Chlorpheniramine, ephedrine, phenylephrine, and carbetapentane (Rynatuss, Tynatuss Pediatric) belladonna, English lavender, henbane, khat

Chlorpheniramine, phenylephrine, and dextromethorphan (Alka-Seltzer Plus Cold and Cough) belladonna, corkwood, henbane, English lavender, khat

Chlorpheniramine, phenylephrine, and methscopolamine (AH-Chew, Extendryl) belladonna, corkwood, henbane, English lavender, khat

Chlorpheniramine, phenylephrine, and phenyltoloxamine (Comhist, Nalex-A) belladonna, corkwood, English lavender, henbane, khat

Chlorpheniramine, phenylephrine, codeine, and potassium iodide (Pediacof) belladonna, corkwood, English lavender, henbane, khat

Chlorpheniramine, pseudoephedrine, and codeine (Dihistine DH, Ryna-C) belladonna, corkwood, English lavender, henbane, khat

Chlorpheniramine, pseudoephedrine, and dextromethorphan (Robitussin Pediatric Night Relief, Vicks Pediatric 44M) belladonna, corkwood, English lavender, henbane, khat

Chlorpromazine (Largactil, Thorazine) angel's trumpet, belladonna, black tea, coffee, corkwood, cowhage, dong quai, evening primrose oil, gotu kola, henbane, jimson weed, kava kava, ma-huang, rauwolfia, riboflavin, valerian, yohimbe

Chlorpropamide (Diabinese, Novo-Propamide) agrimony, aloe, avaram, banaba, barley, basil, bilberry, bitter melon, black tea, bladderwrack, blue cohosh, buchu, bugleweed, burdock, caffeine, chanca piedra, Chinese cucumber root, cinnamon, cocoa, coffee, cola nut, coriander, country mallow, cumin, damiana, dandelion, devil's claw, eucalyptus, fenugreek, flax, garlic, ginger, ginseng (American), ginseng (Panax), ginseng (Siberian), glucomannan, goat's rue, gotu kola, green tea, guar gum, gymnema, horehound, horse chestnut, kudzu, laurel, licorice, Madagascar periwinkle, ma-huang, maitake mushroom, marshmallow, myrrh, niacin, olive, onion, prickly pear cactus, psyllium, psyllium seed, raspberry, senega, Solomon's seal, stevia, St. John's wort

Chlorthalidone (Apo-Chlorthalidone, Thalitone) andrographis, apple cider vinegar, arnica, asa foetida, birch, bishop's weed, black cohosh, black root, bladderwrack, blue cohosh, blue flag, buckthorn, butternut, calotropis, carrageen, cascara sagrada, castor oil plant, cat's claw, catechu, colocynth, corn silk, cowslip, cucumber, dandelion, devil's claw, digitalis, European mistletoe, fo-ti, frangula, gamboge, gossypol, horsetail, Indian hemp, jalap, kelp, khat, licorice, lily-of-the-valley, magnesium, ma-huang, manna, maté, mayapple, parsley, potassium, quassia, rue, senna, sorrel, stevia, stinging nettle, stone root, uva ursi, uzara, wahoo, wallflower, wild carrot, wood betony, yarrow, yellow dock, yohimbe, zinc

Chlorzoxazone (Parafon Forte DSC, Strifion Forte) ethanol, St. John's wort, watercress

Cholestyramine (Prevalite, Questran) beta-carotene, calcium, folic acid, gotu kola, iron, magnesium, niacin, vitamin A, vitamin B_{12}, vitamin D, vitamin E, vitamin K, zinc

Choline magnesium trisalicylate (Trilisate) bog bean, cat's claw, cayenne, dong quai, fever-

few, folic acid, garlic, ginger, ginkgo biloba, gossypol, green tea, heartsease, horse chestnut, iron, licorice, lovage, lungwort, niacin, northern prickly ash, pau d'arco, pineapple, poplar, potassium, red clover, reishi mushroom, safflower, saw palmetto, senega, St. John's wort, tonka bean, turmeric, uva ursi, vitamin C, white willow, wintergreen, yarrow

Choline salicylate (Arthropan, Teejel) bog bean, cayenne, feverfew, folic acid, garlic, ginkgo biloba, gossypol, heartsease, horse chestnut, iron, lovage, lungwort, niacin, northern prickly ash, pau d'arco, pineapple, poplar, potassium, reishi mushroom, safflower, saw palmetto, senega, St. John's wort, tonka bean, turmeric, vitamin C, uva ursi, white willow, wintergreen, yarrow

Ciclopirox (Loprox, Penlac) gossypol

Cidofovir (Vistide) bitter melon, boneset, butterbur, calcium, chaparral, colt's foot, comfrey, echinacea, fenugreek, maté, potassium

Cilazapril (Inhibace) cayenne, dong quai, garlic, pineapple, pomegranate, potassium, St. John's wort, yohimbe

Cilostazol (Pletal) digitalis, Indian squill, squill

Cimetidine (Nu-Cimet, Tagamet) aletris, angelica, belladonna, birthwort, black mustard, black tea, blessed thistle, bog bean, caffeine, calamus, calcium, cocoa, coffee, cola nut, colombo, corkwood, cubeb, dandelion, devil's claw, English lavender, folic acid, ginger, goldenseal, green tea, guarana, henbane, iron, khat, lesser galangal, maté, thiamin, vitamin B_{12}, vitamin D, yellow gentian, zinc

Cinoxacin (Cinobac) biotin, black tea, caffeine, calcium, cocoa, coffee, cola nut, green tea, guarana, iron, magnesium, niacin, riboflavin, thiamin, vitamin B_6, vitamin B_{12}, vitamin K, zinc

Ciprofibrate (Estaprol, Modalim) gotu kola

Ciprofloxacin (Ciloxan, Cipro) agrimony, black tea, caffeine, calcium, celery, cocoa, coffee, cola nut, coriander, dong quai, echinacea, fennel, ginkgo biloba, green tea, guarana, iron, lovage, magnesium, maté, motherwort, niacin, riboflavin, rosemary, thiamin, vitamin B_6, vitamin B_{12}, vitamin K, wild carrot, wormwood, zinc

Cisatracurium (Nimbex) magnesium

Cisplatin (Platinol, Platinol-AQ) black cohosh, calcium, dong quai, magnesium, potassium

Citalopram (Celexa) ergot, gotu kola, kava kava, marijuana, St. John's wort, valerian, yohimbe

Cladribine (Leustatin) ethanol

Clarithromycin (Biaxin, Biaxin XL) biotin, niacin, riboflavin, thiamin, uzara, vitamin B_6, vitamin B_{12}, vitamin K, wahoo

Clemastine (Tavist Allergy) belladonna, corkwood, English lavender, ethanol, henbane, khat

Clidinium and chlordiazepoxide (Apo-Chlorax, Librax) angel's trumpet, areca nut, butterbur, calabar bean, catechu, Chinese club moss, iboga, jimson weed, mandrake, scopolia

Clindamycin (Cleocin, Dalacin C) vitamin K

Clobazam (Alti-Clobazam, Frisium) ashwagandha, bitter almond, California poppy, elecampane, ethanol, German chamomile, gotu kola, kava kava, maté, passion flower, poke, poppy, rauwolfia, scullcap, senega, stinging nettle, St. John's wort, valerian, wild carrot, wild cherry, wild lettuce, yarrow

Clobenzorex (Asenlix) black tea, caffeine, cocoa, coffee, cola nut, green tea

Clodronate (Bonefos, Ostac) calcium, iron, magnesium

Clofibrate (Claripex, Novo-Fibrate) beta-carotene, gotu kola, iron, vitamin B_{12}, vitamin E

Clomipramine (Anafranil, Novo-Clopramine) angel's trumpet, belladonna, black tea, coffee, corkwood, ergot, ethanol, grapefruit, henbane, jimson weed, kava kava, ma-huang, marijuana, rauwolfia, riboflavin, scopolia, St. John's wort, valerian, yohimbe

Clonazepam (Klonopin, Rivotril) ashwagandha, bitter almond, California poppy, catnip, cedar leaf, elecampane, ethanol, evening primrose oil, German chamomile, ginkgo biloba, goldenseal, gotu kola, kava kava, lemon balm, linden, maté, nerve root, passion flower, poke, poppy, rauwolfia, sage, sassafras, scullcap, senega, stinging nettle, St. John's wort, valerian, wild carrot, wild cherry, wild lettuce, wormseed, yarrow

Clonidine (Catapres, Duraclon) andrographis, arnica, asa foetida, bishop's weed, black cohosh, blue cohosh, carrageen, cat's claw, catechu, devil's claw, dong quai, European mistletoe, gotu kola, kava kava, kelp, khat, licorice, ma-huang, parsley, rue, stevia, valerian, wild carrot, wood betony, yarrow, yohimbe

Clopidogrel (Plavix) ajava seeds, allspice, andrographis, angelica, arnica, asa foetida, astragalus, bilberry, bishop's weed, bladderwrack, bog bean, boldo, borage, borage seed oil, bromelain, buchu, carrageen, cat's claw, cayenne, clove, danshen, deer's tongue, dong quai, English hawthorn, evening primrose oil, feverfew, garlic, ginger, ginkgo biloba, ginseng (American), ginseng (Panax), ginseng (Siberian), green tea, horse chestnut, kava kava, licorice, lovage, pau d'arco, quinine, red clover, reishi mushroom, safflower, saw palmetto, sea buckthorn, stinging nettle, sweet clover, sweet vernal grass, turmeric, valerian, vitamin E, white willow, yarrow

Clorazepate (Tranxene, T-Tab) ashwagandha, bitter almond, California poppy, cedar leaf, cowslip, elecampane, English lavender, ethanol, evening primrose oil, German chamomile, ginkgo biloba, gotu kola, kava kava, maté, passion flower, poke, poppy, rauwolfia, sage, scullcap, senega, stinging nettle, St. John's wort, valerian, wild carrot, wild cherry, wild lettuce, wormseed, yarrow

Clotrimazole (Gyne-Lotrimin 3, Mycelex) gossypol

Cloxacillin (Cloxapen, Nu-Cloxi) biotin, niacin, potassium, riboflavin, thiamin, vitamin B$_6$, vitamin B$_{12}$, vitamin K

Clozapine (Clozaril, Gen-Clozapine) black tea, cabbage, caffeine, cocoa, coffee, cola nut, cowhage, gotu kola, green tea, henbane, kava kava, rauwolfia, St. John's wort, valerian

Codeine (Codeine Contin) ashwagandha, bitter almond, California poppy, corkwood, elecampane, English lavender, ethanol, gotu kola, kava kava, maté, parsley, passion flower, poke, poppy, rauwolfia, scullcap, senega, stinging nettle, valerian, wild carrot, wild lettuce, yarrow

Colchicine (ratio-Colchicine) beta-carotene, calcium, colchicum, echinacea, folic acid, magnesium, potassium, vitamin B$_{12}$

Colchicine plus probenecid (ColBenemid) beta-carotene, potassium, vitamin B$_{12}$

Colesevelam (WelChol) beta-carotene, folic acid, gotu kola, iron, vitamin A, vitamin B$_{12}$, vitamin D, vitamin E, vitamin K

Colestipol (Colestid) beta-carotene, calcium, folic acid, gotu kola, iron, niacin, vitamin A, vitamin B$_{12}$, vitamin D, vitamin E, vitamin K

Cortisone (Cortone) adonis, aloe, andrographis, ashwagandha, astragalus, buckthorn, butternut, calcium, cascara sagrada, castor oil plant, folic acid, frangula, Indian squill, larch, licorice, lily-of-the-valley, magnesium, ma-huang, oleander, perilla, potassium, schisandra, squill, strophanthus, vitamin A, vitamin B$_6$, vitamin C, vitamin D, vitamin K, wallflower, zinc

Cyclobenzaprine (Flexeril, Novo-Cycloprine) butterbur, cabbage, catnip, corkwood, ethanol, goldenseal, gotu kola, jimson weed, kava kava, lemon balm, nerve root, sassafras, stinging nettle, valerian

Cyclopentolate (Cyclogyl, Cylate) angel's trumpet, areca nut, butterbur, calabar bean, catechu, Chinese club moss, iboga, jimson weed, mandrake, scopolia

Cyclophosphamide (Cytoxan, Neosar) astragalus, black cohosh, cordyceps, dong quai, potassium, St. John's wort

Cycloserine (Seromycin Pulvules) folic acid, vitamin B_6, vitamin B_{12}

Cyclosporine (Neoral, Sandimmune) alfalfa, andrographis, ashwagandha, astragalus, bitter melon, boneset, butterbur, cat's claw, chaparral, colt's foot, comfrey, echinacea, European mistletoe, fenugreek, grapefruit, larch, licorice, magnesium, maitake mushroom, maté, noni, pill-bearing spurge, potassium, schisandra, scullcap, St. John's wort, turmeric, wild cherry

Cyproheptadine (Periactin) belladonna, corkwood, English lavender, henbane, khat

Cyproterone and ethinyl estradiol (Diane-35) acerola, alfalfa, anise, black cohosh, calcium, dong quai, red clover, senna, St. John's wort, vitamin C, wild cherry, wild yam

Dacarbazine (DTIC, DTIC-Dome) dong quai, ethanol

Daclizumab (Zenapax) andrographis, ashwagandha, astragalus, cat's claw, echinacea, larch, maitake mushroom, schisandra, scullcap, St. John's wort, turmeric

Dactinomycin (Cosmegen) calcium

Dalteparin (Fragmin) ajava seeds, alfalfa, allspice, andrographis, angelica, arnica, asa foetida, astragalus, bilberry, bishop's weed, bladderwrack, bog bean, boldo, borage, borage seed oil, bromelain, buchu, carrageen, cat's claw, cayenne, clove, danshen, deer's tongue, dong quai, evening primrose oil, feverfew, garlic, German chamomile, ginger, ginkgo biloba, ginseng (American), ginseng (Panax), ginseng (Siberian), horse chestnut, kava kava, kelp, licorice, lovage, lungwort, meadowsweet, motherwort, northern prickly ash, papaya, pau d'arco, pineapple, poplar, quinine, red clover, reishi mushroom, safflower, saw palmetto, sea buckthorn, senega, stinging nettle, St. John's wort, sweet clover, sweet vernal grass, tonka bean, turmeric, valerian, vitamin E, white willow, wintergreen, yarrow

Danaparoid (Orgaran) ajava seeds, alfalfa, allspice, andrographis, angelica, arnica, asa foetida, astragalus, bilberry, bishop's weed, bladderwrack, bog bean, boldo, borage, borage seed oil, bromelain, buchu, carrageen, cat's claw, cayenne, clove, danshen, deer's tongue, dong quai, evening primrose oil, feverfew, garlic, German chamomile, ginger, ginkgo biloba, ginseng (American), ginseng (Panax), ginseng (Siberian), green tea, horse chestnut, kava kava, kelp, licorice, lovage, lungwort, meadowsweet, motherwort, northern prickly ash, papaya, pau d'arco, pineapple, poplar, quinine, red clover, reishi mushroom, safflower, saw palmetto, sea buckthorn, senega, stinging nettle, St. John's wort, sweet clover, sweet vernal grass, tonka bean, turmeric, valerian, vitamin E, white willow, wintergreen, yarrow

Dantrolene (Dantrium) gotu kola, kava kava, valerian

Daunorubicin hydrochloride (Cerubidine) ethanol

Deferoxamine (Desferal) calcium

Deflazacort (Calcort, Dezacor) adonis, aloe, andrographis, ashwagandha, astragalus, buckthorn, butternut, cascara sagrada, castor oil plant, frangula, Indian squill, larch, licorice, lily-of-the-valley, ma-huang, oleander, perilla, schisandra, squill, strophanthus, wallflower

Delapril (Adecut, Delakete) cayenne, pineapple, pomegranate, potassium, St. John's wort, yohimbe

Delavirdine (Rescriptor) St. John's wort, vitamin B_{12}, zinc

Demeclocycline (Declomycin) bromelain, calcium, dong quai, folic acid, iron, magnesium, niacin, riboflavin, St. John's wort, thiamin, uzara, vitamin A, vitamin B_6, vitamin B_{12}, vitamin C, vitamin K, wahoo, zinc

Denileukin diftitox (ONTAK) calcium, potassium

Deptropine (Deptropine FNA) belladonna, corkwood, English lavender, henbane, khat

Desipramine (Alti-Desipramine, Norpramin) angel's trumpet, belladonna, black tea, butterbur, catnip, coffee, corkwood, ergot, ethanol, fennel, ginkgo biloba, goldenseal, henbane, jimson weed, kava kava, lemon balm, ma-huang, marijuana, nerve root, rauwolfia, riboflavin, sage, sassafras, scopolia, stinging nettle, St. John's wort, valerian, wormwood, yohimbe

Desloratadine (Aerius, Clarinex) belladonna, corkwood, English lavender, henbane, khat

Dexamethasone (Decadron, Dexasone) adonis, alfalfa, aloe, andrographis, ashwagandha, astragalus, buckthorn, butternut, calcium, cascara sagrada, castor oil plant, cat's claw, country mallow, echinacea, ethanol, European mistletoe, folic acid, frangula, Indian squill, larch, licorice, lily-of-the-valley, magnesium, ma-huang, noni, oleander, perilla, potassium, schisandra, squill, strophanthus, vitamin A, vitamin B_6, vitamin C, vitamin D, vitamin K, wallflower, zinc

Dexbrompheniramine and pseudoephedrine (Drixomed, Drixoral Cold & Allergy) belladonna, corkwood, English lavender, henbane, khat

Dexchlorpheniramine belladonna, corkwood, English lavender, henbane, khat

Dexmedetomidine (Precedex) ashwagandha, bitter almond, California poppy, cowslip, elecampane, English lavender, ethanol, German chamomile, maté, passion flower, poke, poppy, rauwolfia, scullcap, senega, stinging nettle, valerian, wild carrot, wild lettuce, yarrow

Dexmethylphenidate (Focalin) maté

Dextroamphetamine (Dexedrine, Dextrostat) khat, maté, St. John's wort

Dextroamphetamine and amphetamine (Adderall, Adderall XR) khat, maté, St. John's wort

Dextromethorphan (found in various formulations of Alka-Seltzer, Contac, PediaCare, Robitussin, Sudafed, Triaminic, and other over-the-counter medications) bitter orange, ergot, grapefruit

Diazepam (Apo-Diazepam, Valium) ashwagandha, bitter almond, California poppy, catnip, cedar leaf, cowslip, echinacea, elecampane, English lavender, ethanol, evening primrose oil, German chamomile, ginkgo biloba, goldenseal, gotu kola, grapefruit, kava kava, lemon balm, linden, maté, nerve root, passion flower, poke, poppy, rauwolfia, sage, sassafras, scullcap, senega, stinging nettle, St. John's wort, valerian, wild carrot, wild cherry, wild lettuce, wormseed, yarrow

Diazoxide (Hyperstat, Proglycem) andrographis, arnica, asa foetida, bishop's weed, black cohosh, blue cohosh, carrageen, cat's claw, catechu, devil's claw, European mistletoe, kelp, khat, licorice, mahuang, parsley, rue, stevia, wild carrot, wood betony, yarrow

Dibekacin (Debekacyl, Dikacine) magnesium

Dichlorphenamide (Daranide) ma-huang

Diclofenac (Cataflam, Voltaren) bog bean, cat's claw, dong quai, ethanol, feverfew, folic acid, gar-lic, ginger, ginkgo biloba, gossypol, horse chestnut, niacin, red clover, reishi mushroom, saw palmetto, St. John's wort, turmeric, uva ursi, white willow

Diclofenac plus misoprostol (Arthrotec) folic acid

Dicloxacillin (Dycill, Pathocil) biotin, niacin, potassium, riboflavin, thiamin, vitamin B_6, vitamin B_{12}, vitamin K

Dicyclomine (Bentyl, Lomine) angel's trumpet, areca nut, butterbur, calabar bean, catechu, Chinese club moss, iboga, jimson weed, mandrake, scopolia

Didanosine (Videx, Videx EC) ethanol, vitamin B_{12}, zinc

Diethylpropion (Tenuate) black tea, caffeine, cocoa, coffee, cola nut, green tea

Difenoxin and atropine (Motofen) nutmeg

Diflorasone (Florone, Maxiflor) calcium, folic acid, magnesium, potassium, vitamin C, vitamin D, zinc

Diflunisal (Apo-Diflunisal, Dolobid) bog bean, cat's claw, dong quai, ethanol, feverfew, folic acid, garlic, ginger, ginkgo biloba, gossypol, horse chestnut, niacin, red clover, reishi mushroom, saw palmetto, St. John's wort, turmeric, uva ursi, white willow

Digitalis (Digitek, Lanoxin) adonis, aloe, apple cider vinegar, black hellbore, black root, blue flag, buckthorn, butternut, calcium, calotropis, cascara sagrada, castor oil plant, cereus, Chinese rhubarb, colocynth, cucumber, danshen, English hawthorn, English plantain, fenugreek, flax, frangula, fumitory, gamboge, ginger, ginseng (Siberian), goldenseal, guarana, hedge mustard, horsetail, Indian hemp, Indian squill, jalap, khat, kudzu, licorice, lily-of-the-valley, magnesium, ma-huang, motherwort, oleander, pleurisy root, potassium, psyllium, psyllium seed, rauwolfia, rue, sarsaparilla, senna, shepherd's purse, squill, St. John's wort, strophanthus, swamp milkweed, thiamin, uzara, wahoo, wallflower, wild carrot, yellow dock

Digoxin immune fab (Digibind, Digi-Fab) potassium

Dihydrocodeine, aspirin, and caffeine (Synalgos-DC) ashwagandha, bitter almond, California poppy, corkwood, elecampane, English lavender, ethanol, kava kava, maté, parsley, passion flower, poke, poppy, rauwolfia, scullcap, senega, stinging nettle, valerian, wild carrot, wild lettuce, yarrow

Dihydroergotamine (Migranal) country mallow, ergot

Diltiazem (Cardizem, Tiazac) aloe, andrographis, arnica, asa foetida, bishop's weed, black cohosh, blue cohosh, buckthorn, calcium, carrageen, cascara sagrada, cat's claw, catechu, chicory, Chinese rhubarb, devil's claw, dong quai, English hawthorn, ethanol, European mistletoe, fumitory, garlic, ginger, goldenseal, grapefruit, guarana, gymnema, kelp, khat, kudzu, licorice, lily-of-the-valley, magnesium, ma-huang, niacin, parsley, rue, senna, stevia, St. John's wort, wild carrot, wild cherry, wood betony, yarrow, yohimbe

Dimethindene (Fenistil) belladonna, corkwood, English lavender, henbane, khat

Diphenhydramine (Benadryl Allergy, Nytol) ashwagandha, belladonna, bitter almond, butterbur, California poppy, catnip, corkwood, cowslip, elecampane, English lavender, ethanol, German chamomile, goldenseal, gotu kola, henbane, jimson weed, kava kava, khat, lemon balm, maté, nerve root, passion flower, poke, poppy, rauwolfia, sassafras, scullcap, senega, stinging nettle, valerian, wild carrot, wild lettuce, yarrow

Diphenhydramine and pseudoephedrine (Benadryl Allergy/Decongestant, Benadryl Children's Allergy and Sinus) belladonna, corkwood, English lavender, henbane, khat

Diphenoxylate and atropine (Lomotil, Lonox) ethanol, nutmeg

Dipyridamole (Novo-Dipiradol, Persantine) ajava seeds, allspice, andrographis, angelica, arnica, asa foetida, astragalus, bilberry, bishop's weed, black tea, bladderwrack, bog bean, boldo, borage, borage seed oil, bromelain, buchu, caffeine, carrageen, cat's claw, cayenne, clove, cocoa, coffee, cola nut, danshen, deer's tongue, dong quai, English hawthorn, evening primrose oil, feverfew, garlic, ginger, ginkgo biloba, ginseng (American), ginseng (Panax), ginseng (Siberian), green tea, horse chestnut, kava kava, licorice, lovage, pau d'arco, quinine, red clover, reishi mushroom, safflower, saw palmetto, sea buckthorn, stinging nettle, sweet clover, sweet vernal grass, turmeric, valerian, vitamin E, white willow, yarrow

Dipyrone (Analgina, Dinador) bog bean, fever-few, garlic, ginkgo biloba, gossypol, niacin, reishi mushroom, saw palmetto, St. John's wort, turmeric, uva ursi, white willow

Dirithromycin (Dynabac) biotin, niacin, riboflavin, thiamin, uzara, vitamin B_6, vitamin B_{12}, vitamin K, wahoo

Disopyramide (Norpace, Rhythmodan) aloe, buckthorn, cascara sagrada, ethanol, fumitory, khat, kudzu, licorice, potassium, senna

Disulfiram (Antabuse) black tea, caffeine, cocoa, coffee, cola nut, ethanol, green tea, guarana, marijuana

Dobutamine (Dobutrex) digitalis, fever bark, Indian squill, ma-huang, rauwolfia, squill

Docetaxel (Taxotere) boneset, butterbur, chaparral, colt's foot, comfrey, echinacea, ethanol, yew

Docusate (Colace, Ex-Lax Stool Softener) adonis, licorice, lily-of-the-valley, oleander, senna, squill, strophanthus

Docusate and senna (Peri-Colace, Senokot-S) adonis, butternut, calotropis, cascara sagrada, castor oil plant, frangula, gamboge, Indian squill, licorice, lily-of-the-valley, oleander, senna, squill, strophanthus, uzara, wahoo, wallflower

Dofetilide (Tikosyn) aloe, boneset, buckthorn, butterbur, cascara sagrada, chaparral, Chinese rhubarb, colt's foot, comfrey, echinacea, English hawthorn, fumitory, guarana, khat, kudzu, licorice, senna

Donepezil (Aricept) areca nut, Chinese club moss, iboga

Dopamine (Intropin) digitalis, fever bark, Indian squill, ma-huang, rauwolfia, squill

Dopexamine (Dopacard) digitalis, fever bark, Indian squill, ma-huang, rauwolfia, squill

Doxacurium (Nuromax) magnesium

Doxapram (Dopram) maté

Doxazosin (Alti-Doxazosin, Cardura) andrographis, arnica, asa foetida, bishop's weed, black cohosh, blue cohosh, carrageen, cat's claw, catechu, devil's claw, dong quai, European mistletoe, garlic, kelp, khat, licorice, ma-huang, parsley, rue, stevia, wild carrot, wood betony, yarrow, yohimbe

Doxepin (Sinequan, Zonalon) angel's trumpet, belladonna, black tea, butterbur, catnip, coffee, corkwood, cowslip, ergot, ethanol, fennel, ginkgo biloba, goldenseal, henbane, jimson weed, kava kava, lemon balm, ma-huang, marijuana, nerve root, rauwolfia, riboflavin, sassafras, scopolia, stinging nettle, St. John's wort, valerian, wormwood, yohimbe

Doxorubicin (Adriamycin, Rubex) black cohosh, dong quai, riboflavin

Doxorubicin liposomal (Doxil) riboflavin

Doxycycline (Monodox, Vibramycin) agrimony, bromelain, calcium, celery, coriander, dong quai, echinacea, ethanol, fennel, folic acid, iron, lovage, magnesium, motherwort, niacin, riboflavin, rosemary, St. John's wort, thiamin, uzara, vitamin A, vitamin B_6, vitamin B_{12}, vitamin C, vitamin K, wahoo, wild carrot, zinc

Doxylamine and pyridoxine (Diclectin) belladonna, English lavender, ethanol, gotu kola, henbane, kava kava, khat, valerian

Dronabinol (Marinol) ethanol

Droperidol (Inapsine) cowhage, rauwolfia

Drotrecogin alfa (Xigris) cat's claw, dong quai, evening primrose oil, feverfew, garlic, ginger, ginkgo biloba, ginseng (American), ginseng (Panax), ginseng (Siberian), green tea, horse chestnut, red clover

Econazole (Spectazole) gossypol

Edrophonium (Enlon, Reversol) areca nut, Chinese club moss, iboga

Efalizumab (Raptiva) andrographis, ashwagandha, astragalus, cat's claw, echinacea, larch, maitake mushroom, schisandra, scullcap, St. John's wort, turmeric

Efavirenz (Sustiva) ethanol, St. John's wort

Eletriptan (Relpax) St. John's wort

Enalapril (Vasotec) agrimony, andrographis, arnica, asa foetida, bishop's weed, black cohosh, blue cohosh, carrageen, cat's claw, catechu, cayenne, celery, coriander, devil's claw, dong quai, European mistletoe, fennel, garlic, ginger, goldenseal, kelp, khat, licorice, lovage, mahuang, motherwort, parsley, pineapple, pomegranate, potassium, rosemary, rue, stevia, St. John's wort, wild carrot, wood betony, yarrow, yohimbe, zinc

Enalapril plus Felodipine (Lexxel) zinc

Enalapril plus hydrochlorothiazide (Vaseretic) magnesium, potassium, vitamin B_6, zinc

Enoxacin (Penetrex) magnesium, potassium, vitamin B_6, zinc

Enoxaparin (Lovenox) ajava seeds, alfalfa, allspice, andrographis, angelica, anise, arnica, asa foetida, astragalus, bilberry, bishop's weed, bladderwrack, bog bean, boldo, borage, borage seed oil, bromelain, buchu, carrageen, cayenne, clove, danshen, deer's tongue, devil's claw, dong quai, evening primrose oil, fenugreek, feverfew, garlic, German chamomile, ginger, ginkgo biloba, ginseng (American), ginseng (Panax), ginseng (Siberian), goldenseal, grape seed, green tea, horse chestnut, kava kava, licorice, lovage, lungwort, meadowsweet, motherwort, northern prickly ash, onion, papaya, parsley, passion flower, pau d'arco, pineapple, poplar, quinine, red clover, reishi mushroom, rue, safflower, saw palmetto, sea buckthorn, senega, stinging nettle, St. John's wort, sweet clover, sweet vernal grass, tonka bean, turmeric, valerian, vitamin E, white willow, wintergreen, yarrow

Enoximone (Perfan) digitalis, Indian squill, squill

Ephedrine (Pretz-D) black tea, bugleweed, caffeine, cocoa, coffee, cola nut, digitalis, fever bark, goldenseal, green tea, guarana, Indian squill, licorice, ma-huang, maté, rauwolfia, Scotch broom, squill, witch hazel, yohimbe

Epinastine (Elestat) belladonna, corkwood, English lavender, henbane, khat

Epinephrine (Adrenalin, EpiPen) black tea, caffeine, cocoa, coffee, cola nut, green tea, rauwolfia

Epirubicin (Ellence, Pharmorubicin) black cohosh, dong quai, ethanol

Eplerenone (Inspra) andrographis, arnica, asa foetida, bishop's weed, black cohosh, blue cohosh, carrageen, cat's claw, catechu, devil's claw, European mistletoe, kelp, khat, licorice, ma-huang, parsley, rue, stevia, wild carrot, wood betony, yarrow

Epoprostenol (Flolan) potassium

Eprosartan (Teveten) andrographis, arnica, asa foetida, bishop's weed, black cohosh, blue cohosh, carrageen, cat's claw, catechu, devil's claw, dong quai, European mistletoe, garlic, kelp, khat, licorice, ma-huang, parsley, potassium, rue, stevia, wild carrot, wood betony, yarrow, yohimbe

Eptifibatide (Integrillin) ajava seeds, allspice, andrographis, angelica, arnica, asa foetida, astragalus, bilberry, bishop's weed, bladderwrack, bog bean, boldo, borage, borage seed oil, bromelain, buchu, carrageen, cat's claw, cayenne, clove, dan-shen, deer's tongue, dong quai, English hawthorn, evening primrose oil, feverfew, garlic, ginger, ginkgo biloba, ginseng (American), ginseng (Panax), ginseng (Siberian), horse chestnut, kava kava, licorice, lovage, pau d'arco, quinine, reishi mushroom, safflower, saw palmetto, sea buckthorn, stinging nettle, sweet clover, sweet vernal grass, turmeric, valerian, vitamin E, white willow, yarrow

Ergoloid mesylates (Hydergine) country mallow, ergot

Ergonovine country mallow, ergot

Ergotamine (Cafergor, Cafergot) black tea, bugleweed, caffeine, cocoa, coffee, cola nut, country mallow, ergot, goldenseal, green tea, guarana, Scotch broom, witch hazel

Erythromycin (Erythrocin, Staticin) boneset, butterbur, chaparral, colt's foot, comfrey, echinacea, ethanol, folic acid, grapefruit, niacin, pill-bearing spurge, riboflavin, thiamin, uzara, vitamin B_6, vitamin B_{12}, vitamin K, wahoo

Erythromycin and sulfisoxazole (Eryzole, Pediazole) St. John's wort

Esmolol (Brevibloc) aloe, andrographis, arnica, asa foetida, bishop's weed, black cohosh, blue cohosh, buckthorn, butterbur, carrageen, cascara sagrada, cat's claw, catechu, devil's claw, European mistletoe, fumitory, kelp, khat, kudzu, licorice, lily-of-the-valley, ma-huang, motherwort, parsley, rue, senna, stevia, St. John's wort, wild carrot, wood betony, yarrow, yohimbe

Esomeprazole (Nexium) aletris, angelica, birthwort, black mustard, blessed thistle, calamus, colombo, cubeb, dandelion, devil's claw, ginger, iron, lesser galangal, vitamin B₁₂, yellow gentian

Estazolam (ProSom) ashwagandha, bitter almond, California poppy, cowslip, elecampane, English lavender, ethanol, German chamomile, kava kava, maté, passion flower, poke, poppy, rauwolfia, scullcap, senega, stinging nettle, St. John's wort, valerian, wild carrot, wild cherry, wild lettuce, yarrow

Estradiol (Climara, Estrace) acerola, alfalfa, anise, black cohosh, calcium, dong quai, ethanol, red clover, senna, St. John's wort, vitamin C, wild cherry, wild yam

Estradiol and medroxyprogesterone (Lunelle) alfalfa, anise

Estradiol and norethindrone (Activella, Combi-Patch) acerola, alfalfa, anise, calcium, red clover, senna, St. John's wort, vitamin C, wild cherry, wild yam

Estradiol and testosterone (Climacteron) acerola, alfalfa, anise, calcium, red clover, senna, St. John's wort, vitamin C, wild cherry, wild yam

Estrogens (conjugated A/synthetic) (Cenestin) acerola, alfalfa, anise, black cohosh, black tea, caffeine, calcium, Cherokee rosehip, cocoa, coffee, cola nut, dong quai, ethanol, ginseng (Panax), grapefruit, green tea, guarana, red clover, senna, St. John's wort, wild cherry, wild yam

Estrogens (conjugated/equine) (Congest, Premarin) acerola, alfalfa, anise, black cohosh, black tea, caffeine, calcium, Cherokee rosehip, cocoa, coffee, cola nut, dong quai, ethanol, ginseng (Panax), grapefruit, green tea, guarana, red clover, senna, St. John's wort, wild cherry, wild yam

Estrogens (conjugated/equine) and medroxyprogesterone (Premphase, Prempro) acerola, alfalfa, anise, black tea, caffeine, calcium, Cherokee rosehip, cocoa, coffee, cola nut, grapefruit, green tea, guarana, red clover, St. John's wort, wild yam

Estrogens (esterified) (Estratab, Menest) acerola, alfalfa, anise, black cohosh, black tea, caffeine, calcium, Cherokee rosehip, cocoa, coffee, cola nut, dong quai, ethanol, grapefruit, green tea, guarana, red clover, senna, St. John's wort, wild cherry, wild yam

Estrogens (esterified) and methyltestosterone (Estratest, Estratest H.S.) acerola, alfalfa, anise, black tea, caffeine, calcium, Cherokee rosehip, cocoa, coffee, cola nut, grapefruit, green tea, guarana, red clover, senna, St. John's wort, wild cherry, wild yam

Estropipate (Ogen, Ortho-Est) acerola, alfalfa, anise, black cohosh, calcium, dong quai, ethanol, red clover, senna, St. John's wort, wild cherry, wild yam

Ethacrynic acid (Edecrin) aloe, apple cider vinegar, birch, bishop's weed, black root, bladderwrack, blue flag, buckthorn, butternut, calcium, calotropis, cascara sagrada, castor oil plant, colocynth, corn silk, cowslip, cucumber, dandelion, digitalis, fo-ti, frangula, gamboge, gossypol, horsetail, Indian hemp, jalap, licorice, lily-of-the-valley, magnesium, manna, maté, mayapple, potassium, quassia, senna, sorrel, stinging nettle, St. John's wort, stone root, thiamin, uva ursi, uzara, vitamin B_6, vitamin C, wahoo, wallflower, wild carrot, yellow dock, yohimbe, zinc

Ethambutol (Myambutol) zinc

Ethinyl estradiol (Estinyl) acerola, alfalfa, anise, black cohosh, calcium, dong quai, ethanol, red clover, senna, St. John's wort, vitamin C, wild cherry, wild yam

Ethinyl estradiol and desogestrel (Cyclessa, Ortho-Cept) acerola, alfalfa, anise, black tea, caffeine, calcium, chaste tree berry, Cherokee rosehip, cocoa, coffee, cola nut, grapefruit, green tea, guarana, licorice, red clover, senna, St. John's wort, vitamin C, wild cherry, wild yam

Ethinyl estradiol and drospirenone (Yasmin) alfalfa, anise, chaste tree berry, licorice

Ethinyl estradiol and ethynodiol diacetate (Demulen, Zovia) acerola, alfalfa, anise, black cohosh, black tea, caffeine, calcium, chaste tree berry, Cherokee rosehip, cocoa, coffee, cola nut, dong quai, grapefruit, green tea, guarana, licorice, red clover, senna, St. John's wort, vitamin C, wild cherry, wild yam

Ethinyl estradiol and etonogestrel (NuvaRing) acerola, alfalfa, anise, black cohosh, black tea, caffeine, calcium, Cherokee rosehip, cocoa, coffee, cola nut, dong quai, grapefruit, green tea, guarana, red clover, senna, St. John's wort, vitamin C, wild cherry, wild yam

Ethinyl estradiol and levonorgestrel (Alesse, Triphasil) acerola, alfalfa, anise, black cohosh, black tea, caffeine, calcium, chaste tree berry, Cherokee rosehip, cocoa, coffee, cola nut, dong quai, grapefruit, green tea, guarana, licorice, red clover, senna, St. John's wort, vitamin C, wild cherry, wild yam

Ethinyl estradiol and norelgestromin (Evra, Ortho Evra) acerola, alfalfa, anise, black tea, caffeine, calcium, Cherokee rosehip, cocoa, coffee, cola nut, grapefruit, green tea, guarana, red clover, senna, St. John's wort, vitamin C, wild cherry, wild yam

Ethinyl estradiol and norethindrone (Brevicon, Ortho-Novum) acerola, alfalfa, anise, black cohosh, black tea, caffeine, calcium, chaste tree berry, Cherokee rosehip, cocoa, coffee, cola nut, dong quai, ethanol, grapefruit, green tea, guarana, licorice, red clover, senna, St. John's wort, vitamin C, wild cherry, wild yam

Ethinyl estradiol and norgestimate (Cyclen, Ortho Tri-Cyclen) anise, acerola, alfalfa, black cohosh, black tea, caffeine, calcium, chaste tree berry, Cherokee rosehip, cocoa, coffee, cola nut, dong quai, green tea, guarana, grapefruit, licorice, red clover, senna, St. John's wort, vitamin C, wild yam, wild cherry

Ethinyl estradiol and norgestrel (Cryselle, Ovral) acerola, alfalfa, anise, black cohosh, black tea, caffeine, calcium, chaste tree berry, Cherokee rosehip, cocoa, coffee, cola nut, dong quai, grapefruit, green tea, guarana, licorice, red clover, senna, St. John's wort, vitamin C, wild cherry, wild yam

Ethosuximide (Zarontin) biotin, calcium, cedar leaf, evening primrose oil, folic acid, ginkgo biloba, sage, vitamin D, vitamin K, wormseed

Ethotoin (Peganone) folic acid, vitamin D

Etidronate (Didronel) calcium, iron, magnesium, potassium

Etodolac (Lodine, Utradol) agrimony, anise, balsam of Peru, bog bean, boneset, bromelain, butterbur, cat's claw, celery, chaparral, clove, coffee, cola nut, colt's foot, comfrey, coriander, danshen, devil's claw, dong quai, echinacea, ethanol, fennel, fenugreek, feverfew, folic acid, fumitory, garlic, German chamomile, ginger, ginkgo biloba, gossypol, green tea, horse chestnut, juniper, lovage, meadowsweet, motherwort, niacin, oak, onion, parsley, passion flower, red clover, red yeast rice, reishi mushroom, rosemary, rue, saw palmetto, St. John's wort, sweet clover, thunder god vine, turmeric, uva ursi, white willow, wild carrot, wild yam, wintergreen, yohimbe

Etoposide (Toposar, VePesid) ethanol, grapefruit, St. John's wort

Etoposide phosphate (Etopophos) ethanol

Etoricoxib (Arcoxia) bog bean, feverfew, garlic, ginkgo biloba, gossypol, niacin, reishi mushroom,

saw palmetto, St. John's wort, turmeric, uva ursi, white willow

Etozolin (Elkapin) aloe, apple cider vinegar, birch, bishop's weed, black root, bladderwrack, blue flag, buckthorn, butternut, calotropis, cascara sagrada, castor oil plant, colocynth, corn silk, cowslip, cucumber, dandelion, digitalis, fo-ti, frangula, gamboge, gossypol, horsetail, Indian hemp, jalap, licorice, lily-of-the-valley, manna, maté, mayapple, quassia, senna, sorrel, stinging nettle, St. John's wort, stone root, uva ursi, uzara, wahoo, wallflower, wild carrot, yellow dock, yohimbe

Exemestane (Aromasin) black cohosh, dong quai

Famciclovir (Famvir) echinacea

Famotidine (Apo-Famotidine, Pepcid) aletris, angelica, belladonna, birthwort, black mustard, blessed thistle, bog bean, calamus, calcium, colombo, corkwood, cubeb, dandelion, devil's claw, echinacea, English lavender, ethanol, folic acid, ginger, goldenseal, henbane, iron, khat, lesser galangal, thiamin, vitamin B_{12}, vitamin D, yellow gentian, zinc

Famotidine, calcium carbonate, and magnesium hydroxide (Pepcid Complete) aletris, angelica, birthwort, black mustard, blessed thistle, bog bean, buckthorn, calamus, colombo, cubeb, dandelion, devil's claw, ginger, lesser galangal, mahuang, yellow gentian

Felbamate (Felbatol) cedar leaf, ethanol, evening primrose oil, ginkgo biloba, sage, wormseed

Felodipine (Plendil, Renedil) andrographis, arnica, asa foetida, bishop's weed, bitter orange, black cohosh, blue cohosh, calcium, carrageen, cat's claw, catechu, devil's claw, dong quai, English hawthorn, European mistletoe, garlic, ginger, goldenseal, grapefruit, kelp, khat, licorice, lily-of-the-valley, magnesium, ma-huang, niacin, parsley, rue, stevia, St. John's wort, wild carrot, wild cherry, wood betony, yarrow, yohimbe

Fenofibrate (Apo-Fenofibrate, TriCor) gotu kola, potassium, vitamin E

Fenoldopam (Corlopam) andrographis, arnica, asa foetida, bishop's weed, black cohosh, blue cohosh, carrageen, cat's claw, catechu, devil's claw, European mistletoe, kelp, khat, licorice, ma-huang, parsley, potassium, rue, stevia, wild carrot, wood betony, yarrow

Fenoprofen (Nalfon) bog bean, cat's claw, dong quai, ethanol, feverfew, folic acid, garlic, ginger, ginkgo biloba, gossypol, green tea, horse chestnut, niacin, red clover, reishi mushroom, saw palmetto, St. John's wort, turmeric, uva ursi, white willow

Fenoterol (Berotec) black tea, caffeine, cocoa, coffee, cola nut, green tea, yohimbe

Fentanyl (Actiq, Duragesic) ashwagandha, bitter almond, California poppy, corkwood, elecampane, English lavender, ethanol, gotu kola, kava kava, maté, parsley, passion flower, poke, poppy, rauwolfia, scullcap, senega, stinging nettle, valerian, wild carrot, wild lettuce, yarrow

Ferric gluconate (Ferrlecit) artichoke, bilberry, black cohosh, borage, butternut, cascara sagrada, catechu, English lavender, European elder, European mistletoe, eyebright, horehound, horse chestnut, lemon balm, meadowsweet, motherwort, northern prickly ash, oak, poplar, potassium, raspberry, sage, saw palmetto, slippery elm, soybean, stinging nettle, St. John's wort, uva ursi, valerian, witch hazel, wormwood, yarrow, yellow dock

Ferrous fumarate (Femiron, Feostat) artichoke, bilberry, black cohosh, borage, butternut, cascara sagrada, catechu, English lavender, European elder, European mistletoe, eyebright, horehound, horse chestnut, lemon balm, meadowsweet, motherwort, northern prickly ash, oak, poplar, raspberry, sage, saw palmetto, slippery elm, soybean, stinging nettle, St. John's wort, uva ursi, valerian, witch hazel, wormwood, yarrow, yellow dock

Ferrous gluconate (Fergon, Novo-Ferrogluc) artichoke, bilberry, black cohosh, borage, butternut, cascara sagrada, catechu, English lavender, European elder, European mistletoe, eyebright, horehound, horse chestnut, lemon balm, meadowsweet, motherwort, northern prickly ash, oak, poplar, raspberry, sage, saw palmetto, slippery elm, soybean, stinging nettle, St. John's wort, uva ursi, valerian, witch hazel, wormwood, yarrow, yellow dock

Ferrous sulfate (Feratab, Fer-Iron) artichoke, bilberry, black cohosh, borage, butternut, cascara sagrada, catechu, English hawthorn, English lavender, English plantain, European elder, European mistletoe, eyebright, feverfew, German chamomile, gossypol, horehound, horse chestnut, lemon balm, meadowsweet, motherwort, northern prickly ash, oak, oregano, poplar, raspberry, rose hips, sage, saw palmetto, slippery elm, soybean, stinging nettle, St. John's wort, uva ursi, valerian, witch hazel, wormwood, yarrow, yellow dock

Ferrous sulfate and ascorbic acid (Fero-Grad 500, Vitelle Irospan) artichoke, bilberry, black cohosh, borage, butternut, cascara sagrada, catechu, English lavender, European elder, European mistletoe, eyebright, horehound, horse chestnut, lemon balm, meadowsweet, motherwort, northern prickly ash, oak, poplar, raspberry, sage, saw palmetto, slippery elm, soybean, stinging nettle, St. John's wort, uva ursi, valerian, witch hazel, wormwood, yarrow, yellow dock

Fexofenadine (Allegra) belladonna, corkwood, English lavender, grapefruit, henbane, kava kava, khat, sweet orange, valerian, wild cherry

Fexofenadine and pseudoephedrine (Allegra-D) belaldonna, corkwood, English lavender, henbane, khat

Flecainide acetate (Tambocor) aloe, buckthorn, cascara sagrada, Chinese rhubarb, fumitory, guarana, khat, kudzu, licorice, senna

Fluconazole (Apo-Fluconazole, Diflucan) black tea, boneset, butterbur, caffeine, chaparral, cocoa, coffee, cola nut, colt's foot, comfrey, echinacea, gossypol, green tea, guarana, maté, potassium, wild cherry

Flucytosine (Ancobon) calcium, gossypol, magnesium, potassium

Fludarabine (Fludara) ethanol

Fludrocortisone (Florinef) potassium

Flunisolide (AeroBid, Nasarel) adonis, aloe, andrographis, ashwagandha, astragalus, buckthorn, butternut, calcium, cascara sagrada, castor oil plant, folic acid, frangula, Indian squill, larch, licorice, magnesium, ma-huang, perilla, potassium, schisandra, squill, strophanthus, vitamin A, vitamin B_6, vitamin C, vitamin D, vitamin K, wallflower, zinc

Fluocinolone, hydroquinone, and tretinoin (Tri-Luma) vitamin A, dong quai

Fluorometholone (Eflone, Flarex) adonis, aloe, andrographis, ashwagandha, astragalus, buckthorn, butternut, cascara sagrada, castor oil plant, frangula, Indian squill, larch, licorice, ma-huang, perilla, schisandra, squill, strophanthus, wallflower

Fluorouracil (Adrucil, Efudex) black cohosh, dong quai, ethanol, thiamin, vitamin B_6

Fluoxetine (Prozac, Sarafem) catnip, ergot, ethanol, ginkgo biloba, goldenseal, gotu kola, kava kava, lemon balm, marijuana, nerve root, sassafras, stinging nettle, St. John's wort, valerian

Flupenthixol (Fluanxol) cowhage, rauwolfia

Fluphenazine (Modecate, Prolixin) acerola, agrimony, angel's trumpet, belladonna, black tea, boneset, butterbur, catnip, celery, chaparral, Cherokee rosehip, coffee, colt's foot, comfrey, coriander, corkwood, cowhage, dong quai, echinacea, ethanol, evening primrose oil, fennel, goldenseal, gotu kola, henbane, hyssop, jimson weed, kava kava, lemon balm, lovage, ma-huang, motherwort, nerve root, rauwolfia, riboflavin, rose hips, rosemary, sassafras, stinging nettle, valerian, vitamin C, wild carrot, yohimbe

Flurazepam (Apo-Flurazepam, Dalmane) ashwagandha, bitter almond, California poppy, catnip, cowslip, elecampane, English lavender, ethanol, German chamomile, goldenseal, gotu kola, kava kava, lemon balm, linden, maté, nerve root, passion flower, poke, poppy, rauwolfia, sassafras, scullcap, senega, stinging nettle, St. John's wort, valerian, wild carrot, wild cherry, wild lettuce, yarrow

Flurbiprofen (Ansaid, Ocufen) bog bean, cat's claw, dong quai, ethanol, feverfew, folic acid, garlic, ginger, ginkgo biloba, gossypol, green tea, horse chestnut, niacin, red clover, reishi mushroom, saw palmetto, St. John's wort, turmeric, uva ursi, white willow

Fluticasone (Cutivate, Flonase) adonis, aloe, andrographis, ashwagandha, astragalus, buckthorn, butternut, calcium, cascara sagrada, castor oil plant, folic acid, frangula, Indian squill, larch, licorice, magnesium, ma-huang, perilla, potassium, schisandra, squill, strophanthus, vitamin A, vitamin B_6, vitamin C, vitamin D, vitamin K, wallflower, zinc

Fluvastatin (Lescol) boneset, butterbur, chaparral, colt's foot, comfrey, echinacea, ethanol, gotu kola, niacin, oats, pectin, red yeast rice, St. John's wort, wild cherry

Fluvoxamine (Alti-Fluvoxamine, Luvox) black tea, cabbage, caffeine, cocoa, coffee, cola nut, ergot, ethanol, green tea, guarana, kava kava, marijuana, maté, St. John's wort, valerian

Fondaparinux (Arixtra) ajava seeds, alfalfa, allspice, andrographis, angelica, anise, arnica, asa foetida, astragalus, bilberry, bishop's weed, bladderwrack, bog bean, boldo, borage, borage seed oil, bromelain, buchu, carrageen, cat's claw, cayenne, celery, clove, cordyceps, danshen, deer's tongue, dong quai, evening primrose oil, fenugreek, feverfew, garlic, German chamomile, ginger, ginkgo biloba, ginseng (American), ginseng (Panax), ginseng (Siberian), grape seed, green tea, gymnema, horse chestnut, horseradish, kava kava, kelp, licorice, lovage, lungwort, meadowsweet, motherwort, northern prickly ash, papaya, pau d'arco, pineapple, poplar, potassium, quinine, red clover, reishi mushroom, safflower, saw palmetto, sea buckthorn, senega, stinging nettle, St. John's wort, sweet clover, sweet vernal grass, tonka bean, turmeric, valerian, vitamin E, white willow, wintergreen, yarrow

Foscarnet (Foscavir) boneset, butterbur, calcium, chaparral, colt's foot, comfrey, echinacea, magnesium, potassium

Fosfomycin (Monurol) dong quai, garlic, yohimbe

Fosinopril (Monopril) agrimony, andrographis, arnica, asa foetida, bishop's weed, black cohosh, blue cohosh, carrageen, cat's claw, catechu, cayenne, celery, coriander, devil's claw, dong quai, European mistletoe, fennel, ginger, goldenseal, kelp, khat, licorice, lovage, ma-huang, motherwort, parsley, pineapple, pomegranate, potassium, rosemary, rue, stevia, St. John's wort, wild carrot, wood betony, yarrow, yohimbe, zinc

Fosphenytoin (Cerebyx) calcium, cedar leaf, echinacea, evening primrose oil, fennel, folic acid, ginkgo biloba, hyssop, potassium, sage, stinging nettle, thiamin, vitamin B_6, vitamin B_{12}, vitamin D, vitamin K, wormseed, wormwood

Frovatriptan (Frova) calcium, St. John's wort

Furosemide (Apo-Furosemide, Lasix) agrimony, aloe, andrographis, apple cider vinegar, arnica, artichoke, asa foetida, birch, bishop's weed, black cohosh, black root, bladderwrack, blue cohosh, blue flag, buckthorn, butternut, calcium, calotropis, carrageen, cascara sagrada, castor oil plant, cat's claw, catechu, celery, colocynth, coriander, corn silk, cowslip, cucumber, dandelion, devil's claw, digitalis, dong quai, European mistletoe, fennel, fo-ti, frangula, gamboge, garlic, goldenseal, gossypol, horsetail, Indian hemp, jalap, kelp, khat, licorice, lily-of-the-valley, lovage, magnesium, ma-huang, manna, maté, mayapple, motherwort, parsley, potassium, quassia, rosemary, rue, senna, sorrel, stevia, stinging nettle, St. John's wort, stone root, thiamin, uva ursi, uzara, vitamin B_6, vitamin C, wahoo, wallflower, wild carrot, wood betony, yarrow, yellow dock, yohimbe, zinc

Gabapentin (Neurontin, Nu-Gabapentin) cedar leaf, evening primrose oil, ginkgo biloba, gotu kola, kava kava, sage, valerian, wormseed

Galantamine (Razadyne) areca nut, Chinese club moss, ethanol

Ganciclovir (Cytovene, Vitrasert) boneset, butterbur, chaparral, colt's foot, comfrey, echinacea, fennel, ginkgo biloba, wormwood

Gatifloxacin (Tequin, Zymar) agrimony, biotin, black tea, caffeine, calcium, celery, cocoa, coffee, cola nut, coriander, dong quai, fennel, green tea, guarana, iron, lovage, magnesium, motherwort, niacin, riboflavin, rosemary, thiamin, vitamin B_6, vitamin B_{12}, vitamin K, wild carrot, zinc

Gemfibrozil (Apo-Gemfibrozil, Lopid) boneset, butterbur, chaparral, colt's foot, comfrey, echinacea, gotu kola, niacin, potassium, vitamin E

Gemifloxacin (Factive) black tea, caffeine, calcium, cocoa, coffee, cola nut, dong quai, green tea, guarana, iron, magnesium, zinc

Gemtuzumab ozogamicin (Mylotarg) magnesium, potassium

Gentamicin (Gentacidin, Gentak) boneset, butterbur, calcium, chaparral, colt's foot, comfrey, echinacea, magnesium, niacin, potassium, riboflavin, thiamin, vitamin B_6, vitamin B_{12}, vitamin K

Gentian violet gossypol

Gliclazide (Diamicron, Novo-Gliclazide) agrimony, aloe, avaram, banaba, barley, basil, bilberry, bitter melon, black tea, bladderwrack, blue cohosh, buchu, bugleweed, burdock, caffeine, chanca piedra, Chinese cucumber root, cinnamon, cocoa, coffee, cola nut, coriander, country mallow, cumin, damiana, dandelion, devil's claw, ethanol, eucalyptus, fenugreek, flax, garlic, ginger, ginseng (American), ginseng (Panax), ginseng (Siberian), glucomannan, goat's rue, gotu kola, green tea, guar gum, gymnema, horehound, horse chestnut, kudzu, laurel, licorice, Madagascar periwinkle, ma-huang, maitake mushroom, marshmallow, myrrh, olive, onion, prickly pear cactus, psyllium, psyllium seed, raspberry, senega, Solomon's seal, stevia, St. John's wort

Glimepiride (Amaryl) agrimony, aloe, avaram, banaba, barley, basil, bilberry, bitter melon, black tea, bladderwrack, blue cohosh, buchu, bugleweed, burdock, caffeine, chanca piedra, Chinese cucumber root, cinnamon, cocoa, coffee, cola nut, coriander, country mallow, cumin, damiana, dandelion, devil's claw, ethanol, eucalyptus, fenugreek, flax, garlic, ginger, ginseng (American), ginseng (Panax), ginseng (Siberian), glucomannan, goat's rue, gotu kola, green tea, guar gum, gymnema, horehound, horse chestnut, kudzu, laurel, licorice, Madagascar periwinkle, ma-huang, maitake mushroom, marshmallow, myrrh, niacin, olive, onion, prickly pear cactus, psyllium, psyllium seed, raspberry, senega, Solomon's seal, stevia, St. John's wort

Glipizide (Glucotrol) agrimony, aloe, avaram, banaba, barley, basil, bilberry, bitter melon, black tea, bladderwrack, blue cohosh, buchu, bugleweed, burdock, caffeine, chanca piedra, Chinese cucumber root, cinnamon, cocoa, coffee, cola nut, coriander, country mallow, cumin, damiana, dandelion, devil's claw, echinacea, ethanol, eucalyptus, fenugreek, flax, garlic, ginger, ginkgo biloba, ginseng (American), ginseng (Panax), ginseng (Siberian), glucomannan, goat's rue, gotu kola, green tea, guar gum, gymnema, horehound, horse chestnut, kudzu, laurel, licorice, Madagascar periwinkle, ma-huang, maitake mushroom, marshmallow, myrrh, niacin, olive, onion, prickly pear cactus, psyllium, psyllium seed, raspberry, sage, senega, Solomon's seal, stevia, St. John's wort, yarrow

Glipizide and metformin (Metaglip) agrimony, aloe, avaram, banaba, barley, basil, bilberry, bitter melon, black tea, bladderwrack, blue cohosh, buchu, bugleweed, burdock, caffeine, chanca piedra, Chinese cucumber root, cinnamon, cocoa, coffee, cola nut, coriander, country mallow, cumin, damiana, dandelion, devil's claw, eucalyptus, fenugreek, flax, garlic, ginger, ginseng (American), ginseng (Panax), ginseng (Siberian), glucomannan, goat's rue, gotu kola, green tea, guar gum, gymnema, horehound, horse chestnut, kudzu, laurel, licorice, Madagascar periwinkle, ma-huang, maitake mushroom, marshmallow, myrrh, olive, onion, prickly pear cactus, psyllium, psyllium seed, quillaja, raspberry, senega, Solomon's seal, stevia, St. John's wort

Gliquidone (Beglynor, Glurenorm) agrimony, aloe, avaram, banaba, barley, basil, bilberry, bitter melon, black tea, bladderwrack, blue cohosh, buchu, bugleweed, burdock, caffeine, chanca piedra, Chinese cucumber root, cinnamon, cocoa, coffee, cola nut, coriander, country mallow, cumin, damiana, dandelion, devil's claw, eucalyptus, fenugreek, flax, garlic, ginger, ginseng (American), ginseng (Panax), ginseng (Siberian), glucomannan, goat's rue, gotu kola, green tea, guar gum, gymnema, horehound, horse chestnut, kudzu, laurel, licorice, Madagascar periwinkle, ma-huang, maitake mushroom, marshmallow, myrrh, olive, onion, prickly pear cactus, psyllium, psyllium seed, raspberry, senega, Solomon's seal, stevia, St. John's wort

Glutethimide ashwagandha, bitter almond, California poppy, cowslip, elecampane, ethanol, maté, passion flower, poke, poppy, rauwolfia, scullcap, senega, stinging nettle, valerian, wild carrot, wild lettuce, yarrow

Glyburide (DiaBeta, Micronase) agrimony, aloe, avaram, banaba, barley, basil, bilberry, bitter melon, black tea, bladderwrack, blue cohosh, buchu, bugleweed, burdock, caffeine, chanca piedra, Chinese cucumber root, cinnamon, cocoa, coffee, cola nut, coriander, country mallow, cumin, damiana, dandelion, devil's claw, echinacea, ethanol, eucalyptus, fenugreek, flax, garlic, ginger, ginkgo biloba, ginseng (American), ginseng (Panax), ginseng (Siberian), glucomannan, goat's rue, gotu kola, green tea, guar gum, gymnema, horehound, horse chestnut, kudzu, laurel, licorice, Madagascar periwinkle, ma-huang, maitake mushroom, marshmallow, myrrh, niacin, olive, onion, prickly pear cactus, psyllium, psyllium seed, raspberry, sage, senega, Solomon's seal, stevia, St. John's wort, yarrow

Glyburide and metformin (Glucovance) agrimony, aloe, avaram, banaba, barley, basil, bilberry, bitter melon, black tea, bladderwrack, blue

cohosh, buchu, bugleweed, burdock, caffeine, chanca piedra, Chinese cucumber root, cinnamon, cocoa, coffee, cola nut, coriander, country mallow, cumin, damiana, dandelion, devil's claw, eucalyptus, fenugreek, flax, folic acid, garlic, ginger, ginseng (American), ginseng (Panax), ginseng (Siberian), glucomannan, goat's rue, gotu kola, green tea, guar gum, gymnema, horehound, horse chestnut, kudzu, laurel, licorice, Madagascar periwinkle, ma-huang, maitake mushroom, marshmallow, myrrh, olive, onion, prickly pear cactus, psyllium, psyllium seed, quillaja, raspberry, senega, Solomon's seal, stevia, St. John's wort, vitamin B_{12}

Glycopyrrolate (Robinul, Robinul Forte) angel's trumpet, areca nut, butterbur, calabar bean, catechu, Chinese club moss, iboga, jimson weed, mandrake, scopolia

Granisetron (Kytril) horehound

Griseofulvin (Fulvicin, Grifulvin V) gossypol, vitamin K

Guaifenesin and phenylephrine (Endal, Prolex-D) khat

Guaifenesin and pseudoephedrine (Aquatab, Maxifed) khat

Guanabenz (Wytensin) andrographis, arnica, asa foetida, bishop's weed, black cohosh, blue cohosh, carrageen, cat's claw, catechu, devil's claw, European mistletoe, kelp, khat, licorice, ma-huang, parsley, rue, stevia, wild carrot, wood betony, yarrow, yohimbe

Guanadrel (Hylorel) andrographis, arnica, asa foetida, bishop's weed, black cohosh, blue cohosh, carrageen, cat's claw, catechu, devil's claw, European mistletoe, kelp, khat, licorice, ma-huang, parsley, rue, stevia, wild carrot, wood betony, yarrow, yohimbe

Guanfacine (Tenex) andrographis, arnica, asa foetida, bishop's weed, black cohosh, blue cohosh, carrageen, cat's claw, catechu, devil's claw, European mistletoe, kelp, khat, licorice, ma-huang, parsley, rue, stevia, wild carrot, wood betony, yarrow, yohimbe

Halobetasol (Ultravate) calcium, folic acid, magnesium, potassium, vitamin C, vitamin D, zinc

Haloperidol (Haldol, Novo-Peridol) ashwagandha, bitter almond, butterbur, cabbage, California poppy, corkwood, cowhage, cowslip, elecampane, English lavender, ethanol, German chamomile, gotu kola, jimson weed, maté, nutmeg, passion flower, poke, poppy, rauwolfia, Scotch broom, scullcap, senega, stinging nettle, valerian, wild carrot, wild lettuce, yarrow

Heparin (Hepalean, Hep-Lock) ajava seeds, alfalfa, allspice, andrographis, angelica, anise, arnica, asa foetida, astragalus, bilberry, bishop's weed, bladderwrack, bog bean, boldo, borage, borage seed oil, bromelain, buchu, calcium, carrageen, cat's claw, cayenne, clove, danshen, deer's tongue, devil's claw, dong quai, evening primrose oil, fenugreek, feverfew, garlic, German chamomile, ginger, ginkgo biloba, ginseng (American), ginseng (Panax), ginseng (Siberian), goldenseal, grape seed, green tea, horse chestnut, kava, kelp, licorice, lovage, lungwort, meadowsweet, motherwort, northern prickly ash, onion, papaya, parsley, passion flower, pau d'arco, pineapple, poplar, quinine, red clover, reishi mushroom, rue, safflower, saw palmetto, sea buckthorn, senega, stinging nettle, St. John's wort, sweet clover, sweet vernal grass, tonka bean, turmeric, valerian, vitamin C, vitamin D, vitamin E, white willow, wintergreen, yarrow

Homatropine (Isopto Homatropine) angel's trumpet, areca nut, butterbur, calabar bean, catechu, Chinese club moss, iboga, jimson weed, mandrake, scopolia

Hydralazine (Apresoline, Novo-Hylazin) andrographis, arnica, asa foetida, bishop's weed, black cohosh, blue cohosh, carrageen, cat's claw, catechu, devil's claw, dong quai, ethanol, European mistletoe, garlic, kelp, khat, licorice, magnesium, ma-huang, parsley, potassium, rue, stevia, vitamin B_6, wild carrot, wood betony, yarrow, yohimbe, zinc

Hydralazine plus hydrochlorothiazide (Apresazide) magnesium, potassium, vitamin B_6, zinc

Hydrochlorothiazide (Apo-Hydro, Microzide) agrimony, aloe, andrographis, apple cider vinegar, arnica, artichoke, asa foetida, birch, bishop's weed, black cohosh, black root, bladderwrack, blue cohosh, blue flag, buckthorn, butternut, calcium, calotropis, carrageen, cascara sagrada, castor oil plant, cat's claw, catechu, celery, colocynth, coriander, corn silk, cowslip, cucumber, dandelion, devil's claw, digitalis, dong quai, European mistletoe, fennel, fo-ti, frangula, gamboge, garlic, ginkgo biloba, goldenseal, gossypol, horsetail, Indian hemp, jalap, kelp, khat, licorice, lily-of-the-valley, lovage, magnesium, ma-huang, manna, maté, mayapple, motherwort, parsley, potassium, quassia, rosemary, rue, senna, sorrel, stevia, stinging nettle, St. John's wort, stone root, uva ursi, uzara, vitamin D, wahoo, wallflower, wild carrot, wood betony, yarrow, yellow dock, yohimbe, zinc

Hydrochlorothiazide and triamterene (Dyazide, Maxzide) andrographis, asa foetida, birch, bishop's weed, black cohosh, bladderwrack, blue cohosh, calcium, carrageen, cat's claw, catechu, cowslip, cucumber, dandelion, devil's claw, dong quai. European mistletoe, fennel, folic acid, ginkgo biloba, kelp, khat, magnesium, ma-huang, manna, maté, noni, parsley, potassium, rue, sorrel, stevia, stinging nettle, St. John's wort, stone root, uva ursi, vitamin B_6, vitamin D, wild carrot, wood betony, yarrow, yohimbe, zinc

Hydrochlorothiazide plus spironolactone (Aldactazide, Novo-Spirozine) magnesium, zinc

Hydrocodone and acetaminophen (Vicodin, Zydone) ashwagandha, bitter almond, California poppy, corkwood, elecampane, English lavender, ethanol, kava kava, maté, parsley, passion flower, poke, poppy, rauwolfia, scullcap, senega, stinging nettle, valerian, wild carrot, wild lettuce, yarrow

Hydrocodone and aspirin (Damason-P) ashwagandha, bitter almond, California, poppy, cat's claw, corkwood, dong quai, elecampane, English lavender, ethanol, evening primrose oil, feverfew, folic acid, garlic, ginger, ginkgo biloba, ginseng (American), ginseng (Panax), ginseng (Siberian),

green tea, horse chestnut, iron, kava kava, maté, parsley, passion flower, poke, poppy, potassium, rauwolfia, red clover, scullcap, senega, stinging nettle, valerian, vitamin C, wild carrot, wild lettuce, yarrow

Hydrocodone and chlorpheniramine (Tussionex) belladonna, corkwood, English lavender, henbane, khat

Hydrocodone and ibuprofen (Vicoprofen) ashwagandha, bitter almond, California poppy, cat's claw, corkwood, dong quai, elecampane, English lavender, ethanol, evening primrose oil, feverfew, garlic, ginger, ginkgo biloba, ginseng (American), ginseng (Panax), ginseng (Siberian), green tea, horse chestnut, kava kava, maté, parsley, passion flower, poke, poppy, rauwolfia, red clover, scullcap, senega, stinging nettle, valerian, wild carrot, wild lettuce, yarrow

Hydrocodone, carbinoxamine, and pseudoephedrine (Histex HC, Tri-Vent HC) belladonna, corkwood, English lavender, henbane, khat

Hydrocortisone (Anusol-HC, Locoid) adonis, aloe, andrographis, ashwagandha, astragalus, buckthorn, butternut, calcium, cascara sagrada, castor oil plant, cat's claw, echinacea, ethanol, folic acid, frangula, Indian squill, larch, licorice, lily-of-the-valley, magnesium, ma-huang, oleander, perilla, potassium, schisandra, strophanthus, vitamin A, vitamin B_6, vitamin C, vitamin D, wallflower, zinc

Hydroflumethiazide (Diucardin, Saluron) aloe, apple cider vinegar, birch, bishop's weed, black root, bladderwrack, blue flag, buckthorn, butternut, calcium, calotropis, cascara sagrada, castor oil plant, colocynth, corn silk, cowslip, cucumber, dandelion, digitalis, fo-ti, frangula, gamboge, ginkgo biloba, gossypol, horsetail, Indian hemp, jalap, licorice, lily-of-the-valley, manna, maté, mayapple, quassia, senna, sorrel, stinging nettle, St. John's wort, stone root, uva ursi, uzara, vitamin D, wahoo, wallflower, wild carrot, yellow dock, yohimbe

Hydromorphone (Dilaudid, PMS-Hydromorphone) ashwagandha, bitter almond, California poppy, corkwood, elecampane, English lavender, ethanol, gotu kola, kava kava, maté, parsley, passion flower, poke, poppy, rauwolfia, scullcap, senega, stinging nettle, valerian, wild carrot, wild lettuce, yarrow

Hydroxychloroquine (Apo-Hydroxyquine, Plaquenil) ethanol

Hydroxyzine (Atarax, Vistaril) ashwagandha, belladonna, bitter almond, California poppy, corkwood, cowslip, elecampane, English lavender, ethanol, German chamomile, gotu kola, henbane, kava kava, khat, maté, passion flower, poke, poppy, rauwolfia, scullcap, senega, stinging nettle, valerian, wild carrot, wild lettuce, yarrow

Hyoscyamine (Hyosine, Levsin) angel's trumpet, areca nut, butterbur, calabar bean, calcium, catechu, Chinese club moss, iboga, jimson weed, mandrake, scopolia

Hyoscyamine, atropine, scopolamine and phenobarbital (Donnatal, Donnatal Extentabs) angel's trumpet, areca nut, butterbur, calabar bean, catechu, Chinese club moss, iboga, jimson weed, mandrake, scopolia

Ibandronic acid (Bondronat) calcium, iron, magnesium

Ibritumomab (Zevalin) cat's claw, dong quai, evening primrose oil, feverfew, garlic, ginger, ginkgo biloba, ginseng (American), ginseng (Panax), ginseng (Siberian), green tea, horse chestnut, red clover

Ibuprofen (Advil, Motrin) balsam of Peru, agrimony, anise, bogbean, boneset, bromelain, butterbur, cat's claw, celery, chaparral, clove, coffee, cola nut, colt's foot, comfrey, coriander, danshen, devil's claw, dong quai, echinacea, ethanol, fennel, fenugreek, feverfew, folic acid, fumitory, garlic, German chamomile, ginger, ginkgo biloba, gossypol, green tea, horse chestnut, juniper, lovage, meadowsweet, motherwort, niacin, oak, onion, parsley, passion flower, red clover, red yeast rice, reishi mushroom, rosemary, rue, saw palmetto, St. John's wort, sweet clover, tamarind, thunder god vine, turmeric, uva ursi, white willow, wild carrot, wild yam, wintergreen, yohimbe

Ibutilide (Corvert) aloe, buckthorn, cascara sagrada, English hawthorn, fumitory, khat, kudzu, licorice, senna

Imatinib (Gleevec) potassium, St. John's wort

Imidapril (Novarok, Tanatril) cayenne, pineapple, pomegranate, potassium, St. John's wort, yohimbe

Imipramine (Apo-Imipramine, Tofranil) angel's trumpet, belladonna, black tea, butterbur, cabbage, catnip, coffee, corkwood, ergot, ethanol, fennel, ginkgo biloba, goldenseal, henbane, jimson weed, kava kava, lemon balm, ma-huang, marijuana, nerve root, rauwolfia, riboflavin, sassafras, scopolia, stinging nettle, St. John's wort, valerian, wormwood, yohimbe

Inamrinone digitalis, Indian squill, potassium, squill

Indapamide (Lozol, Nu-Indapamide) andrographis, apple cider vinegar, arnica, asa foetida, birch, bishop's weed, black cohosh, black root, bladderwrack, blue cohosh, blue flag, buckthorn, butternut, calotropis, carrageen, cascara sagrada, castor oil plant, cat's claw, catechu, colocynth, corn silk, cowslip, cucumber, dandelion, devil's claw, digitalis, dong quai, European mistletoe, fo-ti, frangula, gamboge, garlic, gossypol, horsetail, Indian hemp, jalap, kelp, khat, licorice, lily-of-the-valley, magnesium, ma-huang, manna, maté, mayapple, parsley, potassium, quassia, rue, senna, sorrel, stevia, stinging nettle, stone root, uva ursi, uzara, wahoo, wallflower, wild carrot, wood betony, yarrow, yellow dock, yohimbe, zinc

Indinavir (Crixivan) boneset, butterbur, chaparral, colt's foot, comfrey, echinacea, garlic, marijuana, St. John's wort, vitamin C

Indobufen (Ibustrin) ajava seeds, allspice, andrographis, angelica, arnica, asa foetida, astragalus, bilberry, bishop's weed, bladderwrack, bog bean, boldo, borage, borage seed oil, bromelain, buchu, carrageen, cat's claw, cayenne, clove, danshen, deer's tongue, dong quai, English hawthorn, evening primrose oil, feverfew, garlic, ginger, ginkgo biloba, ginseng (American), ginseng (Panax), ginseng (Siberian), green tea, horse chestnut, kava kava, licorice, lovage, pau d'arco, quinine, reishi mushroom, safflower, saw palmetto, sea buckthorn, stinging nettle, sweet clover, sweet vernal grass, turmeric, valerian, vitamin E, white willow, yarrow

Indomethacin (Indocin, Novo-Methacin) agrimony, anise, balsam of Peru, bog bean, bromelain, cascara sagrada, cat's claw, celery, clove, coffee, cola nut, coriander, danshen, devil's claw, dong quai, ethanol, fennel, fenugreek, feverfew, folic acid, fumitory, garlic, German chamomile, ginger, ginkgo biloba, gossypol, green tea, horse chestnut, iron, juniper, licorice, lovage, meadowsweet, motherwort, niacin, oak, onion, parsley, passion flower, red clover, red yeast rice, reishi mushroom, rosemary, rue, saw palmetto, St. John's wort, sweet clover, thunder god vine, turmeric, uva ursi, white willow, wild carrot, wild yam, wintergreen, yohimbe

Insulin (Humulin, Novolin R) agrimony, aloe, angelica, apple cider vinegar, avaram, banaba, barley, basil, bilberry, bitter melon, black tea, bladderwrack, blue cohosh, buchu, bugleweed, burdock, caffeine, cascara sagrada, chanca piedra, Chinese cucumber root, Chinese rhubarb, cinnamon, cocoa, coffee, cola nut, country mallow, cumin, damiana, dandelion, devil's claw, eucalyptus, fenugreek, flax, garlic, ginger, ginkgo biloba, ginseng (American), ginseng (Panax), ginseng (Siberian), glucomannan, goat's rue, gotu kola, green tea, guar gum, guarana, gymnema, horehound, horse chestnut, juniper, kudzu, laurel, licorice, Madagascar periwinkle, ma-huang, maitake mushroom, marshmallow, myrrh, olive, onion, prickly pear cactus, psyllium, psyllium seed, raspberry, sage, senega, senna, Solomon's seal, stevia, St. John's wort, yarrow

Interferon Alfa-2a (Roferon-A) calcium

Interferon Alfa-2b (Intron A) calcium

Iodoquinol and hydrocortisone (Dermazene, Vytone) gossypol

Ipecac mayapple

Ipratropium (Atrovent, Nu-Ipratropium) angel's trumpet, areca nut, butterbur, calabar bean, catechu, Chinese club moss, iboga, jimson weed, mandrake, scopolia

Iproniazid (Marsilid) anise, bitter orange, black tea, brewer's yeast, butcher's broom, caffeine, calamus, cayenne, cocoa, coffee, cola nut, country mallow, ergot, ethanol, ginkgo biloba, ginseng (Panax), green tea, guarana, Hawaiian baby woodrose, jimson weed, kava kava, khat, licorice, ma-huang, nutmeg, rauwolfia, Scotch broom, St. John's wort, valerian, yohimbe

Irbesartan (Avapro) andrographis, arnica, asa foetida, bishop's weed, black cohosh, blue cohosh, carrageen, cat's claw, catechu, devil's claw, dong quai, European mistletoe, garlic, kelp, khat, licorice, ma-huang, parsley, potassium, rue, stevia, wild carrot, wood betony, yarrow, yohimbe

Irbesartan plus hydrochlorothiazide (Avalide) magnesium, potassium, zinc

Irinotican (Camptosar) St. John's wort

Iron-dextran complex (Dexferrum, INFeD) artichoke, bilberry, black cohosh, borage, butternut, cascara sagrada, catechu, English hawthorn, English lavender, English plantain, European elder, European mistletoe, eyebright, feverfew, German chamomile, gossypol, horehound, horse chestnut, lemon balm, meadowsweet, motherwort, northern prickly ash, oak, oregano, poplar, raspberry, sage, saw palmetto, slippery elm, soybean, stinging nettle, St. John's wort, uva ursi, valerian, witch hazel, wormwood, yarrow, yellow dock

Isepamicin (Exacin, Isepacine) magnesium

Isoconazole (Fazol, Gyno-Travogen) gossypol

Isoetharine (Beta-2, Bronkosol) digitalis, fever bark, Indian squill, ma-huang, rauwolfia, squill

Isoniazid (Isotamine, Nydrazid) boneset, butterbur, calcium, chaparral, colt's foot, comfrey, echinacea, ethanol, folic acid, niacin, vitamin B_6, vitamin B_{12}, vitamin D

Isoproterenol (Isuprel) digitalis, fever bark, Indian squill, ma-huang, rauwolfia, squill, yohimbe

Isosorbide dinitrate (Dilatrate-SR, Isordil) English hawthorn, ethanol, niacin

Isosorbide mononitrate (Imdur, Ismo) English hawthorn, ethanol, niacin

Isotretinoin (Accutane, Caravis) dong quai, ethanol, vitamin A

Isradipine (DynaCirc) andrographis, arnica, asa foetida, bishop's weed, black cohosh, blue cohosh, calcium, carrageen, cat's claw, catechu, devil's claw, dong quai, English hawthorn, European mistletoe, garlic, ginger, goldenseal, grapefruit, kelp, khat, licorice, lily-of-the-valley, magnesium, ma-huang, niacin, parsley, rue, stevia, St. John's wort, wild carrot, wild cherry, wood betony, yarrow, yohimbe

Itraconazole (Sporanox) calcium, gossypol, grapefruit, potassium, wild cherry

Ivermectin (Stromectol) sweet orange

Kanamycin (Kantrex) biotin, calcium, magnesium, niacin, potassium, riboflavin, thiamin, vitamin B$_6$, vitamin B$_{12}$, vitamin K

Ketoconazole (Apo-Ketoconazole, Nizoral) boneset, butterbur, calcium, chaparral, colt's foot, comfrey, echinacea, gossypol, wild cherry, yew

Ketoprofen (Orudis, Rhodis) balsam of Peru, agrimony, anise, bog bean, boneset, bromelain, butterbur, celery, chaparral, clove, coffee, cola nut, colt's foot, comfrey, coriander, danshen, devil's claw, dong quai, echinacea, fennel, fenugreek, feverfew, folic acid, fumitory, garlic, German chamomile, ginger, ginkgo biloba, gossypol, horse chestnut, juniper, licorice, lovage, meadowsweet, motherwort, niacin, oak, onion, parsley, passion flower, red clover, red yeast rice, reishi mushroom, rosemary, rue, saw palmetto, St. John's wort, sweet clover, thunder god vine, turmeric, uva ursi, white willow, wild carrot, wild yam, wintergreen, yohimbe

Ketorolac (Acular, Toradol) agrimony, anise, balsam of Peru, bog bean, boneset, bromelain, butterbur, cat's claw, celery, chaparral, clove,

coffee, cola nut, colt's foot, comfrey, coriander, danshen, devil's claw, dong quai, echinacea, ethanol, fennel, fenugreek, feverfew, folic acid, fumitory, garlic, German chamomile, ginger, ginkgo biloba, gossypol, green tea, horse chestnut, juniper, licorice, lovage, meadowsweet, motherwort, niacin, oak, onion, parsley, passion flower, red clover, red yeast rice, reishi mushroom, rosemary, rue, saw palmetto, St. John's wort, sweet clover, thunder god vine, turmeric, uva ursi, white willow, wild carrot, wild yam, wintergreen, yohimbe

Ketotifen (Novo-Ketotifen, Zaditor) belladonna, corkwood, English lavender, henbane, khat

Labetalol (Normodyne, Trandate) andrographis, arnica, asa foetida, bishop's weed, black cohosh, blue cohosh, butterbur, carrageen, cat's claw, catechu, devil's claw, dong quai, European mistletoe, fumitory, garlic, ginger, goldenseal, kelp, khat, licorice, lily-of-the-valley, magnesium, ma-huang, motherwort, parsley, rue, saw palmetto, stevia, St. John's wort, wild carrot, wood betony, yarrow, yohimbe

Lacidipine (Aponil, Caldine) bishop's weed, calcium, English hawthorn, grapefruit, khat, lily-of-the-valley, magnesium, niacin, stevia, St. John's wort, wild cherry, yohimbe

Lactobacillus (Kala, Probiotica) nutmeg

Lactulose (Constulose, Enulose) adonis, licorice, lily-of-the-valley, oleander, senna, squill, strophanthus

Lamivudine (Epivir, Heptovir) boneset, butterbur, chaparral, colt's foot, comfrey, echinacea, vitamin B$_{12}$, zinc

Lamotrigine (Lamictal) cedar leaf, ethanol, evening primrose oil, ginkgo biloba, sage, wormseed

Lansoprazole (Prevacid) agrimony, aletris, angelica, beta-carotene, birthwort, black mustard, blessed thistle, bog bean, calamus, celery, colombo, coriander, cubeb, dandelion, devil's claw, dong quai, ethanol, fennel, folic acid, ginger, goldenseal, iron, lesser galangal, lovage, motherwort, rosemary, thiamin, vitamin B_{12}, wild carrot, yellow gentian, zinc

Leflunomide (Arava) potassium

Lepirudin (Refludan) ajava seeds, alfalfa, allspice, andrographis, angelica, arnica, asa foetida, astragalus, bilberry, bishop's weed, bladderwrack, bog bean, boldo, borage, borage seed oil, bromelain, buchu, carrageen, cat's claw, cayenne, clove, danshen, deer's tongue, dong quai, evening primrose oil, feverfew, garlic, German chamomile, ginger, ginkgo biloba, ginseng (American), ginseng (Panax), ginseng (Siberian), green tea, horse chestnut, kava kava, kelp, licorice, lovage, lungwort, meadowsweet, motherwort, northern prickly ash, papaya, pau d'arco, pineapple, poplar, quinine, red clover, reishi mushroom, safflower, saw palmetto, sea buckthorn, senega, stinging nettle, St. John's wort, sweet clover, sweet vernal grass, tonka bean, turmeric, valerian, vitamin E, white willow, wintergreen, yarrow

Lercanidipine (Cardiovasc, Carmen) bishop's weed, calcium, English hawthorn, grapefruit, khat, lily-of-the-valley, magnesium, niacin, stevia, St. John's wort, wild cherry, yohimbe

Levalbuterol (Xopenex) licorice, potassium, Scotch broom, yohimbe

Levamisole (Ergamisol) ethanol

Levetiracetam (Keppra) cedar leaf, ethanol, evening primrose oil, fennel, ginkgo biloba, hyssop, sage, stinging nettle, wormseed, wormwood

Levobetaxolol (Betaxon) butterbur, fumitory, khat, lily-of-the-valley, motherwort, St. John's wort, yohimbe

Levobunolol (Betagan, Novo-Levobunolol) butterbur, fumitory, khat, lily-of-the-valley, motherwort, St. John's wort, yohimbe

Levocabastine (Livostin) belladonna, corkwood, English lavender, henbane, khat

Levodopa (Dopar, Larodopa) chaste tree berry, ethanol, iron, kava kava, potassium, rauwolfia, vitamin B_6

Levodopa-carbidopa (Sinemet, Nu-Levocarb) boneset, butterbur, chaparral, chaste tree berry, colt's foot, comfrey, echinacea, kava kava, potassium, rauwolfia, vitamin B_6

Levofloxacin (Levaquin, Quixin) agrimony, biotin, black tea, caffeine, calcium, celery, cocoa, coffee, cola nut, coriander, dong quai, fennel, green tea, guarana, iron, lovage, magnesium, motherwort, niacin, riboflavin, rosemary, thiamin, vitamin B_6, vitamin B_{12}, vitamin K, wild carrot, zinc

Levomethadyl acetate hydrochloride ashwagandha, bitter almond, California poppy, corkwood, elecampane, English lavender, ethanol, magnesium, maté, parsley, passion flower, poke, poppy, rauwolfia, scullcap, senega, stinging nettle, valerian, wild carrot, wild lettuce, yarrow

Levonorgestrel (Norplant Implant, Plan B) alfalfa, anise, folic acid, magnesium, riboflavin, St. John's wort, vitamin B_6, vitamin B_{12}, vitamin C, zinc

Levorphanol (Levo-Dromoran) ashwagandha, bitter almond, California poppy, corkwood, elecampane, English lavender, ethanol, gotu kola, kava kava, maté, parsley, passion flower, poke, poppy, rauwolfia, scullcap, senega, stinging nettle, valerian, wild carrot, wild lettuce, yarrow

Levothyroxine (Levothroid, Synthroid) bladderwrack, bugleweed, calcium, celery, guggul, horseradish, iron, Scotch broom, shepherd's purse, soybean, yohimbe

Lidocaine (Lidoderm, Xylocaine) aloe, buckthorn, cascara sagrada, fumitory, khat, kudzu, licorice, senna

Linezolid (Zyvox) biotin, ethanol, niacin, riboflavin, thiamin, vitamin B_6, vitamin B_{12}, vitamin K

Liothyronine (Cytomel, Triostat) bladderwrack, bugleweed, soybean

Liotrix (Thyrolar) bladderwrack, bugleweed, soybean

Lisinopril (Prinivil, Zestril) agrimony, andrographis, arnica, asa foetida, bishop's weed, black cohosh, blue cohosh, carrageen, cat's claw, catechu, cayenne, celery, coriander, devil's claw, dong quai, European mistletoe, fennel, garlic, ginger, goldenseal, kelp, khat, licorice, lovage, ma-huang, motherwort, parsley, pineapple, pomegranate, potassium, rosemary, rue, stevia, St. John's wort, wild carrot, wood betony, yarrow, yohimbe, zinc

Lithium (Eskalith, Carbolith) angelica, black tea, buchu, caffeine, cocoa, coffee, cola nut, dandelion, English plantain, green tea, guarana, horsetail, juniper, parsley, psyllium, psyllium seed, stinging nettle, yohimbe

Lofepramine (Feprapax, Gamanil) angel's trumpet, belladonna, black tea, coffee, corkwood, ergot, ethanol, henbane, jimson weed, ma-huang, marijuana, rauwolfia, scopolia, St. John's wort, yohimbe

Lomefloxacin (Maxaquin) biotin, black tea, caffeine, calcium, cocoa, coffee, cola nut, dong quai, green tea, guarana, iron, magnesium, niacin, riboflavin, thiamin, vitamin B_6, vitamin B_{12}, vitamin K, zinc

Loperamide (Diarr-Eze, Imodium A-D) nutmeg, St. John's wort, valerian

Lopinavir and ritonavir (Kaletra) garlic, marijuana, St. John's wort, vitamin C

Loprazolam (Dormonoct, Havlane) ashwagandha, bitter almond, California poppy, elecampane, ethanol, German chamomile, kava kava, maté, passion flower, poke, poppy, rauwolfia, scullcap, senega, stinging nettle, St. John's wort, valerian, wild carrot, wild cherry, wild lettuce, yarrow

Loracarbef (Lorabid) biotin, niacin, riboflavin, thiamin, vitamin B$_6$, vitamin B$_{12}$, vitamin K

Loratadine (Claritin, Alavert) agrimony, belladonna, butterbur, celery, coriander, corkwood, dong quai, English lavender, fennel, henbane, jimson weed, khat, licorice, lovage, motherwort, rosemary, wild carrot

Loratadine and pseudoephedrine (Claritin-D 12 Hour, Claritin-D 24 Hour) belladonna, corkwood, henbane, English lavender, khat

Lorazepam (Ativan, Nu-Loraz) ashwagandha, bitter almond, California poppy, catnip, cedar leaf, cowslip, elecampane, English lavender, ethanol, evening primrose oil, German chamomile, ginkgo biloba, goldenseal, gotu kola, kava kava, lemon balm, linden, maté, nerve root, passion flower, poke, poppy, rauwolfia, sage, sassafras, scullcap, senega, stinging nettle, St. John's wort, valerian, wild carrot, wild cherry, wild lettuce, wormseed, yarrow

Losartan (Cozaar) andrographis, arnica, asa foetida, bishop's weed, black cohosh, blue cohosh, carrageen, cat's claw, catechu, devil's claw, dong quai, European mistletoe, garlic, kelp, khat, licorice, ma-huang, parsley, potassium, rue, stevia, wild carrot, wood betony, yarrow, yohimbe

Losartan plus hydrochlorothiazide (Hyzaar) magnesium, potassium, zinc

Loteprednol (Alrex, Lotemax) adonis, aloe, andrographis, ashwagandha, astragalus, buckthorn, butternut, cascara sagrada, castor oil plant, Indian squill, larch, perilla, schisandra, strophanthus

Lovastatin (Altocor, Mevacor) boneset, butterbur, chaparral, colt's foot, comfrey, echinacea, ethanol, gotu kola, grapefruit, niacin, oats, pectin, red yeast rice, St. John's wort, wild cherry

Loxapine (Loxitane, Nu-Loxapine) cowhage, ethanol, gotu kola, kava kava, rauwolfia

Magaldrate and simethicone (Riopan Plus, Riopan Plus Double Strength) aletris, angelica, birthwort, black mustard, blessed thistle, buckthorn, calamus, colombo, cubeb, dandelion, devil's claw, ginger, lesser galangal, ma-huang, yellow gentian

Magnesium citrate (Citro-Mag) adonis, licorice, lily-of-the-valley, oleander, senna, squill, strophanthus

Magnesium hydroxide (Dulcolax Milk of Magnesia, Phillips' Milk of Magnesia) adonis, aletris, angelica, birthwort, black mustard, blessed thistle, buckthorn, calamus, calcium, colombo, cubeb, dandelion, devil's claw, folic acid, ginger, iron, lesser galangal, licorice, lily-of-the-valley, ma-huang, oleander, senna, squill, strophanthus, vitamin D, yellow gentian, zinc

Magnesium hydroxide and mineral oil (Phillips' M-O) adonis, licorice, lily-of-the-valley, oleander, senna, strophanthus

Magnesium oxide (Mag-Ox 400, Uro-Mag) adonis, aletris, angelica, birthwort, blessed thistle, buckthorn, calamus, calcium, colombo, cubeb, dandelion, devil's claw, ginger, lesser galangal, licorice, lily-of-the-valley, ma-huang, oleander, potassium, senna, squill, strophanthus, yellow gentian

Magnesium salicylate (Doan's, Mobidin) bog bean, feverfew, garlic, ginkgo biloba, gossypol, niacin, reishi mushroom, saw palmetto, St. John's wort, turmeric, uva ursi, white willow

Magnesium sulfate (Epsom salts) adonis, aletris, angelica, birthwort, black mustard, blessed thistle, buckthorn, calamus, calcium, colombo, cubeb, dandelion, devil's claw, ginger, lesser galangal, licorice, lily-of-the-valley, ma-huang, oleander, senna, squill, strophanthus, yellow gentian

Manidipine (Calslot, Iperten) bishop's weed, calcium, English hawthorn, grapefruit, khat, lily-of-the-valley, magnesium, niacin, stevia, St. John's wort, wild cherry, yohimbe

Mannitol (Osmitrol, Resectisol) apple cider vinegar, birch, bishop's weed, black root, bladderwrack, blue flag, buckthorn, butternut, caltropis, cascara sagrada, castor oil plant, colocynth, corn silk, cowslip, cucumber, dandelion, digitalis, fo-ti, frangula, gamboge, gossypol, horsetail, Indian hemp, jalap, licorice, lily-of-the-valley, manna, maté, mayapple, potassium, quassia, senna, sorrel, stinging nettle, stone root, uva ursi, uzara, wahoo, wallflower, wild carrot, yellow dock, yohimbe

Maprotiline (Novo-Maprotiline) ergot

Mebhydrolin (Bexidal, Incidal) belladonna, corkwood, English lavender, henbane, khat

Mecamylamine (Inversine) andrographis, arnica, asa foetida, bishop's weed, black cohosh, blue cohosh, carrageen, cat's claw, catechu, devil's claw, European mistletoe, kelp, khat, licorice, ma-huang, niacin, parsley, rue, stevia, wild carrot, wood betony, yarrow

Mechlorethamine (Mustargen) ethanol

Meclizine (Antivert, Bonine) ethanol

Meclocycline (Meclan Topical) biotin, calcium, iron, magnesium, niacin, riboflavin, thiamin, vitamin B_6, vitamin B_{12}, vitamin K

Meclofenamate (Meclomen) bog bean, ethanol, feverfew, folic acid, garlic, ginkgo biloba, gossypol, niacin, reishi mushroom, saw palmetto, St. John's wort, turmeric, uva ursi, white willow

Medroxyprogesterone (Depo-Provera, Provera) alfalfa, anise, St. John's wort

Medrysone (HMS Liquifilm) adonis, aloe, andrographis, ashwagandha, astragalus, buckthorn, butternut, cascara sagrada, castor oil plant, Indian squill, larch, perilla, schisandra, strophanthus

Mefenamic acid (Ponstan, Ponstel) bog bean, ethanol, feverfew, folic acid, garlic, ginkgo biloba, gossypol, niacin, reishi mushroom, saw palmetto, St. John's wort, turmeric, uva ursi, white willow

Mefruside (Baycaron) andrographis, apple cider vinegar, arnica, asa foetida, birch, bishop's weed, black cohosh, black root, bladderwrack, blue cohosh, blue flag, buckthorn, butternut, caltropis, carrageen, cascara sagrada, castor oil plant, cat's claw, catechu, colocynth, corn silk, cowslip, cucumber, dandelion, devil's claw, digitalis, European mistletoe, fo-ti, frangula, gamboge, gossypol, horsetail, Indian hemp, jalap, kelp, khat, licorice, lily-of-the-valley, ma-huang, manna, maté, mayapple, parsley, quassia, rue, senna, sorrel, stevia, stinging nettle, stone root, uva ursi, uzara, wahoo, wallflower, wild carrot, wood betony, yarrow, yellow dock, yohimbe

Megestrol (Lin-Megestrol, Megace) black cohosh, dong quai

Melitracen (Dixeran) angel's trumpet, belladonna, black tea, coffee, corkwood, ergot, ethanol, henbane, jimson weed, ma-huang, marijuana, rauwolfia, scopolia, St. John's wort, yohimbe

Meloxicam (MOBIC, Mobicox) angelica, anise, bitter melon, bog bean, boneset, butterbur, chaparral, colt's foot, comfrey, danshen, devil's claw, dong quai, echinacea, ethanol, fenugreek, feverfew, folic acid, fumitory, garlic, ginger, ginkgo biloba, gossypol, horse chestnut, juniper, kava kava, licorice, maté, meadowsweet, niacin, oak, passion flower, red clover, reishi mushroom, saw palmetto, St. John's wort, turmeric, uva ursi, white willow, wintergreen, yohimbe

Melphalan (Alkeran) ethanol

Meperidine (Demerol, Meperitab) ashwagandha, bitter almond, California poppy, corkwood, elecampane, English lavender, ergot, ethanol, gotu kola, Hawaiian baby woodrose, kava kava, maté, parsley, passion flower, poke, poppy, rauwolfia, scullcap, senega, stinging nettle, valerian, wild carrot, wild lettuce, yarrow

Meperidine and promethazine ashwagandha, bitter almond, California poppy, corkwood, elecampane, English lavender, ethanol, kava kava, maté, parsley, passion flower, poke, poppy, rauwolfia, scullcap, senega, stinging nettle, valerian, wild carrot, wild lettuce, yarrow

Mephenytoin (Mesantoin) folic acid, vitamin D

Mephobarbital (Mebaral) ashwagandha, bitter almond, California poppy, cedar leaf, cedarwood oil, cowslip, elecampane, English lavender, ethanol, eucalyptus, evening primrose oil, German chamomile, ginkgo biloba, hops, kava kava, lemon balm, marijuana, maté, passion flower, poke, poppy, rauwolfia, sage, scullcap, senega, stinging nettle, St. John's wort, valerian, wild carrot, wild lettuce, wormseed, yarrow

Meprobamate (Miltown, Novo-Mepro) cowslip, ethanol, gotu kola, kava kava, valerian

Mequinol and tretinoin (Solagé) vitamin A

Mesalamine (Asacol Oral, Rowasa Rectal) folic acid

Mesoridazine (Serentil) angel's trumpet, belladonna, black tea, coffee, corkwood, cowhage, ethanol, evening primrose oil, gotu kola, henbane, jimson weed, kava kava, ma-huang, rauwolfia, riboflavin, valerian, yohimbe

Mestranol and norethindrone (Necon 1/50, Ortho-Novum 1/50) acerola, alfalfa, anise, black tea, caffeine, calcium, chaste tree berry, Cherokee rosehip, cocoa, coffee, cola nut, grapefruit, green tea, guarana, licorice, red clover, senna, St. John's wort, wild cherry, wild yam

Metaproterenol (Alupent) digitalis, fever bark, Indian squill, ma-huang, rauwolfia, squill

Metaraminol (Aramine) digitalis, fever bark, Indian squill, ma-huang, rauwolfia, squill

Metformin (Glucophage, Riomet) balsam of Peru, agrimony, aloe, angelica, avaram, banaba, barley, basil, bilberry, bitter melon, black tea, bladderwrack, blue cohosh, buchu, bugleweed, burdock, caffeine, chanca piedra, Chinese cucumber root, cinnamon, cocoa, coffee, cola nut, coriander, country mallow, cumin, damiana, dandelion, devil's claw, ethanol, eucalyptus, fenugreek, flax, folic acid, fumitory, garlic, ginger, ginkgo biloba, ginseng (American), ginseng (Panax), ginseng (Siberian), glucomannan, goat's rue, gossypol, gotu kola, green tea, guar gum, gymnema, horehound, horse chestnut, juniper, kudzu, laurel, licorice, Madagascar periwinkle, ma-huang, maitake mushroom, marshmallow, myrrh, niacin, oak, olive, onion, prickly pear cactus, psyllium, psyllium seed, quillaja, raspberry, red yeast rice, rue, sage, Scotch broom, senega, Solomon's seal, stevia, St. John's wort, thunder god vine, vitamin B_{12}, wintergreen, yarrow, yohimbe

Methacholine (Provocholine) areca nut, Chinese club moss, iboga

Methadone (Dolophine, Methadose) ashwagandha, bitter almond, California poppy, corkwood, elecampane, English lavender, ethanol, gotu kola, kava kava, maté, parsley, passion flower, poke, poppy, rauwolfia, scullcap, senega, stinging nettle, St. John's wort, valerian, wild carrot, wild lettuce, yarrow

Methamphetamine (Desoxyn) ethanol, khat, maté, St. John's wort

Methazolamide (Apo-Methazolamide, Neptazane) apple cider vinegar, birch, bishop's weed, black root, bladderwrack, blue flag, buckthorn, butternut, calotropis, cascara sagrada, castor oil plant, colocynth, corn silk, cowslip, cucumber, dandelion, digitalis, fo-ti, frangula, gamboge, gossypol, horsetail, Indian hemp, jalap, licorice, lily-of-the-valley, manna, maté, mayapple, potassium, quassia, senna, sorrel, stinging nettle, stone root, uva ursi, uzara, wahoo, wallflower, wild carrot, yellow dock, yohimbe

Methocarbamol (Robaxin) ethanol, gotu kola, kava kava, valerian

Methocarbamol plus aspirin (Robaxisal) folic acid, iron, potassium, vitamin C

Methohexital (Brevital, Brevital Sodium) ashwagandha, bitter almond, California poppy, cedarwood oil, elecampane, ethanol, eucalyptus, hops, kava kava, lemon balm, marijuana, maté, passion flower, poke, poppy, rauwolfia, scullcap, senega, stinging nettle, St. John's wort, valerian, wild carrot, wild lettuce, yarrow

Methotrexate (Rheumatrex, Trexall) agrimony, andrographis, ashwagandha, astragalus, beta-carotene, bitter melon, boneset, butterbur, calcium, cat's claw, celery, chaparral, colt's foot, comfrey, coriander, dong quai, echinacea, ethanol, fennel, fenugreek, folic acid, fumitory, gossypol, juniper, kava kava, larch, lovage, maitake mushroom, maté, motherwort, oak, rosemary, schisandra, scullcap, St. John's wort, turmeric, vitamin B_{12}, wild carrot, wintergreen, yohimbe

Methotrimeprazine (Novo-Meprazine, Nozaine) dong quai, ethanol, gotu kola, kava kava, valerian

Methscopolamine (an ingredient in AH-Chew, Extendryl) calcium

Methsuximide (Celontin) calcium, cedar leaf, evening primrose oil, folic acid, ginkgo biloba, sage, vitamin D, vitamin K, wormseed

Methyclothiazide (Aquatensen, Enduron) aloe, andrographis, apple cider vinegar, arnica, asa foetida, birch, bishop's weed, black cohosh, black root, bladderwrack, blue cohosh, blue flag, buckthorn, butternut, calcium, calotropis, carrageen, cascara sagrada, castor oil plant, cat's claw, catechu, colocynth, corn silk, cowslip, cucumber, dandelion, devil's claw, digitalis, European mistletoe, fo-ti, frangula, gamboge, ginkgo biloba, gossypol, horsetail, Indian hemp, jalap, kelp, khat, licorice, lily-of-the-valley, magnesium, ma-huang, manna, maté, mayapple, parsley, potassium, quassia, rue, senna, sorrel, stevia, stinging nettle, St. John's wort, stone root, uva ursi, uzara, vitamin D, wahoo, wallflower, wild carrot, wood betony, yarrow, yellow dock, yohimbe, zinc

Methyldopa (Apo-Methyldopa, Nu-Medopa) andrographis, arnica, asa foetida, bishop's weed, bitter melon, black cohosh, blue cohosh, boneset, butterbur, carrageen, cat's claw, catechu, chaparral, colt's foot, comfrey, devil's claw, echinacea, European mistletoe, fenugreek, iron, kava kava, kelp, khat, licorice, ma-huang, maté, parsley, rue, stevia, vitamin B_{12}, wild carrot, wood betony, yarrow, yohimbe

Methyldopa plus hydrochlorothiazide (Aldoril, PMS-Dopazide) magnesium, potassium, vitamin B_6, zinc

Methylergonovine (Methergine) country mallow, ergot

Methylphenidate (Concerta, Ritalin) ethanol, fennel, ginkgo biloba, kava kava, maté, sage, wormwood, yohimbe

Methylprednisolone (Depoject Injection, Medrol Oral) adonis, alfalfa, aloe, andrographis, ashwagandha, astragalus, buckthorn, butternut, calcium, cascara sagrada, castor oil plant, cat's claw, echinacea, ethanol, European mistletoe, folic acid, frangula, grapefruit, Indian squill, larch, licorice, lily-of-the-valley, magnesium, ma-huang, oleander, perilla, potassium, schisandra, senna, squill, strophanthus, vitamin A, vitamin B_6, vitamin C, vitamin D, vitamin K, wallflower, zinc

Methysergide (Sansert) country mallow, ergot

Metipranolol (OptiPranolol) butterbur, fumitory, khat, lily-of-the-valley, motherwort, St. John's wort, yohimbe

Metoclopramide (Apo-Metoclop, Reglan) catnip, ethanol, fennel, ginkgo biloba, goldenseal, kava kava, lemon balm, nerve root, riboflavin, sassafras, stinging nettle, valerian, wormwood

Metolazone (Mykrox, Zaroxolyn) andrographis, apple cider vinegar, arnica, asa foetida, birch, bishop's weed, black cohosh, black root, bladderwrack, blue cohosh, blue flag, buckthorn, butternut, calotropis, carrageen, cascara sagrada, castor oil plant, cat's claw, catechu, colocynth, corn silk, cowslip, cucumber, dandelion, devil's claw, digitalis, dong quai, European mistletoe, fo-ti, frangula, gamboge, garlic, gossypol, horsetail, Indian hemp, jalap, kelp, khat, licorice, lily-of-the-valley, magnesium, ma-huang, manna, maté, mayapple, parsley, potassium, quassia, rue, senna, sorrel, stevia, stinging nettle, stone root, uva ursi, uzara, wahoo, wallflower, wild carrot, wood betony, yarrow, yellow dock, yohimbe, zinc

Metoprolol (Betaloc, Lopressor) andrographis, arnica, asa foetida, bishop's weed, black cohosh, blue cohosh, butterbur, carrageen, cat's claw, catechu, devil's claw, dong quai, European mistletoe, fumitory, garlic, goldenseal, kelp, khat, licorice, lily-of-the-valley, ma-huang, motherwort, parsley, rue, stevia, St. John's wort, wild carrot, wood betony, yarrow, yohimbe

Metronidazole (Flagyl, Noritate) ethanol, evening primrose oil, fennel, ginkgo biloba, gossypol, vitamin K, wormwood

Mexiletine (Mexitil, Novo-Mexiletine) aloe, black tea, buckthorn, cabbage, caffeine, cascara sagrada, cocoa, coffee, cola nut, fumitory, green tea, guarana, khat, kudzu, licorice, maté, senna

Miconazole (Femizol-M, Monistat 3) gossypol

Midazolam (Apo-Midazolam, Versed) ashwagandha, bitter almond, bitter orange, California poppy, catnip, cowslip, elecampane, English lavender, ethanol, German chamomile, goldenseal, gotu kola, grapefruit, kava kava, lemon balm, linden, maté, nerve root, passion flower, poke, poppy, rauwolfia, sassafras, scullcap, senega, stinging nettle, St. John's wort, valerian, wild carrot, wild cherry, wild lettuce, yarrow

Midecamycin (Macropen, Midecin) uzara, wahoo

Midodrine (Amatine, ProAmatine) ma-huang

Miglitol (Glyset) agrimony, aloe, angelica, avaram, banaba, barley, basil, bilberry, bitter melon, black tea, bladderwrack, blue cohosh, buchu, bugleweed, burdock, caffeine, chanca piedra, Chinese cucumber root, cinnamon, cocoa, coffee, cola nut, coriander, country mallow, cumin, damiana, dandelion, devil's claw, eucalyptus, fenugreek, flax, fumitory, garlic, ginger, ginkgo biloba, ginseng (American), ginseng (Panax), ginseng (Siberian), glucomannan, goat's rue, gossypol, gotu kola, green tea, guar gum, gymnema, horehound, horse chestnut, juniper, kudzu, laurel, licorice, Madagascar periwinkle, ma-huang, maitake mushroom, marshmallow, myrrh, niacin, oak, olive, onion, prickly pear cactus, psyllium, psyllium seed, raspberry, sage, Scotch broom, senega, Solomon's seal, stevia, St. John's wort, wintergreen, yarrow, yohimbe

Milnacipran (Dalcipran, Lixel) ergot

Milrinone (Primacor) digitalis, Indian squill, squill

Mineral oil (Fleet Mineral Oil Enema, Milkinol) beta-carotene, calcium, potassium, vitamin A, vitamin D, vitamin E, vitamin K

Minocycline (Dynacin, Minocin) bromelain, calcium, dong quai, folic acid, iron, magnesium, niacin, riboflavin, St. John's wort, thiamin, uzara, vitamin A, vitamin B_6, vitamin B_{12}, vitamin C, vitamin K, wahoo, zinc

Minoxidil (Loniten, Rogaine) andrographis, arnica, asa foetida, bishop's weed, black cohosh, blue cohosh, carrageen, cat's claw, catechu, devil's claw, European mistletoe, kelp, khat, licorice, ma-huang, parsley, rue, stevia, wild carrot, wood betony, yarrow

Mirtazapine (Remeron) ergot, ethanol, gotu kola, kava kava, valerian

Mitomycin (Mutamycin) black cohosh, dong quai

Mitotane (Lysodren) ethanol

Mitoxantrone (Novantrone) black cohosh, dong quai

Mivacurium (Mivacron) magnesium

Mizolastine (Elina, Mizollen) belladonna, corkwood, English lavender, henbane, khat

Moclobemide (Alti-Moclobemide, Nu-Moclobemide) anise, bitter orange, black tea, brewer's yeast, butcher's broom, caffeine, calamus, cayenne, cocoa, coffee, cola nut, country mallow, ergot, ethanol, ginkgo biloba, ginseng (Panax), green tea, guarana, Hawaiian baby woodrose, jimson weed, kava kava, khat, licorice, ma-huang, nutmeg, rauwolfia, Scotch broom, St. John's wort, valerian, yohimbe

Modafinil (Alertec, Provigil) bitter melon, cocoa, cola nut, fenugreek, green tea, guarana, kava kava, maté, yohimbe

Moexipril (Univasc) andrographis, arnica, asa foetida, bishop's weed, black cohosh, blue cohosh, carrageen, cat's claw, catechu, cayenne, devil's claw, dong quai, European mistletoe, garlic, kelp, khat, licorice, ma-huang, parsley, pineapple, pomegranate, potassium, rue, stevia, St. John's wort, wild carrot, wood betony, yarrow, yohimbe, zinc

Moexipril plus hydrochlorothiazide (Uniretic) magnesium, potassium, zinc

Molindone (Moban) cowhage, ethanol, gotu kola, kava kava, rauwolfia, valerian

Mometasone furoate (Elocom, Nasonex) calcium, folic acid, magnesium, potassium, vitamin A, vitamin B_6, vitamin C, vitamin D, vitamin K, zinc

Moricizine (Ethmozine) aloe, buckthorn, cascara sagrada, fumitory, khat, kudzu, licorice, senna

Morphine hydrochloride bitter melon, boneset, butterbur, catnip, chaparral, colt's foot, comfrey, fenugreek, fumitory, goldenseal, gossypol, juniper, kava kava, lemon balm, maté, nerve root, oak, oats, sassafras, stinging nettle, valerian, wintergreen, yohimbe

Morphine sulfate (Kadian, MS Contin) ashwagandha, bitter almond, bitter melon, boneset, butterbur, California poppy, catnip, chaparral, colt's foot, comfrey, corkwood, elecampane, English lavender, ethanol, fenugreek, fumitory, goldenseal, gossypol, gotu kola, juniper, kava kava, lemon balm, maté, nerve root, oak, oats, parsley, passion flower, poke, poppy, rauwolfia, sassafras, scullcap, senega, stinging nettle, valerian, wild carrot, wild lettuce, wintergreen, yarrow, yohimbe

Moxifloxacin (Avelox, Vigamox) black tea, caffeine, calcium, cocoa, coffee, cola nut, echinacea, evening primrose oil, fennel, ginkgo biloba, green tea, guarana, iron, magnesium, niacin, riboflavin, thiamin, vitamin B_6, vitamin B_{12}, vitamin K, wormwood, zinc

Muromonab-CD3 (Orthoclone OKT 3) andrographis, ashwagandha, astragalus, cat's claw, echinacea, larch, maitake mushroom, schisandra, scullcap, St. John's wort, turmeric

Mycophenolate (CellCept) andrographis, ashwagandha, astragalus, calcium, cat's claw, echinacea, iron, larch, magnesium, maitake mushroom, potassium, schisandra, scullcap, St. John's wort, turmeric

Nabumetone (Relafen) bog bean, cat's claw, dong quai, ethanol, feverfew, folic acid, garlic, ginger, ginkgo biloba, gossypol, green tea, horse chestnut, niacin, red clover, reishi mushroom, saw palmetto, St. John's wort, turmeric, uva ursi, white willow

Nadolol (Apo-Nadol, Corgard) andrographis, arnica, asa foetida, bishop's weed, black cohosh, blue cohosh, butterbur, carrageen, cat's claw, catechu, devil's claw, dong quai, European mistletoe, fumitory, garlic, goldenseal, kelp, khat, licorice, lily-of-the-valley, ma-huang, motherwort, parsley, rue, stevia, St. John's wort, wild carrot, wood betony, yarrow, yohimbe

Nadroparin (Fraxiparine) angelica, arnica, astragalus, bilberry, bladderwrack, borage, cat's claw, cayenne, clove, dong quai, evening primrose oil, feverfew, garlic, ginger, ginkgo biloba, ginseng (Panax), green tea, horse chestnut, kava kava, licorice, red clover, turmeric, valerian, white willow

Nafcillin (Nafcil Injection, Unipen Oral) biotin, khat, niacin, potassium, riboflavin, thiamin, vitamin B_6, vitamin B_{12}, vitamin K

Naftifine (Naftin) gossypol

Nalbuphine (Nubain) ashwagandha, bitter almond, California poppy, corkwood, elecampane, English lavender, ethanol, gotu kola, kava kava, maté, parsley, passion flower, poke, poppy, rauwolfia, scullcap, senega, stinging nettle, valerian, wild carrot, wild lettuce, yarrow

Nalidixic acid (NegGram) biotin, black tea, caffeine, calcium, cocoa, coffee, cola nut, green tea, guarana, iron, magnesium, niacin, riboflavin, thiamin, vitamin B_6, vitamin B_{12}, vitamin K, zinc

Naloxone (Narcan) fever bark, yohimbe

Naltrexone (ReVia) yohimbe

Naphazoline (Allersol, Naphcon) khat

Naproxen (Aleve, Naprosyn) agrimony, angelica, anise, bitter melon, bog bean, boneset, butterbur, cat's claw, celery, chaparral, coffee, cola nut, colt's foot, comfrey, coriander, danshen, devil's claw, dong quai, echinacea, ethanol, fennel, fenugreek, feverfew, folic acid, fumitory, garlic, ginger, ginkgo biloba, gossypol, green tea, horse chestnut, juniper, kava kava, licorice, lovage, maté, meadowsweet, motherwort, niacin, oak, passion flower, red clover, reishi mushroom, rosemary, saw palmetto, St. John's wort, turmeric, uva ursi, white willow, wild carrot, wintergreen, yohimbe

Natamycin (Natacyn) gossypol

Nateglinide (Starlix) agrimony, aloe, avaram, banaba, barley, basil, bilberry, bitter melon, black tea, bladderwrack, blue cohosh, buchu, bugleweed, burdock, caffeine, chanca piedra, Chinese cucumber root, cinnamon, cocoa, coffee, cola nut, coriander, country mallow, cumin, damiana, dandelion, devil's claw, ethanol, eucalyptus, fenugreek, flax, garlic, ginger, ginseng (American), ginseng (Panax), ginseng (Siberian), glucomannan, goat's rue, gotu kola, green tea, guar gum, gymnema, horehound, horse chestnut, kudzu, laurel, licorice, Madagascar periwinkle, ma-huang, maitake mushroom, marshmallow, myrrh, niacin, olive, onion, prickly pear cactus, psyllium, psyllium seed, raspberry, senega, Solomon's seal, stevia, St. John's wort

Nefazodone (Serzone) catnip, ergot, ethanol, goldenseal, kava kava, lemon balm, nerve root, sassafras, stinging nettle, St. John's wort, valerian

Nelfinavir (Viracept) bitter melon, boneset, butterbur, chaparral, colt's foot, comfrey, echinacea, fenugreek, garlic, marijuana, maté, St. John's wort, vitamin C

Neomycin (Mycifradin Sulfate Topical, Neo-Tabs Oral) beta-carotene, calcium, iron, magnesium, potassium, vitamin A, vitamin B_6, vitamin B_{12}, vitamin D, vitamin E, vitamin K

Neostigmine (Prostigmin) areca nut, Chinese club moss, iboga

Nevirapine (Viramune) bitter melon, boneset, butterbur, chaparral, colt's foot, comfrey, fenugreek, kava kava, maté, St. John's wort, vitamin B_{12}, zinc

Niacin (Niacor, Nicotinex) gotu kola

Niacin and lovastatin (Advicor) gotu kola

Nicardipine (Cardene) andrographis, arnica, asa foetida, bishop's weed, black cohosh, blue cohosh, calcium, carrageen, cat's claw, catechu, devil's claw, dong quai, English hawthorn, ethanol, European mistletoe, garlic, grapefruit, kelp, khat, licorice, lily-of-the-valley, magnesium, ma-huang, niacin, parsley, rue, stevia, St. John's wort, wild carrot, wild cherry, wood betony, yarrow, yohimbe

Nicotine (NicoDerm CQ, Nicotrol) niacin

Nifedipine (Nu-Nifed, Procardia) andrographis, arnica, asa foetida, bishop's weed, black cohosh, blue cohosh, calcium, carrageen, cat's claw, catechu, chicory, devil's claw, dong quai, English hawthorn, ethanol, European mistletoe, garlic, ginkgo biloba, ginseng (Panax), goldenseal, grapefruit, kelp, khat, licorice, lily-of-the-valley, magnesium, ma-huang, niacin, parsley, rue, stevia, St. John's wort, wild carrot, wild cherry, wood betony, yarrow, yohimbe

Niflumic acid (Niflam, Nifluril) bog bean, feverfew, garlic, ginkgo, biloba, gossypol, niacin, reishi mushroom, saw palmetto, St. John's wort, turmeric, uva ursi, white willow

Nifuroxazide (Akabar, Diarret) nutmeg

Nilutamide (Anadron, Nilandron) ethanol

Nilvadipine bishop's weed, calcium, English hawthorn, grapefruit, khat, lily-of-the-valley, magnesium, niacin, stevia, St. John's wort, wild cherry, yohimbe

Nimesulide (Areuma, Aulin) bog bean, feverfew, garlic, ginkgo biloba, gossypol, niacin, reishi mushroom, saw palmetto, St. John's wort, turmeric, uva ursi, white willow

Nimodipine (Nimotop) bishop's weed, calcium, dong quai, English hawthorn, garlic, grapefruit, khat, lily-of-the-valley, magnesium, niacin, stevia, St. John's wort, wild cherry, yohimbe

Nisoldipine (Sular) andrographis, arnica, asa foetida, bishop's weed, black cohosh, blue cohosh, calcium, carrageen, cat's claw, catechu, devil's claw, dong quai, English hawthorn, European mistletoe, garlic, grapefruit, kelp, khat, licorice, lily-of-the-valley, magnesium, ma-huang, niacin, parsley, rue, stevia, St. John's

wort, wild carrot, wild cherry, wood betony, yarrow, yohimbe

Nitrendipine bishop's weed, calcium, English hawthorn, grapefruit, khat, lily-of-the-valley, magnesium, niacin, stevia, St. John's wort, wild cherry, yohimbe

Nitrofurantoin (Furadantin, Macrobid) bitter melon, boneset, butterbur, chaparral, colt's foot, comfrey, echinacea, ethanol, fenugreek, fumitory, gossypol, juniper, kava kava, maté, oak, wintergreen, yohimbe

Nitroglycerin (Minitran, Nitro-Dur) andrographis, arnica, asa foetida, bishop's weed, black cohosh, blue cohosh, carrageen, cat's claw, catechu, devil's claw, English hawthorn, European mistletoe, kelp, khat, licorice, ma-huang, niacin, parsley, rue, stevia, wild carrot, wood betony, yarrow

Nitroprusside (Nipride, Nitropress) andrographis, arnica, asa foetida, bishop's weed, black cohosh, blue cohosh, carrageen, cat's claw, catechu, devil's claw, European mistletoe, kelp, khat, licorice, ma-huang, parsley, rue, stevia, wild carrot, wood betony, yarrow

Nitrous oxide folic acid, vitamin B_{12}

Nizatidine (Apo-Nizatidine, Axid) aletris, angelica, belladonna, birthwort, black mustard, blessed thistle, calamus, calcium, colombo, corkwood, cubeb, dandelion, devil's claw, English lavender, ethanol, folic acid, ginger, henbane, iron, khat, lesser galangal, thiamin, vitamin B_{12}, vitamin D, yellow gentian, zinc

Norepinephrine (Levophed) digitalis, fever bark, Indian squill, ma-huang, rauwolfia, squill

Norethindrone (Aygestin, Micronor) folic acid, magnesium, riboflavin, vitamin B_6, vitamin B_{12}, vitamin C, zinc

Norfloxacin (Apo-Norflox, Noroxin) biotin, black tea, caffeine, calcium, cocoa, coffee, cola nut, green tea, guarana, iron, magnesium, niacin, riboflavin, thiamin, vitamin B_6, vitamin B_{12}, vitamin K, zinc

Norgestrel (Ovrette) alfalfa, anise, black cohosh, chaste tree berry, dong quai

Nortriptyline (Aventyl, Pamelor) agrimony, angel's trumpet, belladonna, black tea, catnip, celery, coffee, coriander, dong quai, ergot, ethanol, evening primrose oil, fennel, ginkgo biloba, goldenseal, henbane, jimson weed, kava kava, lemon balm, lovage, ma-huang, marijuana, motherwort, nerve root, rauwolfia, riboflavin, rosemary, sage, sassafras, scopolia, Scotch broom, stinging nettle, St. John's wort, valerian, wild carrot, wormwood, yohimbe

Nystatin (Mycostatin, Nystat-RX) gossypol

Octreotide (Sandostatin) beta-carotene, nutmeg

Ofloxacin (Floxin, Ocuflox) agrimony, black tea, caffeine, calcium, celery, cocoa, coffee, cola nut, coriander, dong quai, echinacea, evening primrose oil, fennel, fumitory, ginkgo biloba, gossypol, green tea, guarana, iron, juniper, kava kava, lovage, magnesium, motherwort, niacin, oak, riboflavin, rosemary, thiamin, vitamin B_6, vitamin

B_{12}, vitamin K, wild carrot, wintergreen, wormwood, yohimbe, zinc

Olanzapine (Zyprexa, Zyprexa Zydis) cabbage, catnip, cowhage, dong quai, ethanol, evening primrose oil, fennel, ginkgo biloba, goldenseal, gotu kola, kava kava, lemon balm, nerve root, nutmeg, rauwolfia, sage, sassafras, stinging nettle, valerian, wormwood

Olmesartan (Benicar) andrographis, arnica, asa foetida, bishop's weed, black cohosh, blue cohosh, carrageen, cat's claw, catechu, devil's claw, European mistletoe, garlic, kelp, khat, licorice, ma-huang, parsley, potassium, rue, stevia, wild carrot, wood betony, yarrow, yohimbe

Olmesartan and hydrochlorothiazide (Benicar HCT) aloe, apple cider vinegar, birch, bishop's weed, black root, bladderwrack, blue flag, buckthorn, butternut, calcium, caltropis, cascara sagrada, castor oil plant, colocynth, corn silk, cowslip, cucumber, dandelion, digitalis, fo-ti, frangula, gamboge, ginkgo biloba, gossypol, horsetail, Indian hemp, jalap, licorice, lily-of-the-valley, manna, maté, mayapple, potassium, quassia, senna, sorrel, stinging nettle, St. John's wort, stone root, uva ursi, uzara, vitamin D, wahoo, wallflower, wild carrot, yellow dock, yohimbe

Olopatadine (Patanol) belladonna, corkwood, English lavender, henbane, khat

Olsalazine (Dipentum) folic acid

Omeprazole (Losec, Prilosec) agrimony, aletris, angelica, beta-carotene, birthwort, black mustard, blessed thistle, bog bean, calamus, celery, colombo, coriander, cubeb, dandelion, devil's claw, dong quai, ethanol, fennel, folic acid, ginger, goldenseal, iron, lesser galangal, lovage, motherwort, rosemary, thiamin, vitamin B_{12}, wild carrot, yellow gentian, yew, zinc

Omoconazole (Afongan, Fongamil) gossypol

Ondansetron (Zofran) bitter melon, boneset, butterbur, chaparral, colt's foot, comfrey, echinacea, fenugreek, horehound, kava kava, maté, potassium

Opium tincture ashwagandha, bitter almond, California poppy, corkwood, elecampane, English lavender, ethanol, kava kava, maté, nutmeg, parsley, passion flower, poke, poppy, rauwolfia, scullcap, senega, stinging nettle, valerian, wild carrot, wild lettuce, yarrow

Orlistat (Xenical) beta-carotene, vitamin A, vitamin D, vitamin E, vitamin K

Oxaliplatin (Eloxatin) potassium

Oxaprozin (Apo-Oxaprozin, Daypro) bog bean, cat's claw, dong quai, ethanol, feverfew, folic acid, garlic, ginger, ginkgo biloba, gossypol, green tea, horse chestnut, niacin, red clover, reishi mushroom, saw palmetto, St. John's wort, turmeric, uva ursi, white willow

Oxatomide (Cenacert, Tinset) belladonna, corkwood, English lavender, henbane, khat

Oxazepam (Novoxapam, Serax) cabbage, catnip, cedar leaf, cowslip, ethanol, evening primrose oil, German chamomile, ginkgo biloba, goldenseal, gotu kola, kava kava, lemon balm, nerve root, sage, sassafras, stinging nettle, St. John's wort, valerian, wormseed, yohimbe

Oxcarbazepine (Trileptal) calcium, catnip, cedar leaf, ethanol, evening primrose oil, fennel, folic acid, ginkgo biloba, goldenseal, gotu kola, hyssop, kava kava, lemon balm, nerve root, sage, sassafras, stinging nettle, valerian, vitamin D, wormseed, wormwood

Oxiconazole (Oxistat) gossypol

Oxitropium (Oxivent, Tersigat) angel's trumpet, areca nut, butterbur, calabar bean, catechu, Chinese club moss, iboga, jimson weed, mandrake, scopolia

Oxprenolol (Slow-Trasicor, Trasicor) andrographis, arnica, asa foetida, bishop's weed, black cohosh, blue cohosh, butterbur, carrageen, cat's claw, catechu, devil's claw, dong quai, ethanol, European mistletoe, fumitory, kelp, khat, licorice, lily-of-the-valley, mahuang, motherwort, parsley, rue, stevia, St. John's wort, wild carrot, wood betony, yarrow, yohimbe

Oxybutinin (Ditropan, Oxytrol) ethanol, henbane

Oxycodone (OxyContin, Roxicodone) ashwagandha, bitter almond, California poppy, corkwood, elecampane, English lavender, ethanol, gotu kola, kava kava, maté, parsley, passion flower, poke, poppy, rauwolfia, scullcap, senega, stinging nettle, valerian, wild carrot, wild lettuce, yarrow

Oxycodone and acetaminophen (Endocet, Percocet) ashwagandha, bitter almond, California poppy, corkwood, elecampane, English lavender, ethanol, kava kava, maté, parsley, passion flower, poke, poppy, rauwolfia, scullcap, senega, stinging nettle, valerian, wild carrot, wild lettuce, yarrow

Oxycodone and aspirin (Endodan, Percodan) ashwagandha, bitter almond, California poppy, corkwood, elecampane, English lavender, ethanol, folic acid, iron, kava kava, maté, parsley, passion flower, poke, poppy, potassium, rauwolfia, scullcap, senega, stinging nettle, valerian, vitamin C, wild carrot, wild lettuce, yarrow

Oxymorphone (Numorphan) ashwagandha, bitter almond, California poppy, corkwood, elecampane, English lavender, ethanol, gotu kola, kava kava, maté, parsley, passion flower, poke, poppy, rauwolfia, scullcap, senega, stinging nettle, valerian, wild carrot, wild lettuce, yarrow

Oxytetracycline (Terramycin, Terramycin IM) bromelain, calcium, iron, magnesium, St. John's wort, uzara, vitamin A, wahoo, zinc

Oxytocin (Pitocin, Syntocinon) ma-huang

Paclitaxel (Onxol, Taxol) bitter melon, black cohosh, boneset, butterbur, chaparral, colt's foot, comfrey, dong quai, echinacea, fenugreek, gotu kola, kava kava, maté, St. John's wort, valerian, yew

Pamidronate (Aredia) calcium, iron, magnesium, potassium

Pancuronium magnesium

Pantoprazole (Pantoloc, Protonix) aletris, angelica, beta-carotene, birthwort, bitter melon, black mustard, blessed thistle, bog bean, boneset, butterbur, calamus, chaparral, colombo, colt's foot, comfrey, cubeb, dandelion, devil's claw, echinacea, ethanol, fenugreek, ginger, goldenseal, iron, lesser galangal, maté, thiamin, vitamin B_{12}, yellow gentian, yew

Papaverine (Para-Time S.R.) ginkgo biloba

Paregoric ashwagandha, bitter almond, California poppy, corkwood, elecampane, English lavender, ethanol, maté, nutmeg, parsley, passion flower, poke, poppy, rauwolfia, scullcap, senega, stinging nettle, valerian, wild carrot, wild lettuce, yarrow

Paroxetine (Paxil) ergot, ethanol, kava kava, marijuana, St. John's wort, valerian, yohimbe

Pefloxacin (Peflacine, Perflox) black tea, caffeine, calcium, cocoa, coffee, cola nut, green tea, guarana, iron, magnesium, zinc

Peginterferon alfa-2a (Pegasys) ethanol

Peginterferon alfa-2b (PEG-Intron) ethanol

Pemoline (Cylert, PemADD) ethanol, maté

Penicillamine (Cuprimine, Depen) iron, magnesium, vitamin B_6, zinc

Penicillin (Pfizerpen, Wycillin) fumitory, gossypol, juniper, khat, oak, wintergreen, yohimbe

Penicillin G Benzathine (Bicillin L-A, Permapen) biotin, niacin, potassium, riboflavin, thiamin, vitamin B_6, vitamin B_{12}, vitamin K

Penicillin G Benzathine plus Penicillin G Procaine (Bicicillin C-R) biotin, niacin, potassium, riboflavin, thiamin, vitamin B_6, vitamin B_{12}, vitamin K

Penicillin G Procaine (Pfizerpen-AS, Wycillin) biotin, niacin, potassium, riboflavin, thiamin, vitamin B_6, vitamin B_{12}, vitamin K

Penicillin V Potassium (Suspen, Truxcillin) biotin, niacin, potassium, riboflavin, thiamin, vitamin B_6, vitamin B_{12}, vitamin K

Pentamidine (NebuPent, Pentacarinat) calcium, ethanol, folic acid, magnesium

Pentazocine (Talwin) ashwagandha, bitter almond, cabbage, California poppy, corkwood, cowslip, elecampane, English lavender, ergot, ethanol, German chamomile, Hawaiian baby woodrose, kava kava, maté, parsley, passion flower, poke, poppy, rauwolfia, scullcap, senega, stinging nettle, valerian, wild carrot, wild lettuce, yarrow

Pentobarbital (Nembutal) ashwagandha, bitter almond, California poppy, cedar leaf, cedarwood oil, cowslip, elecampane, English lavender, ethanol, eucalyptus, evening primrose oil, ginkgo biloba, hops, kava kava, lemon balm, marijuana, maté, passion flower, poke, poppy, rauwolfia, sage, scullcap, senega, stinging nettle, St. John's wort, valerian, wild carrot, wild lettuce, wormseed, yarrow

Pentoxifylline (Pentoxil, Trental) country mallow, digitalis, Indian squill, squill

Pergolide (Permax) chaste tree berry, ergot, ethanol, kava kava

Perindopril erbumine (Aceon, Coversyl) andrographis, arnica, asa foetida, bishop's weed, black cohosh, blue cohosh, carrageen, cat's claw, catechu, cayenne, devil's claw, garlic, kelp, khat, licorice, ma-huang, mistletoe, parsley, pineapple, pomegranate, potassium, rue, stevia, St. John's wort, wild carrot, wood betony, yarrow, yohimbe, zinc

Perphenazine (Apo-Perphenazine, Trilafon) angel's trumpet, belladonna, black tea, coffee, corkwood, cowhage, ethanol, evening primrose oil, gotu kola, henbane, jimson weed, kava kava, ma-huang, rauwolfia, riboflavin, valerian, yohimbe

Phenelzine (Nardil) anise, bitter orange, black tea, brewer's yeast, butcher's broom, caffeine, calamus, cayenne, cocoa, coffee, cola nut, country mallow, cowhage, ergot, ethanol, ginkgo biloba, ginseng (Panax), green tea, guarana, Hawaiian baby woodrose, jimson weed, kava kava, khat, licorice, ma-huang, nutmeg, rauwolfia, Scotch broom, St. John's wort, valerian, vitamin B_6, yohimbe

Phenobarbital (Luminal Sodium, PMS-Phenobarbital) ashwagandha, bitter almond, calcium, California poppy, cedar leaf, cedarwood oil, cowslip, elecampane, English lavender, ethanol, eucalyptus, evening primrose oil, folic acid, German chamomile, ginkgo biloba, gotu kola, hops, kava kava, lemon balm, marijuana, maté, passion flower, poke, poppy, rauwolfia, sage, scullcap, senega, stinging nettle, St. John's wort, valerian, vitamin B_6, vitamin B_{12}, vitamin D, vitamin K, wild carrot, wild lettuce, wormseed, wormwood, yarrow

Phenoperidine ashwagandha, bitter almond, California poppy, corkwood, elecampane, English lavender, ethanol, kava kava, maté, parsley, passion flower, poke, poppy, rauwolfia, scullcap, senega, stinging nettle, valerian, wild carrot, wild lettuce, yarrow

Phenoxybenzamine (Dibenzyline) andrographis, arnica, asa foetida, bishop's weed, black cohosh, blue cohosh, carrageen, cat's claw, catechu, devil's claw, European mistletoe, kelp, khat, licorice, mahuang, parsley, rue, stevia, wild carrot, wood betony, yarrow

Phentermine (Adipex-P, Ionamin) black tea, caffeine, cocoa, coffee, cola nut, green tea

Phentolamine (Regitine, Rogitine) andrographis, arnica, asa foetida, bishop's weed, black cohosh, blue cohosh, carrageen, cat's claw, catechu, devil's claw, European mistletoe, kelp, khat, licorice, mahuang, milk thistle, parsley, rue, stevia, wild carrot, wood betony, yarrow

Phenylephrine (Neo-Synephrine Extra Strength, Vicks Sinex Nasal Spray) digitalis, fever bark, Indian squill, ma-huang, rauwolfia, squill, yohimbe

Phenytoin (Dilantin, Phenytek) agrimony, aloe, bitter melon, black pepper, boneset, buckthorn, butterbur, calcium, cascara sagrada, cedar leaf, celery, chaparral, colt's foot, comfrey, coriander, dong quai, echinacea, ethanol, evening primrose oil, fennel, fenugreek, folic acid, fumitory, ginkgo biloba, gotu kola, hyssop, Indian long pepper, kava kava, khat, kudzu, licorice, lovage, maté, motherwort, rosemary, sage, senna, stinging nettle, St. John's wort, thiamin, valerian, vitamin B_6, vitamin

B_{12}, vitamin D, vitamin K, wild carrot, wormseed, wormwood

Physostigmine (Eserine) areca nut, Chinese club moss, iboga

Pilocarpine (Isopto Carpine, Salagen) areca nut, Chinese club moss, iboga

Pimecrolimus (Elidel) andrographis, ashwagandha, astragalus, cat's claw, echinacea, larch, maitake mushroom, schisandra, scullcap, St. John's wort, turmeric

Pimozide (Orap) cowhage, rauwolfia

Pinaverium (Dicetel) bishop's weed, calcium, English hawthorn, grapefruit, khat, lily-of-the-valley, magnesium, niacin, stevia, St. John's wort, wild cherry, yohimbe

Pindolol (Apo-Pindol, Novo-Pindol) andrographis, arnica, asa foetida, bishop's weed, black cohosh, blue cohosh, butterbur, carrageen, cat's claw, catechu, devil's claw, dong quai, European mistletoe, fumitory, kelp, khat, licorice, lily-of-the-valley, ma-huang, motherwort, parsley, rue, stevia, St. John's wort, wild carrot, wood betony, yarrow, yohimbe

Pioglitazone (Actos) agrimony, aloe, angelica, avaram, banaba, barley, basil, bilberry, bitter melon, black tea, bladderwrack, blue cohosh, boneset, buchu, bugleweed, burdock, butterbur, caffeine, chanca piedra, chaparral, Chinese cucumber root, cinnamon, cocoa, coffee, cola nut, colt's foot, comfrey, coriander, country mallow, cumin, damiana, dandelion, devil's claw, ethanol, eucalyptus, fenugreek, flax, garlic, ginger, ginkgo biloba, ginseng (American), ginseng (Panax), ginseng (Siberian), glucomannan, goat's rue, gotu kola, green tea, guar gum, gymnema, horehound, horse chestnut, juniper, kudzu, laurel, licorice, Madagascar periwinkle, ma-huang, maitake mushroom, marshmallow, maté, myrrh, niacin, olive, onion, prickly pear cactus, psyllium, psyllium seed, raspberry, sage, Scotch broom, senega, Solomon's seal, stevia, St. John's wort, yarrow

Pipamperone (Dipiperon, Piperonil) cowhage, rauwolfia

Piperacillin (Pipracil) biotin, niacin, potassium, riboflavin, thiamin, vitamin B_6, vitamin B_{12}, vitamin K

Piperacillin plus tazobactam sodium (Zosyn) biotin, niacin, potassium, riboflavin, thiamin, vitamin B_6, vitamin B_{12}, vitamin K

Piracetam (Geram, Piracetam Verla) cowhage, rauwolfia

Piroxicam (Feldene, Nu-Pirox) agrimony, angelica, anise, bitter melon, bog bean, boneset, butterbur, cat's claw, celery, chaparral, coffee, cola nut, colt's foot, comfrey, coriander, danshen, devil's claw, dong quai, echinacea, ethanol, fennel, fenugreek, feverfew, folic acid, fumitory, garlic, ginger, ginkgo biloba, gossypol, green tea, horse chestnut, juniper, licorice, lovage, maté, meadowsweet, motherwort, niacin, oak, passion flower, red clover, reishi mushroom, rosemary, saw palmetto, St. John's wort, turmeric, uva ursi,

white willow, wild carrot, wild yam, wintergreen, yohimbe

Pizotifen (Sandomigran) ethanol, gotu kola, kava kava, valerian

Plicamycin (Mithracin) calcium, potassium

Polyestradiol acerola, alfalfa, anise, calcium, senna, St. John's wort, wild cherry, wild yam

Polyethylene glycol-electrolyte solution (Colyte, MiraLax) adonis, licorice, lily-of-the-valley, oleander, senna, squill, strophanthus

Polysaccharide-iron complex (Hytinic, Niferex) artichoke, bilberry, black cohosh, borage, butternut, cascara sagrada, catechu, English lavender, European elder, European mistletoe, eyebright, horehound, horse chestnut, lemon balm, meadowsweet, motherwort, northern prickly ash, oak, poplar, raspberry, sage, saw palmetto, slippery elm, soybean, stinging nettle, St. John's wort, uva ursi, valerian, witch hazel, wormwood, yarrow, yellow dock

Polythiazide (Renese) aloe, andrographis, apple cider vinegar, arnica, asa foetida, birch, bishop's weed, black cohosh, black root, bladderwrack, blue cohosh, blue flag, buckthorn, butternut, calcium, calotropis, carrageen, cascara sagrada, castor oil plant, cat's claw, catechu, colocynth, corn silk, cowslip, cucumber, dandelion, devil's claw, digitalis, European mistletoe, fo-ti, frangula, gamboge, ginkgo biloba, gossypol, horsetail, Indian hemp, jalap, kelp, khat, licorice, lily-of-the-valley, magnesium, ma-huang, manna, maté, mayapple, parsley, potassium, quassia, rue, senna, sorrel, stevia, stinging nettle, St. John's wort, stone root, uva ursi, uzara, vitamin D, wahoo, wallflower, wild carrot, wood betony, yarrow, yellow dock, yohimbe, zinc

Potassium and sodium phosphates (K-Phos Neutral, Uro-KP-Neutral) calcium, magnesium

Potassium chloride (Apo-K, Micro-K) magnesium, vitamin B$_{12}$

Povidone-iodine (Betadine, Vagi-Gard) gossypol

Pramipexole (Mirapex) chaste tree berry, ethanol, kava kava, valerian

Pravastatin (Novo-Pravastatin, Pravachol) bitter melon, boneset, butterbur, chaparral, colt's foot, comfrey, echinacea, ethanol, fenugreek, gotu kola, maté, niacin, oats, pectin, red yeast rice, St. John's wort, wild cherry

Prazepam ashwagandha, bitter almond, California poppy, elecampane, ethanol, German chamomile, gotu kola, kava kava, maté, passion flower, poke, poppy, rauwolfia, scullcap, senega, stinging nettle, St. John's wort, valerian, wild carrot, wild cherry, wild lettuce, yarrow

Praziquantel (Biltricide) grapefruit

Prazosin (Minipress, Nu-Prazo) andrographis, arnica, asa foetida, bishop's weed, black cohosh, blue cohosh, butcher's broom, carrageen, cat's claw, catechu, devil's claw, dong quai, ethanol, European mistletoe, fenugreek, garlic, goldenseal, kelp, khat,

licorice, ma-huang, parsley, rue, saw palmetto, stevia, wild carrot, wood betony, yarrow, yohimbe

Prazosin plus polythiazide (Minizide) magnesium, potassium, zinc

Prednisolone (Inflamase Forte, Pediapred) adonis, aloe, andrographis, ashwagandha, astragalus, buckthorn, butternut, calcium, cascara sagrada, castor oil plant, cat's claw, cordyceps, echinacea, ethanol, folic acid, frangula, Indian squill, larch, licorice, lily-of-the-valley, magnesium, ma-huang, oleander, perilla, potassium, schisandra, squill, strophanthus, vitamin A, vitamin B$_6$, vitamin C, vitamin D, vitamin K, wallflower, zinc

Prednisone (Apo-Prednisone, Deltasone) adonis, alfalfa, aloe, andrographis, ashwagandha, astragalus, buckthorn, butternut, calcium, cascara sagrada, castor oil plant, cat's claw, echinacea, ethanol, European mistletoe, folic acid, frangula, Indian squill, larch, licorice, lily-of-the-valley, magnesium, ma-huang, noni, oleander, perilla, potassium, schisandra, senna, squill, strophanthus, vitamin A, vitamin B$_6$, vitamin C, vitamin D, vitamin K, wallflower, zinc

Prifinium (Padrin, Riabel) angel's trumpet, areca nut, butterbur, calabar bean, catechu, Chinese club moss, iboga, jimson weed, mandrake, scopolia

Primaquine ethanol

Primidone (Apo-Primidone, Mysoline) ashwagandha, bitter almond, calcium, California poppy, cedar leaf, cedarwood oil, elecampane, ethanol, eucalyptus, evening primrose oil, folic acid, ginkgo biloba, gotu kola, hops, kava kava, lemon balm, marijuana, maté, passion flower, poke, poppy, rauwolfia, sage, scullcap, senega, stinging nettle, St. John's wort, valerian, vitamin B$_6$, vitamin B$_{12}$, vitamin D, vitamin K, wild carrot, wild lettuce, wormseed, yarrow

Probucol gotu kola

Procainamide (Procanbid, Pronestyl-SR) aloe, belladonna, buckthorn, cascara sagrada, ethanol, fumitory, henbane, khat, kudzu, licorice, senna

Procarbazine (Matulane, Natulan) ethanol

Prochlorperazine (Compazine, Compro) agrimony, angel's trumpet, belladonna, bitter melon, black tea, boneset, butterbur, catnip, celery, chaparral, coffee, colt's foot, comfrey, coriander, corkwood, cowhage, dong quai, echinacea, ethanol, evening primrose oil, fennel, fenugreek, ginkgo biloba, goldenseal, gotu kola, henbane, jimson weed, kava kava, lemon balm, lovage, ma-huang, maté, motherwort, nerve root, nutmeg, rauwolfia, riboflavin, rosemary, sage, sassafras, stinging nettle, valerian, wild carrot, wormwood, yohimbe

Procyclidine (Kemadrin, Procyclid) angel's trumpet, areca nut, butterbur, calabar bean, catechu, Chinese club moss, iboga, jimson weed, mandrake, scopolia

Progesterone (Crinone, Prometrium) red clover

Promethazine (Phenergan) angel's trumpet, ashwagandha, belladonna, bitter almond, black tea, California poppy, coffee, corkwood, cowslip, elecampane, English lavender, ethanol, evening primrose oil, German chamomile, gotu kola, hen-

bane, jimson weed, kava kava, khat, ma-huang, maté, passion flower, poke, poppy, rauwolfia, riboflavin, scullcap, senega, stinging nettle, valerian, wild carrot, wild lettuce, yarrow, yohimbe

Promethazine and codeine (Phenergan with Codeine) belladonna, corkwood, English lavender, henbane, khat

Promethazine and dextromethorphan (Promatussin DM) belladonna, corkwood, English lavender, henbane, khat

Promethazine and phenylephrine belladonna, corkwood, English lavender, henbane, khat

Promethazine, phenylephrine, and codeine belladonna, corkwood, English lavender, henbane, khat

Propafenone (Gen-Propafenone, Rhythmol) aloe, buckthorn, cascara sagrada, fumitory, khat, kudzu, licorice, senna

Propantheline (Propanthel) angel's trumpet, areca nut, butterbur, calabar bean, catechu, Chinese club moss, iboga, jimson weed, mandrake, scopolia

Propofol (Diprivan) ashwagandha, bitter almond, California poppy, cowslip, elecampane, English lavender, ethanol, German chamomile, maté, passion flower, poke, poppy, rauwolfia, scullcap, senega, stinging nettle, valerian, wild carrot, wild lettuce, yarrow

Propoxyphene (Darvon, Darvon-N) ashwagandha, bitter almond, bitter melon, boneset, butterbur, California poppy, catnip, chaparral, colt's foot, comfrey, corkwood, elecampane, English lavender, ethanol, fenugreek, fumitory, goldenseal, gossypol, juniper, kava kava, lemon balm, maté, nerve root, oak, parsley, passion flower, poke, sassafras, scullcap, senega, stinging nettle, valerian, wild carrot, wild lettuce, wintergreen, yarrow, yohimbe

Propoxyphene and acetaminophen (Darvocet-N 50, Darvocet-N 100) ashwagandha, bitter almond, California poppy, corkwood, elecampane, English lavender, ethanol, kava kava, maté, parsley, passion flower, poke, poppy, rauwolfia, scullcap, senega, stinging nettle, valerian, wild carrot, wild lettuce, yarrow

Propoxyphene, aspirin, and caffeine (Darvon Compound) ashwagandha, bitter almond, California poppy, corkwood, elecampane, English lavender, ethanol, kava kava, maté, parsley, passion flower, poke, poppy, rauwolfia, scullcap, senega, stinging nettle, valerian, wild carrot, wild lettuce, yarrow

Propranolol (Inderal, InnoPran XL) aloe, andrographis, arnica, asa foetida, bishop's weed, black cohosh, black pepper, blue cohosh, buckthorn, butterbur, cabbage, carrageen, cascara sagrada, cat's claw, catechu, devil's claw, dong quai, ethanol, European mistletoe, fumitory, garlic, goldenseal, guggul, Indian long pepper, kelp, khat, kudzu, licorice, lily-of-the-valley, ma-huang, motherwort, parsley, rue, senna, stevia, St. John's wort, wild carrot, wood betony, yarrow, yohimbe

Propranolol plus hydrochlorothiazide (Inderide) magnesium, potassium, zinc

Protriptyline (Vivactil) angel's trumpet, belladonna, black tea, coffee, corkwood, ergot, ethanol, henbane, jimson weed, kava kava, ma-huang, marijuana, rauwolfia, riboflavin, scopolia, St. John's wort, valerian, yohimbe

Pseudoephedrine (Dimetapp Decongestant, Sudafed) black tea, caffeine, cocoa, coffee, cola nut, digitalis, fever bark, green tea, Indian squill, khat, ma-huang, rauwolfia, scotch broom, squill, yohimbe

Pseudoephedrine plus ibuprofen (Advil Cold & Sinus Caplets, Dimetapp Sinus Caplets) folic acid

Psyllium (Metamucil, Reguloid) adonis, licorice, lily-of-the-valley, nutmeg, oleander, senna, squill, strophanthus

Pyridostigmine (Mestinon) areca nut, Chinese club moss, iboga

Pyrimethamine (Daraprim) folic acid

Quazepam (Doral) ashwagandha, bitter almond, California poppy, cowslip, elecampane, English lavender, ethanol, German chamomile, kava kava, maté, passion flower, poke, poppy, rauwolfia, scullcap, senega, stinging nettle, St. John's wort, valerian, wild carrot, wild cherry, wild lettuce, yarrow

Quetiapine (Seroquel) catnip, cowhage, ethanol, evening primrose oil, fennel, ginkgo biloba, goldenseal, gotu kola, kava kava, lemon balm, nerve root, nutmeg, rauwolfia, sage, sassafras, stinging nettle, valerian, wormwood

Quinapril (Accupril) agrimony, andrographis, arnica, asa foetida, bishop's weed, black cohosh, blue cohosh, carrageen, cat's claw, catechu, cayenne, celery, coriander, devil's claw, dong quai, European mistletoe, fennel, garlic, goldenseal, kelp, khat, licorice, lovage, ma-huang, motherwort, parsley, pineapple, pomegranate, potassium, rosemary, rue, stevia, St. John's wort, wild carrot, wood betony, yarrow, yohimbe, zinc

Quinidine (Quinaglute Dura-Tabs, Novo-Quinidin) adonis, aloe, belladonna, buckthorn, cascara sagrada, Chinese rhubarb, digitalis, fumitory, guarana, henbane, Indian squill, khat, kudzu, licorice, lily-of-the-valley, oleander, quinine, scopolia, Scotch broom, senna, squill, strophanthus, wallflower

Quinine (Quinine-Odan) digitalis, strophanthus, uzara, wahoo, wallflower

Rabeprazole (Aciphex, Pariet) aletris, angelica, beta-carotene, birthwort, black mustard, blessed thistle, calamus, colombo, cubeb, dandelion, devil's claw, ethanol, folic acid, ginger, iron, lesser galangal, thiamin, vitamin B$_{12}$, yellow gentian, zinc

Raloxifene (Evista) ethanol, magnesium, vitamin B$_6$

Raltitrexed (Tomudex) folic acid

Ramipril (Altace) andrographis, arnica, asa foetida, bishop's weed, black cohosh, blue cohosh, carrageen, cat's claw, catechu, cayenne, devil's claw, dong quai, European mistletoe, garlic, kelp, khat, licorice, ma-huang, parsley, pineapple, pomegranate, potassium, rue, stevia, St. John's

wort, wild carrot, wood betony, yarrow, yohimbe, zinc

Ranitidine (Alti-Ranitidine, Zantac) aletris, angelica, belladonna, birthwort, black mustard, blessed thistle, bog bean, calamus, calcium, colombo, corkwood, cubeb, dandelion, devil's claw, English lavender, ethanol, folic acid, ginger, goldenseal, henbane, iron, khat, lesser galangal, thiamin, vitamin B$_{12}$, vitamin D, yellow gentian, yew, zinc

Reboxetine (Davedax, Integrex) ergot

Remifentanil (Ultiva) ashwagandha, bitter almond, California poppy, corkwood, elecampane, English lavender, ethanol, kava kava, maté, parsley, passion flower, poke, poppy, rauwolfia, scullcap, senega, stinging nettle, valerian, wild carrot, wild lettuce, yarrow

Repaglinide (GlucoNorm, Prandin) agrimony, aloe, angelica, avaram, banaba, barley, basil, bilberry, bitter melon, black tea, bladderwrack, blue cohosh, boneset, buchu, bugleweed, burdock, butterbur, caffeine, chanca piedra, chaparral, Chinese cucumber root, cinnamon, cocoa, coffee, cola nut, colt's foot, comfrey, coriander, country mallow, cumin, damiana, dandelion, devil's claw, ethanol, eucalyptus, fenugreek, flax, garlic, ginger, ginkgo biloba, ginseng (American), ginseng (Panax), ginseng (Siberian), glucomannan, goat's rue, gotu kola, green tea, guar gum, gymnema, horehound, horse chestnut, juniper, kudzu, laurel, licorice, Madagascar periwinkle, ma-huang, maitake mushroom, marshmallow, maté, myrrh, niacin, olive, onion, prickly pear cactus, psyllium, psyllium seed, raspberry, sage, Scotch broom, senega, Solomon's seal, stevia, St. John's wort, yarrow

Reserpine andrographis, arnica, asa foetida, bishop's weed, black cohosh, blue cohosh, carrageen, cat's claw, catechu, devil's claw, European mistletoe, kelp, khat, licorice, ma-huang, parsley, rue, stevia, St. John's wort, wild carrot, wood betony, yarrow, yohimbe

Reteplase (Retavase) angelica, arnica, astragalus, bilberry, bladderwrack, borage, cat's claw, cayenne, clove, dong quai, evening primrose oil, feverfew, garlic, ginger, ginkgo biloba, ginseng (Siberian), horse chestnut, kava kava, licorice, pineapple, red clover, turmeric, valerian, white willow

Rifabutin (Mycobutin) echinacea, vitamin D

Rifampin (Rifadin, Rimactane) bitter melon, boneset, butterbur, calcium, chaparral, colt's foot, comfrey, echinacea, ethanol, fenugreek, fumitory, gossypol, juniper, maté, oak, vitamin D, wintergreen, yohimbe

Rifampin plus isoniazid (Rifamate) calcium, niacin, vitamin B_6, vitamin D

Rifapentine (Priftin) bitter melon, boneset, butterbur, chaparral, colt's foot, comfrey, echinacea, fenugreek, maté, vitamin D

Riluzole (Rilutek) black tea, caffeine, cocoa, coffee, cola nut, ethanol, green tea, guarana

Rimexolone (Vexol) adonis, aloe, andrographis, ashwagandha, astragalus, buckthorn, butternut, cascara sagrada, castor oil plant, Indian squill, larch, perilla, schisandra, strophanthus

Risedronate (Actonel) calcium, ethanol, iron, magnesium

Risperidone (Risperdal) agrimony, catnip, celery, coriander, cowhage, dong quai, ethanol, fennel, goldenseal, gotu kola, kava kava, lemon balm, lovage, motherwort, nerve root, nutmeg, rauwolfia, rosemary, sassafras, stinging nettle, valerian, wild carrot

Ritonavir (Norvir) bitter melon, boneset, butterbur, chaparral, colt's foot, comfrey, echinacea, fenugreek, garlic, marijuana, maté, St. John's wort, vitamin C

Rivastigmine (Exelon) areca nut, Chinese club moss, ethanol, iboga

Rizatriptan benzoate (Maxalt) bugleweed, feverfew, goldenseal, horehound, Scotch broom, witch hazel

Rocuronium (Zemuron) magnesium

Rofecoxib (Vioxx) agrimony, angelica, anise, bitter melon, bog bean, boneset, borage seed oil, butterbur, celery, chaparral, coffee, cola nut, colt's foot, comfrey, coriander, danshen, devil's claw, dong quai, fennel, fenugreek, feverfew, folic acid, garlic, ginger, ginkgo biloba, gossypol, horse chestnut, licorice, lovage, maté, meadowsweet, motherwort, niacin, passion flower, red clover, reishi mushroom, rosemary, saw palmetto, St. John's wort, turmeric, uva ursi, white willow, wild carrot, wild yam

Ropinirole (Requip) chaste tree berry, ethanol, gotu kola, kava kava, valerian

Rosiglitazone (Avandia) agrimony, aloe, angelica, avaram, banaba, barley, basil, bilberry, bitter melon, black tea, bladderwrack, blue cohosh, boneset, buchu, bugleweed, burdock, butterbur, caffeine, chanca piedra, chaparral, Chinese cucumber root, cinnamon, cocoa, coffee, cola nut, colt's foot, comfrey, coriander, country mallow, cumin, damiana, dandelion, devil's claw, ethanol, eucalyptus, fenugreek, flax, garlic, ginger, ginkgo biloba, ginseng (American), ginseng (Panax), ginseng (Siberian), glucomannan, goat's rue, gotu kola, green tea, guar gum, gymnema, horehound, horse chestnut, juniper, kudzu, laurel, licorice, Madagascar periwinkle, ma-huang, maitake mushroom, marshmallow, maté, myrrh, niacin, olive, onion, prickly pear cactus, psyllium, psyllium seed, raspberry, sage, Scotch broom, senega, Solomon's seal, stevia, St. John's wort, yarrow

Rosiglitazone and metformin (Avandamet) agrimony, aloe, avaram, banaba, barley, basil, bilberry, bitter melon, black tea, bladderwrack, blue cohosh, buchu, bugleweed, burdock, caffeine, chanca piedra, Chinese cucumber root, cinnamon, cocoa, coffee, cola nut, coriander, country mallow, cumin, damiana, dandelion, devil's claw, eucalyptus, fenugreek, flax, garlic, ginger, ginseng (American), ginseng (Panax), ginseng (Siberian), glucomannan, goat's rue, gotu kola, green tea, guar gum, gymnema, horehound, horse chestnut, kudzu, laurel, licorice, Madagascar periwinkle, ma-huang, maitake mushroom, marshmallow, myrrh, niacin, olive, onion, prickly pear cactus, psyllium, psyllium seed, raspberry, senega, Solomon's seal, stevia, St. John's wort

Rosuvastatin (Crestor) ethanol, gotu kola, niacin, oats, pectin, red yeast rice, St. John's wort, wild cherry

Roxithromycin (Claramid, Roxibeta) uzara, wahoo

Salsalate (Amgesic, Salflex) bog bean, cat's claw, cayenne, dong quai, ethanol, feverfew, folic acid, garlic, ginger, ginkgo biloba, gossypol, green tea, heartsease, horse chestnut, lovage, lungwort, niacin, northern prickly ash, pau d'arco, pineapple, poplar, potassium, red clover, reishi mushroom, safflower, saw palmetto, senega, St. John's wort, tonka bean, turmeric, uva ursi, white willow, wintergreen, yarrow

Saquinavir (Fortovase, Invirase) bitter melon, boneset, butterbur, chaparral, colt's foot, comfrey, echinacea, fenugreek, garlic, grapefruit, marijuana, maté, St. John's wort, vitamin C

S-citalopram (Lexapro) ergot, ethanol, gotu kola, kava kava, marijuana, St. John's wort, valerian

Scopolamine (Scopace, Transderm Scop) angel's trumpet, areca nut, black root, butterbur, calabar bean, catechu, Chinese club moss, grapefruit, iboga, jimson weed, mandrake, scopolia

Secobarbital (Seconal) ashwagandha, bitter almond, California poppy, cedarwood oil, cowslip, elecampane, English lavender, ethanol, eucalyptus, German chamomile, hops, kava kava, lemon balm, marijuana, maté, passion flower, poke, poppy, rauwolfia, scullcap, senega, stinging nettle, St. John's wort, valerian, wild carrot, wild lettuce, yarrow

Selegiline (Eldepryl) anise, bitter orange, black tea, brewer's yeast, butcher's broom, caffeine, calamus, cayenne, cocoa, coffee, cola nut, country mallow, ergot, ethanol, ginkgo biloba, ginseng (Panax), green tea, guarana, Hawaiian baby woodrose, jimson weed, kava kava, khat, licorice, ma-huang, nutmeg, parsley, passion flower, rauwolfia, Scotch broom, St. John's wort, valerian, yohimbe

Sertraline (Apo-Sertraline, Zoloft) ergot, ethanol, gotu kola, kava kava, marijuana, St. John's wort, valerian, yohimbe

Sevelamer (Renagel) folic acid, vitamin D, vitamin E, vitamin K

Sibutramine (Meridia) yohimbe

Sildenafil (Viagra) aloe, black cohosh, cascara sagrada, Chinese rhubarb, digitalis, grapefruit, guarana, Indian squill, licorice, senna, squill

Simvastatin (Apo-Simvastatin, Zocor) beta-carotene, bitter melon, boneset, butterbur, chaparral, colt's foot, comfrey, echinacea, ethanol, fenugreek, gotu kola, grapefruit, maté, niacin, oats, pectin, red yeast rice, St. John's wort, vitamin E, wild cherry

Sirolimus (Rapamune) andrographis, ashwagandha, astragalus, cat's claw, echinacea, larch, maitake mushroom, schisandra, scullcap, St. John's wort, turmeric

Sodium bicarbonate (Brioschi, Neut) aletris, angelica, birthwort, black mustard, blessed thistle, buckthorn, calamus, calcium, colombo, cubeb, dandelion, devil's claw, ginger, lesser galangal, ma-huang, potassium, yellow gentian

Sodium chloride (Nasal Moist, Simply Saline) potassium

Sodium oxybate (Xyrem) California poppy, ethanol, gotu kola, kava kava, passion flower, poke, poppy, rauwolfia, scullcap, senega, stinging nettle, valerian, wild carrot, wild lettuce

Sodium phosphate (Fleet Enema, Fleet Phospho-Soda) calcium, magnesium, potassium

Sodium polystyrene sulfonate (Kayexalate) calcium, potassium

Sorbitol (Sorbilax) adonis, licorice, lily-of-the-valley, oleander, senna, squill, strophanthus

Sotalol (Betapace, Sorine) aloe, black cohosh, buckthorn, butterbur, cascara sagrada, Chinese rhubarb, English hawthorn, fumitory, guarana, khat, kudzu, licorice, lily-of-the-valley, motherwort, senna, St. John's wort, yohimbe

Sparfloxacin (Zagam) biotin, black tea, caffeine, calcium, cocoa, coffee, cola nut, dong quai, green tea, guarana, iron, magnesium, niacin, riboflavin, thiamin, vitamin B_6, vitamin B_{12}, vitamin K, zinc

Spiramycin (Rovamycine) uzara, wahoo

Spirapril cayenne, pineapple, pomegranate, potassium, St. John's wort, yohimbe

Spironolactone (Aldactone, Novo-Spiroton) andrographis, arnica, asa foetida, birch, bishop's weed, black cohosh, bladderwrack, blue cohosh, carrageen, cat's claw, catechu, cowslip, cucumber, dandelion, devil's claw, European mistletoe, kelp, khat, magnesium, ma-huang, maté, noni, parsley, potassium, rue, sorrel, stevia, stinging nettle, stone root, wild carrot, wood betony, yarrow, yohimbe

Stanzolol (Winstrol) iron

Stavudine (Zerit) bitter melon, boneset, chaparral, colt's foot, comfrey, echinacea, fenugreek, gossypol, juniper, maté, oak, vitamin B_{12}, wintergreen, yohimbe, zinc

Streptokinase (Streptase) angelica, arnica, astragalus, bilberry, bladderwrack, borage, cat's claw, cayenne, clove, dong quai, evening primrose oil, feverfew, garlic, ginger, ginkgo biloba, ginseng (Panax), ginseng (Siberian), green tea, horse chestnut, kava kava, licorice, pineapple, red clover, turmeric, valerian, white willow

Streptomycin calcium, magnesium, potassium

Succinylcholine (Quelicin) magnesium

Sucralfate (Carafate, Sulcrate) aletris, black mustard, blessed thistle, bog bean, calcium, cayenne, fumitory, ginger, goldenseal, gossypol, juniper, oak, vitamin A, vitamin D, vitamin E, vitamin K, wintergreen, yarrow, yew, yohimbe

Sufentanil (Sufenta) ashwagandha, bitter almond, California poppy, corkwood, elecampane, English lavender, ethanol, kava kava, maté, parsley, passion flower, poke, poppy, rauwolfia, scullcap, senega, stinging nettle, valerian, wild carrot, wild lettuce, yarrow

Sulconazole (Exelderm) gossypol

Sulfacetamide (Bleph-10, Klaron) St. John's wort

Sulfadiazine (Coptin, Microsulfon) biotin, dong quai, niacin, riboflavin, St. John's wort, thiamin, vitamin B_6, vitamin B_{12}, vitamin K

Sulfamethoxazole and trimethoprim (Bactrim, Septra) dong quai, St. John's wort

Sulfasalazine (Azulfidine, Salazopyrin) calcium, dong quai, folic acid, iron, vitamin B_6, vitamin B_{12}

Sulfinpyrazone (Apo-Sulfinpyrazone, Nu-Sulfinpyrazone) dong quai

Sulfisoxazole (Gantrisin, Sulfizole) dong quai, niacin, riboflavin, St. John's wort, thiamin, vitamin B_6, vitamin B_{12}, vitamin K

Sulfur and sulfacetamide (Nocosyn, Rosanil) St. John's wort

Sulindac (Clinoril, Nu-Sundac) bog bean, cat's claw, dong quai, ethanol, feverfew, folic acid, garlic, ginger, ginkgo biloba, gossypol, green tea, horse chestnut, niacin, red clover, reishi mushroom, saw palmetto, St. John's wort, turmeric, uva ursi, white willow

Sumatriptan (Imitrex) horehound

S-zopiclone (Lunesta) elecampane, ethanol, German chamomile, maté, passion flower, poke, poppy, rauwolfia, scullcap, senega, stinging nettle, valerian, wild carrot, wild lettuce, yarrow

Tacrine (Cognex) areca nut, cabbage, Chinese club moss, iboga

Tacrolimus (Prograf, Protopic) andrographis, ashwagandha, astragalus, calcium, cat's claw, echinacea, larch, magnesium, maitake mushroom, potassium, schisandra, scullcap, St. John's wort, turmeric

Tadalafil (Cialis) digitalis, ethanol, Indian squill, squill

Tamoxifen (Nolvadex, Tamofen) anise, bitter melon, black cohosh, boneset, butterbur, chaparral, colt's foot, comfrey, dong quai, echinacea, fenugreek, maté, red clover, soybean, St. John's wort, yew

Telmisartan (Micardis) andrographis, arnica, asa foetida, bishop's weed, black cohosh, blue cohosh, carrageen, cat's claw, catechu, devil's claw, dong quai, European mistletoe, garlic, kelp, khat, licorice, ma-huang, parsley, potassium, rue, stevia, wild carrot, wood betony, yarrow, yohimbe

Telmisartan plus hydrochlorothiazide (Micardis HCT, Micardis Plus) magnesium, potassium, zinc

Temazepam (Novo-Temazepam, Restoril) ashwagandha, bitter almond, California poppy, catnip, cowslip, echinacea, elecampane, English lavender, ethanol, German chamomile, goldenseal, gotu kola, kava kava, lemon balm, linden, maté, nerve root, passion flower, poke, poppy, rauwolfia, sassafras, scullcap, senega, stinging nettle, St. John's wort, valerian, wild carrot, wild cherry, wild lettuce, yarrow

Tenecteplase (TNKase) angelica, arnica, astragalus, bilberry, bladderwrack, borage, cat's claw, cayenne, clove, dong quai, evening primrose oil, feverfew, garlic, ginger, ginkgo biloba, ginseng (Siberian), horse chestnut, kava kava, licorice, pineapple, red clover, turmeric, valerian, white willow

Tenoxicam (Dolmen, Mobiflex) bog bean, feverfew, garlic, ginkgo biloba, gossypol, niacin, reishi mushroom, saw palmetto, St. John's wort, turmeric, uva ursi, white willow

Terazosin (Alti-Terazosin, Hytrin) andrographis, arnica, asa foetida, bishop's weed, black cohosh, blue cohosh, carrageen, cat's claw, catechu, devil's claw, dong quai, European mistletoe, garlic, kelp, khat, licorice, ma-huang, parsley, rue, stevia, wild carrot, wood betony, yarrow, yohimbe

Terbinafine (Lamisil, Lamisil AT) black tea, caffeine, cocoa, coffee, cola nut, gossypol, green tea, guarana

Terbutaline (Brethine) digitalis, fever bark, Indian squill, ma-huang, rauwolfia, squill, yohimbe

Terconazole (Terazol 3, Terazol 7) gossypol

Teriparatide (Forteo) ethanol

Testosterone (Androderm, Testoderm) licorice

Tetracycline (Novo-Tetra, Sumycin) agrimony, bromelain, calcium, celery, coriander, dong quai, echinacea, fennel, folic acid, iron, lovage, magnesium, motherwort, niacin, riboflavin, rosemary, St. John's wort, thiamin, uzara, vitamin A, vitamin

B$_6$, vitamin B$_{12}$, vitamin C, vitamin K, wahoo, wild carrot, zinc

Tetrazepam (Mobiforton, Musapam) ashwagandha, bitter almond, California poppy, elecampane, ethanol, German chamomile, kava kava, maté, passion flower, poke, poppy, rauwolfia, scullcap, senega, stinging nettle, St. John's wort, valerian, wild carrot, wild cherry, wild lettuce, yarrow

Thalidomide (Thalomid) andrographis, ashwagandha, astragalus, cat's claw, echinacea, ethanol, larch, maitake mushroom, schisandra, scullcap, St. John's wort, turmeric

Theophylline (Elixophyllin, Theochron) black pepper, black tea, cabbage, caffeine, cayenne, cocoa, coffee, cola nut, country mallow, digitalis, grapefruit, green tea, guarana, horsetail, Indian long pepper, Indian squill, marijuana, squill, St. John's wort, thiamin, vitamin B$_6$

Theophylline and guaifenesin (Elixophyllin-GC, Quibron) country mallow, digitalis, Indian squill, squill

Thiethylperazine (Torecan) angel's trumpet, belladonna, black tea, coffee, corkwood, ethanol, evening primrose oil, gotu kola, henbane, jimson weed, kava kava, ma-huang, riboflavin, valerian, yohimbe

Thiopental (Pentothal) ashwagandha, bitter almond, California poppy, cedar leaf, cedarwood oil, cowslip, elecampane, English lavender, ethanol, eucalyptus, evening primrose oil, German cham-

omile, ginkgo biloba, hops, kava kava, lemon balm, marijuana, maté, passion flower, poke, poppy, rauwolfia, sage, scullcap, senega, stinging nettle, St. John's wort, valerian, wild carrot, wild lettuce, wormseed, yarrow

Thioridazine (Mellaril) angel's trumpet, belladonna, black tea, coffee, corkwood, cowhage, dong quai, ethanol, evening primrose oil, gotu kola, henbane, jimson weed, kava kava, ma-huang, rauwolfia, riboflavin, valerian, yohimbe

Thiotepa (Thioplex) black cohosh, dong quai, ethanol

Thiothixene (Navane) angel's trumpet, belladonna, black tea, coffee, corkwood, cowhage, ethanol, evening primrose oil, gotu kola, henbane, jimson weed, kava kava, ma-huang, rauwolfia, valerian, yohimbe

Thyroid (Nature-Throid NT, Westhroid) bladderwrack, bugleweed

Tiagabine (Gabitril) cedar leaf, ethanol, evening primrose oil, ginkgo biloba, gotu kola, kava kava, sage, valerian, wormseed

Tiaprofenic acid (Dom-Tiaprofenic, Surgam) bog bean, cat's claw, dong quai, ethanol, feverfew, garlic, ginger, ginkgo biloba, gossypol, green tea, horse chestnut, niacin, red clover, reishi mushroom, saw palmetto, St. John's wort, turmeric, uva ursi, white willow

Ticarcillin (Ticar) biotin, niacin, potassium, riboflavin, thiamin, vitamin B$_6$, vitamin B$_{12}$, vitamin K

Ticarcillin and clavulanate potassium (Timentin) biotin, niacin, potassium, riboflavin, thiamin, vitamin B_6, vitamin B_{12}, vitamin K

Ticlopidine (Alti-Ticlopidine, Ticlid) ajava seeds, allspice, andrographis, angelica, anise, arnica, asa foetida, astragalus, bilberry, bishop's weed, bladderwrack, bog bean, boldo, borage, borage seed oil, bromelain, buchu, calcium, carrageen, cat's claw, cayenne, clove, danshen, deer's tongue, devil's claw, dong quai, English hawthorn, evening primrose oil, feverfew, garlic, ginger, ginkgo biloba, ginseng (American), ginseng (Panax), ginseng (Siberian), grape seed, green tea, horse chestnut, kava kava, licorice, lovage, meadowsweet, onion, passion flower, pau d'arco, quinine, red clover, reishi mushroom, safflower, saw palmetto, sea buckthorn, stinging nettle, sweet clover, sweet vernal grass, turmeric, valerian, vitamin E, white willow, yarrow

Tiludronate (Skelid) calcium, iron, magnesium

Timolol (Betimol, Timoptic) andrographis, arnica, asa foetida, bishop's weed, black cohosh, blue cohosh, butterbur, carrageen, cat's claw, catechu, devil's claw, European mistletoe, fumitory, goldenseal, kelp, khat, licorice, lily-of-the-valley, ma-huang, motherwort, parsley, rue, stevia, St. John's wort, wild carrot, wood betony, yarrow, yohimbe

Tinzaparin (Innohep) ajava seeds, alfalfa, allspice, andrographis, angelica, arnica, asa foetida, astragalus, bilberry, bishop's weed, bladderwrack, bog bean, boldo, borage, borage seed oil, bromelain, buchu, carrageen, cat's claw, cayenne, clove, danshen, deer's tongue, dong quai, evening primrose oil, feverfew, garlic, German chamomile, ginger, ginkgo biloba, ginseng (American), ginseng (Panax), ginseng (Siberian), horse chestnut, kava kava, kelp, licorice, lovage, lungwort, meadowsweet, motherwort, northern prickly ash, papaya, pau d'arco, pineapple, poplar, quinine, red clover, reishi mushroom, safflower, saw palmetto, sea buckthorn, senega, stinging nettle, St. John's wort, sweet clover, sweet vernal grass, tonka bean, turmeric, valerian, vitamin E, white willow, wintergreen, yarrow

Tioconazole (1-Day, Vagistat) gossypol

Tiotropium (Spiriva) angel's trumpet, areca nut, butterbur, calabar bean, catechu, Chinese club moss, iboga, jimson weed, mandrake, scopolia

Tirofiban (Aggrastat) ajava seeds, allspice, andrographis, angelica, arnica, asa foetida, astragalus, bilberry, bishop's weed, bladderwrack, bog bean, boldo, borage, borage seed oil, bromelain, buchu, carrageen, cat's claw, cayenne, clove, danshen, deer's tongue, dong quai, English hawthorn, evening primrose oil, feverfew, garlic, ginger, ginkgo biloba, ginseng (American), ginseng (Panax), ginseng (Siberian), horse chestnut, kava kava, licorice, lovage, pau d'arco, quinine, reishi mushroom, safflower, saw palmetto, sea buckthorn, stinging nettle, sweet clover, sweet vernal grass, turmeric, valerian, vitamin E, white willow, yarrow

Tizanidine (Zanaflex) ethanol, gotu kola, kava kava, valerian

Tobramycin (Nebcin, Tobrex) biotin, calcium, magnesium, niacin, potassium, riboflavin, thiamin, vitamin B_6, vitamin B_{12}, vitamin K

Tocainide (Tonocard) aloe, buckthorn, cascara sagrada, fumitory, khat, kudzu, licorice, senna

Tolazamide (Tolinase) agrimony, aloe, avaram, banaba, barley, basil, bilberry, bitter melon, black tea, bladderwrack, blue cohosh, buchu, bugleweed, burdock, caffeine, chanca piedra, Chinese cucumber root, cinnamon, cocoa, coffee, cola nut, coriander, country mallow, cumin, damiana, dandelion, devil's claw, eucalyptus, fenugreek, flax, garlic, ginger, ginseng (American), ginseng (Panax), ginseng (Siberian), glucomannan, goat's rue, gotu kola, green tea, guar gum, gymnema, horehound, horse chestnut, kudzu, laurel, licorice, Madagascar periwinkle, ma-huang, maitake mushroom, marshmallow, myrrh, niacin, olive, onion, prickly pear cactus, psyllium, psyllium seed, raspberry, senega, Solomon's seal, stevia, St. John's wort

Tolbutamide (Apo-Tolbutamide, Tol-Tab) agrimony, aloe, avaram, banaba, barley, basil, bilberry, bitter melon, black tea, bladderwrack, blue cohosh, buchu, bugleweed, burdock, caffeine, chanca piedra, Chinese cucumber root, cinnamon, cocoa, coffee, cola nut, coriander, country mallow, cumin, damiana, dandelion, devil's claw, eucalyptus, fenugreek, flax, garlic, ginger, ginseng (American), ginseng (Panax), ginseng (Siberian), glucomannan, goat's rue, gotu kola, green tea, guar gum, gymnema, horehound, horse chestnut, kudzu, laurel, licorice, Madagascar periwinkle, ma-huang, maitake mushroom, marshmallow,

myrrh, niacin, olive, onion, prickly pear cactus, psyllium, psyllium seed, raspberry, senega, Solomon's seal, stevia, St. John's wort

Tolcapone (Tasmar) ethanol, gotu kola, kava kava, valerian

Tolciclate (Fungifos, Tolmicol) gossypol

Tolmetin (Tolectin) bog bean, cat's claw, dong quai, ethanol, feverfew, folic acid, garlic, ginger, ginkgo biloba, gossypol, green tea, horse chestnut, niacin, red clover, reishi mushroom, saw palmetto, St. John's wort, turmeric, uva ursi, white willow

Tolnaftate (Gold Bond Antifungal, Tinactin Antifungal Jock Itch) gossypol

Tolterodine (Detrol, Detrol LA) angel's trumpet, areca nut, butterbur, calabar bean, catechu, Chinese club moss, iboga, jimson weed, mandrake, scopolia

Topiramate (Topamax) cedar leaf, ethanol, evening primrose oil, ginkgo biloba, sage, wormseed

Topotecan (Hycamtin) ethanol

Torsemide (Demadex) aloe, andrographis, apple cider vinegar, arnica, asa foetida, birch, bishop's weed, black cohosh, black root, bladderwrack, blue cohosh, blue flag, buckthorn, butternut, calcium, calotropis, carrageen, cascara sagrada, castor oil plant, cat's claw, catechu, colocynth, corn silk, cowslip, cucumber, dandelion, devil's claw, digitalis, dong quai, European mistletoe, fo-ti, frangula, gamboge, garlic, gossypol, horsetail, Indian hemp, jalap, kelp, khat, licorice, lily-of-the-valley, magnesium, ma-huang, manna, maté, mayapple, parsley, potassium, quassia, rue, senna, sorrel, stevia, stinging nettle, St. John's wort, stone root, thiamin, uva ursi, uzara, vitamin B_6, vitamin C, wahoo, wallflower, wild carrot, wood betony, yarrow, yellow dock, yohimbe, zinc

Tramadol (Ultram) bitter melon, boneset, butterbur, catnip, chaparral, colt's foot, comfrey, ergot, ethanol, evening primrose oil, fennel, fenugreek, fumitory, ginkgo biloba, goldenseal, gossypol, gotu kola, Hawaiian baby woodrose, kava kava, lemon balm, maté, nerve root, oak, sage, sassafras, stinging nettle, valerian, wintergreen, wormwood, yohimbe

Trandolapril (Mavik) andrographis, arnica, asa foetida, bishop's weed, black cohosh, blue cohosh, calcium, carrageen, cat's claw, catechu, cayenne, devil's claw, dong quai, European mistletoe, garlic, kelp, khat, licorice, ma-huang, parsley, pineapple, pomegranate, potassium, rue, stevia, St. John's wort, wild carrot, wood betony, yarrow, yohimbe, zinc

Trandolapril plus verapamil (Tarka) calcium, zinc

Tranylcypromine (Parnate) anise, bitter orange, black tea, brewer's yeast, butcher's broom, caffeine, calamus, cayenne, cocoa, coffee, cola nut, country mallow, cowhage, ergot, ethanol, ginkgo biloba, ginseng (Panax), green tea, guarana, Hawaiian baby woodrose, jimson weed, kava kava, khat, licorice, ma-huang, nutmeg, rauwolfia, Scotch broom, St. John's wort, valerian, yohimbe

Trazodone (Desyrel, Novo-Trazodone) ergot, ethanol, kava kava, St. John's wort, valerian

Tretinoin, oral (Vesanoid) dong quai, ethanol, vitamin A

Triamcinolone (Aristocort, Trinasal) adonis, aloe, andrographis, ashwagandha, astragalus, buckthorn, butternut, calcium, cascara sagrada, castor oil plant, cat's claw, echinacea, ethanol, folic acid, frangula, Indian squill, larch, licorice, lily-of-the-valley, magnesium, ma-huang, oleander, perilla, potassium, schisandra, squill, strophanthus, vitamin A, vitamin B_6, vitamin C, vitamin D, vitamin K, wallflower, zinc

Triamterene (Dyrenium) andrographis, arnica, asa foetida, birch, bishop's weed, black cohosh, bladderwrack, blue cohosh, calcium, carrageen, cat's claw, catechu, cowslip, cucumber, dandelion, devil's claw, European mistletoe, folic acid, kelp, khat, magnesium, ma-huang, maté, noni, parsley, potassium, rue, sorrel, stevia, stinging nettle, stone root, wild carrot, wood betony, yarrow, yohimbe, zinc

Triazolam (Apo-Triazo, Halcion) ashwagandha, bitter almond, California poppy, catnip, cowslip, echinacea, elecampane, English lavender, ethanol, German chamomile, goldenseal, gotu kola, grapefruit, kava kava, lemon balm, linden, maté, nerve root, passion flower, poke, poppy, rauwolfia, sassafras, scullcap, senega, stinging nettle, St. John's wort, valerian, wild carrot, wild cherry, wild lettuce, yarrow

Trichlormethiazide (Metatensin, Naqua) aloe, andrographis, apple cider vinegar, arnica, asa foetida, birch, bishop's weed, black cohosh, black root, bladderwrack, blue cohosh, blue flag, buckthorn, butternut, calcium, calotropis, carrageen, cascara sagrada, castor oil plant, cat's claw, catechu, colocynth, corn silk, cowslip, cucumber, dandelion, devil's claw, digitalis, European mistletoe, fo-ti, frangula, gamboge, ginkgo biloba, gossypol, horsetail, Indian hemp, jalap, kelp, khat, licorice, lily-of-the-valley, magnesium, ma-huang, manna, maté, mayapple, parsley, potassium, quassia, rue, senna, sorrel, stevia, stinging nettle, St. John's wort, stone root, uva ursi, uzara, vitamin D, wahoo, wallflower, wild carrot, wood betony, yarrow, yellow dock, yohimbe, zinc

Trifluoperazine (Novo-Trifluzine, Stelazine) angel's trumpet, belladonna, black tea, coffee, corkwood, cowhage, cowslip, dong quai, ethanol, evening primrose oil, gotu kola, henbane, jimson weed, kava kava, ma-huang, rauwolfia, riboflavin, valerian, yohimbe

Trihexyphenidyl (Apo-Trihex) angel's trumpet, areca nut, butterbur, calabar bean, catechu, Chinese club moss, ethanol, iboga, jimson weed, mandrake, scopolia

Trimebutine (Apo-Trimebutine, Modulon) ethanol

Trimethobenzamide (Tigan) angel's trumpet, areca nut, butterbur, calabar bean, catechu, Chinese club moss, iboga, jimson weed, mandrake, scopolia

Trimethoprim (Primsol, Trimpex) biotin, folic acid, niacin, riboflavin, thiamin, vitamin B_6, vitamin B_{12}, vitamin K

Trimipramine (Apo-Trimip, Surmontil) angel's trumpet, belladonna, black tea, coffee, corkwood, ergot, ethanol, henbane, jimson weed, kava kava, ma-huang, marijuana, rauwolfia, riboflavin, scopolia, St. John's wort, valerian, yohimbe

Tripelennamine (PBZ, PBZ-SR) belladonna, corkwood, English lavender, henbane, khat

Triprolidine and pseudoephedrine (Actifed Cold and Allergy, Silafed) belladonna, corkwood, English lavender, henbane, khat

Triprolidine, pseudoephedrine, and codeine (CoActifed, Covan) belladonna, corkwood, English lavender, henbane, khat

Troleandomycin (Tao) uzara, wahoo

Trovafloxacin (Trovan) biotin, black tea, caffeine, calcium, cocoa, coffee, cola nut, dong quai, green tea, guarana, iron, magnesium, niacin, riboflavin, thiamin, vitamin B_6, vitamin B_{12}, vitamin K, zinc

Tulfisoxazole (Gantrisin) biotin

Urea (Amino-Cerv, UltraMide) apple cider vinegar, birch, bishop's weed, black root, bladderwrack, blue flag, buckthorn, butternut, calotropis, cascara sagrada, castor oil plant, colocynth, corn silk, cowslip, cucumber, dandelion, digitalis, fo-ti, frangula, gamboge, gossypol, horsetail, Indian hemp, jalap, licorice, lily-of-the-valley, manna, maté, mayapple, quassia, senna, sorrel, stinging nettle, stone root, uva ursi, uzara, wahoo, wall-flower, wild carrot, yellow dock, yohimbe

Urokinase (Abbokinase) angelica, anise, arnica, astragalus, bilberry, bladderwrack, borage, borage seed oil, cat's claw, cayenne, clove, danshen, devil's claw, dong quai, evening primrose oil, feverfew, garlic, ginger, ginkgo biloba, ginseng (Siberian), grape seed, horse chestnut, kava kava, licorice, meadowsweet, onion, passion flower, pineapple, red clover, turmeric, valerian, white willow

Valacyclovir (Valtrex) fumitory, gossypol, juniper, oak, wintergreen, yohimbe

Valdecoxib (Bextra) bog bean, cat's claw, dong quai, ethanol, feverfew, garlic, ginger, ginkgo biloba, gossypol, green tea, horse chestnut, niacin, red clover, reishi mushroom, saw palmetto, St. John's wort, turmeric, uva ursi, white willow

Valganciclovir (Valcyte) echinacea, fumitory, oak, wintergreen, yohimbe

Valproic acid (Depacon, Depakote) cedar leaf, ethanol, evening primrose oil, folic acid, ginkgo biloba, sage, vitamin B_{12}, vitamin D, wormseed, yohimbe

Valsartan (Diovan) andrographis, arnica, asa foetida, bishop's weed, black cohosh, blue cohosh, carrageen, cat's claw, catechu, devil's claw, dong quai, European mistletoe, garlic, goldenseal, kelp, khat, licorice, ma-huang, parsley, potassium, rue, stevia, wild carrot, wood betony, yarrow, yohimbe

Valsartan plus hydrochlorothiazide (Diovan HCT) magnesium, potassium, zinc

Vancomycin (Vancocin) fumitory, gossypol, juniper, oak, wintergreen, yohimbe

Vardenafil (Levitra) digitalis, Indian squill, squill

Vecuronium (Norcuron) magnesium

Venlafaxine (Effexor) ergot, ethanol, evening primrose oil, fennel, ginkgo biloba, kava kava, sage, Scotch broom, St. John's wort, valerian, wormwood, yohimbe

Verapamil (Calan, Isoptin) aloe, andrographis, arnica, asa foetida, bishop's weed, black cohosh, black tea, blue cohosh, buckthorn, caffeine, calcium, carrageen, cascara sagrada, cat's claw, catechu, chicory, Chinese rhubarb, cocoa, coffee, cola nut, devil's claw, dong quai, English hawthorn, ethanol, European mistletoe, fumitory, garlic, goldenseal, grapefruit, green tea, guarana, kelp, khat, kudzu, licorice, lily-of-the-valley, magnesium, ma-huang, maté, niacin, parsley, rue, senna, stevia, St. John's wort, wild carrot, wild cherry, wood betony, yarrow, yohimbe

Vigabatrin (Sabril) cedar leaf, ethanol, evening primrose oil, ginkgo biloba, gotu kola, kava kava, sage, valerian, wormseed

Vinblastine (Velban) black cohosh, dong quai

Voriconazole (VFEND) gossypol, magnesium, potassium, wild cherry

Warfarin (Coumadin, Jantoven) acerola, ajava seeds, alfalfa, allspice, andrographis, angelica, anise, arnica, asa foetida, astragalus, bilberry, bishop's weed, bladderwrack, bog bean, boldo, borage, borage seed oil, bromelain, buchu, cabbage, carrageen, cat's claw, cayenne, Cherokee rosehip, chlorella, clove, corn silk, danshen, deer's tongue, devil's claw, dong quai, ethanol, evening primrose oil, feverfew, garlic, German chamomile, ginger, ginkgo biloba, ginseng (American), ginseng (Panax), ginseng (Siberian), grapefruit, grape seed, green tea, horse chestnut, kava kava, kelp, licorice, lovage, lungwort, meadowsweet, motherwort, niacin, northern prickly ash, onion, papaya, passion flower, pau d'arco, pineapple, poplar, psyllium, psyllium seed, quinine, red clover, reishi mushroom, rose hips, safflower, saw palmetto, sea buckthorn, senega, soybean, spinach, stinging nettle, St. John's wort, sweet clover, sweet vernal grass, tonka bean, valerian, vitamin A, vitamin C, vitamin E, vitamin K, watercress, white willow, wintergreen, yarrow

Xipamide (Diurexan, Lumitens) aloe, apple cider vinegar, birch, bishop's weed, black root, bladderwrack, blue flag, buckthorn, butternut, calcium, calotropis, cascara sagrada, castor oil plant, colocynth, corn silk, cowslip, cucumber, dandelion, digitalis, fo-ti, frangula, gamboge, ginkgo biloba, gossypol, horsetail, Indian hemp, jalap, licorice, lily-of-the-valley, manna, maté, mayapple, quassia, senna, sorrel, stinging nettle, St. John's wort, stone root, uva-ursi, uzara, vitamin D, wahoo, wallflower, wild carrot, yellow dock, yohimbe

Zalcitabine (Hivid) calcium, magnesium, vitamin B_{12}, zinc

Zaleplon (Sonata, Stamoc) ashwagandha, bitter almond, California poppy, cowslip, elecampane, ethanol, gotu kola, kava kava, maté, passion flower, poke, poppy, rauwolfia, scullcap, senega, stinging nettle, valerian, wild carrot, wild lettuce, yarrow

Zidovudine (Retrovir, Novo-AZT) bitter melon, boneset, butterbur, chaparral, colt's foot, comfrey, echinacea, fenugreek, fumitory, gossypol, juniper, maté, oak, vitamin B_{12}, wintergreen, yohimbe, zinc

Zidovudine plus lamivudine (AZT + 3TC) vitamin B_{12}, zinc

Zidovudine plus lamivudine plus abacavir (Trizivir) vitamin B_{12}, zinc

Zileuton (Zyflo) cabbage, ethanol

Ziprasidone (Geodon) cowhage, ethanol, rauwolfia, valerian

Zoledronic acid (Zometa) calcium, iron, magnesium, potassium

Zolmitriptan (Zomig) bugleweed, cabbage, ethanol, feverfew, goldenseal, Scotch broom, witch hazel

Zolpidem (Ambien) ashwagandha, bitter almond, California poppy, catnip, cowslip, elecampane, English lavender, ethanol, German chamomile, goldenseal, gotu kola, kava kava, lemon balm, maté, nerve root, passion flower, poke, poppy, rauwolfia, sassafras, scullcap, senega, stinging nettle, valerian, wild carrot, wild lettuce, yarrow

Zonisamide (Zonegran) calcium, cedar leaf, ethanol, evening primrose oil, folic acid, ginkgo biloba, sage, thiamin, wormseed

Zopiclone (Alti-Zopiclone, Gen-Zopiclone) ashwagandha, bitter almond, California poppy, cowslip, elecampane, ethanol, gotu kola, kava kava, maté, passion flower, poke, poppy, rauwolfia, scullcap, senega, stinging nettle, valerian, wild carrot, wild lettuce, yarrow

Zuclopenthixol (Clopixol) cowhage, dong quai, ethanol, gotu kola, rauwolfia, valerian

Which Are the Most Popular Herbs?

To be honest, nobody can say with absolute certainty which herbs are the most popular. We can make very educated guesses, however, by looking at the sales figures. Unfortunately, herbs are sold through a great many channels, including natural food stores, doctor's offices, Wal-Mart, Asian markets, multilevel marketing companies, and vitamin stores. No one has yet gathered together all the sales data from the myriad sources to come up with figures covering all the sales of herbs in the United States.

Here are the top-ten-selling herbal supplements in the United States, according to HerbalGram.* These figures are for 2004, the latest year for which information is available. These figures include sales of herbs in food, drug, and mass market retail channels for 2004. They do not include sales made at natural food stores, health stores, multilevel marketing companies, health professionals, convenience stores, Wal-Mart, and warehouse-

Herb	2004 Sales Figures
1. Garlic	$27,013,000
2. Echinacea	$23,783,000
3. Saw palmetto	$20,334,000
4. Ginkgo biloba	$19,334,000
5. Soy	$17,420,000
6. Cranberry	$13,446,000
7. Ginseng	$12,165,000
8. Black cohosh	$11,985,000
9. St. John's wort	$9,088,000
10. Milk thistle	$7,776,000

*M. Blumenthal, "Herbal Sales Down 7.4 Percent in Mainstream Market," *HerbalGram* 66 (2005): 63. Accessible at www.herbalgram.org/herbalgram/articleview.asp?a=2828. Viewed February 22, 2006.

style buying clubs. And these figures track the sales of individual herbal supplements, not multiherb combination products that contain two or more herbs.

After these ten come, in order, evening primrose, valerian, green tea, bilberry, grape seed, horny goat weed, yohimbe, horse chestnut, eleuthero, and ginger.

Properties of Various Herbs and Supplements

These lists, while not exhaustive, will give you an idea of which herbs and supplements have various medicinal properties or contain substances you should be aware of.

Herbs and Other Substances That Contain High Levels of Alkaloids Include . . .

Coffee, colchicum, goldenseal, ma-huang, mandrake, schisandra, Scotch broom, tea

Herbs with Alpha-Agonist Properties Include . . .

Bitter orange, ma-huang

Herbs with Alpha-Antagonist Properties Include . . .

Saw palmetto, yohimbe

Herbs and Supplements with Anticholinergic Effects Include . . .

Belladonna, henbane, jimson weed, mandrake, scopolia

Herbs and Supplements with Anticoagulant/ Antiplatelet Potential Include . . .

Angelica, anise, bogbean, danshen, garlic, ginger, ginkgo biloba, horse chestnut, red clover, turmeric, white willow

Herbs Containing Anthraquinone Include . . .

Aloe, alder buckthorn, buckthorn, cascara sagrada, frangula, rhubarb, senna

Herbs from the Asteraceae (Daisy) Family Include . . .

Arnica, boneset, burdock, butterbur, chicory, colt's foot, daisy, dandelion, echinacea, elecampane, feverfew, German chamomile, milk thistle, safflower, saw palmetto, stevia, tansy, wild lettuce, wormwood, yarrow

Herbs and Supplements That Lower Blood Glucose Include . . .

Bilberry, bitter melon, devil's claw, fenugreek, garlic, ginseng (Panax and Siberian), goat's rue, guar gum, horse chestnut, kudzu, psyllium, white willow

Herbs, Foods, and Supplements That Contain Caffeine Include . . .

Black or green tea, many soft drinks, cocoa, coffee, cola nut, guarana, maté

Herbs and Supplements That Contain Cardiac Glycosides Include . . .

Adonis, black hellebore, calotropis, digitalis, hedge mustard, Indian hemp, jalap, lily-of-the-valley, motherwort, oleander, pleurisy root, squill, strophanthus, swamp milkweed, uzara, wahoo, wallflower

Herbs and Supplements with Cardioactive Properties Include . . .

Adonis, calamus, cereus, cola nut, colt's foot, devil's claw, digitalis, English hawthorn, European mistletoe, fenugreek, fumitory, ginger, ginseng (Panax), horehound, lily-of-the-valley, parsley, quassia, Scotch broom, shepherd's purse, squill, wild carrot

Herbs and Supplements That Lower Cholesterol Include . . .

Flax, garlic, guar gum, niacin, oats, psyllium, red yeast rice

Herbs with Diuretic Properties Include . . .

Agrimony, artichoke, buchu, burdock, celery, corn silk, juniper, poke, Scotch broom, shepherd's purse, squill, stone root, uva ursi, yarrow

Herbs and Supplements with Estrogenic Activity Include . . .

Alfalfa, black cohosh, chaste tree berry, flax, hops, licorice, red clover, soy

Herbs and Supplements That Can Cause Hepatotoxicity (Destructive Effects on the Liver) Include . . .

Bishop's weed, borage, chaparral, coenzyme Q_{10}, comfrey, niacin, red yeast rice, uva ursi, valerian

Herbs and Supplements with Hypotensive (Blood-Sugar-Lowering) Activity Include . . .

Black cohosh, celery seed, danshen, ginger, ginseng (Panax), turmeric, valerian

Herbs and Supplements with Monoamine Oxidase Inhibiting (MAOI) Potential Include . . .

Butcher's broom, California poppy, chaste tree berry, ginseng (American and Panax), goldenseal, kava kava, licorice, ma-huang, mace, passion flower, St. John's wort, yohimbe

Herbs and Supplements That Increase Photosensitivity Include . . .

Bitter orange, dong quai, northern prickly ash, rosemary, St. John's wort

Herbs That Deplete Potassium Include . . .

Adonis, black hellebore, cascara sagrada, horsetail, licorice, strophanthus

Herbs That Contain Unsaturated Pyrrolizidine Alkaloids (UPAs) Include . . .

Borage, butterbur, colt's foot, comfrey, golden ragwort, lungwort

Herbs and Supplements That Contain Safrole Include . . .

Basil, cinnamon, nutmeg, sassafras

Herbs and Supplements with Sedative Properties Include . . .

Calamus, California poppy, catnip, German chamomile, hops, kava kava, lemon balm, scullcap, St. John's wort, valerian

Herbs and Supplements with Serotonergic Properties Include . . .

Hawaiian baby woodrose, St. John's wort

Herbs and Supplements with Stimulant Laxative Properties Include . . .

Aloe, black root, blue flag, buckthorn, butternut, cascara sagrada, castor oil plant, Chinese rhubarb, colocynth, cucumber, frangula, gamboge, jalap, manna, mayapple, senna, wahoo, wallflower, yellow dock

Herbs and Supplements with Stimulant Properties Include . . .

Bitter orange, caffeine, coffee, cola nut, ginseng (American, Panax, and Siberian), green tea, guarana, ma-huang, maté

Herbs and Supplements with Sympathomimetic Activity Include . . .

Bitter orange, caffeine, country mallow, guarana, ma-huang

Herbs and Supplements That Contain High Amounts of Tannin Include . . .

Avarum, bilberry, black walnut, horse chestnut, oak, pomegranate, raspberry, sorrel, white willow, wood betony

Herbs That Affect Thyroid Function Include . . .

Bugleweed, kelp, motherwort, shepherd's purse

Herbs and Supplements That Contain Vitamin K Include . . .

Alfalfa, cabbage, parsley, English plantain, stinging nettle, watercress

Medicines by Brand Name

A

Abbokinase urokinase

Abelcet amphotericin b lipid complex

Abilify aripiprazole

Accupril quinapril

Accutane isotretinoin

Acemetacin Heumann acemetacin

Acemetacin Sandoz acemetacin

Aceon perindopril erbumine

Aciphex rabeprazole

Acipimox acipimox

Actifed Cold and Allergy triprolidine and pseudoephedrine

Actiq fentanyl

Activase alteplase

Activella estradiol and norethindrone

Actonel risedronate

Actos pioglitazone

Acular ketorolac

Adderall, Adderall XR dextroamphetamine and amphetamine

Adecut, Delakete delapril

Adenocard adenosine

Adenoscan adenosine

Adipex-P phentermine

Adrenalin epinephrine

Adriamycin doxorubicin

Adrucil fluorouracil

Advicor niacin and lovastatin

Advil ibuprofen

Advil Cold & Sinus Caplets pseudoephedrine plus ibuprofen

Aerius desloratadine

AeroBid flunisolide

Afongan omoconazole

Agenerase amprenavir

Aggrastat tirofiban

Aggrenox aspirin and dipyridamole

AH-Chew chlorpheniramine, phenylephrine, and methscopolamine

Akabar nifuroxazide

Alavert loratadine

Albenza albendazole

Aldactazide hydrochlorothiazide plus spironolactone

Aldactone spironolactone

Aldoril methyldopa plus hydrochlorothiazide

Alertec modafinil

Alesse ethinyl estradiol and levonorgestrel

Aleve naproxen

Alfenta alfentanil

Alka-Seltzer Plus Cold and Cough chlorpheniramine, phenylephrine, and dextromethorphan

Alka-Seltzer Plus Flu Liqui-Gels acetaminophen, dextromethorphan, and pseudoephedrine

Alkeran melphalan

Allegra fexofenadine

Allegra fexofenadine hydrochloride

Allegra-D fexofenadine and pseudoephedrine

Allersol naphazoline

Aloprim allopurinol

Alphagan P brimonidine

Alrex loteprednol

Altace ramipril

AlternaGel aluminum hydroxide

Alti-Acyclovir acyclovir
Alti-Clobazam clobazam
Alti-Despiramine desipramine
Alti-Doxazosin doxazosin
Alti-Fluvoxamine fluvoxamine
Alti-Moclobemide moclobemide
Alti-Ranitidine ranitidine
Alti-Terazosin terazosin
Alti-Ticlopidine ticlopidine
Alti-Zopiclone zopiclone
Altocor lovastatin
Alu-Cap aluminum hydroxide
Alupent metaproterenol
Amaryl glimepiride
Amatine midodrine
Ambien zolpidem
AmBisome amphotericin b liposomal
Amgesic salsalate
Amikin amikacin
Amino-Cerv urea
Amoxil amoxicillin
Ampamet aniracetam
Amphocin amphotericin b
Amphotec amphotericin b cholesteryl sulfate complex
Amycor bifonazole
Amytal amobarbital
Anadron nilutamide
Anafranil clomipramine
Analgina dipyrone
Ancef cefazolin
Ancobon flucytosine
Androderm testosterone
Angiomax bivalirudin
Anquil benperidol
Ansaid flurbiprofen
Antabuse disulfiram
Antivert meclizine
Anusol-HC hydrocortisone
Apo-Acetazolamide acetazolamide
Apo-Alpraz alprazolam
Apo-Atenol atenolol
Apo-Benztropine benztropine
Apo-Bromazepam bromazepam
Apo-Bromocriptine bromocriptine
Apo-Butorphanol butorphanol
Apo-Chlorax clidinium and chlordiazepoxide
Apo-Chlordiazepoxide chlordiazepoxide
Apo-Chlorthalidone chlorthalidone
Apo-Diazepam diazepam
Apo-Diflunisal diflunisal
Apo-Famotidine famotidine
Apo-Fenofibrate fenofibrate
Apo-Fluconazole fluconazole

Apo-Flurazepam flurazepam
Apo-Furosemide furosemide
Apo-Gemfibrozil gemfibrozil
Apo-Hydro hydrochlorothiazide
Apo-Hydroxyquine hydroxychloroquine
Apo-Imipramine imipramine
Apo-K potassium chloride
Apo-Ketoconazole ketoconazole
Apo-Methazolamide methazolamide
Apo-Methyldopa methyldopa
Apo-Metoclop metoclopramide
Apo-Midazolam midazolam
Apo-Nadol nadolol
Aponil lacidipine
Apo-Nizatidine nizatidine
Apo-Norflox norfloxacin
Apo-Oxaprozin oxaprozin
Apo-Perphenazine perphenazine
Apo-Pindol pindolol
Apo-Prednisone prednisone
Apo-Primidone primidone
Apo-Sertraline sertraline
Apo-Simvastatin simvastatin
Apo-Sulfinpyrazone sulfinpyrazone
Apo-Tolbutamide tolbutamide
Apo-Triazo triazolam
Apo-Trihex trihexyphenidyl
Apo-Trimebutine trimebutine
Apo-Trimip trimipramine
Apresazide hydralazine plus hydrochlorothiazide
Apresoline hydralazine
Aquachloral Supprettes chloral hydrate
Aquatab guaifenesin and pseudoephedrine
Aquatensen methyclothiazide
Aralen chloroquine
Aramine metaraminol
Arava leflunomide
Arcoxia etoricoxib
Aredia pamidronate
Areuma nimesulide
Aricept donepezil
Arimidex anastrozole
Aristocort triamcinolone
Arixtra fondaparinux
Aromasin exemestane
Arthropan choline salicylate
Arthrotec diclofenac plus misoprostol
Asacol Oral mesalamine
Asendin amoxapine
Asenlix clobenzorex
Astelin azelastine
Atacand candesartan
Atacand HCT candesartan plus hydrochlorothiazide

Atarax   hydroxyzine
Atgam   antithymocyte globulin equine
Ativan   lorazepam
Atrovent   ipratropium
Aulin   nimesulide
Avalide   irbesartan plus hydrochlorothiazide
Avandamet   rosiglitazone and metformin
Avandia   rosiglitazone
Avapro   irbesartan
Avelox   moxifloxacin
Aventyl   nortriptyline
Axert   almotriptan
Axid   nizatidine
Aygestin   norethindrone
Azdone   hydrocodone plus aspirin
AZT + 3TC   zidovudine plus lamivudine
Azulfidine   sulfasalazine

B
B&O Supprettes   belladonna and opium
Bactrim   sulfamethoxazole and trimethoprim
Baycaron   mefruside
Beconase   beclomethasone
Beglynor   gliquidone
Bellamine S   belladonna, phenobarbital, and
   ergotamine
Bel-Tabs   belladonna, phenobarbital, and
   ergotamine
Benadryl Allergy   diphenhydramine
**Benadryl Allergy/Decongestant, Benadryl Children's
   Allergy and Sinus**   diphenhydramine and
   pseudoephedrine
Benicar   olmesartan
Benicar HCT   olmesartan and hydrochlorothiazide
Bentos   befunolol
Bentyl   dicyclomine
Berotec   fenoterol
Beta-2   isoetharine
Betaclar   befunolol
Betadine   povidone-iodine
Betagan   levobunolol
Betaloc   metoprolol
Betapace   sotalol
Betatrex   betamethasone
Betaxon   levobetaxolol
Betimol   timolol
Betoptic S   betaxolol
Bexidal   mebhydrolin
Bextra   valdecoxib
Bezalip   bezafibrate
Biaxin, Biaxin XL   clarithromycin
Bicicillin C-R   penicillin G benzathine plus penicillin
   G procaine

Bicillin L-A   penicillin G benzathine
Biltricide   praziquantel
Biocef   cephalexin
Bleph-10   sulfacetamide
Bondronat   ibandronic acid
Bonefos   clodronate
Bonine   meclizine
Botox, Botox Cosmetic   botulinum toxin type A
Brethine   terbutaline
Brevibloc   esmolol
Brevicon   ethinyl estradiol and norethindrone
Brevital, Brevital Sodium   methohexital
Brioschi   sodium bicarbonate
Bronkosol   isoetharine
Bufferin   aspirin
Buprenex   buprenorphine
BuSpar   buspirone
Busulfex   busulfan
Butalan   butabarbital
Butisol, Butisol Sodium   butabarbital

C
Cafergot   ergotamine
Calan   verapamil
Calcort, Dezacor   deflazacort
Caldine   lacidipine
Calslot   manidipine
Camptosar   irinotican
Cancidas   caspofungin
Canesten   bifonazole
Capoten   captopril
Carafate   sucralfate
Caravis   isotretinoin
Carbastat   carbachol
Carbatrol   carbamazepine
Carbolith   lithium
Cardene   nicardipine
Cardiovasc   lercanidipine
Cardizem   diltiazem
Cardura   doxazosin
Carmen   lercanidipine
Carter's Little Pills   bisacodyl
Cartrol   carteolol
Cataflam   diclofenac
Catapres   clonidine
Cathflo Activase   alteplase
Caverject   alprostadil
Ceclor   cefaclor
Cedax   ceftibuten
Cefadyl   cephapirin
Cefizox   ceftizoxime
Cefobid   cefoperazone
Cefotan   cefotetan

Ceftin   cefuroxime
Cefzil   cefprozil
Celebrex   celecoxib
Celexa   citalopram
CellCept   mycophenolate
Celontin   methsuximide
Cenacert   oxatomide
Cenestin   estrogens conjugated a/synthetic
Ceporacin   cephalothin
Ceptaz   ceftazidime
Cerebyx   fosphenytoin
Cerubidine   daunorubicin hydrochloride
Cetacort   hydrocortisone
Charcoal Plus DS   charcoal
Children's Dimetapp Elixir Cold & Allergy
    brompheniramine and pseudoephedrine
Children's Tylenol Plus Cold   acetaminophen,
    chlorpheniramine, and pseudoephedrine
Cialis   tadalafil
Ciloxan   ciprofloxacin
Cinobac   cinoxacin
Cipro   ciprofloxacin
Citro-Mag   magnesium citrate
Claforan   cefotaxime
Claramid   roxithromycin
Clarinex   desloratadine
Claripex   clofibrate
Claritin   loratadine
Claritin-D 24 Hour   loratadine and pseudoephedrine
Cleocin   clindamycin
Climacteron   estradiol and testosterone
Climara   estradiol
Clinoril   sulindac
Clopixol   zuclopenthixol
Cloxapen   cloxacillin
Clozaril   clozapine
Clozeril   clozapine
CoActifed   triprolidine, pseudoephedrine, and codeine
Cogentin   benztropine
Cognex   tacrine
Colace   docusate
Colazal   balsalazide
ColBenemid   colchicine plus probenecid
Colestid   colestipol
Colyte   polyethylene glycol-electrolyte solution
CombiPatch   estradiol and norethindrone
Comhist   chlorpheniramine, phenylephrine, and
    phenyltoloxamine
Compazine   prochlorperazine
Compro   prochlorperazine
Concerta   methylphenidate
Codeine Contin   codeine
Congest   estrogens conjugated/equine

Constulose   lactulose
Coptin   sulfadiazine
Cordarone   amiodarone
Coreg   carvedilol
Corgard   nadolol
Coricidin HBP Col and Flu   chlorpheniramine and
    acetaminophen
Corlopam   fenoldopam
Cortone   cortisone
Corvert   ibutilide
Coryphen Codeine   aspirin and codeine
Cosmegen   dactinomycin
Coumadin   warfarin
Covan   triprolidine, pseudoephedrine, and codeine
Coversyl   perindopril erbumine
Cozaar   losartan
Crestor   rosuvastatin
Crinone   progesterone
Crixivan   indinavir
Cryselle   ethinyl estradiol and norgestrel
Cuprimine   penicillamine
Cutivate   fluticasone
Cyclen   ethinyl estradiol and norgestimaté
Cyclessa   ethinyl estradiol and desogestrel
Cyclogyl   cyclopentolate
Cylate   cyclopentolate
Cylert   pemoline
Cytomel   liothyronine
Cytovene   ganciclovir
Cytoxan   cyclophosphamide

D

Dalacin C   clindamycin
Dalcipran   milnacipran
Dalmane   flurazepam
Damason-P   hydrocodone and aspirin
Dantrium   dantrolene
Daranide   dichlorphenamide
Daraprim   pyrimethamine
Darvocet-N 50, Darvocet-N 100   propoxyphene and
    acetaminophen
Darvon Compound   propoxyphene, aspirin, and
    caffeine
Darvon, Darvon-N   propoxyphene
Davedax   reboxetine
Daypro   oxaprozin
Debekacyl   dibekacin
Decadron   dexamethasone
Declomycin   demeclocycline
Defecton   carpipramine
Deltasone   prednisone
Demadex   torsemide
Demerol   meperidine

Demulen   ethinyl estradiol and ethynodiol diacetate
Depacon   valproic acid
Depakote   valproic acid
Depen   penicillamine
Depoject Injection   methylprednisolone
Depo-Provera   medroxyprogesterone
Deptropine FNA   deptropine
Dermazene   iodoquinol and hydrocortisone
Desferal   deferoxamine
Desoxyn   methamphetamine
Desyrel   trazodone
Detrol, Detrol LA   tolterodine
Dexasone   dexamethasone
Dexedrine   dextroamphetamine
Dexferrum, INFeD   iron-dextran complex
Dextrostat   dextroamphetamine
DiaBeta   glyburide
Diabinese   chlorpropamide
Diamicron   gliclazide
Diamox Sequels   acetazolamide
Diane-35   cyproterone and ethinyl estradiol
Diarret   nifuroxazide
Diarr-Eze   loperamide
Diat   azosemide
Dibenzyline   phenoxybenzamine
Dicetel   pinaverium
Diclectin   doxylamine and pyridoxine
Didronel   etidronate
Diflucan   fluconazole
Digibind   digoxin immune fab
Digi-Fab   digoxin immune fab
Digitek   digitalis
Dihistine DH   chlorpheniramine, pseudoephedrine, and codeine
Dikacine   dibekacin
Dilantin   phenytoin
Dilatrate-SR   isosorbide dinitrate
Dilaudid   hydromorphone
Dimetapp Decongestant   pseudoephedrine
Dimetapp Sinus Caplets   pseudoephedrine plus ibuprofen
Dinador   dipyrone
Diochloram   chloramphenicol
Diovan   valsartan
Diovan HCT   valsartan plus hydrochlorothiazide
Dipentum   olsalazine
Dipiperon   pipamperone
Diprivan   propofol
Ditropan   oxybutinin
Diucardin   hydroflumethiazide
Diurexan   xipamide
Diuril   chlorothiazide
Dixeran   melitracen

Doan's   magnesium salicylate
Dobutrex   dobutamine
Dolmen   tenoxicam
Dolobid   diflunisal
Dolophine   methadone
Dom-Tiaprofenic   tiaprofenic acid
Donnatal, Donnatal Extentabs   hyoscyamine, atropine, scopolamine, and phenobarbital
Dopacard   dopexamine
Dopar   levodopa
Dopram   doxapram
Doral   quazepam
Dormonoct   loprazolam
Dostinex   cabergoline
Doxil   doxorubicin liposomal
Draganon   aniracetam
Drixomed   dexbrompheniramine and pseudoephedrine
Drixoral Cold & Allergy   dexbrompheniramine and pseudoephedrine
DTIC-Dome, DTIC   dacarbazine
Dulcolax   bisacodyl
Duraclon   clonidine
Duragesic   fentanyl
Duricef   cefadroxil
Duvoid   bethanechol
Dyazide   hydrochlorothiazide and triamterene
Dycill   dicloxacillin
Dynabac   dirithromycin
Dynacin   minocycline
DynaCirc   isradipine
Dyrenium   triamterene

E
Ecotrin   aspirin
Edecrin   ethacrynic acid
Effexor   venlafaxine
Eflone   fluorometholone
Efudex   fluorouracil
Elavil   amitriptyline
Eldepryl   selegiline
Elestat   epinastine
Elidel   pimecrolimus
Elina   mizolastine
Elixophyllin   theophylline
Elixophyllin-GC   theophylline and guaifenesin
Elkapin   etozolin
Ellence   epirubicin
Elocom   mometasone furoate
Eloxatin   oxaliplatin
Endal   guaifenesin and phenylephrine
Endocet   oxycodone and acetaminophen
Endodan   oxycodone and aspirin

Enduron methyclothiazide
Enlon edrophonium
Entocort budesonide
Enulose lactulose
EpiPen epinephrine
Epivir lamivudine
Epsom salts magnesium sulfate
Equagesic, 292 MEP aspirin and meprobamate
Ergamisol levamisole
Erythrocin erythromycin
Eryzole erythromycin and sulfisoxazole
Eserine physostigmine
Esgic butalbital, acetaminophen, and caffeine
Esidrix hydrochlorothiazide
Eskalith lithium
Estaprol ciprofibrate
Estinyl ethinyl estradiol
Estrace estradiol
Estratab estrogens esterified
Estratest, Estratest H.S. estrogens esterified and methyltestosterone
Ethmozine moricizine
Ethyol amifostine
Etopophos etoposide phosphate
Etrafon amitriptyline and perphenazine
Evista raloxifene
Evoxac cevimeline
Evra ethinyl estradiol and norelgestromin
Exacin isepamicin
Exelderm sulconazole
Exelon rivastigmine
ExLax Stool Softener docusate
Extendryl chlorpheniramine, phenylephrine, and methscopolamine
EZ-Char charcoal

F
Factive gemifloxacin
Famvir famciclovir
Fazol isoconazole
Felbatol felbamaté
Feldene piroxicam
Femiron ferrous fumarate
Femizol-M miconazole
Fenistil dimethindene
Feostat ferrous fumarate
Feprapax lofepramine
Feratab ferrous sulfate
Fergon ferrous gluconate
Fer-Iron ferrous sulfate
Fero-Grad 500 ferrous sulfate and ascorbic acid
Ferrlecit ferric gluconate
Fioricet butalbital, acetaminophen, and caffeine

Fiorinal butalbital, aspirin, and caffeine
Flagyl metronidazole
Flarex fluorometholone
Fleet Enema sodium phosphate
Fleet Mineral Oil Enema mineral oil
Fleet Phospho-Soda sodium phosphate
Flexeril cyclobenzaprine
Flolan epoprostenol
Flonase fluticasone
Florinef fludrocortisone
Florone diflorasone
Floxin ofloxacin
Fluanxol flupenthixol
Fludara fludarabine
Focalin dexmethylphenidate
Fongamil omoconazole
Fortaz ceftazidime
Forteo teriparatide
Fortovase saquinavir
Fosamax alendronate
Foscavir foscarnet
Fragmin dalteparin
Fraxiparine nadroparin
Frisium clobazam
Fulvicin griseofulvin
Fungifos tolciclate
Fungizone amphotericin b
Furadantin nitrofurantoin

G
Gabitril tiagabine
Gamanil lofepramine
Gantrisin sulfisoxazole
Gantrisin tulfisoxazole
Gaviscon Extra Strength, Gaviscon Liquid aluminum hydroxide and magnesium carbonate
Gaviscon Tablet aluminum hydroxide and magnesium trisilicate
Genapap acetaminophen
Gen-Bromazepam bromazepam
Gen-Clozapine clozapine
Gen-Propafenone propafenone
Gentacidin gentamicin
Gentak gentamicin
Gen-Zopiclone zopiclone
Geocillin carbenicillin
Geodon ziprasidone
Geram piracetam
Gleevec imatinib
Glianimon benperidol
GlucoNorm repaglinide
Glucophage metformin
Glucotrol glipizide

Glucovance   glyburide and metformin
Glurenorm   gliquidone
Glyset   miglitol
Gold Bond Antifungal   tolnaftate
Grifulvin V   griseofulvin
Gynazole-1   butoconazole
Gyne-Lotrimin 3   clotrimazole
Gyno-Travogen   isoconazole

H
Halcion   triazolam
Haldol   haloperidol
Havlane   loprazolam
Helidac   bismuth subsalicylate, metronidazole, and tetracycline
Hepalean   heparin
Hep-Lock   heparin
Heptovir   lamivudine
Histatab Plus   chlorpheniramine and phenylephrine
Histex CT, Histex PD   carbinoxamine
Histex HC   hydrocodone, carbinoxamine, and pseudoephedrine
Hivid   zalcitabine
HMS Liquifilm   medrysone
Humulin   insulin
Hycamtin   topotecan
Hydergine   ergoloid mesylates
Hylorel   guanadrel
Hyosine   hyoscyamine
Hyperstat   diazoxide
Hytinic   polysaccharide-iron complex
Hytrin   terazosin
Hyzaar   losartan plus hydrochlorothiazide

I
Ibustrin   indobufen
Imdur   isosorbide mononitrate
Imitrex   sumatriptan
Imodium A-D   loperamide
Impromen   bromperidol
Imuran   azathioprine
Inapsine   droperidol
Incidal   mebhydrolin
Inderal   propranolol
Inderide   propranolol plus hydrochlorothiazide
Indocin   indomethacin
Inflamase Forte   prednisolone
Inhibace   cilazapril
Innohep   tinzaparin
InnoPran XL   propranolol
Inspra   eplerenone
Integrex   reboxetine

Integrillin   eptifibatide
Intron A   interferon alfa-2b
Intropin   dopamine
Inversine   mecamylamine
Invirase   saquinavir
Ionamin   phentermine
Iperten   manidipine
Isepacine   isepamicin
Ismo   isosorbide mononitrate
Isoptin   verapamil
Isopto Atropine   atropine
Isopto Carbachol   carbachol
Isopto Carpine   pilocarpine
Isopto Homatropine   homatropine
Isordil   isosorbide dinitrate
Isotamine   isoniazid
Isuprel   isoproterenol

J
Jantoven   warfarin

K
Kadian   morphine sulfate
Kala   lactobacillus
Kaletra   lopinavir and ritonavir
Kantrex   kanamycin
Kaopectate   bismuth
Kayexalate   sodium polystyrene sulfonate
Keftab   cephalexin
Kefurox   cefuroxime
Kefzol   cefazolin
Kemadrin   procyclidine
Keppra   levetiracetam
Kerlone   betaxolol
Klaron   sulfacetamide
Klonopin   clonazepam
K-Phos Neutral   potassium and sodium phosphates
Kytril   granisetron

L
Lamictal   lamotrigine
Lamisil, Lamisil AT   terbinafine
Lanoxin   digitalis
Largactil   chlorpromazine
Larodopa   levodopa
Lasix   furosemide
Lendorm   brotizolam
Lescol   fluvastatin
Leustatin   cladribine
Levaquin   levofloxacin
Levate   amitriptyline
Levitra   vardenafil

Levo-Dromoran   levorphanol
Levophed   norepinephrine
Levothroid   levothyroxine
Levsin   hyoscyamine
Levulan Kerastick   aminolevulinic acid
Lexapro   s-citalopram
Lexxel   enalapril plus felodipine
Librax   clidinium and chlordiazepoxide
Librium   chlordiazepoxide
Lidoderm   lidocaine
Limbitrol   amitriptyline and chlordiazepoxide
Lin-Megestrol   megestrol
Lioresal   baclofen
Lipitor   atorvastatin
Livostin   levocabastine
Lixel   milnacipran
Loceryl   amorolfine
Locetar   amorolfine
LoCHOLEST   cholestyramine
Locoic   hydrocortisone
Locoid   hydrocortisone
Lodine   etodolac
Lodrane   brompheniramine and pseudoephedrine
Lodsoyn   carbidopa
Lomine   dicyclomine
Lomotil   diphenoxylate and atropine
Loniten   minoxidil
Lonox   diphenoxylate and atropine
Lopid   gemfibrozil
Lopressor   metoprolol
Loprox   ciclopirox
Lorabid   loracarbef
Lortab ASA   hydrocodone plus aspirin
Losec   omeprazole
Lotemax   loteprednol
Lotensin   benazepril
Lotrimin Ultra   butenafine
Lovenox   enoxaparin
Loxitane   loxapine
Lozol   indapamide
Luminal Sodium   phenobarbital
Lumitens   xipamide
Lunelle   estradiol and medroxyprogesterone
Lunesta   s-zopiclone
Luvox   fluvoxamine
Lysodren   mitotane

M
Maalox   aluminum hydroxide, magnesium hydroxide, and simethicone
Macrobid   nitrofurantoin
Macropen   midecamycin
Mag-Ox 400   magnesium oxide

Maliasin   barbexaclone
Mandol   cefamandole
Marinol   dronabinol
Marsilid   iproniazid
Matulane   procarbazine
Mavik   trandolapril
Maxalt   rizatriptan benzoate
Maxaquin   lomefloxacin
Maxifed   guaifenesin and pseudoephedrine
Maxiflor   diflorasone
Maxipime   cefepime
Maxivate   betamethasone
Maxzide   hydrochlorothiazide and triamterene
Mebaral   mephobarbital
Meclan Topical   meclocycline
Meclomen   meclofenamate
Medrol Oral   methylprednisolone
Mefoxin   cefoxitin
Megace   megestrol
Mellaril   thioridazine
Menest   estrogens esterified
Mentax   butenafine
Meperitab   meperidine
Meridia   sibutramine
Mesantoin   mephenytoin
Mestinon   pyridostigmine
Metaglip   glipizide and metformin
Metamucil   psyllium
Metatensin   trichlormethiazide
Methadose   methadone
Methergine   methylergonovine
Mevacor   lovastatin
Mexitil   mexiletine
Micardis   telmisartan
Micardis HCT, Micardis Plus   telmisartan plus hydrochlorothiazide
Micro-K   potassium chloride
Micronase   glyburide
Micronor   norethindrone
Microsulfon   sulfadiazine
Microzide   hydrochlorothiazide
Midamor   amiloride
Midecin   midecamycin
Migranal   dihydroergotamine
Milkinol   mineral oil
Miltown   meprobamate
Minipress   prazosin
Minitran   nitroglycerin
Minizide   prazosin plus polythiazide
Minocin   minocycline
Miochol-E   acetylcholine
MiraLax   polyethylene glycol-electrolyte solution
Mirapex   pramipexole

Mithracin plicamycin
Mivacron mivacurium
Mizollen mizolastine
Moban molindone
MOBIC meloxicam
Mobicox meloxicam
Mobidin magnesium salicylate
Mobiflex tenoxicam
Mobiforton tetrazepam
Modalim ciprofibrate
Modecate fluphenazine
Modulon trimebutine
Moduret amiloride plus hydrochlorothiazide
Monistat 3 miconazole
Monocid cefonicid
Monocor bisoprolol
Monodox doxycycline
Monopril fosinopril
Monurol fosfomycin
Motofen difenoxin and atropine
Motrin ibuprofen
MS Contin morphine sulfate
Mucopront carbocysteine
Musapam tetrazepam
Muse alprostadil
Mustargen mechlorethamine
Mutamycin mitomycin
Myambutol ethambutol
Mycelex clotrimazole
Mycelex-3 butoconazole
Mycifradin Sulfate Topical neomycin
Mycobutin rifabutin
Mycostatin nystatin
Mykrox metolazone
Mylanta aluminum hydroxide plus magnesium
   hydroxide
Mylanta Children calcium carbonate
Mylanta Gelcaps calcium carbonate and magnesium
   hydroxide
Mylanta Liquid aluminum hydroxide, magnesium
   hydroxide, and simethicone
Myleran busulfan
Mylotarg gemtuzumab ozogamicin
Myobloc botulinum toxin type B
Mysoline primidone

N
Nafcil Injection nafcillin
Naftin naftifine
Nalex-A chlorpheniramine, phenylephrine, and
   phenyltoloxamine
Nalfon fenoprofen
Naphcon naphazoline

Naprosyn naproxen
Naqua trichlormethiazide
Narcan naloxone
Nardil phenelzine
Nasal Moist sodium chloride
Nasarel flunisolide
Nasonex mometasone furoate
Natacyn natamycin
Natulan procarbazine
Nature-Throid NT thyroid
Navane thiothixene
Nebcin tobramycin
NebuPent pentamidine
Necon 1/50 mestranol and norethindrone
NegGram nalidixic acid
Nemasol Sodium aminosalicylic acid
Nembutal pentobarbital
Neoral cyclosporine
Neosar cyclophosphamide
Neo-Synephrine Extra Strength phenylephrine
Neo-Tabs Oral neomycin
Neptazane methazolamide
Neurontin gabapentin
Neut sodium bicarbonate
Nexium esomeprazole
Niacor niacin
NicoDerm CQ nicotine
Nicotinex niacin
Nicotrol nicotine
Niferex polysaccharide-iron complex
Niflam niflumic acid
Nifluril niflumic acid
Nilandron nilutamide
Nimbex cisatracurium
Nimotop nimodipine
Nipride nitroprusside
Nitro-Dur nitroglycerin
Nitropress nitroprusside
Nizoral ketoconazole
Nocosyn sulfur and sulfacetamide
Nolvadex tamoxifen
Norcuron vecuronium
Noritate metronidazole
Normodyne labetalol
Noroxin norfloxacin
Norpace disopyramide
Norplant Implant levonorgestrel
Norpramin desipramine
Norvasc amlodipine
Norvir ritonavir
Novamoxin amoxicillin
Novantrone mitoxantrone
Novarok imidapril

Novo-Acebutolol   acebutolol
Novo-Alendronate   alendronate
Novo-AZT   zidovudine
Novo-Captopril   captopril
Novo-Clopate   clorazepate
Novo-Clopramine   clomipramine
Novo-Cycloprine   cyclobenzaprine
Novo-Dipiradol   dipyridamole
Novo-Ferrogluc   ferrous gluconate
Novo-Fibrate   clofibrate
Novo-Gliclazide   gliclazide
Novo-Hylazin   hydralazine
Novo-Ketotifen   ketotifen
Novo-Levobunolol   levobunolol
Novo-Maprotiline   maprotiline
Novo-Meprazine   methotrimeprazine
Novo-Mepro   meprobamate
Novo-Methacin   indomethacin
Novo-Mexiletine   mexiletine
Novo-Peridol   haloperidol
Novo-Pindol   pindolol
Novo-Pravastatin   pravastatin
Novo-Propamide   chlorpropamide
Novo-Quinidin   quinidine
Novo-Spiroton   spironolactone
Novo-Spirozine   hydrochlorothiazide plus
    spironolactone
Novo-Temazepam   temazepam
Novo-Tetra   tetracycline
Novo-Trazodone   trazodone
Novo-Trifluzine   trifluoperazine
Novoxapam   oxazepam
Nozain   methotrimeprazine
Nu-Amilzide   amiloride plus hydrochlorothiazide
Nu-Baclo   baclofen
Nubain   nalbuphine
Nu-Buspirone   buspirone
Nu-Cimet   cimetidine
Nu-Cloxi   cloxacillin
Nu-Gabapentin   gabapentin
Nu-Indapamide   indapamide
Nu-Ipratropium   ipratropium
Nu-Levocarb   levodopa-carbidopa
Nu-Loraz   lorazepam
Nu-Loxapine   loxapine
Nu-Medopa   methyldopa
Nu-Moclobemide   moclobemide
Numorphan   oxymorphone
Nu-Nifed   nifedipine
Nu-Pirox   piroxicam
Nu-Prazo   prazosin
Nuromax   doxacurium
Nu-Sulfinpyrazone   sulfinpyrazone

Nu-Sundac   sulindac
NuvaRing   ethinyl estradiol and etonogestrel
Nydrazid   isoniazid
Nystat-RX   nystatin
Nytol   diphenhydramine

O
Ocufen   flurbiprofen
Ocuflox   ofloxacin
Ocupress   carteolol
Ogen   estropipate
Olbetam   acipimox
Omnicef   cefdinir
Omnipen   ampicillin
1-Day   tioconazole
ONTAK   denileukin diftitox
Onxol   paclitaxel
Optimine   azatadine
OptiPranolol   metipranolol
Optivar   azelastine
Orap   pimozide
Orgaran   danaparoid
Ortho Evra   ethinyl estradiol and norelgestromin
Ortho Tri-Cyclen   ethinyl estradiol and
    norgestimaté
Ortho-Cept   ethinyl estradiol and desogestrel
Orthoclone OKT 3   muromonab-cd3
Ortho-Est   estropipate
Ortho-Novum   ethinyl estradiol and
    norethindrone
Ortho-Novum 1/50   mestranol and norethindrone
Orudis   ketoprofen
Osmitrol   mannitol
Ostac   clodronate
Osteocit   calcium citrate
Ovral   ethinyl estradiol and norgestrel
Ovrette   norgestrel
Oxistat   oxiconazole
Oxivent   oxitropium
OxyContin   oxycodone
Oxytrol   oxybutinin

P
Pacerone   amiodarone
Padrin   prifinium
Pamelor   nortriptyline
Panretin   alitretinoin
Pantoloc   pantoprazole
Parafon Forte DSC   chlorzoxazone
Paraplatin, Paraplatin-AQ   carboplatin
Para-Time S.R.   papaverine
Pariet   rabeprazole
Parlodel   bromocriptine

Parnate   tranylcypromine
Paser   aminosalicylic acid
Patanol   olopatadine
Pathocil   dicloxacillin
Paxil   paroxetine
PBZ, PBZ-SR   tripelennamine
Pediacof   chlorpheniramine, phenylephrine, codeine, and potassium iodide
Pediapred   prednisolone
Pediazole   erythromycin and sulfisoxazole
Peflacine   pefloxacin
Peganone   ethotoin
Pegasys   peginterferon alfa-2a
PEG-Intron   peginterferon alfa-2b
PemADD   pemoline
Penetrex   enoxacin
Penlac   ciclopirox
Pentacarinat   pentamidine
Pentamycetin   chloramphenicol
Pentothal   thiopental
Pentoxil   pentoxifylline
Pepcid Complete   famotidine, calcium carbonate, and magnesium hydroxide
Pepcid   famotidine
Pepto-Bismol   bismuth
Percocet   oxycodone and acetaminophen
Percodan   oxycodone and aspirin
Perfan   enoximone
Perflox   pefloxacin
Periactin   cyproheptadine
Peri-Colace, Senokot-S   docusate and senna
Permapen   penicillin g benzathine
Permax   pergolide
Persantine   dipyridamole
Pfizerpen   penicillin
Pfizerpen-AS   penicillin g procaine
Pharmorubicin   epirubicin
Phenergan   promethazine
Phenytek   phenytoin
Phillips Milk of Magnesia   magnesium hydroxide
Phillips M-O   magnesium hydroxide and mineral oil
PhosLo   calcium acetate
Piperonil   pipamperone
Pipracil   piperacillin
Piracetam Verla   piracetam
Pitocin   oxytocin
Plan B   levonorgestrel
Plaquenil   hydroxychloroquine
Platinol, Platinol-AQ   cisplatin
Plavix   clopidogrel
Plendil   felodipine
Pletal   cilostazol

PMS-Bezafibrate   bezafibrate
PMS-Brimonidine Tartrate   brimonidine
PMS-Dopazide   methyldopa plus hydrochlorothiazide
PMS-Hydromorphone   hydromorphone
PMS-Phenobarbital   phenobarbital
Ponstan   mefenamic acid
Ponstel   mefenamic acid
Prandase   acarbose
Prandin   repaglinide
Pravachol   pravastatin
Pravigard PAC   aspirin and pravastatin
Prazinil   carpipramine
Precedex   dexmedetomidine
Precose   acarbose
Premarin   estrogens conjugated/equine
Premphrase   estrogens conjugated/equine and medroxyprogesterone
Prempro   estrogens conjugated/equine and medroxyprogesterone
Pretz-D   ephedrine
Prevacid   lansoprazole
Prevalite   cholestyramine
Priftin   rifapentine
Prilosec   omeprazole
Primacor   milrinone
Primsol   trimethoprim
Prinivil   lisinopril
ProAmatine   midodrine
Probiotica   lactobacillus
Procanbid   procainamide
Procardia   nifedipine
Procyclid   procyclidine
Proglycem   diazoxide
Prograf   tacrolimus
Proleukin   aldesleukin
Prolex-d   guaifenesin and phenylephrine
Prolixin   fluphenazine
Promatussin DM   promethazine and dextromethorphan
Prometrium   progesterone
Pronestyl-SR   procainamide
Propanthel   propantheline
Prorazin   prochlorperazine
ProSom   estazolam
Prostigmin   neostigmine
Protonix   pantoprazole
Protopic   tacrolimus
Proventil   albuterol
Provera   medroxyprogesterone
Provigil   modafinil
Provocholine   methacholine
Prozac   fluoxetine

Q

Quelicin   succinylcholine
Questran   cholestyramine
Quibron   theophylline and guaifenesin
Quinaglute Dura-Tabs   quinidine
Quinine-Odan   quinine
Quixin   levofloxacin

R

Rapamune   sirolimus
Raptiva   efalizumab
Razadyne   galantamine
Reactine   cetirizine
Refludan   lepirudin
Regitine   phentolamine
Reglan   metoclopramide
Reguloid   psyllium
Relafen   nabumetone
Relpax   eletriptan
Remeron   mirtazapine
Renagel   sevelamer
Renedil   felodipine
Renese   polythiazide
ReoPro   abciximab
Requip   ropinirole
Rescriptor   delavirdine
Resectisol   mannitol
Restoril   temazepam
Retavase   reteplase
Retrovir   zidovudine
Reversol   edrophonium
ReVia   naltrexone
Rheumatrex   methotrexate
Rhinatiol   carbocysteine
Rhinocort   budesonide
Rhodis   ketoprofen
Rhythmol, Gen-Propafenone   propafenone
Riabel   prifinium
Rifadin   rifampin
Rifamaté   rifampin plus isoniazid
Rilutek   riluzole
Rimactane   rifampin
Riomet   metformin
Riopan Plus, Riopan Plus Double Strength
    magaldrate and simethicone
Risperdal   risperidone
Ritalin   methylphenidate
Rivotril   clonazepam
Robaxin   methocarbamol
Robaxisal   methocarbamol plus aspirin
Robinul, Robinul Forte   glycopyrrolate
Robitussin Pediatric Night Relief   chlorpheniramine,
    pseudoephedrine, and dextromethorphan

Rocephin   ceftriaxone
Roferon-A   interferon alfa 2a
Rogaine   minoxidil
Rogitine   phentolamine
Rolaids Extra Strength   calcium carbonate and
    magnesium hydroxide
Rondec Drops   carbinoxamine and
    pseudoephedrine
Rondec-DM Drops   carbinoxamine, pseudoephedrine,
    and dextromethorphan
Rosanil   sulfur and sulfacetamide
Rovamycine   spiramycin
Rowasa Rectal   mesalamine
Roxibeta   roxithromycin
Roxicodone   oxycodone
Rubex   doxorubicin
Rulox   aluminum hydroxide and magnesium
    hydroxide
Ryna-C   chlorpheniramine, pseudoephedrine, and
    codeine
Rynatan   chlorpheniramine and phenylephrine
Rynatan Tablet   azatadine and pseudoephedrine
Rynatuss   chlorpheniramine, ephedrine,
    phenylephrine, and carbetapentane
Rythmodan   disopyramide

S

Sabril   vigabatrin
Salagen   pilocarpine
Salazopyrin   sulfasalazine
Salflex   salsalate
Sal-Tropine   atropine
Saluron   hydroflumethiazide
Sandimmune   cyclosporine
Sandomigran   pizotifen
Sandostatin   octreotide
Sansert   methysergide
Sarafem   fluoxetine
Scopace   scopolamine
Seconal   secobarbital
Sectral   acebutolol
Semprex-D   acrivastine and pseudoephedrine
Septra   sulfamethoxazole and trimethoprim
Serax   oxazepam
Serentil   mesoridazine
Seromycin Pulvules   cycloserine
Seroquel   quetiapine
Serzone   nefazodone
Silafed   triprolidine and pseudoephedrine
Sildec   carbinoxamine and pseudoephedrine
Simply Saline   sodium chloride
Simulect   basiliximab
Sinemet   levodopa-carbidopa

Sinequan doxepin
Sintonal brotizolam
Sinutab Sinus Allergy Maximum Strength
    acetaminophen, chlorpheniramine, and
    pseudoephedrine
Skelid tiludronate
Slow-Trasicor oxprenolol
Solagé mequinol and tretinoin
Soma Compound carisoprodol plus aspirin
Somnote chloral hydrate
Sonata zaleplon
Sorbilax sorbitol
Soriatane acitretin
Sorine sotalol
Spectazole econazole
Spectracef cefditoren
Spiriva tiotropium
Sporanox itraconazole
Stadol butorphanol
Stamoc zaleplon
Starlix nateglinide
Staticin erythromycin
Stelazine trifluoperazine
Stemetil prochlorperazine
Streptase streptokinase
Strifon Forte chlorzoxazone
Stromectol ivermectin
Suboxone buprenorphine and naloxone
Subutex buprenorphine
Sudafed pseudoephedrine
Sudafed Severe Cold acetaminophen,
    dextromethorphan, and pseudoephedrine
Sufenta sufentanil
Sular nisoldipine
Sulcrate sucralfate
Sulfizole sulfisoxazole
Sumycin tetracycline
Surgam tiaprofenic acid
Surmontil trimipramine
Suspen penicillin v potassium
Sustiva efavirenz
Symbicort budesonide and formoterol
Symmetrel amantadine
SynalogsDC dihydrocodeine, aspirin, and caffeine
Synthroid levothyroxine
Syntocinon oxytocin

T
Tagamet cimetidine
Talwin pentazocine
Tambocor flecainide acetate
Tamofen tamoxifen
Tanatril imidapril

Tao troleandomycin
Targretin bexarotene
Tarka trandolapril plus verapamil
Tasmar tolcapone
Tavist Allergy clemastine
Taxol paclitaxel
Taxotere docetaxel
Teejel choline salicylate
Tegretol carbamazepine
Tenex guanfacine
Tenoretic atenolol plus chlorthalidone
Tenormin atenolol
Tenuate diethylpropion
Tequin gatifloxacin
Terazol 3, Terazol 7 terconazole
Terramycin, Terramycin IM oxytetracycline
Tersigat oxitropium
Tesoprel bromperidol
Testoderm testosterone
Teveten eprosartan
Thalitone chlorthalidone
Thalomid thalidomide
Theochron theophylline
Thioplex thiotepa
Thorazine chlorpromazine
Thrombate III antithrombin iii
Thymoglobulin antithymocyte globulin rabbit
Thyrolar liotrix
Tiazac diltiazem
Ticar ticarcillin
Ticlid ticlopidine
Tigan trimethobenzamide
Tikosyn dofetilide
Timentin ticarcillin and clavulanate potassium
Timoptic timolol
Tinactin Antifungal Jock Itch tolnaftate
Tinset oxatomide
TNKase tenecteplase
Tobrex tobramycin
Tofranil imipramine
Tolectin tolmetin
Tolinase tolazamide
Tolmicol tolciclate
Tol-Tab tolbutamide
Tomudex raltitrexed
Tonocard tocainide
Topamax topiramate
Toposar etoposide
Toradol ketorolac
Torecan thiethylperazine
Totacillin ampicillin
Tracrium atracurium
Trandate labetalol

Transderm Scop scopolamine
Tranxene clorazepate
Trasicor oxprenolol
Trental pentoxifylline
Trexall methotrexate
Triavil amitriptyline and perphenazine
TriCor fenofibrate
Trilafon perphenazine
Trileptal oxcarbazepine
Trilisate choline magnesium trisalicylate
Tri-Luma fluocinolone, hydroquinone, and tretinoin
Trimpex trimethoprim
Trinalin azatadine and pseudoephedrine
Trinasal triamcinolone
Triostat liothyronine
Triphasil ethinyl estradiol and levonorgestrel
Trisenox arsenic trioxide
Tri-Vent HC hydrocodone, carbinoxamine, and pseudoephedrine
Trizivir zidovudine plus lamivudine plus abacavir
Trovan trovafloxacin
Truxcillin penicillin v potassium
TTab clorazepate
Tuinal amobarbital and secobarbital
Tums calcium carbonate
Tussafed carbinoxamine, pseudoephedrine, and dextromethorphan
Tussionex hydrocodone and chlorpheniramine
Tylenol acetaminophen
Tynatuss Pediatric chlorpheniramine, ephedrine, phenylephrine, and carbetapentane

U
Ultiva remifentanil
Ultram tramadol
UltraMide urea
Ultravate halobetasol
Unipen Oral nafcillin
Uniretic moexipril plus hydrochlorothiazide
Univasc moexipril
Urecholine bethanechol
Uro-KP-Neutral potassium and sodium phosphates
Uro-Mag magnesium oxide
Utradol etodolac

V
Vagi-Gard povidone-iodine
Vagistat tioconazole
Valcyte valganciclovir
Valium diazepam
Valtrex valacyclovir

Vanceril beclomethasone
Vancocin vancomycin
Vantin cefpodoxime
Vascor bepridil
Vaseretic enalapril plus hydrochlorothiazide
Vasotec enalapril
Velban vinblastine
Velosef cepharadine
Ventolin albuterol
VePesid etoposide
Versed midazolam
Vesanoid tretinoin, oral
Vexol rimexolone
VFEND voriconazole
Viagra sildenafil
Vibramycin doxycycline
Vicks Pediatric 44m chlorpheniramine, pseudoephedrine, and dextromethorphan
Vicks Sinex Nasal Spray phenylephrine
Vicodin hydrocodone and acetaminophen
Vicoprofen hydrocodone and ibuprofen
Videx, Videx EC didanosine
Vigamox moxifloxacin
Vioxx rofecoxib
Viracept nelfinavir
Viramune nevirapine
Vistaril hydroxyzine
Vistide cidofovir
Vitelle Irospan ferrous sulfate and ascorbic acid
Vitrasert ganciclovir
Vivactil protriptyline
Voltaren diclofenac
Vytone iodoquinol and hydrocortisone

W
WelChol colesevelam
Wellbutrin bupropion
Westhroid thyroid
Winstrol stanzolol
Wycillin penicillin
Wytensin guanabenz

X
Xanax alprazolam
Xenical orlistat
Xigris drotrecogin alfa
Xopenex levalbuterol
Xylocaine lidocaine
Xyrem sodium oxybate

Y
Yasmin ethinyl estradiol and drospirenone

Z

Zaditor   ketotifen
Zagam   sparfloxacin
Zanaflex   tizanidine
Zantac   ranitidine
Zarontin   ethosuximide
Zaroxolyn   metolazone
Zebeta   bisoprolol
Zemuron   rocuronium
Zenapax   daclizumab
Zerit   stavudine
Zestril   lisinopril
Zevalin   ibritumomab
Ziagen   abacavir
Zithromax   azithromycin
Zocor   simvastatin
Zofran   ondansetron

Zoloft   sertraline
Zometa   zoledronic acid
Zomig   zolmitriptan
Zonalon   doxepin
Zonegran   zonisamide
Zosyn   piperacillin plus tazobactam sodium
Zovia   ethinyl estradiol and ethynodiol diacetate
Zovirax   acyclovir
Zyban   bupropion
Zydone   hydrocodone and acetaminophen
Zyflo   zileuton
Zyloprim   allopurinol
Zymar   gatifloxacin
Zyprexa, Zyprexa Zydis   olanzapine
Zyrtec   cetirizine
Zyvox   linezolid

ABOUT THE AUTHORS

GEORGE T. GROSSBERG, M.D., is a professor of geriatric psychiatry at St. Louis University School of Medicine. As a specialist who works with older patients, Dr. Grossberg sees the effects of herb-drug interactions firsthand. Dr. Grossberg has been cited online by his peers in Best Doctors in America and in *America's Top Docs* since their inception. His work has been highlighted in *People, Reader's Digest, Good Housekeeping,* and *USA Today,* and he has appeared on CNN, Lifetime Television, *The Sally Jessy Raphael Show, 48 Hours,* and elsewhere.

BARRY FOX, PH.D., is the bestselling author, coauthor, or ghostwriter of numerous health books, including the number-one bestselling *The Arthritis Cure, The Side Effects Bible,* and *Alternative Cures That Really Work.* He lives in Calabasas, California.